COLLABORATE®

for Professional Case Management: A Universal Competency-Based Paradigm

Teresa M. Treiger, RN-BC, MA, CHCQM-CM/TOC, CCM
Principal of Ascent Care Management, LLC
Holbrook, Massachusetts

Ellen Fink-Samnick, MSW, ACSW, LCSW, CCM, CRP
Principal of EFS Supervision Strategies, LLC
Burke, Virginia

Wolters Kluwer

Philadelphia • Baltimore • New York • London
Buenos Aires • Hong Kong • Sydney • Tokyo

Acquisitions Editor: Shannon W. Magee
Product Development Editor: Maria M. McAvey
Developmental Editor: Lisa Marshall
Senior Marketing Manager: Mark Wiragh
Editorial Assistant: Kathryn Leyendecker
Production Project Manager: Bridgett Dougherty
Design Coordinator: Joan Wendt
Manufacturing Coordinator: Kathleen Brown
Prepress Vendor: S4Carlisle Publishing Services

9 8 7 6 5 4 3 2 1

Printed in China (or the United States of America)
Library of Congress Cataloging-in-Publication Data
Cataloging-in-Publication data available on request from the Publisher

ISBN 13: 978-1-4511-9342-8
ISBN 10: 1-4511-9342-4

LWW.com

RRS1503

Dedication

To Dave: You are my love and soul mate, my most trusted friend and companion.
May we circle the globe together for many years to come.

To Steven and Kevin: Your love empowers me to go from wishing on stars to achieving beyond what I ever think is possible. I cherish you both more than words can express.

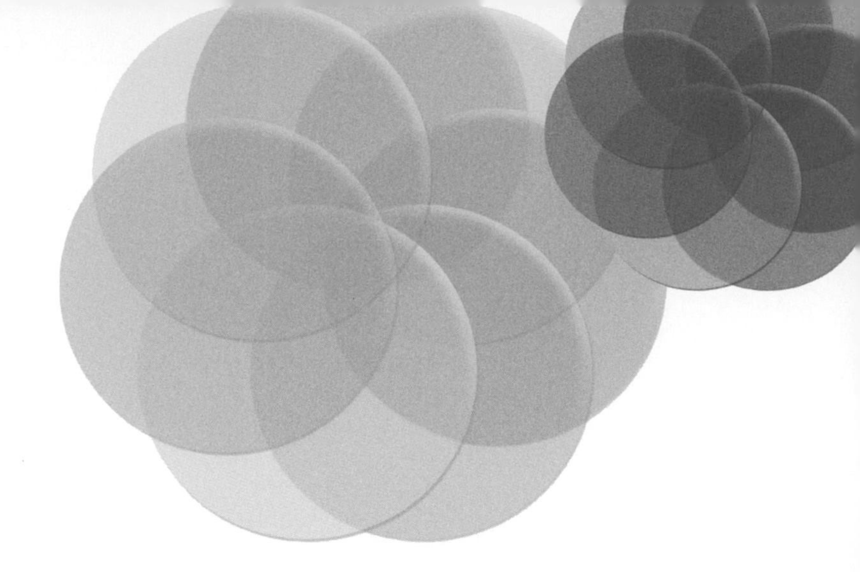

FOREWORD

Every once in a while, a fresh and promising approach is defined for case management. This book represents that new model. This book is *not* the same discussion on the current models of case management. Health care has changed and, in order to remain relevant, so must case management. We must remain open minded and nimble in order to reconcile ongoing changes in health care laws. Case Management's collective success in managing change will enhance our value no matter what obstacles present on the horizon (e.g. massive epidemic, data breach).

Yet some things remain the same. Patient advocacy will always be the cornerstone of case management. And our fundamental, heartfelt goal has always been to serve as stewards of health care resources, performing well-coordinated activities that move the patients into their next phase, yielding quality and safety.

Still, there are many gaps (perhaps chasms) and confusion between what case management purports to be and case management best practice. There are fewer resources that walk us through a method to achieve goals of consistency in training and in practice. This book *is* about a new paradigm that is fluid enough to fit into all settings and one that transcends professional practices. It pushes us to answer the fundamental question: How is a competent case manager defined?

The book contains thoughtful discussions on the history of case management, the influences, models attempted, and reasons why some of those models were less than successful. Influencers of case management must, realistically, include the history and evolution, the regulations we must adhere to, accreditation bodies, credentialing agencies, etc.—all addressed within these pages.

Necessarily, updated terminology is used which includes an interprofessional perspective, one that is not discipline-specific. *Transdisciplinary* is a term that transcends professional disciplines, moves across teams and across the continuum, and is all-inclusive. Theory is included (such as change management); however, the book is not all history and theory; it has real-world application, as well. There are unique, action-oriented competencies that move case managers to practicing better and more uniformly. In addition, you will find the following:

- A framework for developing a purposeful job description that aligns with setting meaningful performance management and expectations;
- Guidance of competency-based assessment tools and skills, identification training, and development of strategies; and
- Intent-driven performance management and interview principles.

Peter Drucker, sometimes called the man who invented management, stated, "The greatest danger in times of turbulence is not the turbulence—it is to act with yesterday's logic." Case management is getting more complex and, it seems, will always be on a fast-changing trajectory. When I started case management in the 1980s, we had regulations, but fewer. We had early clinical criteria, but milder (much milder). We had social problems, but more resources. A new approach is needed now: COLLABORATE, a competency-based paradigm that contains new wisdom for a new health care world.

Suzanne K. Powell
Editor in Chief, Professional Case Management Journal

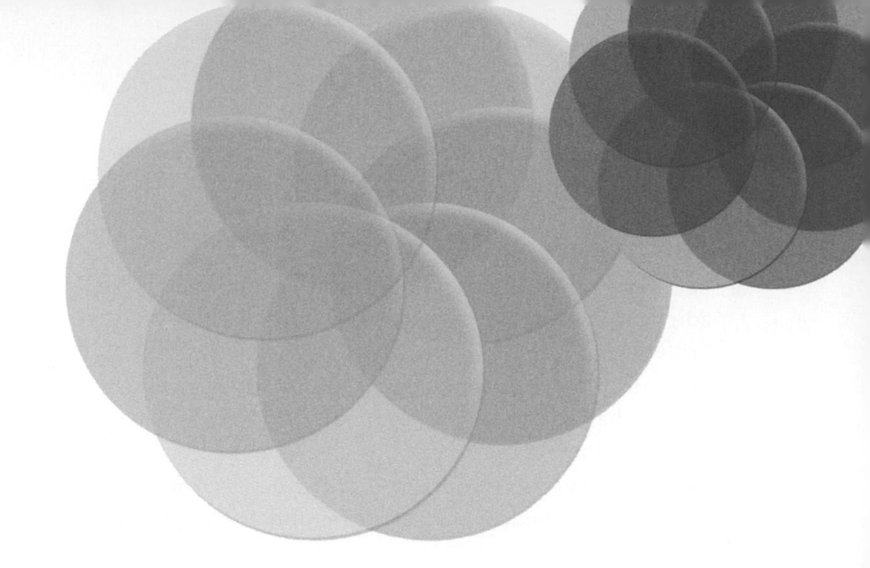

PREFACE

This book is about the progressive improvement of case management beyond that which exists to that of a practice specialty focused on professionalism and collegiality across all practice settings. Our desire to produce a framework for such practice began when we connected several years ago. It was a result of a dialogue, the sharing of our stories and experiences. Separately, we were already passionate about and committed to case management excellence. Together, our vision coalesced to form this competency-based framework for advancing case management captured by an acronym that defined the essence of professional practice—COLLABORATE.

We spent hours discussing the implications of a perceived epidemic involving less-than-productive interactions between individuals working under the title of case manager and consumers, providers, and clinical colleagues. These accumulated experiences heightened our commitment to lead the much-needed change. Our conversation endured over many months as we realized a shared

- respect for case management's rich heritage in health care, across professional disciplines and practice settings;
- concern for those factors that devalue case management's professional standing;
- agreement that while the practice of case management transcends many representative professional disciplines and educational levels, each stakeholder continues to cling to their respective stake in the ground; and
- belief of the importance for case management to move from advanced practice to profession once and for all.

COLLABORATE was born from a vision, the mandate to solidify a foundation for case management practice that combines unique action-oriented competencies, transcends professional disciplines, crosses over practice settings, and recognizes educational levels. The ultimate focus is on improving the client's health care experience through the promotion of effective transdisciplinary collaboration.

COLLABORATE recognizes the hierarchy of competencies and practice behaviors defined by the educational levels of all professionals engaged: associates and bachelor's, master's, and doctoral degree holders across practice disciplines. Through this approach, every qualified health and human service professional has a valued place setting at the case management's ever-expanding table.

Each of the competencies is presented as mutually exclusive and uniquely defined; however, all are complementary and call on the practitioner to conduct work processes in a wholly integrated manner. Although appearing in order for the acronym's sake, they are not necessarily sequential. Ultimately, case management is an iterative process.

When united in a comprehensive and strategic effort, the COLLABORATE competencies comprise a purpose-driven, powerful case management paradigm. The agility of this model extends to the use of key concepts that include both action-oriented verbs and nouns, which are significant elements in any professional case management endeavor. To date, case management practice models have been driven by care setting and business priorities. Unfortunately, this exclusivity has contributed to a lack of practice consistency due to shifting organizational and regulatory priorities. However, this is only one reason for a fragmented case management identity. COLLABORATE recognizes and leverages these important influencers as critical to successful practice and quality client outcomes.

Interprofessional education and teamwork are beginning to emerge as the means to facilitate relationship-building in the workplace. Through this approach, health care practitioners absorb the theoretical underpinning of intentionally working together in a mutually respectful manner that acknowledges the value of expertise of each care team stakeholder. This educational approach provides the opportunity to engage in clinical practice that incorporates the professional standards to which we hold ourselves accountable.

Innovative and emerging care coordination models, defined by evidence-based initiatives, appear across the industry. Each promotes attention to interprofessional practice in order to achieve quality patient-centered care. Herein lies an opportunity to demonstrate the value drawn from diverse expertise of case managers constituting the collective workforce. However, a critical prefacing stage of this endeavor involves defining a core practice paradigm highlighting case management as a profession.

The diverse and complex nature of population health mandates that case management intervene from an interprofessional and collaborative stance. Although inherent value is derived from the variety of disciplines, this advanced model unifies case management's unique identity. Now is the time to define and adopt a competency-based model for professional case management. COLLABORATE provides this framework.

This text is presented in four sections:

- **Section 1:** Historical validation of why this practice paradigm is critical for case management to advance to a profession
- **Section 2**: Presentation of the COLLABORATE paradigm, with a chapter devoted to each distinct competency and the key elements
- **Section 3**: Practical application of the book's content for use by the individual case manager and at the organizational level
- **The Epilogue**: Summary of the COLLABORATE approach in a forward-looking context

For the reader with limited time, reviewing section 2 provides the substantive meat associated with each of the competencies.

Our ultimate desire is that the COLLABORATE approach provides an impetus for all stakeholders (e.g., practitioners, educational institutions, professional organizations) to take the necessary steps toward unified practice in order to facilitate the transition of case management considered as a task-driven job to its recognition as being a purpose-driven profession.

With deep gratitude and respect,
Teresa M. Treiger and Ellen Fink-Samnick

ACKNOWLEDGMENTS

We thank our colleagues, families, and friends who supported us during the entire process of researching and writing this book. Their patience and generosity raised us up during very challenging times. We also thank Lisa, Shannon, and the team at Wolters Kluwer for support and understanding as the project progressed. There are people who deserve special recognition for going above and beyond the call of duty.

- Please know that your support has been the world to me, especially Dave for your keen eye and unfailing support. Although 2014 will not go down as our favorite year, we survived it and came out the other side stronger than ever. My heartfelt thanks also to my sibs P, M, T, and A; J.G., who told me very long ago I was destined to do great things; R.G. for confidence and the opportunities to succeed; A.L. for encouragement and publishing my first article; S.K.P. for insights and inspiration; C.L. for support through all sorts of weather; M.E.M., G.A.H., D.C., G.P., T.N.H., M.E.F., and G.J.M. for the many ways in which you contributed to my life and to my success; and finally, my parents LCDR Norman and Eva Frates, for their unconditional love, support, and belief in me.—**Teresa M. Treiger**
- My sincere appreciation to those who provided their unconditional love, guidance, and wisdom, especially M.J.F. for the impetus to grow my passion in all I do; L.B.D. for empowering me to define my legacy; C.S.U., L.V., and J.B. for your ethical mentoring; M.O. for the professional respect, "hugs" and "kumbaya" sessions; S.K.P. for your consummate vision and candor; L.G. and C.M. for igniting my writing flame for those first articles; B.L. for challenging me to grow and learn; J.R. for your quality lens plus looking beyond credentials to competencies; my irreplaceable village, you know who you are and how you each inspire me to soar; and my parents Dr. and Mrs. Herbert Fink for teaching me so many lessons and allowing me to always define my unique path in life. —**Ellen Fink-Samnick**

Finally, to professional case managers past, present, and future . . . Thank you for supporting your clients and each other. Our strength has been and always will be our dedication to excellence.

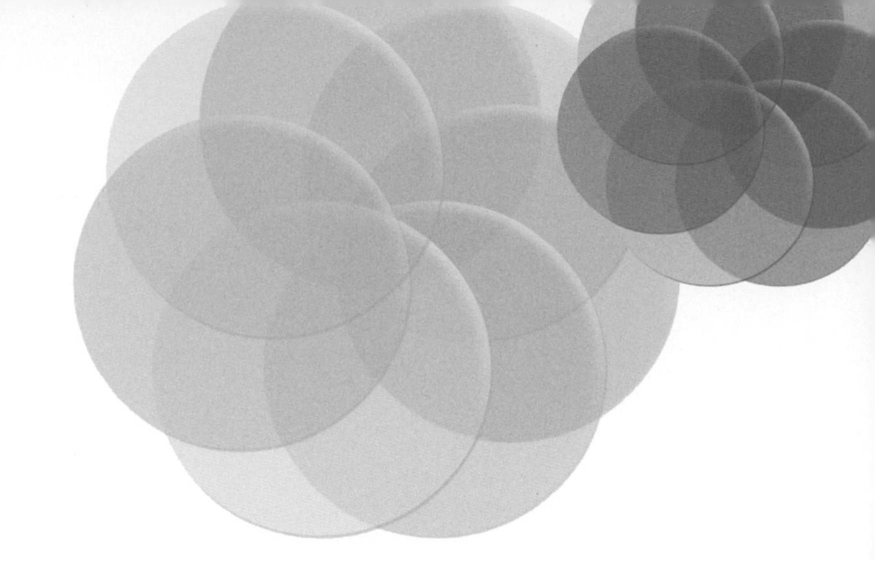

CONTENTS

SECTION 1

Grounding the COLLABORATE Paradigm

1 HISTORICAL PERSPECTIVE

OBJECTIVES

After studying this chapter, you will be able to:

1. Discuss the historical underpinnings of current case management practice.
2. Identify pioneers and their contributions to case management development.
3. Discuss historical precursors to present-day utilization management.
4. Describe the various sections of the Social Security Act of 1935 and their importance to current case management.
5. Describe the impact of case management on workers' compensation and veterans' health care coordination.
6. Describe the impact of corporate-driven priorities on case management programs.

KEY TERMS

Boards of Charity
Charity Organization Societies
Demonstration projects
Health Maintenance Organization Act
Older Americans Act
Public health nursing
Settlement House
Social Security Act
Waiver programs

Case management grew out of the social and human service sectors through a chain of social developments and historical events to address the needs of the disadvantaged, ill, and injured populations through the identification and provision of social services and coordination of care. Although initially not labeled as case management, this history provides a context for understanding how case management evolved. This chapter provides a historical perspective of health care coordination and other precursors that contributed to what was subsequently identified as case management practice from the 19th century through the 1960s.

EARLY EFFORTS IN CARE COORDINATION

Beginning in the 19th century and prior to government-sponsored interventions, charitable and community-based organizations recognized that basic human needs were not being addressed by formal government programs. The U.S. government had not yet expanded into areas of social support or health care realms, and so efforts to provide social assistance and supportive services for individuals in need were humanitarian and grassroots in nature. The history of caring for the disadvantaged arose from the context of social–political–industrial changes, which piqued more liberal attitudes of social consciousness.

Boards of Charity

In 1863, the Commonwealth of Massachusetts established a board of charity, the first of its kind in the nation (Weil & Karls, 1985). The Board was formed in order to coordinate limited assistance resources among the poor and infirmed. Although the Board's scope of work was not equivalent to present-day case management, passage of the law demonstrated a shift toward defining responsibility for evaluation of individuals and coordination of available services and housing. As described in Chapter 240, An Act in Relation to State Charitable and Correctional Institutions, the Board was charged with "examination of paupers and lunatics, to ascertain their places of settlement and means of support, or who may be responsible therefor; the removal of paupers and lunatics to their usual homes" (Commonwealth of Massachusetts, 1863).

The intent of the Board was articulated in the 1867 annual report in which Chairman Dr. Samuel Gridley Howe stated, "[T]he purpose of charity in New England has been to diminish the number of the helpless, to make them sounder, stronger, more hopeful and self-reliant. Justice, no less than mercy, has been in the thoughts of our people; a justice not satisfied with almsgiving, but seeking zealously to establish a social condition in which alms would be less and less needed." (Massachusetts State Hospitals: A Social History, 1867).

Boards of Charity preceded the formation of **Charity Organization Societies** (COS), which arose in the late 1870s in an effort to coordinate available resources across multiple agencies.

Settlement Houses

The settlement movement was a social reform undertaking that began in the 1880s and continued into the early 1900s. The better known of these were Hull House, the Henry Street Settlement, and the University Settlement (Table 1-1). Settlement houses were established in disadvantaged urban settings with the desire that members of higher social class would become more involved and supportive of improving the plight of the poor through closer living arrangements. These houses provided services such as day care, education, and health care (Wade, 1967; Weil & Karls, 1985).

The **settlement house** concept was imported from England. The first established house, Toynbee Hall, was a cooperative effort between Oxford and Cambridge Universities, founded in 1884. Students volunteered to participate in the program in order to gain a better understanding of the conditions faced by the poor. The founders, Canon Samuel and Henrietta Barnett, envisioned Toynbee Hall as a living laboratory affording a unique opportunity for participants to develop practical solutions to address the challenges of poverty. It was Toynbee Hall that sparked the creation of the settlement house movement in the United States (Wade, 1967).

Arguably, the most influential settlement initiative was the Hull House, located in Chicago, IL. Hull House was founded by Laura Jane Addams (see Box 1-1) and Ellen Gates Starr in 1889, following a visit to Toynbee Hall in England. Hull House evolved into a community that provided social and educational opportunities. The volunteer workers, referred to as *residents*, were responsible to identify the needs of the population and engage services to help address these needs. A system of index cards was used to document each family's situation as well as to track the utilization of services. Recipients were mostly immigrants and low-income families (Johnson, 2005; Wade, 1967; Weil & Karls, 1985).

Resident workers provided instructional classes, performed concerts, and gave lectures. Children's services, such as day care and social clubs, were also available. From its original single building, Hull House expanded into a compound of several structures that operated under the auspices of the Jane Addams Hull House Association until 2012.

Charity Organization Societies

Focus on coordination of cost-effective and efficient service to the deserving needy was behind the **Charity Organization Societies** (COS), which came into being around 1877 and continued until the 1920s (Lewis, 2008). The industrialization and growth of urban areas gave rise to the COS movement. This period in history saw increases in work-related accidents, poor living conditions, rapid disease spread, and social and economic problems, including unemployment, aging, disability, and lack of family support systems. There were few options aside from begging, private charities, or application for public relief.

TABLE 1-1 Early U.S. Settlement Houses

Name	Location	Founding Details
Friendly Inn Settlement House	Cleveland, OH	Established in 1874 by the Women's Temperance Union League
The University Settlement (aka The Neighborhood Guild)	New York, NY	Established in 1886 by Stanton Coit and Charles Bunstein Stover
Hull House	Chicago, IL	Established in 1889 by Laura Jane Addams and Ellen Gates Starr
The Henry Street Settlement	New York, NY	Established in 1893 by Lillian Wald and Marion Brewster
Lenox Hill Neighborhood House	New York, NY	Established in 1894 by the Alumnae Association of Normal College (now known as Hunter College of the City University of New York)

BOX 1-1 Laura "Jane" Addams (1860–1935)

Laura Jane Addams is worthy of specific mention with regard to her influence in the development of social services and case management (see Table 1-2, Early Pioneers of Modern-Day Case Management). Born in 1860, Jane was the youngest child of nine born into a prominent and well-to-do family. Her parents were John and Sarah (née Weber); both influenced her views of social obligation to serve the poor. John was a successful businessman and cofounder of the Republican Party and a personal friend of Abraham Lincoln. Jane was just two years old when her mother, weakened by the premature birth of her ninth child, passed away. At age 4, Jane contracted tuberculosis (of the spine) and was diagnosed with Pott disease, which resulted in a spinal curvature. The subsequent disability left her unable to keep up with other children; so instead, she focused on reading and education pursuits (Linn, 1935; Lundblad, 1995).

In 1868, John H. Addams remarried. The second Mrs. Addams, Anna H. Haldeman, was an interesting and accomplished person in her own right. She was a skilled musician and a voracious reader. She often read plays aloud, a habit that was introduced and practiced at Hull House years later. A widow, Anna also brought sons George and Harry into the Addams household. Harry would subsequently become a gifted surgeon who actually operated on Jane to correct her spinal curvature (Linn, 1935). Although she preferred to attend Smith College in Massachusetts to obtain a formal degree, she deferred to her father's wish that she remain close to home and attended Rockford Seminary, graduating as valedictorian with a plan to continue into medical school (Lane, 1963).

Following her father's sudden death in 1881, Jane became depressed. Although she completed one semester of medical school, the rigors of training proved too demanding in light of her physical disabilities. These factors, in combination with the decline in her stepmother's health, prompted her return to Illinois. Over time, her desire to return to medical school waned. However, in spite of being able to live comfortably from proceeds of the inheritance from her father's estate, Jane became increasingly disillusioned by the lack of meaning and purpose in her life. Her stepbrother recommended rest, which sparked travel abroad. It was on one visit to England that she witnessed the alarming poverty and wretched living conditions of the poor embodied in a street auction of rotten food. It was this, and similar experiences, that solidified her belief that something needed to be done to improve the horrible situations some people were unfortunately facing. A subsequent trip to Europe in 1887 brought her to Toynbee House, which would eventually become the model for the settlement house concept in Illinois (Lane, 1963; Linn, 1935; Lundblad, 1995).

Over the ensuing years, Addams was involved in a number of social movements in addition to continuing work at Hull House: the development of ethical principles (pertaining to settlement homes), children's services, documenting the spread of typhoid, feminism, and the peace movement. Despite her views being branded as unpatriotic, she dedicated her life to service to others and was recognized as the first woman in the United States to be awarded the Nobel Peace Prize, in 1931. Addams is applauded for her "expression of an essentially American democracy" (Lane, 1963; Linn, 1935; Lundblad, 1995).

The COS approach emphasized taking a methodical approach to the investigation, registration, and supervision of applicants eligible for charity. Community-wide efforts were undertaken in order to coordinate the resources and activities of decentralized organizations and bureaus created to register and collect information from recipients (Hansan, n.d.). Another important development of the COS movement was the recognition that understanding and developing a relationship with the client would enhance understanding of the client and the specific causative factor(s) of his or her needs.

There was a point of view that individuals receiving aid that was not truly deserved fostered their becoming dependent on the system. This perspective was foundational to COS philosophy which initially focused on seeking out fraud and misuse of services in an effort to ensure equitable resource distribution. Detecting abuse was aided by improvements in record-keeping which allowed for verification that recipients did not receive more than their share of assistance from the multiple participating agencies. The COS focused more on the needs of the organization than on the development or coordination of services to the client. What were considered innovative practices in their time became precursors of modern-day case management and utilization management (Table 1-2; Box 1-2).

Public and Community Health

The history of **public health nursing** provides yet another glimpse into the beginnings of modern-day case management. It began in the United States as a small undertaking in which a few socially conscious wealthy individuals hired nurses to visit the sick poor in their homes (Buhler-Wilkerson, 1985). By 1910, efforts expanded beyond care of the sick to include health education, including programs aimed at illness prevention. Responsibility for the prevention programs subsequently shifted to the purview of public health departments or boards of education. However, care of the sick continued as work done by voluntary organizations, supported primarily by philanthropy. The seeds of dividing sick care from health education were sown, the growth from which continues to affect the perception of present-day case

TABLE 1-2 Early Pioneers of Modern-Day Case Management

Era	Name	Impact on Modern Case Management
1820–1910	Florence Nightingale	Pioneer of modern nursing practice, advocate of nursing education and nurses as health educators
1860–1935	Laura "Jane" Addams	Pioneer of social worker identity and practice standards, peace activist, suffrage activist, founder of Hull House, Nobel laureate
1861–1928	Mary E. Richmond	Distinguished social worker identity, practice standards, and client-focused assessment in place
1867–1940	Lillian Wald	Established Public Health Nursing specialty, founder of Henry Street Settlement and Visiting Nurse Service of New York
1866–1954	Annie W. Goodrich	Advocate of nursing education, U.S. Army hospitals chief nursing inspector, founded U.S. Army School of Nursing, director of Visiting Nurse Service of New York, 1st dean of Yale University School of Nursing

BOX 1-2 Mary E. Richmond (1861–1928)

Another pioneer in the evolution of what would eventually become case management is Mary E. Richmond. Richmond was born in Belleville, IL. Upon the death of her parents, Henry and Lavinia (née Harris), she moved to Baltimore to be raised by her maternal grandmother and two aunts. An active suffragette, her grandmother raised Richmond immersed in an environment of political and intellectual discussions on topics such as racial inequality, spiritualism, and women's right to vote among other issues important to social activism of the time. Initially home-schooled, Richmond was eventually enrolled in public school and graduated high school at the age of 16. Subsequently, she moved to New York City with one of her aunts and began working at a publishing house. Within a year's time, her aunt returned to Baltimore because of illness, leaving Mary behind. Eventually, she returned to Baltimore, where Richmond worked as a bookkeeper and became involved with the Unitarian Church before working at the Baltimore COS as treasury assistant (Murdach, 2011; The Social Welfare History Project, n.d.).

Richmond expanded the concept of social service beyond that of fraud-focused investigation and into client-oriented service coordination (Weil & Karls, 1985) by highlighting the concept that the efforts of a dedicated person, referred to as the friendly visitor, could bring about a change in the circumstance of another person when the needs of that person were identified, understood, and addressed in the context of their living and family situation. Her concept of care coordination was articulated in the 1901 Proceedings of the National Conference on Charities and Correction in recognition of the lack of coordination and communication across agencies of the time (Weil & Karls, 1985).

Richmond continued to pave the way for what eventually would be known as case management. She described a model of case coordination, depicted in Figure 1-1, as concentric circles beginning at the center with Family Forces, followed by Personal Forces, Neighborhood Forces, Civic Forces, Private Charitable Forces, and, finally, Public Relief Force. The Richmond model identified forces that the charitable worker addressed when working with a client. As part of a more systematic approach, Richmond advocated using a checklist approach to ensure consistency in the process of identification and documentation of impact: "It sometimes seemed worthwhile, in puzzling cases, to advise the agent to go to work as deliberately as this: Taking the list of forces in each circle, to check off each one that had been tried, and then make a note of ways in which to use the others" (Richmond, 1901).

Following her work in Baltimore, Richmond worked in Philadelphia and eventually returned to New York City to lead the Russell Sage Foundation's Charity Organizational Department in 1909 and published multiple books, including *Friendly Visiting among the Poor*, *Social Diagnosis*, and *What Is Social Case Work*. Richmond's work was built on the belief that the origins of social failure could often be uncovered by examining the circumstances of the individual and family unit and that there was great importance of evaluating a client's strengths as part of the process of determining assistance needed rather than simply affixing blame or focusing on situational weaknesses as the cause and assigning random interventions and services to resolve the current situation.

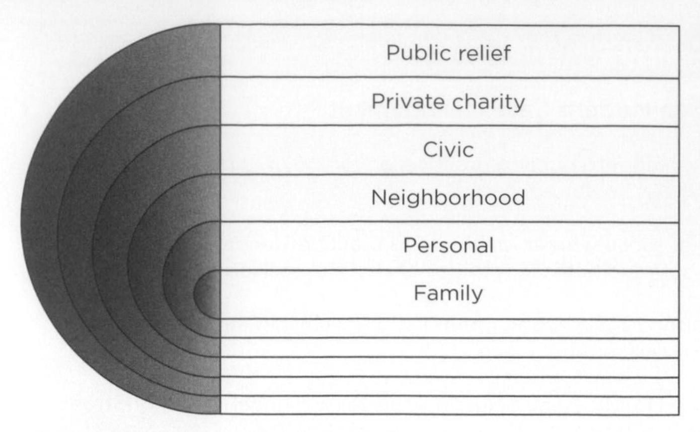

Figure 1-1. Richmond's forces model.

management as being applicable to the confined space of complex illness and injury care management versus disease management, where the focus has been on health condition education and risk reduction.

As was the circumstance with philanthropic activities of that time, public health nurses were charged not only with care for the sick but also to provide instruction in personal hygiene and morality. The image of the visiting nurse climbing the tenement stairs to save the indigent from illness and bad habits struck the fancy of a wide variety of social reformers (Buhler-Wilkerson, 1985). An anonymous quote from the turn of the century regarding visiting nurses characterizes expectations of those working in this capacity: "There is no form of organized philanthropy that demonstrates more clearly the present progressive ideas of social and economic work among the less fortunate" (Fulmer, 1902).

Another influence that public health nursing made on the progression of case management practice was also an echo from the COS. The visiting worker was considered a gatekeeper, preventing abuses of health care utilization, specifically hospital admissions. As hospitals were attempting to shed the perception of existing solely as charitable organizations, the visiting nurse was charged with care of the poor in the community order to keep hospital beds available for those who were able to pay for care. While the dynamics of health care payment have changed over the years, the inclusion of utilization gatekeeping by case managers continues through to the present day.

At the turn of the last century, American cities were petri dishes for infectious diseases. This reality was associated with poor public sanitation and gross residential overcrowding. Although those living in these conditions were at highest risk, it was also perceived as a hazard for those of higher social station who lived in close proximity within urban areas (Leavitt & Numbers, 1997). These and other socioeconomic inequities weighed on the conscience of Lillian Wald, which spurred her on as a pioneer of public health nursing practice (Box 1-3). Wald cofounded and developed the Henry Street Settlement in New York's Lower East Side in order to address the gaps in health care and social services needed to support the disadvantaged (Buhler-Wilkerson, 1993).

BOX 1-3 Lillian Wald (1867-1940)

Lillian Wald was born into a middle-class family in Cincinnati, OH. In 1878, she moved with her family to Rochester, NY, attending Miss Cruttenden's English-French Boarding and Day School for Young Ladies before attending New York Hospital's School of Nursing and subsequently graduating from the New York Hospital Training School for Nurses in 1891. She pursued further study at the Women's Medical College (Buhler-Wilkerson, 1993; Feld, 2008). By 1893, she left medical school and began teaching home nursing to immigrants at a Sabbath school and working as a visiting nurse.

Wald shared a room with fellow nurse Mary Brewster in order to be closer to the people for whom she cared. It was during this time that she had an experience that changed the course of her work. She arrived at a patient's home, the route taken to which led through living conditions so horrible that it drove the establishment of the Henry Street Settlement, "Wald and Brewster moved to the lower East Side in July 1893, thus joining the growing ranks of "new women." Described as a revolutionary demographic and political phenomenon, the new woman was typically single, educated, and economically independent, a champion of professional visibility for women and an advocate of economic and social reform" (Buhler-Wilkerson, 1993). Wald began using the term *public health nurse* to describe her duties as an integrated member of the community in which she worked.

In 1893, Wald founded Henry Street Settlement with financial support from philanthropists Mrs. Solomon Loeb and Jacob Schiff. This funding afforded Wald the ability to provide services to clients in her neighborhood. Within 2 years, a building was purchased, providing the space to develop the services she envisioned (Buhler-Wilkerson, 1993). By 1913, Henry Street Settlement expanded its programs as well as its service area beyond the Lower East Side. The Henry Street Settlement eventually incorporated as two entities, the Visiting Nurse Service of New York and the Henry Street Settlement, which focused on social services (Social Welfare History Archives, n.d.; Wald, 1915/1991); this seemed to reinforce a separation of sick care from health education. However, although the opportunity for specialization in nursing practice expanded with public health, Wald opposed breaking out health teaching from sick care. Her view was that public health nursing was a link across a client's physical health, social and economic needs, and the services necessary to recover from illness and establish health (Wales, 1941). Today, the most widely accepted, cross-continuum case management standards of practice reinforce the fusion of these roles by highlighting the importance of the whole person orientation when undertaking the case management process, inclusive of assessment, care planning, implementation, monitoring, and advocacy

(Case Management Society of America, 2010). Wald's work continued the spirit of work initiated by Florence Nightingale and other "new women" who were revolutionizing the delivery of social services and health care as part of contemporary economic and social reforms.

HISTORIC LEGISLATION HAVING IMPACT ON PRESENT-DAY CASE MANAGEMENT

Another major area of influence on the development of case management practice was a stream of socially motivated legislation that positioned federal and state governments and subsequently created regulatory agencies in a position of responsibility for support and care of the general population. Accompanying these major pieces of legislation was the demand for accountability, service quality, and consumer protection. The role of case manager (also identified as a service coordinator) was first seen in the school setting (Education of All Handicapped Children Act in 1975). Subsequent passage of federal and state laws mandated case management services for elders (the **Older Americans Act**), the mentally ill (the Community Mental Health Centers Act), and the developmentally disabled (the Developmentally Disabled Assistance and Bill of Rights Act) (Weil & Karls, 1985).

The Social Security Act

Enacted on August 14, 1935, the **Social Security Act** (SSA) was drafted by President Franklin D. Roosevelt and passed as part of the New Deal. The SSA was intended to provide for general welfare by establishing a system of federal old-age benefits and enabling states to improve provisions for aged persons, blind persons, dependent and crippled children, maternal and child welfare, public health, and the administration of their unemployment compensation laws; to establish a social security board; to raise revenue; and for other purposes (SSA of 1935 Legislative History, 2013).

The SSA provided grants, funded by taxes applied to both individual wages and employer payroll, to states that demonstrated compliance with program requirements, including the administration, delivery, and reporting of services for the aged, maternal and child welfare, crippled children, the blind, and the unemployed. In addition, the Act funded education and training for staff, vocational training, and family health programs (Our Documents, 2012). Table 1-3 provides a title-by-title description of the original SSA sections that had, and continue to have, an impact on case management.

The SSA provided funding for the creation and administration of programs that relied on knowledgeable and experienced individuals to ensure these new programs were developed and administered in a way that addressed the needs of aid recipients. In addition, qualification standards for each program were needed. The reliance on charitable donations as the primary source of funding for community-based care was coming to a close. Although the COS movement previously attempted to exert control mechanisms on resource utilization, the efforts were local in nature. The SSA signaled federal government involvement in health care and social assistance, raising the bar on accountability and resource conservation.

As new programs were created and rolled out, the effect on those working in care coordination was just beginning to be realized. One example to consider is found within Title II's disability benefits. As possibly qualified individuals became known, the need to involve someone to shepherd the application and monitoring process arose. These were often individuals facing complex biopsychosocial issues, which affected their disability and health status. Eventually, it was recognized that the person involved in administering the health care benefits of these programs would need diverse knowledge in order to understand the influence of an individual's health condition(s) and disability status, be able to clearly document the qualification requirements, and incorporate the necessary skills into efficiently reconnoitering the business processes. This individual also needed the knowledge and experience to manage the benefits on an ongoing basis. Administrative staff lacked the necessary clinical knowledge. Medical staff possessed clinical knowledge but were more focused on diagnosis and treatment. Nurses, social workers, and other trained health care professionals were well suited and thus began to filter into these midlevel positions.

The SSA was repeatedly amended multiple times over the years following its initial passage. In 1956, monthly disability payments to disabled workers between the ages of 50 and 65 were approved. In addition, benefits were made available for disabled, dependent children of retired or deceased workers. Subsequent protections were broadened at the same time that other provisions were eliminated. These ongoing modifications are too numerous to discuss for the purpose of this chapter, and the reader is encouraged to become acquainted with the current status of SSA provisions for both national and state-based programs in order to best serve clients.

Arguably, the SSA amendment, which had the most lasting impact on health and social welfare, was passed in 1965. President Lyndon B. Johnson signed H.R. 6675 into law on July 30, 1965. This legislation created the Medicare and Medicaid programs. Medicare was composed of hospital insurance and medical insurance plans covering payments for physicians' services and other medical and health services to cover certain areas not covered by the hospital insurance plan, and Medicaid provided health insurance for poor families (Cohen & Ball, 1965).

In October 1972, the then president Richard M. Nixon signed Public Law 92-336, amending the SSA once again. This piece of legislation contained a number of modifications (Ball, 1973), including the following:

- Increase in monthly cash payment benefit
- Decrease in waiting period for disability benefit
- Change in blind and childhood disability benefits

TABLE 1-3 The Social Security Act of 1935

Title	Title Name	Purpose
I	Grants to States for Old-Age Assistance	Enables each state to furnish financial assistance, as far as practicable under the conditions in such state, to aged needy individuals.
II	Federal Old-Age Benefits	Establishes an "old age benefit" for qualified individuals beginning on the date they attain the age of 65 and ending on the date of their death.
III	Grants to States for Unemployment Compensation Administration	Establishes assistance to states for the administration of unemployment compensation laws.
IV	Grants to States for Aid to Dependent Children	Enables each State to furnish financial assistance to needy dependent children.
V	Grants to States for Maternal and Child Welfare	Part 1 Maternal and Child Health Services Extend and improve services for promoting the health of mothers and children, especially in rural areas and in areas suffering from severe economic distress.
		Part 2 Services for Crippled children Locate crippled children and provide medical, surgical, corrective, and other services and care, and facilities for diagnosis, hospitalization, and aftercare, for children who are crippled or who are suffering from conditions that lead to crippling.
		Part 3 Child Welfare Services Establish, extend, and strengthen public-welfare services for the protection and care of homeless, dependent, and neglected children and children in danger of becoming delinquent, especially in predominantly rural areas.
		Part 4 Vocation Rehabilitation Extend and strengthen vocational rehabilitation programs for the physically disabled and provide for the promotion of vocational rehabilitation of persons disabled in industry or otherwise and their return to civil employment.
VI	Public Health Work	Establishes and maintains adequate public-health services, including the training of personnel for state and local health work.

- Extension of Medicare coverage to qualified individuals under the age of 65 diagnosed with chronic kidney disease
- Allowance of Health Maintenance Organization coverage option extended to Medicare
- Establishment of Professional Standards Review Organizations (PSRO)
- Definition of broadened Medicare-covered extended-care services and extension of the same definition to skilled nursing facility services under Medicaid
- Authorization for experiments and **demonstration projects** to test various payment and delivery programs.

Demonstration projects focus on testing the efficiency and effectiveness of care options outside of institutional settings of care. Identified as waivers under Section 222 in Medicare, these test projects often featured case management as an integral program component. In Medicaid, waivers fall under Section 1115. Waivers are exceptions to program requirements that foster testing of research in health care delivery. The value of testing new concepts on a limited scale is to allow for real-life results to be produced and analyzed prior to enacting permanent program changes or mandating widespread implementation. Federal law permits the Secretary of Health and Human Services to waive certain provisions of the Social Security Act and/or regulations to allow for demonstration projects in Medicare, Medicaid, or both. Performance incentives and other forms of financial reimbursement or payment are included in such **waiver programs**, making them more attractive to health care providers to become a program participant. While Medicaid waivers are state-based, Medicare demonstrations may be either national or state-specific. Additional limitations include provider type, population, and geographic region. In addition, programs may be limited to only a certain number of participants (e.g., providers, beneficiaries) (Ball, 1973).

Waiver projects may be proposed by any organization or individual (e.g., providers, health plans, state-based Medicaid agencies). Although there is an open invitation for project proposals, most Medicare demonstration projects are mandated by Congress or initiated from within the Centers for Medicare and Medicaid in response to orders from the Secretary of Health and Human Services, the Executive Branch, the Office of the Inspector General, or the Medicare Advisory Commission (MedPAC) (Ball, 1973). Following these changes, legislation to conduct case management research was passed at the state level in California, Pennsylvania, Washington, Utah, and Arkansas. These projects focused on community-based and in-home programs for individuals receiving public assistance (Weil & Karls, 1985).

The Education for All Handicapped Children Act of 1975

The Education for All Handicapped Children Act (EHA or EAHCA) was the first federal legislation which mandated appropriate and free education for students with disabilities. It was signed into law by the then president Gerald Ford in November 1975 as an amendment of the Education for All Handicapped Act of 1974 (Education for All Handicapped Children Act, 1975; U.S. Department of Education, n.d.). This law served as the foundation of special education. Although a number of regulatory mandates originated with this legislation, key elements that impacted the development of case management included the following:

Nondiscriminatory Identification and Evaluation

To ensure a fair process for identification and placement into special education programs, assessments were required to be administered in a child's primary language, overseen by qualified staff, focused to enable assessment of specific need areas, nondiscriminatory of a child's handicap, and administered by a multidisciplinary team representing all specialties related to the assumed disability (Hunt & Kirk, 2005; Turnbull & Turnbull, 2000).

Individualized Education Program (IEP)

Each identified student was required to have a documented IEP. A multidisciplinary team was required to develop and/or update the IEP for each recipient student at a minimum annual interval. This team included professionals, parents, and child, each of whom was identified as appropriate and necessary to address the recipient's individualized needs. IEPs included the following: current performance status, measurable annual and interim goals, objective evaluation criteria and procedure, specification of special education and services to be utilized, the extent of participation in general population education and rationale for use of special education services, necessary accommodations to be used within the general population environment, anticipated start and stop dates for necessary services, and an annual progress evaluation (Hunt & Kirk, 2005; Turnbull & Turnbull, 2000).

Due Process

Due process represented a check and balance system to ensure fair treatment of students and families as well as accountability of administrators, staff, and professionals who were involved in the design, implementation, and administration of the program. These procedures included the requirements and rights associated with program access, including an appeals process and expectation of confidentiality (Hunt & Kirk, 2005; Turnbull & Turnbull, 2000).

Parental Participation

This ensured parental rights of inclusion in the decision, evaluation, and IEP planning process. Schools were responsible to collaborate and communicate consistently with appropriate family members. Parents had the right to access their children's educational records (Hunt & Kirk, 2005; Turnbull & Turnbull, 2000).

The EHA emphasized that a collaborative process be undertaken as is noted in the evaluation and IEP sections earlier. This multidisciplinary approach extended to the makeup of these teams. Individuals from a variety of professional backgrounds were to be included on the basis of the recipient's needs. Team membership included teachers, administrators, related service personnel, students, parents, and advocates. Team members were expected to leverage their specialized resources and expertise to advocate and improve the education and subsequent outcomes of handicapped students. In addition, communication that was both ongoing and collaborative across the team was expected to occur. All of these noted elements have been carried forward in shaping current case management process and practice (Slavin, 2006; Turnbull & Turnbull, 2000; Weil & Karls, 1985).

The Older Americans Act

Although individual initiatives existed prior to this, President Lyndon Johnson signed the Older Americans Act (OAA) into law on July 1965. The OAA established the Administration on Aging to reside within the Department of Health, Education and Welfare. It also mandated the creation of state-based efforts. The OAA created a means to organize, coordinate, and deliver community-based services and opportunities to older Americans (OAA, 1965).

In the Older Americans Act Comprehensive Services Amendments passed in 1973, the Area Agencies on Aging were established. This amendment also included Title V authorizing grants to local community agencies for multipurpose senior centers (U.S. Department of Health and Human Services, 2014). The year 1974 saw passage of the Title XX amendment which authorized social service grants for protective, homemaker, transportation, and adult day care services. Also included were employment training, nutrition assistance, and health support. In 1978, amendments included funding specifically aimed at case management projects. These demonstration projects allowed these programs and their case managers to maintain control over expenditure and reimbursement. Subsequent amendments followed over the ensuing decades inclusive of creating various ombudsman roles, elder abuse prevention, elder rights, legal assistance, and outreach, counseling, and assistance programs (U.S. Department of Health and Human Services, 2014). Each development brought emphasis to the need for cross-program collaboration. Areas Agencies on Aging were established to create community-based support networks in order to provide services to the local population. Often, case management included nurse/social worker dyads to provide care and service coordination (Netting, 1992; Tahan, 1998; Weil & Karls, 1985).

THE HISTORY AND IMPACT OF HEALTH CARE INSURANCE AND MANAGED CARE

The federal government did not mandate insurance of any kind until the passage of the SSA in 1935. The SSA altered the perception of the insurance concept as a means to realize a level of financial protection that was otherwise not readily available to the individual, thus triggering a market boom following World War II. Beginning with coverage programs for home and mortgage, life and health insurance programs also expanded. Payment for health care services rendered prior to medical insurance required an individual to bear the cost out of pocket or, in some instances, in exchange for goods or services. This form of payment is referred to as fee-for-service. Although there are known to be very early policies, these were actually accident and disability insurance focused on income replacement, not health care coverage (Health Insurance Association of America, 1997b). Policies specific to health and medical care would not become common until the mid- to late 20th century.

Hospitals began offering direct-to-consumer, prepaid services in the 1920s. Baylor University Hospital was the first of this kind of prepaid group plan. The "Baylor Plan" was developed to help teachers afford hospital care. This program was a precursor to employer-sponsored insurance and served as a predecessor of Blue Cross (Health Insurance Association of America, 1997a). Around the same time, physician groups began offering prepay medical and surgical care programs, subsequently evolving into Blue Shield. Initially, plans provided services that were rendered by participating hospitals and physicians, whereas today's Blue Cross and Blue Shield plans provide reimbursement for services delivered by contracted providers.

The informal concept of a health maintenance organization (HMO) is believed to have begun at the Ross-Loos Clinic in Los Angeles, California, in 1929 (Bodenheimer & Grumbach, 2009). Henry J. Kaiser went on to organize a network of hospitals and clinics in order to provide prepaid health benefits to his shipyard workers during World War II, representing another employer-sponsored coverage effort. This program transformed into what is now known as the Kaiser Permanente HMO (Bodenheimer & Grumbach, 2009). These developments, in addition to rapidly inflating health care costs, influenced passage of the **Health Maintenance Organization Act** of 1973, discussed later in this chapter.

In the 1960s, as insurance companies initiated programs focused on workers' compensation and return-to-work strategies, the Insurance Company of North America, which would eventually become CIGNA, launched a vocational rehabilitation program employing nurse case managers on the basis of the success of preceding programs (Powell & Tahan, 2008). The successes of these case management efforts were the impetus for creating case management and utilization review departments in commercial health insurance companies and HMO. Models of case management practice are discussed later in this book.

Employer-Sponsored Health Insurance

Historically, employers played an important role in financing individual health care. The provision of health insurance through the workplace has important implications apart from its role as the source of health care financing (Buchmueller & Monheit, 2009). The impetus of employer-sponsored health insurance stemmed from post–World War II market influences of high demand for goods, coupled with a limited pool of workers and controlled wages and prices. The worker pool shortage was related to federal restrictions on wage increases as a means of attracting workers (Buchmueller & Monheit, 2009). When health insurance was determined not to be considered as part of earned wages, employers were left with few other options of attracting workers, and thus, benefits became an even stronger magnet. The implication of employer-supported benefits was that it affected an individual's decisions regarding where to work as well as the number of hours to work because of tiered benefit systems that affected the percentage contribution of the employer toward benefit coverage due the employee.

The Health Maintenance Organization Act of 1973

Although this section could have been included under the Historic Legislation section, the authors opted to cover the topic of HMOs herein. The HMO Act of 1973 was the federal government's response to growth in the health care delivery industry, providing consumers the option of traditional coverage. HMOs offered prepaid coverage and service option as a change from the existing provider fee-for-service model. Although the HMO Act of 1973 established certain federal standards for HMOs that elected to operate under federal law, almost all other aspects of regulatory authority over the business of health insurance remained with the states (Fuchs, 1997). This created substantial variation in the regulation over managed care organizations across the United States. Although a number of state-based HMO laws and regulations were based on the National Association of Insurance Commissioner's (NAIC) HMO Model Act, some states used the model act only as a starting point on which to build more restrictive regulations. The NAIC responded to the variation in types of risk-bearing entities with additional model law language pertaining to quality assessment and improvement, provider credentialing, network adequacy, grievance procedures, and standards for utilization review (Fuchs, 1997). In the 2006 version of the model act, case management is contained within the definition of utilization review as "Utilization review means a set of formal techniques utilized by or on behalf of the health maintenance organization designed to monitor the use of or evaluate the clinical necessity, appropriateness, efficacy or efficiency of health care services, procedures, providers or facilities. Techniques may include ambulatory review, prospective review, second opinion, certification, concurrent review, case management, discharge planning or retrospective review" (National Association of Insurance Commissioners, 2003). From this placement, it appeared as though the insurance industry viewed case management simply as a tool to achieve plan administration and care delivery to its members. However, placed in the larger historical context, the limited scope of this definition ignores the rich history of case management's development and reduces its activity to a mere business tactic.

In terms of health care insurance and its influence on case management's growth, Liberty Mutual began to leverage case management strategies in an effort to control the cost of rehabilitation care for injured workers. Following World War II, returning injured soldiers suffering catastrophic injuries required an intensive, multidisciplinary treatment. This approach to care required coordinated support from nurses and social workers who were best qualified to provide oversight to their complex clinical care needs (Lowery, 2009).

Two additional pieces of legislation passed in the late 1900s continue to influence health care coverage beyond the turn of the century. The Consolidated Omnibus Budget Reconciliation Act of 1985, popularly known as COBRA, allowed certain individuals covered by an employer-sponsored health plan to continue their coverage under certain conditions, termed as "qualifying events." Although possibly required to bear the full cost of coverage, the individuals would not lose their health care coverage altogether. COBRA applies to companies with 20 or more employees and affords this continued coverage protection only for a limited length of time. In addition, some states passed modified COBRA-like legislation for companies with fewer than 20 employees (Fuchs, 1997; Health Insurance Association of America, 1997a, 1997b).

The Health Insurance Portability and Accountability Act of 1996, known as HIPAA, provided additional protections by allowing "group-to-group" and "group-to-individual" health coverage portability. In the situation when an individual changed health plans at the same employer, the new plan had to include the previous coverage when tracking time toward fulfillment of any preexisting condition waiting period (assuming there was no break in coverage over 63 days). Another example of portability was that when qualified individuals lost group coverage, they were guaranteed access to some form of individual coverage, assuming they met qualifying conditions such as length of continuous coverage. States determined the conditions and details of cost and coverage. Coordination of continuing coverage and benefits to covered individuals with complex conditions came under the purview of each plan's case management department (Fuchs, 1997; Health Insurance Association of America, 1997a, 1997b).

A solid historical footing is essential to develop understanding as to how case management came about. It was not merely the outcome of a single event, piece of legislation, or professional affiliation but rather an organic development where growth was fostered by history and the insightful response to biologic, psychological, and sociologic needs of a growing and complex population.

References

Ball, R. M. (1973). Social Security Amendments of 1972: Summary and legislative history. *Social Security Bulletin, 36*(3), 3–25.

Bodenheimer, T., & Grumbach, K. (2009). *Understanding health policy: A clinical approach* (6th ed.). New York, NY: McGraw Hill Medical.

Buchmueller, T. C., & Monheit, A. C. (2009). *Employer-sponsored health insurance and the promise of health insurance reform* (Working Paper 14839). Cambridge, MA: National Bureau of Economic Research. Retrieved from http://www.nber.org/papers/w14839

Buhler-Wilkerson, K. (1985). Public health nursing: In sickness or in health? *American Journal of Public Health, 75*(10), 1155–1161.

Buhler-Wilkerson, K. (1993). Bringing care to the people: Lillian Wald's legacy to public health nursing. *American Journal of Public Health, 83*(12), 1778–1786.

Case Management Society of America. (2010). *CMSA Standards of practice for case management* (Rev.). Retrieved from http://www.cmsa.org/portals/0/pdf/memberonly/StandardsOfPractice.pdf

Cohen, W. J., & Ball, R. M. (1965). Social Security Amendments of 1965: Summary and legislative history. *Social Security Bulletin, 28*(9), 3–21.

Commonwealth of Massachusetts. (1863). *An act in relation to state charitable and correctional institutions* (Chapter 240). Retrieved from http://archives.lib.state.ma.us/actsResolves/1863/1863acts0240.pdf

Education for All Handicapped Children Act of 1975. 20 U.S.C. §1401 (1975). Retrieved from http://www.gpo.gov/fdsys/pkg/STATUTE-89/pdf/STATUTE-89-Pg773.pdf

Feld, M. N. (2008). *Lillian Wald: A biography*. New York, NY: The University of North Carolina Press.

Fuchs, B. (1997). *Managed health care: Federal and state regulation*. Library of Congress—Congressional Research Service, Series 97-938 EPW. Retrieved from http://research.policyarchive.org/485.pdf

Fulmer, H. (1902). History of visiting nurse work in America. *American Journal of Nursing, 2*(6), 411–425.

Hansan, J. E. (n.d.). *Charity organization societies: 1877–1893*. The Social Welfare History Project. Retrieved from http://www.socialwelfarehistory.com/organizations/charity-organization-societies-1877-1893

Health Insurance Association of America. (1997a). *Fundamentals of health insurance: Part A*. Washington, DC: Author.

Health Insurance Association of America. (1997b). *Fundamentals of health insurance: Part B*. Washington, DC: Author.

Hunt, N., & Kirk, S. (2005). *The Education for All Handicapped Children Act (PL 94-142) 1975*. Houghton Mifflin College Division. Retrieved from http://college.hmco.com/education/resources/res_prof/students/spec_ed/legislation/pl_94-142.html

Johnson, M. A. (2005). Hull House. In *The Electronic Encyclopedia of Chicago*. Retrieved from www.encyclopedia.chicagohistory.org/pages/615.html

Lane, L. C. (1963). *Jane Addams as social worker, the early years at Hull House* (Doctoral dissertation). Retrieved from ProQuest Dissertations and Theses. (Accession No. AAI6307514)

Leavitt, J. W., & Numbers, R. L. (Eds.). (1997). *Sickness and health in America: Readings in the history of medicine and public health* (pp. 3–10). Madison: University of Wisconsin Press.

Lewis, L. (2008). Discussion and recommendations: Nurses and social workers supporting family caregivers. *Journal of Social Work Education, 44*(3), 129–136.

Linn, J. W. (1935). *Jane Addams: A biography* [Kindle version]. Retrieved from http://www.amazon.com/Jane-Addams-James-Weber-Linn-ebook/dp/B00CIX2USC/ref=tmm_kin_title_popover

Lowery, S. (2009). Overview of case management. In S. Powell & H. Tahan (Eds.), *Case management: A practical guide for education and practice* (3rd ed.). Philadelphia, PA: Lippincott Williams & Wilkins.

Lundblad, K. S. (1995). Jane Addams and social reform: A role model for the 1990s. *Social Work, 40*(5), 661–669.

Massachusetts State Hospitals: A social history. (1867). Retrieved from http://www.1856.org/socialhistory.html

Murdach, A. D. (2011). Mary Richmond and the image of social work. *Social Work, 56*(1), 92–94.

National Association of Insurance Commissioners. (2003). *Health maintenance organization model act*. Retrieved from http://naic.org/store/free/MDL-430.pdf

Netting, F. E. (1992). Case management: Service or symptom? *Social Work, 37*(2), 160–164.

Older Americans Act of 1965, 42 U.S.C. 3056 (1965). Retrieved from http://www.gpo.gov/fdsys/pkg/STATUTE-79/pdf/STATUTE-79-Pg218.pdf

Our Documents. (2012). An act to provide for the general welfare by establishing a system of Federal old-age benefits, and by enabling the several States to make more adequate provision for aged persons, blind persons, dependent and crippled children, maternal and child welfare, public health, and the administration of their unemployment compensation laws; to establish a Social Security Board; to raise revenue; and for other purposes, August 14, 1935; Enrolled Acts and Resolutions of Congress, 1789-; General Records of the United States Government; Record Group 11; National Archives. Retrieved from http://www.ourdocuments.gov/doc.php?flash=true&doc=68

Powell, S., & Tahan, H. (2008). *CMSA core curriculum for case management* (2nd ed.). Philadelphia, PA: Lippincott Williams & Wilkins.

Richmond, M. E. (1901). Charitable co-operation. In I. C. Barrows (Ed.). *Proceedings of the national conference of charities and correction*. Retrieved from https://archive.org/stream/proceedingsnati13sessgoog#page/n319/mode/2up

Slavin, R. (2006). *Educational psychology* (8th ed.). Boston, MA: Allyn & Bacon.

Social Security Act of 1935 Legislative History. (2013). Retrieved from http://www.ssa.gov/history/35act.html

Social Welfare History Archives. (n.d.). *Henry Street Settlement Records*. Retrieved from http://special.lib.umn.edu/findaid/xml/sw0058.xml

The Social Welfare History Project. (n.d.). *Mary Ellen Richmond (1861–1928)—Social work pioneer, administrator, researcher and author*. Retrieved from http://www.socialwelfarehistory.com/people/richmond-mary

Tahan, H. (1998). Case management: A heritage more than a century old. *Nursing Case Management, 3*(2), 55–60.

Turnbull, H. R., III, & Turnbull, A. P. (2000). *Free and appropriate public education: The law and children with disabilities* (6th ed.). Denver, CO: Love Publishing.

U.S. Department of Education. (n.d.). *History twenty five years of programs in educating children with disabilities through IDEA* (archived). Washington, DC: Office of Special Education and Rehabilitative Services.

U.S. Department of Health and Human Services. (2014). *Historical evolution of programs for older americans. Administration on Aging*. Retrieved from http://www.aoa.gov/AOA_programs/OAA/resources/History.aspx

Wade, L. (1967). The heritage from Chicago's early settlement houses. *Journal of the Illinois State Historical Society, 60*(4), 411–441. Retrieved from http://www.jstor.org/stable/40190170

Wald, L. D. (1991). *The house on Henry Street*. New Brunswick, NJ: Transaction Publishers. (Original work published 1915).

Wales, M. (1941). *The public health nurse in action*. New York, NY: Macmillan.

Weil, M., & Karls, J. M. (1985). *Case management in human service practice* (1st ed.). San Francisco, CA: Jossey-Bass.

2 CONTEMPORARY INFLUENCES OF CASE MANAGEMENT PRACTICE

OBJECTIVES

After studying this chapter, you will be able to:

1. Identify contemporary influences on case management practice.
2. Recognize issues relating to professional licensure recognition between states.
3. Understand the three branches of government, the balance of powers, and how each branch relates to health care.
4. Recognize federal agencies involved in health care administration.

KEY TERMS

Accreditation
Coinsurance
Co-payment
Deductible
Endorsement
Home state
Licensure
Model Social Work Practice Act
Nurse Licensure Compact
Party state
Qualification
Reciprocity
Remote state
Standards of Practice

Since the 1970s, health care witnessed the proliferation of case management programs across a variety of care settings. It is important to recognize that although these programs were referred to as case management, the actual functions and activities of both program and staff were not always clearly defined, nor did they adhere to a legal or regulatory standard. The advent of credentialing programs and practice standards provided structure and expectations of program and role definition and scope of service, thus improving, but not perfecting, consistency. This chapter looks at some of the contemporary issues affecting the practice of case management.

HOW GOVERNMENT INFLUENCES CASE MANAGEMENT

Federal Government

There are three distinct branches of the U.S. federal government system: executive, judicial, and legislative. Each maintains a defined scope of power and responsibility in accordance with the Constitution. The checks and balances concept ensures that no single branch of the government overpowers the other branches through definition and interrelational nature of their respective powers.

Executive Branch

The executive branch of the government includes the president, vice president, executive offices, and various federal agencies. Article II of the Constitution grants presidential powers. The president is responsible to execute and enforce laws created by Congress, serves as the head of state, and is the commander in chief of the armed forces. In addition, the president appoints the heads of the federal agencies, including the cabinet (The White House, 2014a). The president's responsibility for health care lies mostly in his or her ability to define the national policy and/or agenda, and legislative action and make appointments to important leadership positions.

The cabinet is the president's key advisory body. Although appointed by the president, cabinet members undergo confirmation by the Senate. Each cabinet member bears responsibility for major federal agencies, many of which are involved in the administration of health care services (The White House, 2014a). Cabinet members serve at the pleasure of the president, who may dismiss them at will. The cabinet consists of the departments depicted in Figure 2-1. Many of these departments oversee aspects of health care services, the U.S. Department of Health and Human Services (DHHS) being the most recognizable.

Judicial Branch

The judicial branch of the government was established in Article III of the Constitution. The president appoints, and the Senate confirms, many of its members. Congress also maintains significant influence over the structure and shape of the federal judicial system, establishing both the district and appeals courts (The White House, 2014b). The highest authority court is the Supreme Court of the United States, sometimes referred to as SCOTUS or the Supreme Court (see Figure 2-2).

The Judicial Branch influences health care policy through the legal process. When a party (referred to as a litigant) loses a case in the lower court system, he or she may petition SCOTUS to review the case by filing a "writ of certiorari." SCOTUS maintains the option to accept or reject the cases it reviews; usually based on its importance to defining new legal principle, in situations when lower court interpretation of a law is contradictory, or if mandated to do so (The White House, 2014b). The Patient Protection and Affordable Care Act (PPACA) is an example of such a case and is discussed later in this chapter.

Legislative Branch

The legislative branch of the government, established by Article I of the Constitution, is also referred to as the U.S. Congress. It consists of two chambers: the Senate and the House of Representatives. Congress has authority to enact legislation, declare war, and confirm or reject a number of presidential appointments, and retains significant investigative powers (The White House, 2014c). Congress influences health care policy through the legislation it passes and, in some cases, the proposals and/or bills on which it chooses not to act. Members of Congress are elected by popular vote, which is one way in which the citizenry (as well as special interest groups) influences public policy through participation in the election process. Understanding the legislative process is essential if one is to effectively contribute to its outcome (see Figure 2-3).

Regulatory Agencies

Federal regulation is one of the basic tools the government uses to define and carry out public policy. Agencies issue, administer, and enforce regulations in order to operationalize the laws passed by Congress.

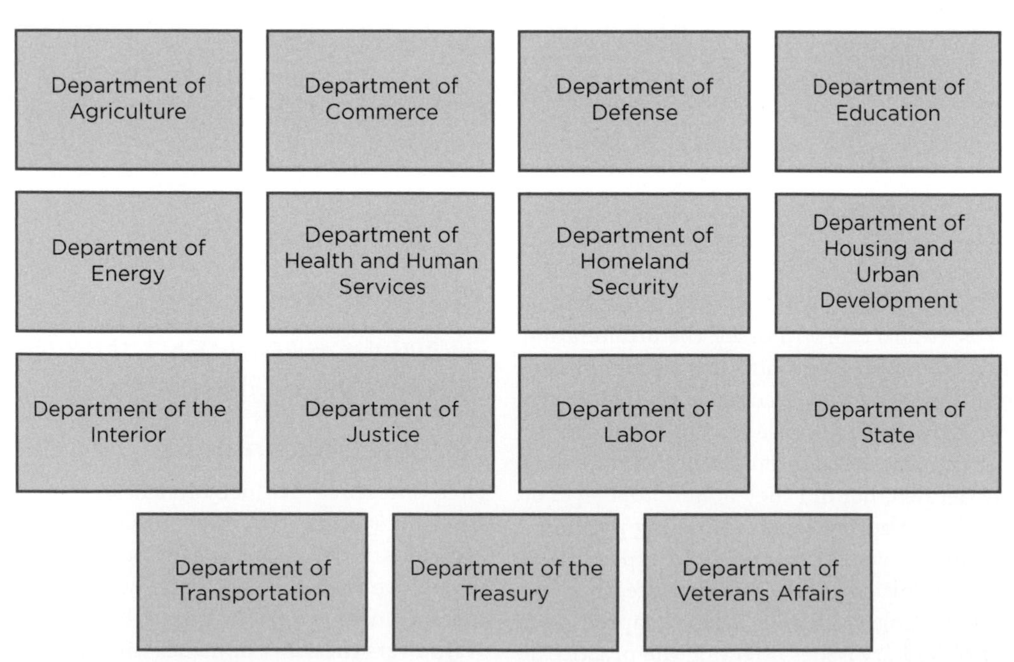

Figure 2-1. Cabinet-level departments.

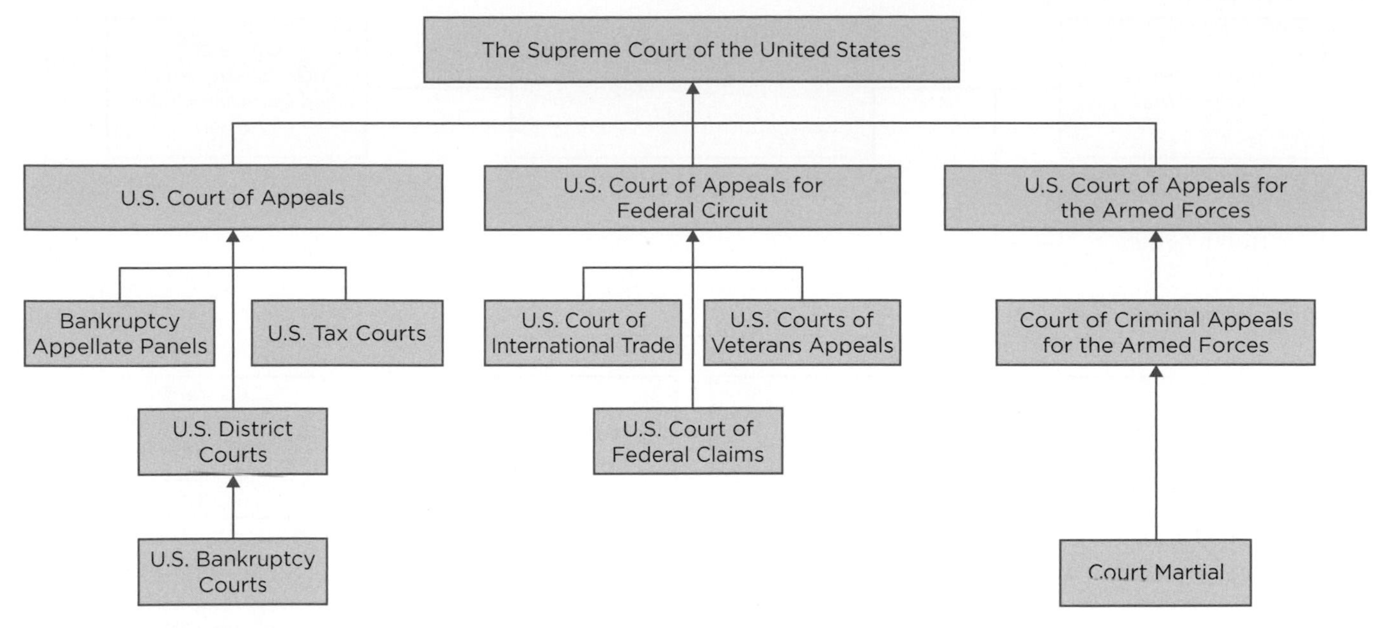

Figure 2-2. U.S. Federal Court system.

Department of Health and Human Services

The DHHS is the federal agency with the most health care-related responsibilities. Its mission is to help provide the building blocks that Americans need to live healthy, successful lives (DHHS, 2014). Agencies and departments falling within DHHS are shown in Figure 2-4. A number of agencies that play a role in health care delivery and/or policy are mentioned below.

Centers for Medicare and Medicaid Services

The Centers for Medicare and Medicaid Services (CMS) administers the Medicare program, partners with state governments to administer Medicaid and the State Children's Health Insurance Program (SCHIP), and has administrative oversight of health insurance portability standards. CMS affects case management practice in a variety of ways, not only providing and administering health care insurance but also

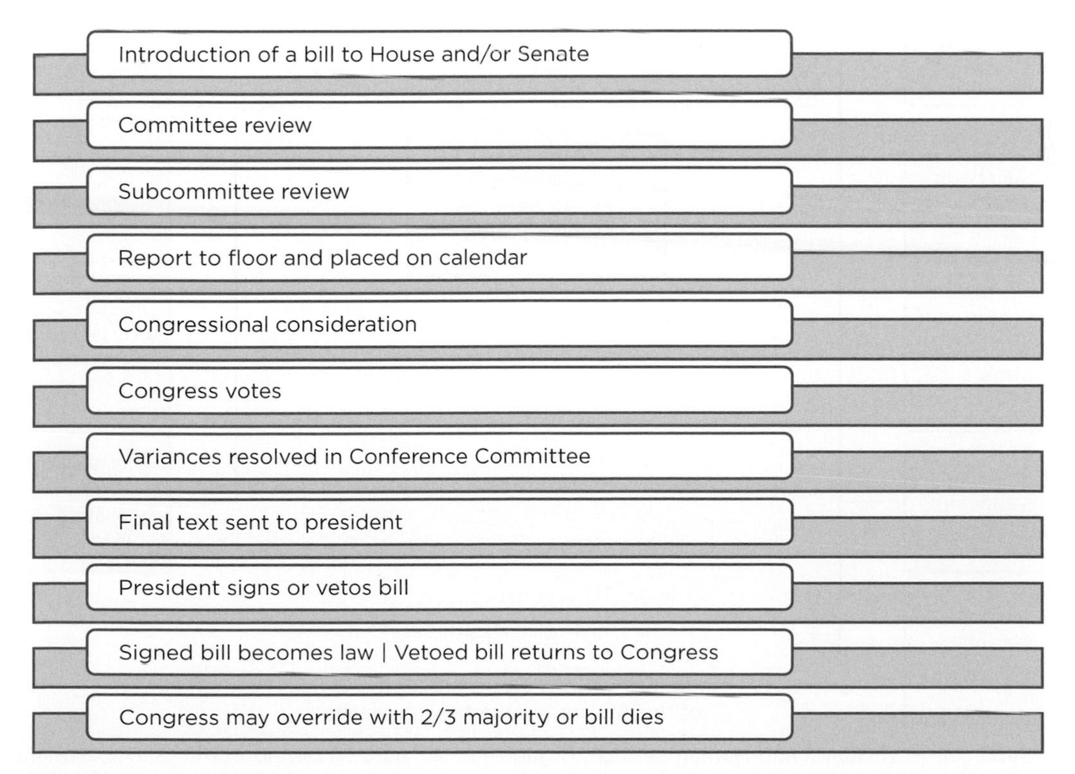

Figure 2-3. Federal legislative process.

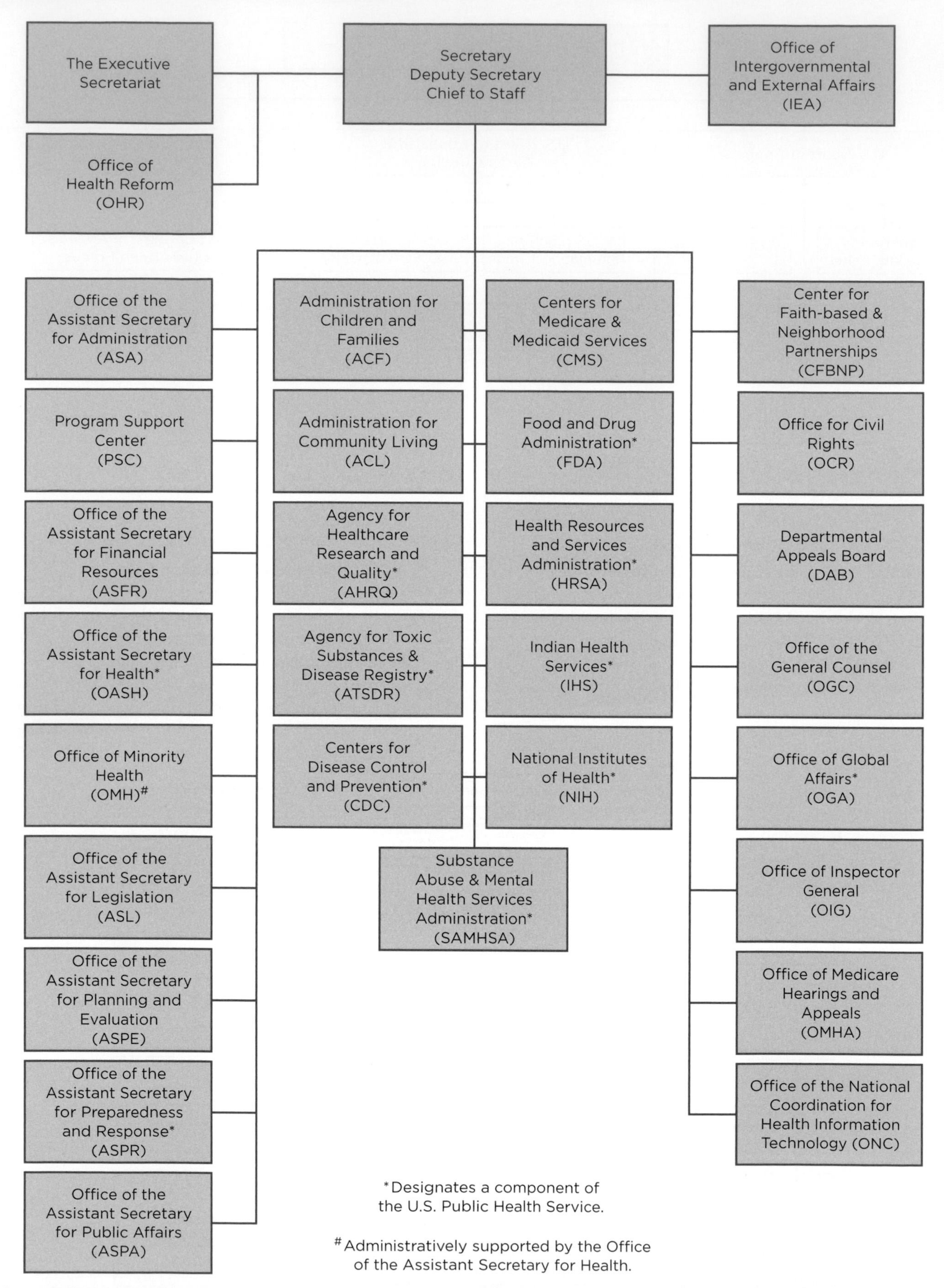

Figure 2-4. U.S. Department of Health and Human Services organizational chart. (Adapted from U.S. Department of Health and Human Services. (2014b). *Organizational chart.* Retrieved from http://www.hhs.gov/about/orgchart)

through its support of various programs, which include a case management service component.

Food and Drug Administration

The Food and Drug Administration (FDA) protects the public health through assuring the safety, efficacy, and security of drugs, biological products, medical devices, the food supply, cosmetics, and products that emit radiation (DHHS—FDA, 2014). Case managers intersect the FDA through accessing the website for information and adhering to regulations and mandates impacting client and population care delivery and quality.

Agency for Health Care Research and Quality

The Agency for Healthcare Research and Quality (AHRQ) produces evidence which improves health care delivery, quality, and safety. AHRQ ensures communication and utilization of evidence through ongoing communication with health care industry stakeholders and consumers (DHHS—AHRQ, 2013). The case management industry provides expert feedback through various means, including the Effective Healthcare Program Key Questions, and in meetings with AHRQ officials. Case managers utilize AHRQ resources for professional education, evidence-based care guidelines from the National Guidelines Clearinghouse, as well as ready-to-use consumer-friendly education materials.

Substance Abuse and Mental Health Services Administration

The Substance Abuse and Mental Health Services Administration (SAMHSA) leads public health efforts to advance the behavioral health of the nation. SAMHSA's mission is to reduce the impact of substance abuse and mental illness on America's communities (DHHS—SAMHSA, 2014). Case managers working with complex, dual-diagnosis clients and those working primarily in mental health care settings access SAMHSA resources to bring up-to-date care coordination information and benefits to the client and the care team.

Office of the National Coordinator for Health Information Technology

The Office of the National Coordinator for Health Information Technology (ONC) focuses on the use and implementation of health information technology and the electronic exchange of health information. Legislation mandated the creation of the ONC as part of Health Information Technology for Economic and Clinical Health Act implementation (DHHS—ONC, 2014). Case managers feel the ONC's impact through use of technology and electronic health records.

Department of Defense

The Department of Defense (DOD) is America's oldest and largest government agency. The DOD provides direct health care services and support to over 3.5 million individuals (DOD, 2014a), including active-duty military personnel and their dependents, military retirees and their families, and those eligible for DOD benefits (Sultz & Young, 2014).

Today, the Military Health Service (MHS) falls under the DOD umbrella, operating hospitals and outpatient clinics around the world. The MHS began prior to the Civil War; however, progress has moved it forward from lone regimental surgeons caring for ill and injured soldiers in tents to mobile surgical units in the field to centralized brick-and-mortar facilities. The improvements in communication and transportation infrastructure were essential to MHS advancements (DOD, 2014b).

Department of Veterans Affairs

The Department of Veterans Affairs (VA) traces back to 1636, when the Pilgrims of Plymouth Colony passed a law stating that soldiers disabled in the war with the Pequot Indians were to be supported by the colony. Today, the VA offers a variety of health care services through information, benefits, and educational opportunities. It is the nation's largest integrated health care system, operating more than 1,700 sites of care (e.g., medical centers, community clinics, community living centers, domiciliary, readjustment counseling centers) serving 8.76 million veterans each year (VA, 2014). The VA provides treatment to active-duty military and is affiliated with medical, dental, and other health care-related schools across the nation. Approximately 90,000 individuals receive training at VA facilities each year (Sultz & Young, 2014).

An asset of the VA system is that most veterans have established primary and specialty care, allowing the opportunity to build lifelong relationships and a comprehensive medical record (Sultz & Young, 2014). Case managers working for the VA are members of interdisciplinary teams who work face-to-face and/or in virtual environments with the interdisciplinary care team, including the veteran and their caregiver(s). In addition to working at facilities, there are opportunities to working with veterans through telemedicine. This model of case management is especially helpful for reaching individuals living in geographically remote areas, when there is no VA facility within a reasonable distance, and for veterans who face transportation and/or mobility barriers.

It is important to note that the wars in Iraq and Afghanistan placed tremendous stress on the capacity and resources of both the DOD and VA health care systems. This was evidenced by the quality-of-care issues brought to light through focus groups, interviews with patients and their families, as well as a presidential commission charged with evaluating the care of returning soldiers. In the report Serve, Support, Simplify (2007), the job title of case manager was specifically targeted as problematic in care coordination efforts. It was noted that many were undertrained and did not understand the complexities of the issues faced by injured soldiers. Unfortunately, the qualifications and responsibilities associated with these positions were not addressed in the report. Ultimately, it was the combination of various recommendations (e.g., base closure, quality of care) which led to realignment and consolidation of resources into modern treatment facilities capable of meeting the needs of returning military and veterans.

Department of Commerce

The Department of Commerce (DOC) promotes job creation, economic growth, sustainable development, and improved standards of living for all Americans. The DOC's influence over health care policy comes into play when issues cross into the areas within the department's purview, such as telemedicine and telehealth (DOC, 2014).

In 2009, the DOC issued the report Telemedicine: An Important Force in the Transformation of Healthcare. In it, the DOC recognized the importance of telemedicine in addressing barriers to successful implementation. The report identified a number of areas that would benefit from telemedicine, many of which are often primary responsibilities of case management, including chronic condition management and monitoring, care management for elders and home-bound individuals, and patient empowerment. An important barrier identified was that of the variation and exclusivity of state **licensure** requirements (Hein, 2009). The issues of licensure and interstate practice have been addressed by the DOC and are discussed later in this chapter.

State Government

General Overview of State Impact

Sultz and Young (2014) point out that since Medicare and Medicaid were established, the government has played an essential role in health care, serving to regulate, pay, and provide benefits and services. The Constitution provides state's governing authority over areas not clearly defined under federal jurisdiction. States are major stakeholders in health care, serving as regulators, payers, and providers. Services are chiefly funded through taxation and various other sources (e.g., grants).

Since the 1960s, cost containment has been the chief methodology for controlling health care expenditure. Medicaid is the federal/state program providing health care services to low-income children, the elderly, the blind, and individuals with disabilities. Table 2-1 provides a timeline for major milestones within the Medicaid program from 1965 to 2005. Each of these events affected case management due to the resulting expansion or contraction of both eligibility thresholds and/or benefits. State budgets felt the impact of

TABLE 2-1 Medicaid Milestones (1965-2005)

Year	Milestone
1965	The Medicare and Medicaid programs were signed into law on July 30, 1965.
1967	The Early and Periodic Screening, Diagnostic, and Treatment (EPSDT) established.
1972	Federal Supplemental Security Income program (SSI).
1981	Freedom of choice waivers (1915b) and home and community-based care waivers (1915c) mandated. States required to pay hospitals treating a disproportionate share of low-income patients additional payments.
1986	Medicaid coverage for pregnant women and infants established.
1988	The Qualified Medicare Beneficiary (QMB) eligibility rule.
1989	EPSDT requirements were expanded.
1990	The Medicaid prescription drug rebate program was enacted.
1991	DSH spending controls established. Provider donations banned. Provider taxes capped.
1996	The Aid to Families with Dependent Children (AFDC) entitlement program replaced by the Temporary Assistance for Needy Families (TANF) block grant.
1997	The Balanced Budget Act (BBA) of 1997 created the State Children's Health Insurance Program (SCHIP).
1999	The Ticket to Work and Work Incentives Improvement Act (TWWIIA) The Medicare, Medicaid, and SCHIP Balanced Budget Refinement Act stabilized the SCHIP allotment formula and modified the Medicaid DSH program.
2000	The Benefits Improvement and Protection Act (BIPA) modified the DSH program and modified SCHIP allotments.
2001	Section 1115 waiver initiative, Health Insurance Flexibility and Accountability (HIFA), allowed states to demonstrate comprehensive state approachesthat would expand coverage.

Year	Milestone
2003	The Jobs and Growth Tax Relief Reconciliation Act raised state Medicaid matching rates by 2.95 percentage points as temporary federal fiscal relief.
2003	The Medicare Prescription Drug, Improvement, and Modernization Act established Medicare Part D prescription drug coverage.
2003	Congress raises state-specific DSH allotments by 16% for FY 2004 for all states, through FY 2009 for low-DSH states.
2005	The U.S. Congress budget resolution requiring $10 billion in cost savings from Medicaid.
2005	Medicaid Commission established to report on cost savings and service improvements recommendations to help ensure the long-term sustainability.

Adapted from U.S. Department of Health and Human Services—Center for Medicare and Medicaid. (2013). Medicaid Milestones. Retrieved from http://www.cms.gov/About-CMS/Agency-Information/History/index.html?redirect=/History and The Henry J. Kaiser Family Foundation. (2008). Medicaid: A timeline of key developments. Retrieved from http://kff.org/medicaid/timeline/medicaid-a-timeline-of-key-developments

these changes, turning to grants and special funding opportunities to supplement shortfalls or through reductions in services.

The organizational structure of each state is individualized based on the population's needs; however, the three-branch model of government is used. Regulatory and administration responsibility for health care services is spread across a number of agencies. The reader is urged to learn more about how health care is administered at both state and local levels within their licensure jurisdiction(s).

HOW ACCREDITATION ORGANIZATIONS INFLUENCE CASE MANAGEMENT

To accredit something means to give it an official authorization or approval to an entity, such as a program or institution (Merriam-Webster, 2014a). In health care, **accreditation** demonstrates conformance with a prescribed set of expectations, often referred to as standards, and allows organizations to display specific credentials in association with the approval. Some accreditation programs maintain different levels of recognition, which may affect the period of time for which accreditation has been granted.

Accreditation differs from certification, which generally applies to an individual who meets prescribed criteria, including education, knowledge, and experience as set forth by the certifying body (Case Management Society of America, 2014). The impact of accreditation and/or certification depends on regulatory mandated status, as well as the acceptance by the industry and/or community served.

In the United States, the process of accreditation is voluntary. However, reimbursement is often tied an organization's accreditation status, making it, for all intents and purposes, mandatory if an organization or provider wishes to be reimbursed for its services. Accreditation granted by reputable and recognized organizations is a means to establish market credibility for a program, product, or service. In health care, there are numerous accreditation organizations, many of which include case management within its institutional and/or program recognitions.

The Joint Commission

The Joint Commission (JC) is an independent, not-for-profit organization that accredits and/or certifies health care organizations and programs in the United States. Founded in 1951, The JC evaluates and accredits more than 20,000 health care organizations and programs. It is the nation's oldest health care accreditation body (The JC, 2014).

In order to achieve accredited status, an organization undergoes an extensive survey of its operations, including documentation and physical site(s) at a minimum of every 3 years. As of January 2014, there were no case management-specific standards in use; however, there are transition of care measures which impact case managers working in acute care institutional settings (The JC, 2014).

URAC

Due to the rising trepidation regarding inconsistencies in utilization review activities, URAC was established in the latter part of the 1980s. Originally incorporated under the name, Utilization Review Accreditation Commission, the organization opted to abbreviate its name to the acronym as a result of expansion in the types of organizations it accredited (e.g., health plans, preferred provider organizations) beginning in 1996 (URAC, 2014a).

Utilization review (UR) is the process to determine the medical necessary of a health care service or product for a particular patient. Initially URAC's mission was to improve the quality and accountability of health care organizations leveraging UR as a means of cost containment. As accreditation offerings expanded, so too did URAC's mission.

Today, URAC has over 30 accreditation and certification programs in its portfolio (URAC, 2014a). Where case management is concerned, URAC offers a program accreditation

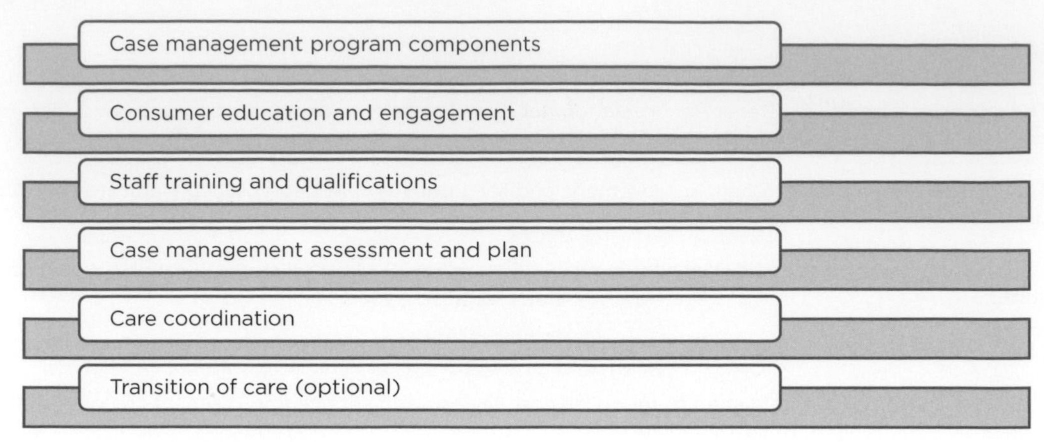

Figure 2-5. URAC case management domains.

as well as includes case management and care coordination standards within other accreditation programs. The URAC Case Management Standards, version 5.0 (2014b), address various domains, which are highlighted in Figure 2-5. In addition to the domain standards, organizations seeking recognition are required to submit measurement reports in the following areas:

- Medical readmissions
- Percentage of participants who were medically released to return to work
- Disability and workers' compensation only
- Complaint response timeliness
- Overall consumer satisfaction
- Excludes disability and workers' compensation
- Percentage of individuals who refused case management services
- Three-item care transition measure (optional—exploratory measure)
- Patient activation measure (optional—exploratory measure)

Commission on Accreditation of Rehabilitation Facilities

Founded in 1966, the Commission on Accreditation of Rehabilitation Facilities (CARF) is an international, nonprofit accreditation organization for health and human services. There are almost 50,000 programs and services in over 22,000 locations (CARF, 2014a) currently recognized by CARF. The scope of products and services surveyed by CARF include:

- Aging Services,
- Behavioral Health,
- Business and Services Management Networks,
- Child and Youth Services,
- Employment and Community Services, and
- Medical Rehabilitation.

CARF accredits case management within the purview of its Medical Rehabilitation program. Identified as a proactive service, the recognition of case management activities includes coordinating, facilitating, and advocating for services to patients with impairments, activity limitations, and participation restrictions. Included in case management program review are initial and ongoing assessment, knowledge and awareness of care options and linkages, effective and efficient use of resources, individualized care plans, achievement of predicted outcomes, and recognition of regulatory, legislative, and financial implications (CARF, 2014b).

National Committee for Quality Assurance

Founded in 1990, the National Committee for Quality Assurance (NCQA) continues to be a driving force committed to quality improvement across the health care continuum. NCQA's accreditation portfolio includes programs for health plans, provider organizations, health plan contracting organizations, and health/wellness promotion (NCQA, 2014a).

NCQA recognizes that case management programs exist within many care settings (e.g., provider offices, managed care, community-based organizations). The scope of case management program review includes documentation as well as processes that address: identification of case management candidates, personalized care planning, monitoring and adjusting care plans to individual needs, outcome/goal orientation, getting the appropriate services to the right people, communication and information sharing, transition planning, consumer protection, qualified staff, and protection of health information (NCQA, 2014b).

The NCQA accreditation program for health plans also includes standards pertaining to complex case management. Requirements within the Quality Management and Improvement section address areas such as assessment of member population characteristics and needs, program description, identification of candidates for complex case management, evidence-based practice, information system support, appropriate documentation, performance measures, and member satisfaction (NCQA, 2014c).

HOW LICENSURE AFFECTS CASE MANAGEMENT PRACTICE

Generically speaking, licensure is a process by which an authority grants permission to an individual to undertake an activity. The process of licensure is defined through legislation and regulation. Because the Constitution does not specify federal jurisdiction over licensure, governance falls to individual states, which has resulted in variances as to definition, scope, and oversight of practice. The issue of licensure pertains to individual qualifications to work in a case management position. **Qualification** is defined as "a special skill or type of experience or knowledge that makes someone suitable to do a particular job or activity or something that is necessary in order for you to do, have, or be a part of something" (Merriam-Webster, 2014b).

In case management, qualifications are frequently defined within job descriptions. However, qualifications may also be located in professional **standards of practice** and/or certification eligibility requirements.

The CMSA Standards of Practice include a qualification standard that sets an expectation to preparatory education and training which a case manager should attain. The language regarding case manager qualification is important as a point of consumer protection because when an individual identifies her or himself as a case manager, the consumer should have a reasonable expectation that the person meets a minimum level of education and training.

According to the CMSA Standards of Practice for Case Management, the qualification standard states that a case manager must have "current, active, and unrestricted licensure or certification in a health or human services discipline that allows the professional to conduct an assessment independently as permitted within the scope of practice of the discipline" (2010). The standard includes language pertaining to instances in which licensure or certification is not required by the granting authority (e.g., State Board of Registration), which is discussed later in the chapter. An examination of practice standards from two other case management organizations showed neither specifically addressing the point of qualification to be a case manager. The National Association of Professional Geriatric Care Managers (2013) addresses certification without discussion of education or training. The American Case Management Association (2013) standards include a certification requirement but do not specify the predicating education or training requirements within the standard.

Why is a qualification standard important? Individuals who do not meet minimum requirements of qualification are not deemed able to perform certain aspects of the role in the absence of specific education, training, and licensure. With regard to vocational or licensed practical nurses, neither of these levels of nursing recognition is within their scope of licensure to conduct an independent assessment; therefore, they should not qualify to work as case managers (according to the CMSA standard). Baccalaureate-level social workers face similar challenges with respect to licensure scope. Although most health care providers and institutions understand the importance of hiring qualified clinical professionals into case management positions, some do not. An example of this was a health system in Illinois. This organization hired licensed practical nurses into case manager positions. Subsequently, the organization acknowledged these individuals could not perform independent assessments within the scope of their licensure and took steps to correct the situation.

Standards of practice for case management are voluntary. There is no legal recourse available for enforcement or failure to adhere. However, standards have been referenced during legal action to demonstrate that an act or omission of an act was outside of the normal and expected practice. The situation previously described serves as an opportunity for educating employers to appropriately apply the case manager job title, specify accurate qualifications, and understand the scope of responsibility that authentic case management positions require. It also presents an opportunity to discourage the use of the case manager job title in instances when the full scope and responsibility of the position does not encapsulate professional case management practice.

Registered Nurse Licensure

The National Council of State Boards of Nursing (NCSBN) (2014) defines licensure as the process by which a Board of Nursing (BON) grants permission to engage in nursing practice after determining that the applicant has attained the competency necessary to perform a unique scope of practice.

Traditional Licensure Model

Traditionally, licensure is granted on a state-by-state basis. BONs, also identified as Boards of Registration, are state government agencies responsible for regulating practice. Each state's BON defines its mission, vision, goals, and priorities. The BON identifies the process and qualifications for attaining licensed status, as well as the scope and standards for safe nursing practice at various levels of qualification (e.g., licensed practical, advanced practice). The BON serves as the reporting agency in the event of assumed breaches of standard practice and defines disciplinary action in accordance with state laws and regulations. According to the NCSBN (2014), the usual authority and duties of a BON include the enforcement of the Nurse Practice Act and nurse licensure, accreditation/approval of nurse education programs in schools and universities, the development of practice standards, and the development of policies, administrative rules, and regulations governing practice. Though practice acts vary, Figure 2-6 identifies common elements found in nurse practice acts in the United States.

A few industry stakeholders believe that case management is not a practice of nursing (or of another clinical discipline). If one examines accurately titled position descriptions, it is not difficult to see that there is a consistent inclusion of a clinical licensure requirement in order to qualify for the position. Hence, the requirement for a predicate, unrestricted

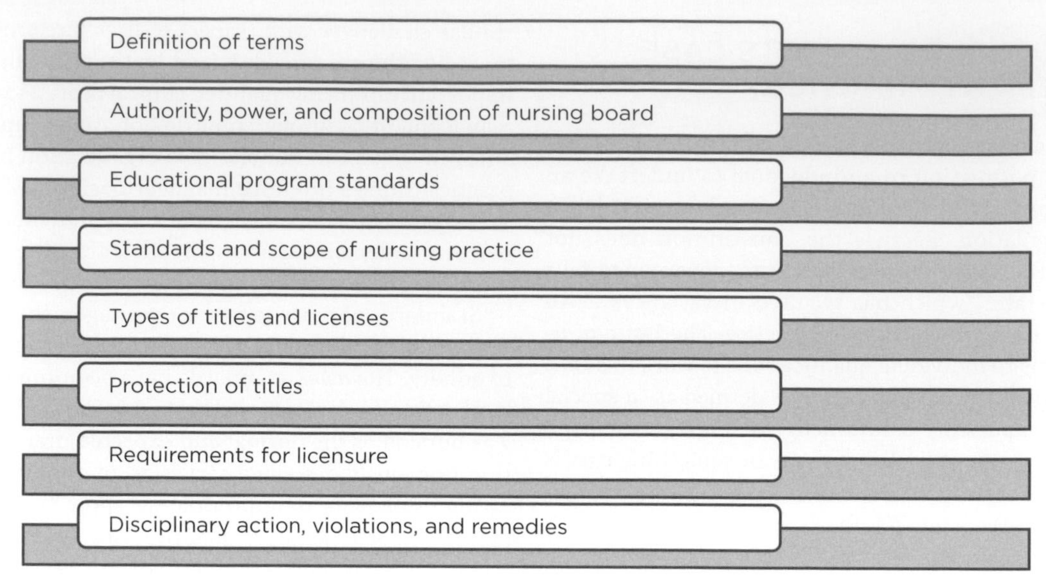

Figure 2-6. Common elements in nurse practice acts in the United States. (Adapted from Russell, K. A. (2012). Nurse practice acts guide and govern nursing practice. *Journal of Nursing Regulation, 3*(3), 36–40. Retrieved from https://www.ncsbn.org/2012_JNR_NPA_Guide.pdf)

clinical license sits in direct opposition to that opinion. When a nurse works as a case manager, she or he applies clinical education and experience throughout the case management process. In order to remain qualified for the case management position into which one was hired, it is essential to maintain one's licensure. A registered nurse is effectively practicing outside the scope of his or her licensure when responsibilities include working with clients who are physically located outside the borders of their state of licensure. In order to practice within the scope of one's license, the nurse obtains licensure in the state where the client(s) resides. The most frequently encountered exceptions to this apply to nurses serving in the military, working in the Veterans Administration system, working for the MHS, and those living in a state that is a party to the **Nurse Licensure Compact (NLC)**.

Nurse Licensure Compact

Health care professionals no longer need to be in the same physical location as their patient. There are a number of factors that influence the delivery of health care services, including insurance contract terms, transportation, and communication technology.

Employers provide health benefits for individuals residing across the country as well as internationally. Modern transportation has resulted in expanded mobility and people travel more extensively than ever before. In addition, telehealth is transforming clinical practice from strictly face-to-face visits to encounters using a wide variety of audio, video, and computer technologies. The NLC addresses the advances in care delivery, as well as simplifies the expense and bureaucratic complexity of maintaining licensure in more than one jurisdiction.

The NLC is a mutual recognition licensure model. For a licensed, registered nurse residing in a Compact state, it allows for recognition of primary licensure by other states that are also a party to the Compact, thereby allowing that individual to practice in other participating state(s) without having to obtain separate licenses. This recognition allows for physical and virtual practice according to the state's laws and regulations in which nursing practice occurs (Poe, 2008). Figures 2-7 A–C depict common scenarios in which nursing practice is affected by a state's adoption of the Compact. It is important to note that there are Compacts applicable to licensed practical/vocational and advanced practice nurses. However, for simplicity's sake this chapter focuses on the RN version of the NLC.

The NCSBN (2014) provides a helpful example demonstrating application of the Compact principles. Mary is a licensed registered nurse who has declared primary residence in Colorado. She holds a nursing license in Colorado. She lives near the four corners (Utah, Arizona, New Mexico, and Colorado) area. Because each of these states adopted the Compact, Mary may cross borders to practice nursing, either physically or electronically, without incurring additional applications or fees, assuming she follows the appropriate procedure for notification of each state in which she chooses to work. However, if Mary moves her primary residence to New Mexico, she must change her state of residence and have a new license issued by the BON in New Mexico. In this example, each of these states is a **party state**, one that has adopted the Compact. Mary's **home state** is Colorado. Utah, Arizona, and New Mexico are **remote states**, party states other than the nurse's home state.

There have been issues relating to state adoption of the NLC. The Health Resource and Services Administration (HRSA) submitted a report to Congress relating to clinical licensure which included discussion of the NLC. In the report, the common reasons for state opposition to the NLC include the loss of control or authority, lack of uniform standards, loss of revenue/incurrence of cost, fear among unions and state nurse associations that the NLC would facilitate strike breaking, and misinformation about the Compact and the lack of independent evaluation (DHHS—HRSA, 2011).

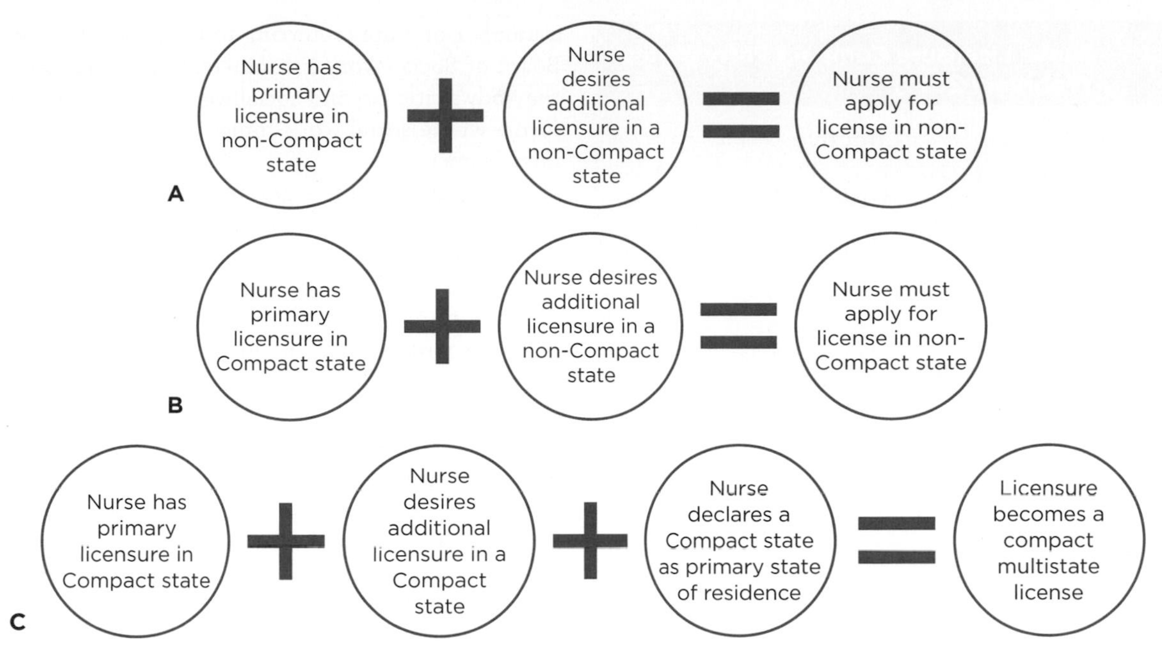

Figure 2-7. A: Nurse Licensure Compact scenario 1. **B**: Nurse Licensure Compact scenario 2. **C**: Nurse Licensure Compact scenario 3.

The NCSBN works to address and/or resolve misunderstandings and misapplications of the Compact. In an August 2013 memorandum, the NCSBN addressed the matter of employer mandates for nurses in Compact states to apply for licensure in the state in which the organization is located, as a condition of employment. This was noted as a direct violation of the Compact language specifying that a licensed registered nurse would only hold licensure in one party state at a time, their home state being their primary state of residence (Masters, 2013a).

In a previous matter within the state of Oklahoma, the NCSBN issued a statement with regard to the Attorney General's opinion of the state's sovereign power. The Attorney General concluded that the Compact represented an unlawful delegation of power as it related to the authorization of other states to determine a nurse's qualification to work within the state of Oklahoma in the absence of adopting its standards. In the NCSBN memorandum (Masters, 2013b), the following points were articulated:

- The Compact provides that nurses subject to the Compact are only licensed to practice nursing in their home state and that said license will be recognized by each Compact member state "as authorizing a multi-state licensure privilege to practice as a registered nurse in the Compact member states."
- The Compact limits the delegated power by reserving to Party states the authority to "limit or revoke the multistate licensure privilege of any nurse to practice in their state and may take any other actions under their applicable state laws necessary to protect the health and safety of their citizens."
- The Compact requires that nurses practicing in a party state must comply with the state practice laws in the state in which the patient is located at the time the care is rendered.
- The Compact recognizes that the practice of nursing is not limited to patient care, but includes all forms of nursing practice as defined by the state practice laws of a party state.

As of January 2014, the Compact has passed into law in 24 states. There are bills before the legislatures of five additional states (Massachusetts, Minnesota, Illinois, New York, and Oklahoma) slated for the 2013 to 2014 session (see Table 2-2). Clearly, a state's interpretation of Compact provisions greatly influenced its chances for adoption into law. However, there are other barriers to passage, including the strong opposition of collective bargaining units, which represent the concerns of nurses working in acute care and institutional settings. It is important that legislators, regulators, and employers receive current and accurate information as to the implications of Compact passage and that case managers remain vigilant to ensure their practice remains within the limitations as set forth by their respective nurse practice act.

Social Work Licensure

Inconsistency Across the States

Licensure for social workers is granted by each state. However, the regulations pertaining to social work practice are more complex. Intricacies underlie every element of licensure. This extends from how the state boards are organized to which levels of practice are recognized, how those levels are regulated, and their respective scopes of practice. This results in confusion across the industry as professionals and stakeholders wrestle to comprehend the similarities

TABLE 2-2 Nurse Licensure Compact Party States (February 2014)

State	Effective
Arizona	July 1, 2002
Arkansas	July 1, 2000
Colorado	October 1, 2007
Delaware	July 1, 2000
Idaho	July 1, 2001
Iowa	July 1, 2000
Kentucky	June 1, 2007
Maine	July 1, 2001
Maryland	July 1, 1999
Mississippi	July 1, 2001
Missouri	June 1, 2010
Nebraska	January 1, 2001
New Hampshire	January 1, 2006
New Mexico	January 1, 2004
North Carolina	July 1, 2000
North Dakota	January 1, 2004
Rhode Island	July 1, 2008
South Carolina	February 1, 2006
South Dakota	January 1, 2001
Tennessee	July 1, 2003
Texas	January 1, 2000
Utah	January 1, 2000
Virginia	January 1, 2005
Wisconsin	January 1, 2000

and differences among social workers throughout the country. Although it is common practice to refer professionals to board websites and select established resources for the purpose of obtaining current information about licensure, it is absolutely the most advisable manner for social work stakeholders to proceed.

Each state has an administrative body tasked with regulatory oversight of social workers practicing within the jurisdiction. However, not all of these bodies are referred to as Boards of Social Work. Texas and Maryland are among a number of states referring to their oversight body as the Board of Social Work Examiners. Still other states broaden the body's title beyond social work. Such is the case in California where social work comes under the Board of Behavioral Sciences.

Each state's entity is granted administrative oversight to define the eligibility requirements and scopes of practice for the levels of licensure offered. Not all offer the same licensure levels. However, the Clinical Social Work level is always licensed. In most states, Masters-level social workers are licensed regardless of their clinical practice status. Many, but not all, states license baccalaureate-level social workers (SocialWorkLicensure.org, 2014a).

Some states exempt certain types of social workers from licensure, such as those employed in specific care settings (e.g., hospitals, nursing homes, schools) (Fink-Samnick, 2012). As it pertains to case management, these exemptions may pose as an additional challenge for individuals seeking certification. This is related to the eligibility requirements of certain credentials which specifically include licensure.

The credentials applied to social work licensure levels are equally varied. For example, in Virginia the clinical licensure designated credential is Licensed Certified Social Worker (LCSW). The equivalent designation in the District of Columbia is Licensed Independent Clinical Social Worker (LICSW), and in Maryland it is LCSW-C (Fink-Samnick, 2011). Box 2-1 provides a comparison of states to further demonstrate how complex social work licensure presents across jurisdictions.

Efforts to Standardize Social Work Licensure

There have been several attempts to define a more uniform approach to social work licensure. In 1960, the National Association of Social Workers (NASW) created the Academy of Certified Social Workers (ACSW). Before enacting state licensing requirements, the ACSW served as the source to qualify social workers for independent practice (Kelly, 2010). Some in the industry viewed this credential as the profession's way to set a national standard for practice amid the lack of a consistent licensure structure. Although the ACSW remains one of the most recognized social work certifications, it is not the same as licensing and grants no legal authority to practice (SocialWorkLicensure.org, 2014a).

In 1996, the Association of Social Work Boards (ASWB) developed the **Model Social Work Practice Act**. The ASWB is the nonprofit organization composed of and owned by the social work regulatory boards and colleges of 49 U.S. states, the District of Columbia, the U.S. Virgin Islands, and all 10 Canadian provinces. Similar to the NCSBN, they serve a number of oversight functions for the profession with their mission to strengthen protection of the public by providing support and services to the social work regulatory community to advance safe, competent, and ethical practices (ASWB, 2014).

Recognizing the disparity in social work legislation and regulation, the Model Social Work Practice Act established standards of minimal social work competence and methods of fairly and objectively addressing consumer complaints. The Act also contributed to increased public and professional

BOX 2-1 Social Work Licensure Comparison

Alabama: Board of Social Work

Three levels of licensure and one additional certification.

One may be licensed as a social worker with either a bachelor's or a master's degree from an accredited institution.

Licensed Bachelor Social Worker (LBSW) is granted to social workers with bachelor's degrees.

Licensed Graduate Social Worker (LGSW), Licensed Certified Social Worker (LCSW), and Private Independent Practice (PIP) all require the minimum of a master's-level education.

The Board recognizes distinct practice areas, including

- social casework,
- clinical social work,
- social work administration, and
- social work research.

New Hampshire: Board of Mental Health Practice

One social work license offered.

Licensed Independent Clinical Social Worker (LICSW) is granted to professionals at the highest level of practice.

The credentialing process includes graduate level education, post-degree supervised work experience, a licensing exam, and a rigorous application process.

Oklahoma: State Board of Licensed Social Workers

Five social work licenses offered.

Licensed Social Worker Associate (LSWA) is granted to individuals with baccalaureate education and supervised work experience.

All other licensure designations require a master's degree.

A person is eligible for the Licensed Master's Social Worker (LMSW) immediately after graduation. After a period of supervised practice the individual may earn one of the following designations:

A. Licensed Social Worker (LSW),

B. Licensed Clinical Social Worker (LCSW), or

C. Licensed Social Worker—Administration (LSW-ADM).

The Board has a well-defined scope of practice for each level. A distinction is made between independent practice and private practice. Only LCSWs are permitted to go into private practice, but LSWs and LSW-ADMs are allowed to practice independently.

Adapted from SocialWorkLicensure.org. (2014b). Social work licensure requirement state map. Retrieved from http://www.socialworklicensure.org

understanding of social work through advancing the consistency in legal decisions related to licensure, renewal, discipline, and other board activities (ASWB, 2013).

The Model Social Work Practice Act continues to serve a pivotal role in promoting more consistent terminology and regulation from jurisdiction to jurisdiction. Figure 2-8 shows the key areas recommended for adoption by all state boards.

Social work licensure standardization, across all states, would provide an invaluable asset to those working as case managers. Not only would this enhance an employer's ability to ascertain a social worker's qualifications, it would also address a certification challenge. This challenge pertains to an element of the Model Social Work Practice Act, Independent Practice. Although it is generally understood that social workers licensed at the clinical level may practice independently, the inclusion of this defining language may be noticeably absent, or lack necessary clarity, in state regulation. For example, a state may equate independent practice with private practice, and fail to clarify that a social worker is allowed to conduct an independent assessment. This gray area contributes to difficulties experienced by individuals wishing to become certified. As a result, the application process becomes unduly complicated for the certification review committee and results in rejection of the application.

The Social Work Examination

Among the various responsibilities of the ASWB is to maintain the examinations which test an individual's competence to ethically and safely practice social work (ASWB, 2014). There are four categories of social work examinations: Bachelors, Masters, Advanced Generalist, and Clinical. Each examination encompasses a well-defined scope of knowledge, the current details of which may be accessed on the ASWB website. However, as noted earlier in this chapter, not all recognition levels are available in every state. Those offered are delineated according to the licensure designations that each state regulates (ASWB, 2014).

Endorsement and Reciprocity

The practice issues resulting from increased mobility and technologic advances are causing ripples across the ranks of social workers, as is the case for other health care professionals. Despite these evolving societal advances, social work does not have a licensure compact or true **reciprocity**, whereby the virtue of possessing licensure in one state means an individual can automatically practice at that licensure level in another state. Although there is no existing social work licensure compact, there are exemptions to licensure for clinical social workers employed for government agencies. This applies to those serving in the military or employed as a military contractors.

Presently, a social worker must register for **endorsement**, assuming the option is available, for each state in which the individual wishes to practice. This represents a significant expense as well as an administrative burden to the individual. It also represents a barrier to employment. A social worker who must undergo an endorsement review faces the prospect of processing delays, added expense of multiple

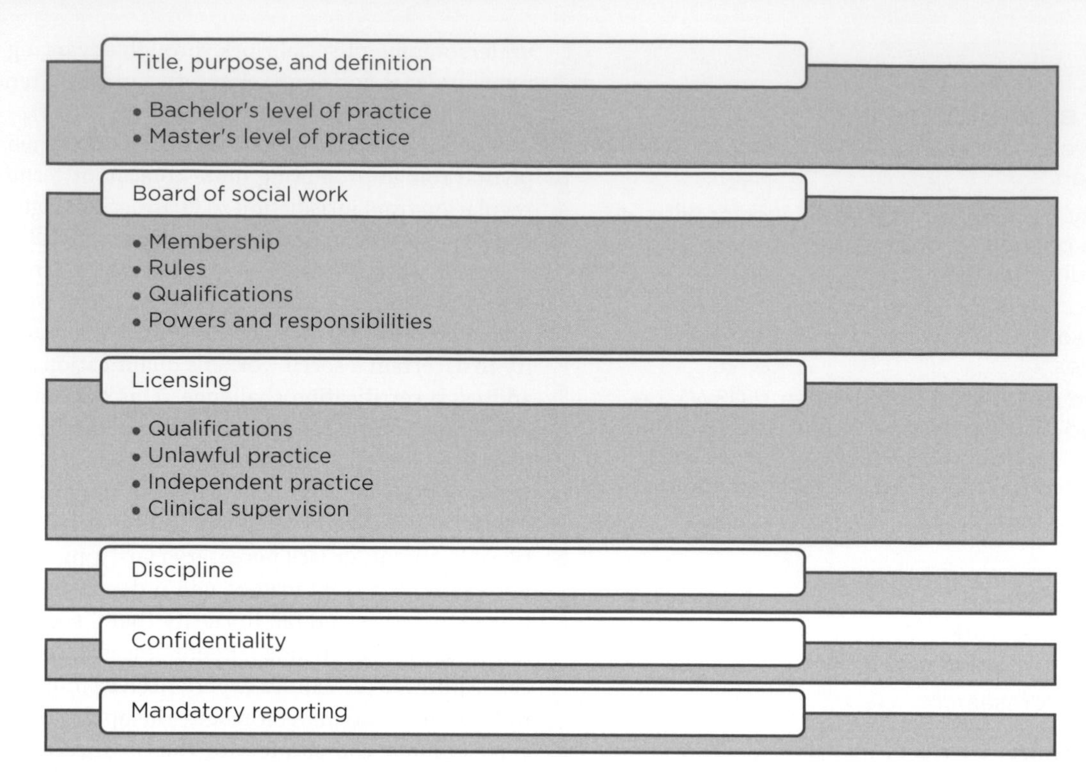

Figure 2-8. ASWB-recommended elements for Social Work Practice Acts.

state fees, the administrative burden associated with tracking multiple credentials, and the manifesting inconvenience to potential employers (Fink-Samnick, 2011).

HOW PAYERS AFFECT CASE MANAGEMENT PRACTICE

Case managers today need a working knowledge of the U.S. health care financing system in order to optimize benefit utilization and to access other sources of care funding when appropriate. This nontraditional curriculum content calls for expansion of undergraduate education in nursing and social work as well as the other disciplines, which feed the working pool of case management. This section provides an overview of existing health care finance mechanisms. The reader is advised to investigate additional resources in their practice setting and jurisdiction.

Health Care Spending in the United States

It is important to understand that health care finance affects case management practice. The amount of money spent on health care in the United States is staggering. Consider the percentage of health care expenditure in terms of our nation's gross domestic product (GDP). The GDP is the monetary measure of a country's total economic production. Health care outstrips the costs of education and national defense combined. In the 1950s, the percentage of GDP for health care cost was less than 5%. By the year 2020, that percentage is anticipated to be just less than 20%.

According to the CMS's Office of the Actuary, health care spending in 2012 broke down as follows:

- Medicare spending totaled $572.5 billion
- Medicaid spending reached $421.2 billion
- Private health insurance premiums reached $917.0 billion
- Out-of-pocket spending amounted to $328.2 billion

Major Factors Influencing Health Care Cost

Although many factors influence the cost of care, for the purpose of this textbook, the three impacts discussed are inflation, advancing technology, and service demand.

In economic terms, inflation is the percentage change in the value of a price index on a year-over-year basis (Economic Times.com, 2014). In plain English, inflation measures the change in the price of a basket of goods and services and is expressed as a percentage. Inflation is an indicator of how many dollars it takes to purchase that same basket of goods and services. When the economy experiences inflation, the value of currency is effectively reduced; hence, it buys less. For example, in January 2013 a basket of goods and services costs $1.00. When inflation applies, that same basket costs $1.03 in January 2014. The year-over-year inflation rate is 3%. Although this may not sound significant, over a 10-year period, a 3% annual inflation rate results in a $1.00 cost becoming $1.34. This is a loss in currency value of over one third.

Inflation affects the case manager's ability to stretch benefit dollars in order to obtain products and services required by a client. Today's $1,500 benefit limit does not go as far as it did 5 to 10 years ago. Case managers must remain informed of factors such as pharmaceutical **co-payments** (discussed later in this section). For a client on a fixed income, the difference between paying a $10 versus a $50 medication co-payment could make having nutritious food on the table quite challenging or may delay paying a utility bill. In these instances, the case manager needs to be mindful of various forms of financial assistance and also be efficient in completing any application processes in order to qualify a client for a given benefit. In addition, maintaining knowledge of available generic versions of medication and advising the prescriber of less expensive options may help to alleviate financial burden and improve adherence because the client is able to afford buying the medication and not forced to make a choice between medication and food.

Advances in health care technology abound, including hardware (e.g., diagnostic equipment), pharmaceuticals, and biologics, as well as the procedures used to treat illness. Both information technology and computer-assisted innovation require extensive investment of time and money in development and testing prior to market use. There is also the need of skilled technicians to operate and maintain systems and equipment after deployment (Sultz and Young, 2014).

Demand is a business term and a basic principle of economics. It describes the consumer desire for goods or service, as well as the willingness to pay a given price for it. In health care, the changing age demographic is a significant influencer of demand. Consider demand as expressed as a waiting line. The number of adults over 65 years of age represents over 13% or about 1 in every 8 Americans. This reflects an increase by 6.3 million people or 18% since 2000. To place this into context, the under-65 population increased 9.4% during the same period (DHHS—AOA, 2012). The waiting line demanding health care services is lengthening.

HEALTH CARE FINANCE MECHANISMS

There are a variety of financing mechanisms at play in the health care system. This creates tremendous complexity and cost in processing the billing and payment of goods and services.

Self-Payment

Out-of-pocket coverage of health care expenses is classified as self-payment. Today, this is not a common option as a sole means of payment due to the existence of health insurance, the unpredictability of health status, and the related variability in the cost of care. However, there is a degree of self-payment through the requirement of **coinsurance**, **deductible**, and co-payment. Coinsurance is a type of cost sharing where the insured party and insurer share a payment of the approved charge for covered services in a specified ratio after payment of the deductible by the insured (Dasco & Dasco, 1999). A deductible is a minimum threshold payment that must be reached by an enrollee each year before the plan begins to make payments on a full or partial basis (Dasco & Dasco, 1999). A co-payment is a type of sharing under which the insured party is responsible for paying a fixed dollar amount for a product or service (Dasco & Dasco, 1999). Each of these mechanisms carries the potential of financial hardship based on the health insurance coverage choices of the individual. Case managers must be mindful of the particulars associated with each client's health insurance coverage.

Private Health Insurance

Insurance for payment of health care services has been part of the landscape since the 19th century; however, it was more a functional income replacement or death benefit mechanism than it was a means to pay health care costs and did not resemble today's insurance (Sultz & Young, 2014). Refer to the discussion of health insurance and health maintenance organization development in chapter 1.

Publicly Funded Health Care Programs

Creation of Medicare and Medicaid was discussed in chapter 1. Together, these programs provide a significant portion of health care coverage and service to populations at greatest risk and need (e.g., aged, disabled, financially disadvantaged).

Medicare is funded through payroll deduction. Both employer and employee contribute equally to the fund, which has become a major payer source. Approximately 30% of payments to hospitals and 22% of payments to providers come through Medicare. There are four distinct parts of Medicare: Part A is hospital insurance, Part B is supplemental medical insurance, Part C is managed Medicare referred to as Medicare Advantage, and Part D is prescription drug coverage. Although initially popular, enrollment in Part C declined as cuts were made to reimbursements, causing providers to withdraw from participation (Sultz & Young, 2014). With the reduction in provider selection, many beneficiaries returned to traditional Medicare coverage.

The impact on the case manager is in remaining abreast of Medicare coverage for each programs. Each client's covered benefits, benefit limits, and out-of-pocket expense ramifications must be understood in order to optimize benefits and minimize adverse financial impact. One example of a significant financial impact to a beneficiary is the 3-day inpatient admission rule. Coverage of the skilled nursing facility (SNF) benefit requires a 3-day inpatient admission to a hospital setting. When a traditional Medicare beneficiary enters an acute care hospital, it is important to know if the encounter is classified as inpatient or observation. If an observation stay, the beneficiary would be wholly responsible for the per diem cost of an SNF admission. This classification schema has resulted in unexpected out-of-pocket expenses for numerous beneficiaries who did not understand their financial responsibility of SNF days following observation stays. In the situation where a beneficiary elects Part C (Medicare Advantage), this rule is not applicable.

Medicaid is a grant program funding medical assistance to low-income groups through a partnership of state and federal funding although states administer their respective

Medicaid programs. Medicaid does not provide consistent coverage to low-income individuals. Exclusions include single individuals, couples without children, or disability. Qualification criteria varies according to each state. States were allowed to offer a managed care plan option since 1993. A majority of recipients have enrolled in a managed care plan.

Case managers must maintain current knowledge of Medicaid eligibility and coverage for the state where the beneficiary is receiving benefits. Coverage such as Temporary Assistance for Needy Families (TANF) is not assured, and there may be a need to spend down assets in order to meet qualification requirements.

Patient Protection and Affordable Care Act

Few pieces of legislation have had the impact on health care in the United States that PPACA triggered. It has the potential to deliver the most extensive overhaul of the health care system since the creation of Medicare and Medicaid in 1965. Ultimately, PPACA is anticipated to provide health coverage for an additional 32 million uninsured Americans with provisions that continually highlight the focus on improving coordination and transitions of care.

However, there has been ongoing opposition to some of the provisions in PPACA, the most notable to date was the individual coverage mandate. Because the mandate involved coverage through Medicaid or health care exchanges, states had legal standing (sufficient connection to and/or harm relating to the law) to mount challenges to its constitutionality. Cases in multiple states made their way through the lower courts challenging the mandate and other provisions. Eventually, the case reached SCOTUS. In their June 2012 ruling, the mandate was upheld. However, the Court rejected a provision that would have penalized states not complying with expanded Medicaid eligibility requirements (Cauchi, 2014a).

In January 2014, SCOTUS issued an injunction, which suspended the implementation of a provision requiring faith-based organizations to offer birth control coverage in employee health insurance (Cauchi, 2014b). PPACA is in a continuous state of change and the student is strongly advised to conduct thorough research in order to learn up-to-date details of these and other issues relating to this legislation.

SUMMARY

Contemporary issues affecting the practice of case management are numerous and multidimensional. There will continue to be an endless stream of challenges to the structure and expectations placed on case management programs determined by reproducible outcomes expressed in objective terms. Hence, it becomes critically important for case management practitioners and stakeholders to define themselves and the practice in order to unite behind accepted expectations, scope of responsibility, to lead legislative and regulatory advocacy initiatives toward the improvement of health care access and quality of care.

References

American Case Management Association. (2013). *Standards of practice & scope of services for health care delivery system case management and transitions of care (TOC) professionals*. Retrieved from http://www.acmaweb.org/forms/2013SoPBrochure_FINAL_Online.pdf

Association of Social Work Boards. (2013). *Modal Social Work Practice Act*. Retrieved from http://www.aswb.org/wp-content/uploads/2013/10/Model_law.pdf

Association of Social Work Boards. (2014). *About the ASWB*. Retrieved from http://www.aswb.org/about/

Case Management Society of America. (2010). *Standards of practice for case management*. Retrieved from http://www.cmsa.org/Individual/MemberToolkit/StandardsofPractice/tabid/69/Default.aspx

Case Management Society of America. (2014). *Definition of certification*. Retrieved from http://www.cmsa.org/Individual/Education/Accreditation

Cauchi, R. (2014a). *State laws and actions challenging certain health reforms*. National Conference of State Legislatures. Retrieved from http://www.ncsl.org/research/health/state-laws-and-actions-challenging-ppaca.aspx

Cauchi, R. (2014b). *State laws and actions challenging certain health reforms. National Conference of State Legislatures*. Retrieved from http://www.ncsl.org/research/health/state-laws-and-actions-challenging-ppaca.aspx#Contraception

Commission on Accreditation of Rehabilitation Facilities. (2014a). *About CARF*. Retrieved from http://www.carf.org/About

Commission on Accreditation of Rehabilitation Facilities. (2014b). *Medical rehabilitation*. Retrieved from http://www.carf.org/Programs/Medical

Dasco, S. T., & Dasco, C. C. (1999). *Managed Care Answer Book* (3rd ed.). Gaithersburg, NY: Aspen Publishers

The Economic Times.com. (2014). Definition of inflation. Retrieved from http://economictimes.indiatimes.com/definition/Inflation

Fink-Samnick, E. (2011). Today's case manager and the state of the licensing dilemma. *Professional Case Management, 16*(2), 89–92.

Fink-Samnick, E. (2012). Aligning ethics and innovation: Licensure portability's predicament. *CMSA Today*, (2), 10–13.

Hein, M. A. (2009). *Telemedicine: An important force in the transformation of healthcare. Department of Commerce*. Retrieved from http://www.ita.doc.gov/td/health/telemedicine_2009.pdf

The Joint Commission. (2014). *History*. Retrieved from http://www.jointcommission.org/about_us/history.aspx

Kelly, J. (2010). Celebrating 50 years of ACSW. *NASW News, 55*(2). Retrieved from http://www.socialworkers.org/pubs/news/2010/02/kelly.asp

Masters, R. (2013a). *Compact requirement of acceptance of multistate license*. Memorandum issued August 2, 2013. Retrieved from https://www.ncsbn.org/Memo2Employers_PSOR.Requirements.pdf

Masters, R. (2013b). *Rebuttal to Oklahoma Attorney General opinion*. Memorandum issued February 18, 2013. Retrieved from https://www.ncsbn.org/OK_AG_Opinion_with_Rebuttal_for_web.pdf

Merriam-Webster Online Dictionary. (2014a). *Definition of accredit*. Retrieved from http://www.merriam-webster.com/dictionary/accredit

Merriam-Webster Online Dictionary. (2014b). *Definition of qualification*. Retrieved from http://www.merriam-webster.com/dictionary/qualification.

National Association of Professional Geriatric Care Managers. (2013). *Standards of practice*. Retrieved from http://www.caremanager.org/about/standards-of-practice/#s11

National Commission of Quality Assurance. (2014a). *About NCQA*. Retrieved from http://www.ncqa.org/AboutNCQA.aspx

National Commission of Quality Assurance. (2014b). *Case management accreditation*. Retrieved from http://www.ncqa.org/Programs/Accreditation/CaseManagementCM.aspx

National Commission of Quality Assurance. (2014c). *Health plan accreditation*. Retrieved from http://www.ncqa.org/Programs/Accreditation/HealthPlanHP.aspx

National Council of State Boards of Nursing. (2014). *Nurse licensure compact*. Retrieved from https://www.ncsbn.org/nlc.htm

Poe, L. (2008). Nursing regulation, the nurse licensure compact, and nurse administrators working together for patient safety. *Nursing Administration Quarterly*, *32*(4), 267–272.

Serve, Support, Simplify: Report of the President's Commission on Care for America's Returning Wounded Warriors. (July 2007). Retrieved from http://www.veteransforamerica.org/wp-content/uploads/2008/12/presidents-commission-on-care-for-americas-returning-wounded-warriors-report-july-2007.pdf

Sultz, H. A., & Young, K. M. (2014). *Health care USA: Understanding its organization and delivery*. Burlington, MA: Jones and Bartlett.

SocialWorkLicensure.org. (2014a). *Social work license requirements*. Retrieved from http://www.socialworklicensure.org/articles/social-work-license-requirements.html

URAC. (2014a). *History of URAC*. Retrieved from https://www.urac.org/about-urac/frequently-asked-questions

URAC. (2014b). *Case management standards, version 5.0*. Retrieved from https://www.urac.org/wp-content/uploads/CaseMgmt-Standards-At-A-Glance-10-9-2013.pdf

U.S. Department of Commerce. (2014). *About the department of commerce*. Retrieved from http://www.commerce.gov/about-department-commerce

U.S. Department of Defense. (2014a). *About the department of defense*. Retrieved from http://www.defense.gov/about

U.S. Department of Defense. (2014b). *Military health service history*. Retrieved http://www.health.mil/About_MHS/History.aspx

U.S. Department of Health and Human Services. (2014). *About HHS*. Retrieved from http://www.hhs.gov/about

U.S. Department of Health and Human Services–Administration on Aging. (2012). *Profile of older Americans: 2012*. Retrieved from http://www.aoa.gov/Aging_Statistics/Profile/2012/docs/2012profile.pdf

U.S. Department of Health and Human Services—Agency for Healthcare Research and Quality. (2013). *AHRQ at a glance*. Retrieved from http://www.ahrq.gov/about/index.html

U.S. Department of Health and Human Services—Center for Medicare and Medicaid. (2013). *Medicaid Milestones*. Retrieved from http://www.cms.gov/About-CMS/Agency-Information/History/index.html?redirect=/History

U.S. Department of Health and Human Services—Food and Drug Administration. (2014). *About the FDA*. Retrieved from http://www.fda.gov/AboutFDA/WhatWeDo/default.htm

U.S Department of Health and Human Services—Health Resources and Services Association. (2011). Health Licensing Board Report to Congress by M. Wakefield. Requested by Senate Report 111–86. Retrieved from www.hrsa.gov/ruralhealth/about/telehealth/licenserpt10.pdf

U.S. Department of Health and Human Services—Office of the National Coordinator. (2014). *About ONC*. Retrieved from http://www.healthit.gov/newsroom/about-onc

U.S. Department of Health and Human Services—Substance Abuse and Mental Health Services Administration. (2014). *About SAMHSA*. Retrieved from http://beta.samhsa.gov/about-us

U.S. Department of Veterans Affairs. (2014). *Veterans affairs history*. Retrieved from http://www.va.gov/about_va/vahistory.asp

The White House. (2014a). *The executive branch*. Retrieved from http://www.whitehouse.gov/our-government/executive-branch

The White House. (2014b). *The judicial branch*. Retrieved from http://www.whitehouse.gov/our-government/judicial-branch

The White House. (2014c). *The legislative branch*. Retrieved from http://www.whitehouse.gov/our-government/legislative-branch

3 PATHS TO CASE MANAGEMENT

OBJECTIVES

After studying this chapter, you will be able to:

1. Recognize the impacts relating to maintaining multiple case management definitions.
2. Identify research pertaining to case management role ambiguity and confusion.
3. Appreciate the variety of personal perspectives from individuals working in case management.

KEY TERMS

Case management
Case Management Model Act
Certificate of completion
Certification
Continuing education
Role ambiguity
Training

As discussed in chapter 2, there are multiple educational and work experience paths that lead into case management careers. This chapter delves into the issues of personal motivations and general concerns relating to work in the area of case management through the eyes of experienced case managers who participated in the Case Manager Histories Survey. The topics of job title, definition, transition issues, job satisfaction, and role-related issues of case management are examined.

THE USE AND MISUSE OF CASE MANAGEMENT AND CASE MANAGER

In recent decades, case management has become a standard component of health care delivery in virtually every segment of the care continuum. Unfortunately, the misuse of the terms **case management** and *case manager* have increased as recognition flourishes. The use of the Case Management Society of America's case management definition as the point of reference for this text was previously noted in chapter 2 (Box 3-1).

Assessing the accurate use of the case management and case manager as a percentage of job postings first requires agreement on both definition and appropriate application of the terms themselves. However, this is not to say that one definition is any better or worse than the next. The purpose and the intended audience of the definition play an important part in its wording. However, when organiziations create definitions in which differences are barely detectable from existing ones, it begs questions about its utility in the advancement of case management practice as well as to the reason it was created.

When scanning job listings that feature the case manager job title, one obtains results as far-flung as the following:

- an administrative coordinator for a medical practice,
- a complaint and grievance coordinator for an employee health care support team,

> **BOX 3-1** Case Management Society of America's Definition of Case Management
>
> Case management is a collaborative process of assessment, planning, facilitation, care coordination, evaluation, and advocacy for options and services to meet an individual's and family's comprehensive health needs through communication and available resources to promote quality cost-effective outcomes.
>
> ***Case Management Society of America, 2009***

- an acute hospital utilization reviewer for a licensed practical nurse,
- a case worker for a prerelease center of a women's correctional facility, and
- a registered nurse case manager on an organ transplant team.

This simple search demonstrates the wide variety of positions that include case manager in the job title. Clearly, the job title has been liberally applied to many situations, and it leaves one to ask why. Could it be a complete lack of creativity or a lackadaisical approach on the part of the hiring official? Perhaps it is that having *case manager* in the job title is assumed to be desirable or eye catching to the job seeker? The end result is confusion for the job seeker and misconceptions as to what case management means for the health care industry.

At the crux of the misuse of these terms is the absence of a unified case management definition accepted and that is embraced and utilized across both case management and health care industries. However, if case management experts cannot agree upon a definition, it is unreasonable to expect the health care industry to choose one from the numerous options. Employers rely on the case management industry and subject-matter experts; unfortunately, case management industry leaders have not offered clear guidance.

A review of available definitions conducted by Tahan (1999) demonstrated both disparities and commonalities. The lack of consensus was observed, as were a number of basic concepts which had gone unresolved, including "whether case management services are a care-based continuum, promoting a continuity in care delivery, or whether a specific health care professional is necessary to coordinate these services." Furthermore, it was noted that a portion of the definitions listed essential activities, others did not. It did not appear that any of the cited definitions included all of what were generally considered to be all essential case management activities. A sampling of case management definitions from professional organizations is listed in Box 3-2 and from credentialing organizations in Box 3-3.

The reasons behind the discrepancies have multiplied and/or changed over the years, as have the sources of definitions. In the absence of industry cohesion, definitions have been created by individual authors, at the local level (e.g., state- and community-based care coordination programs), by professional organizations (e.g., setting-of-care-specific, population-specific), and by companies employing case managers. Depending on the research skills of an individual, any of these sources may be repeated in subsequent citations. The failure to coalesce around a unified definition contributes to the "one-offing" and blending of various definitions to suit the needs of any given program or organization. Although many statements were revised over the years, the issue of having a unified definition must be reexamined in light of rampant confusion across the health care industry. Perhaps understanding the impact of having numerous, disparate definitions may lead to collective wisdom and creation of a consensus definition.

BOX 3-2 Professional Associations and Societies' Definitions of Case Management

Case Management in Hospital/Health Care Systems is a collaborative practice model including patients, nurses, social workers, physicians, other practitioners, caregivers and the community. The Case Management process encompasses communication and facilitates care along a continuum through effective resource coordination. The goals of Case Management include the achievement of optimal health, access to care and appropriate utilization of resources, balanced with the patient's right to self-determination.

American Case Management Association, 2002

A systematic process merging counseling and managerial concepts and skills through the application of techniques derived from intuitive and researched methods, thereby advancing efficient and effective decision-making for functional control of self, client, setting, and other relevant factors for anchoring a proactive practice. In case management, the counselor's role is focused on interviewing, counseling, planning rehabilitation programs, coordinating services, interacting with significant others, placing clients and following up with them, monitoring progress, and solving problems.

American Rehabilitation Counseling Association, n.d.

The Association of Rehabilitation Nurses supports the following definition of case management: the process of assessing, planning, organizing, coordinating, implementing, monitoring and evaluating the services and resources needed to respond to an individual's healthcare needs.

Association of Rehabilitation Nurses, 2010

Case managers work with people to get the health care and other community services they need, when they need them, and for the best value.

Case Management Leadership Coalition, 2006

Case management is a collaborative process of assessment, planning, facilitation, care coordination, evaluation, and advocacy for options and services to meet an individual's and family's comprehensive health needs through communication and available resources to promote quality, cost-effective outcomes.

Case Management Society of America, 2009

Professional geriatric care management is a holistic, client-centered approach to caring for older adults or others facing ongoing health challenges. Working with families, geriatric care manager expertise provides the answers at a time of uncertainty. Their guidance leads families to the actions and decisions that ensure quality care and an optimal life for those they love, thus reducing worry, stress and time off of work for family caregivers through: Assessment and monitoring, Planning

(continued)

BOX 3-2 Professional Associations and Societies' Definitions of Case Management (*Continued*)

and problem-solving, Education and advocacy, and Family caregiver coaching.

National Association of Professional Geriatric Care Managers, 2013

A process to plan, seek, advocate for, and monitor services from different social services or health care organizations and staff on behalf of a client. The process enables social workers in an organization, or in different organizations, to coordinate their efforts to serve a given client through professional teamwork, thus expanding the range of needed services offered. Case management limits problems arising from fragmentation of services, staff turnover, and inadequate coordination among providers. Case management can occur within a single, large organization or within a community program that coordinates services among settings.

National Association of Social Workers, 2013

or

Social work case management is a method of providing services whereby a professional social worker assesses the needs of the client and the client's family, when appropriate. The case manager arranges, coordinates, monitors, evaluates, and advocates for a package of multiple services to meet the specific client's complex needs. A professional social worker is the primary provider of social work case management. Distinct from other forms of case management, social work case management addresses the individual client's biopsychosocial status as well as the state of the social system in which case management operates. Social work case management is both micro and macro in nature. Intervention occurs at both the client and system levels.

National Association of Social Workers, 2002

BOX 3-3 Certification Programs' Definitions of Case Management

Occupational Health Nursing case management is the process of coordinating the individual employee's health care services to achieve optimal quality care delivered in a cost effective manner. The case manager establishes or qualifies a provider network, recommends treatment plans, monitors outcomes, and maintains a strong communication link among all the parties.

American Board of Occupational Health Nurses, 2008

Nursing Case Management is a dynamic and systematic collaborative approach to providing and coordinating healthcare services to a defined population. It is a participative process to identify and facilitate options and services for meeting individuals' health needs, while decreasing fragmentation and duplication of care, and enhancing quality, cost-effective clinical outcomes. The framework for nursing case management includes five components: assessment, planning, implementation, evaluation, and interaction.

American Association of Nurse Credentialing, 2012

Case management is a collaborative process that assesses, plans, implements, coordinates, monitors, and evaluates the options and services required to meet the client's health and human service needs. It is characterized by advocacy, communication, and resource management and promotes quality and cost-effective interventions and outcomes.

Commission for Case Manager Certification, n.d.

A systematic process merging counseling and managerial concepts and skills through the application of techniques derived from intuitive and researched methods, thereby advancing efficient and effective decision-making for functional control of self, client, setting, and other relevant factors for anchoring a proactive practice. In case management, the counselor's role is focused on interviewing, counseling, planning rehabilitation programs, coordinating services, interacting with significant others, placing clients and following up with them, monitoring progress, and solving problems.

Commission on Rehabilitation Counselor Certification, n.d.

A unified definition and guidance as to the use of the terms *case management* and *case manager* are but steps in the process of heightening the understanding and recognition of case management. Another is the enactment of legislation and/or regulatory mandates in order to establish and enforce title protection. Without control over use of title, health care consumers are left with no assurance as to the level or quality of service received from someone using the title of case manager. Without the bite of law or regulation, the impact of a unified definition is akin to a lion without teeth or claws; the definition continues to be voluntary and is likely to be overlooked.

In 2009, the **Case Management Model Act** was drafted as a means to educate legislators and regulators regarding case management's essential elements at a program and individual level. The ultimate desire is for all or part of the Model Act's language to be adopted into law and/or regulation at local, state, and/or federal levels. The Model Act was a result of collaborative stakeholder effort between the National Association of Social Workers and the Case Management Society of America. Endorsement of other professional and credentialing organizations stalled. The Model Act continues to be used in national and local education efforts; however, in light of numerous entities pushing organization-specific priorities to legislators and regulators, the individual messages drown each other out. No other model legislation pertaining to cross-continuum case management has been widely touted for general industry review or adoption since the original draft was released.

LACK OF CLARITY AND ROLE AMBIGUITY

Adding to the need of a consensus definition is the downstream impact of challenges facing case managers relating to the **role ambiguity** and resulting lack of clarity. Dierdorff and Rubin (2007) noted that work roles encompass the expectations pertaining to the perceived responsibilities or requirements associated with specific jobs. The lack of a clear definition of case management has created barriers to accurate performance of important activities which precede and follow a new hire (e.g., writing a meaningful job description, setting appropriate performance goals, assessing individual performance). It also creates difficulty for the individual case manager seeking to define a career path or identify and achieve personal goals. Be that as it may, work has been done to address basic elements of practice, such as roles, functions, level of effort, role ambiguity, and the challenges of transitioning into case management positions from other work environments.

As far back as 1998, Zander cited the evolving nature of case management not only as a career for nurses to consider but also as being problematic in terms of practice concepts and job satisfaction. These and other implications were investigated by Bergen (1992), Lamb (1992), and Schutt et al. (2010). Role and function definition was undertaken in two studies conducted under the auspices of the Commission for Case Management Certification (Tahan et al., 2006; Tahan & Campagna, 2010). Capturing consistent practice elements and level of effort was investigated (Reimanis et al., 2001; Huber et al., 2003; Park & Huber, 2009; Park et al., 2009). Schmitt (2005 and 2006) recognized ethical considerations and lack of educational preparation as contributors to job strain and unanticipated conflicts of interest for nurses transitioning from bedside practice to case management in the payor setting. Waterman et al. (1996) noted the lack of preparation related to workload, issues with coworkers, and environment as contributors to anxiety and role confusion during role transition. O'Donnell (2007a, 2007b) identified ethical dilemmas over cost containment responsibilities and a lack of preparatory orientation to job responsibilities as problematic, and Smith (2011) highlighted the issues of role ambiguity and conflict as being pivotal and ones which individuals transitioning into case management positions should prepare to address. Research in social work also identified role ambiguity as caused by uncertainty or a lack of information pertintent to job responsibilities (Pasupuleti et al., 2009), and this lack of information caused an impact on an individual's understanding of their job role requirements (Dierdorff & Rubin, 2007).

Research on job-related self-enhancing behavior conducted by Yun et al. (2007) found that "when role ambiguity is high, self-set specific and challenging goals can impress others, including the supervisor, because a self-set goal that is specific and challenging indicates the self-efficacy of the employees and implies that they care about the organization and its performance." Also acknowledged is the other end of the performance spectrum, individuals with "low motivation to enhance their self-image may take advantage of the role ambiguity as a justification for their modest task performance." Yun et al. went on to state, "When role ambiguity is high, there is much more room for employees to develop different interpretations of their job requirements. This can be considered a weak situation in which there are few situational constraints on the incumbents and they have a high degree of discretion about how they do their job." Role ambiguity and how it applies to case management was discussed by Gray and White (2012). In their analysis, it was concluded that role confusion occurs when there is no defined expectations for the nurse case manager; however, the authors also acknowledged that there is insufficient research on the issue specific to nursing case management.

Schmitt's work relating to nurses entering case management is especially on point with results from the Case Manager Histories survey. In Schmitt's study, participants believed that case management jobs would afford a measure of relief from perceived undesirable working conditions, which included schedule flexibility, physical demand, workload, compensation, and job security. Schmitt (2006) also described unexpected feelings of inadequacy and incompetence for which existing clinical knowledge and previous work experience had not prepared them. It is not discussed if these beliefs were established as a result of information provided by colleagues when positions became available, nor were factors which may have influenced the information provided to job candidates (e.g., existence of a recruitment bonus for each new hire) disclosed.

CASE MANAGER HISTORIES—YOUR PATH TO PRACTICE SURVEY

Survey Background, Demographic, and Content

Case Manager Histories was an informal, small-scale informal survey conducted between December 1 and 31, 2013. The intent of the survey was to provide a means for experienced case managers to share their personal history regarding initial interest and continued work in case management. A total of 54 invitations were e-mailed to practicing case managers known to the authors. Information was gathered using an online collection tool, and participation was voluntary. Authors acknowledge the small survey size and informal methodology. Although commonalities were noted, it is recommended that additional study be conducted in order to confirm and generalize the results.

Thirty-one individuals responded, with 24 fully completed and 7 partially completed surveys. Responders were predominantly female (94%), between the ages of 40 and

69 years, residing within the United States (94%). The level of educational preparation query revealed that participants achieved the following: graduate degree (55%), baccalaureate degree (32%), associate degree (6%), and nursing school diploma (6%); some reported multiple degrees in the comments section. Educational background included nursing (74%) and social work (13%), with smaller representation from occupational health, psychology, and unspecified behavioral health degrees. Some reported having a degree (e.g., business, psychology, health care administration) in addition to a clinical degree. Although invitations were sent to individuals reflecting a wide range of professional affiliations (e.g., medicine, pharmacy, occupational therapy, physical therapy), it was concluded that individuals either did not respond or did not identify a specific professional affiliation in order to allow categorization.

Motivations for Working in Case Management

Survey Findings—Starting to Work in Case Management

Within case management circles, many factors are generally accepted as contributing to the variation in the paths to case management practice, not the least of which is an individual's personal motivation. In the survey, respondents were invited to complete the sentence "I started working in case management because __________." Participant responses are listed in Table 3-1.

Survey Findings—Personal Stories of Working in Case Management

Participants were given an opportunity to share their personal stories in an open-ended manner by answering, "Please share the story of how you started working in case management." Box 3-4 highlights participant responses.

Related Research and Information

In 2006, Schmitt studied issues encountered when transitioning from previous roles into case management positions. The motivation for making a career change frequently stemmed from dissatisfaction with a current work situation. Participants noted what they considered to be intolerable working conditions (e.g., inflexible schedules, poor staff/patient ratios, job insecurity, inadequate compensation, physically taxing activities). Schmitt stated that survey participants were generally not aware of aspects of the new role which would prove to be problematic in light of personal expectations of relief from their current undesirable work situations. Participants also admitted that there were unanticipated situations that previous experience and education did not prepare them to handle (e.g., technical demands). The resulting internal tension contributed to feeling inadequate or incompetence which further contributed to individual role strain. Four themes emerged including time-task orientation, interactions and relationships, business culture and objectives, and professional identity and self-image (Schmitt, 2006). This study was limited to practicing nurse case managers with a minimum 3 years of hospital- or

TABLE 3-1 Reasons Why Individuals Began Working in Case Management

I Started Working in Case Management Because	Response Percent
A friend/family member recruited me to work in the same department.	4.2
I could no longer physically perform the responsibilities associated with clinical practice.	4.2
I did not have a choice, my employer reassigned me.	4.2
I only wanted to work during regular business hours (e.g., no weekends, no holidays).	8.3
I had a strong desire to work in the field of case management.	33.3
I was mentally/emotionally burned out from my previous job(s) and needed a change.	8.3
It looked easy.	0.0
Someone I respected suggested that I would be good at it.	20.8
Other: (fill in)	16.7
Please note that this space is provided for use only if your circumstance is vastly different than one of the options provided. • Looking for a new adventure • I was already doing it but not getting the recognition • I was interested in being able to use my skills from my psychiatric nursing and management background • I was interested in furthering my career	

BOX 3-4 Case Manager Stories of Starting to Work in Case Management

After working in the acute care setting for 16 years, I desperately wanted to do something different. I was unable to provide patient care according to the way I was trained and in keeping with my personal commitment to the care of patients. After interviewing for several positions, I literally "fell" into a case management position providing oncology and transplant case management.

I initially worked for the military in utilization management, which evolved into medical management. Case management is under medical management in the military setting. The first case I managed was for one of our military doctors who suffered a brain injury due to an aneurysm. It was difficult as he was not only a colleague but also a friend. I continued to attend case management training but also became ANCC certified and obtained my master's in Nursing Case Management.

My graduate work was focused on Home Health/Case Management at the University of Virginia. Since I had been a preceptor for these graduate students, prior to pursuing my MSN full-time, I was familiar with the degree and the opportunities it offered. During my studies, I was able to experience case management roles in the community setting and home care. This included facilitating transitions from hospital to home as well as an introduction to financial issues, which were not a function of my direct care/bedside role. When I look back, over 20 years, and consider the evolution, or revolution, in American health care, I am extremely appreciative of the fundamentals emphasized in my graduate program. After graduation, I worked part-time for a hospice followed by a full-time role as a case manager with a rehabilitation facility.

I was actually hurt on the job and was not able to return to the clinical setting. I was 31. I learned about case management when I read a want ad asking "Are you a nurse wanting to work from home?" This was 1995. It was a worker's compensation field nurse. I did not have a case manager helping me during my injury and it was very tough doing it alone when I was so sick. I never wanted this to happen to another person, so I became their advocate during their worker's compensation. I love being a case manager. I became certified in 1999. I have learned other aspects of case management during my time as a case manager. I worked in worker compensation for 12 years. Now, I have experience working in disease management, hospital case management, and utilization review.

I wanted to practice occupational therapy in an injury prevention/return-to-work context. The pathway to do that was through the state's worker compensation system, which had mandated disability case management as part of worker compensation statutes.

I went to an insurance company and my job was performing behavioral health utilization review. The case management position opened and I wanted to expand my job skills and began in case management for a major group health carrier in my state.

I have 20 years of experience as a hospital social worker and discharge planner. Essentially, as case management became a recognized field and our department merged social workers and nurses to develop a more comprehensive set of services, it became evident that case management was what we were providing. I took the seminar and prepared to take the exam to set the example for my department (I was the director at the time) and to obtain recognition for myself, and my department, regarding our mission and work.

I was working full-time as a clinical specialist in psychiatry and saw the opportunity to work as a team lead in acute rehab. It was not called case management but the job entailed coordinating the care for the patients, collaborating and managing the multiple providers, family, insurance liaison, and discharge planning. The company then transformed the team leads and social workers into one area called Case Management. I had the opportunity to participate in that development.

A friend of mine who had an LCSW degree inspired me. She was in private practice at the time. Being practical, I chose the MSW degree because in California, it offered 3rd party reimbursement. I was an intensive care nurse at the time and wanted a mommy-friendly job. After my kids were born, I left healthcare and then decided against being a therapist. My family moved a few years ago. I applied for a case manager position. I am quite good at it and I enjoy working. I was in sales for a few years; they call this motivational interviewing now. I work in an acute care hospital; it is fast-paced and challenging. It is becoming more challenging all the time as we are expected to do more with less people.

A friend introduced me to an independent case manager who was looking for someone to do case management. I was hired and mentored by this case manager because of my diverse background. I shadowed her for about a month and then started seeing patients. I read everything I could get my hands on about case management and, after 1 year, sat for my certification. I networked with other case managers in order to find out how they did their jobs, what worked, and what did not.

clinic-based nursing experience in addition to nursing education and **training** prior entering case management. Individuals having worked within their case management roles for 1 to 3 years were included. In addition, only payer-based case managers were included.

CASE MANAGEMENT TRAINING AND EDUCATION

An aging workforce, low enrollment rates in nursing programs, and the exploding over-65 population are recognized as influencers on the adequacy of health care workforce in the United States (Institutes of Medicine, 2010; American Association of Colleges of Nursing, 2014). Enrollment into nursing programs is further affected by the low number of qualified nursing instructors at college/university level. Assuming an adequate number of qualified individuals applied, admission offices are forced to restrict the number of incoming degree candidates in order to preserve the integrity of the student/instructor ratio and the quality of education. Because nurses make up the bulk of the case management workforce, the trickle-down effect of these factors is a cause for concern: "The case management field must be prepared to deal with the reality of smaller pools of professionals from which to draw the case managers of the future. We cannot count on the typical career progression as practitioners gain experience and pursue case management as advanced practice. Instead, a concerted effort must be made to expand the education and training of all health and human services professionals in the principles of case management, starting with undergraduates" (Stanton, 2009).

Survey Findings—Training and Educational Preparation

Respondents were asked "What education or training did you receive in order to begin working as a case manager?" On-the-job training dominated the responses, although there was variation as to the type of training received (Table 3-2). The opportunity to provide a personal response was utilized by two responders, one of which was reclassified into an existing category and the second remained classified as other.

Respondents were also asked "Since beginning your case management career, how have you remained current as to your practice specialty?" Multiple answers were allowed for this query. Joining professional associations for access to educational content, attending multiday conferences, attending online webinars, and reading professional journals were virtually tied for frequency. These were followed by attending employer-sponsored education sessions, taking online courses, and attending evening seminars.

Related Research and Information

The issues relating to case management-specific formal education have been studied previously. In a 2002 study, Scheyett and Blyer recognized that individuals come to their positions with little formal education specific to case management. Tholcken et al. (2004) examined the design of one case management course in an undergraduate nursing program. In 2005, Kuric and White attempted to identify essential concepts and skills relevant to case management in various degree level (e.g., associate, baccalaureate, graduate) nursing education. As of 2014, there are a number of graduate level programs emphasizing nursing case management (Table 3-3). However, although the necessity for inclusion of case management principles in undergraduate nursing education has been recognized (Institutes of Medicine, 2010), the change in curriculum at the undergraduate level is slower to materialize.

In addition to formal education and in accordance with applicable definitions, qualifications, and practice standards, case managers maintain current knowledge through completion of **continuing education** (CE). Common means for obtaining CEs include seminars, work shops, online courses,

TABLE 3-2 What Education or Training Did You Receive in Order to Begin Working as a Case Manager?

Answer Options	Response Percent
Attended a seminar (one day, in person) not employer-specific	4.2
Attended a continuing education program (multiple days, in person) not employer-specific	12.5
On-the-job training ("trial-by-fire," no formal training received)	37.5
On-the-job training (job-specific training by supervisor)	20.8
On-the-job training (job-specific training and buddy-preceptor)	33.3
Took an online course (not specific to my employer)	4.2
I read a book or manual (self-educated)	4.2
I never received training or education to begin working in case management, I just started doing it	4.2
Other (fill in) —I attended seminars and training through DoD as well as CMSA —I obtained an MSW, my first degree was BS in Nursing	

TABLE 3-3 Graduate Degree Programs in Case Management

Institution	Location	Degree
American Sentinel University	An online university	Master of science in Nursing*
Grantham University	Kansas City, MO, and online	Master of science in Nursing*
Loyola University	New Orleans, LA, and online	Master of science in Nursing†
Samuel Merritt University	Oakland and Sacramento, CA	Master of science in Nursing†
Seton Hall University	South Orange, NJ, and online	Master of science in Nursing/Health Administration†
University of Alabama	Tuscaloosa, AL, and online	Master of science in Nursing†

*Accredited by the Accrediting Commission of the Distance Education and Training Council.
†Accredited by the Accreditation Commission for Education in Nursing.

and conference sessions. On completion of the content or event, the individual receives a **certificate of completion** providing a preapproved number of CE credits which are approved by specific granting authorities (e.g., board of registration, **certification** entity). CE credits are required to maintain licensure and/or certification.

Training is defined as "a process by which someone is taught the skills that are needed for an art, profession, or job" (Merriam-Webster Dictionary, 2013); however, for the purpose of clinical professionals, it is related to hands-on experience needed to learn new skills and refine existing ones. Case management training is frequently associated with on-the-job skills (e.g., computer systems, patient care) or college-credit course internships and cooperative field learning experiences.

Though traditionally delivered face-to-face, today's CE programs are increasingly transitioning to delivery formats which are accessed and completed via the Internet (e.g., webinar, recorded slide deck). The benefits of web-based delivery are the focus on user convenience and flexibility. In light of various personal and professional demands, users may log in to the course content from anywhere with Internet connectivity. Face-to-face classes require participants to be in a specific physical location for a given period of time. Another consideration is cost. The production costs associated with live delivery are substantial, not only for course materials but also for speaker time, travel to the site, accomodations, food service, and administration.

It is also important to point out the difference between receiving a certificate upon completion of a particular program or course and becoming certified and obtaining a credential in case management. A certificate simply acknowledges that an individual attended an event. It may or may not award CE credit, the type of which is identified on the certificate document. But certification is a type of a personal credential intended to demonstrate a basic competence in a given topic, subject, or activity and usually includes a verification process and an examination. Please refer to chapter 4 for a thorough examination of case management certifications.

CASE MANAGERS GAIN INSPIRATION FROM DOING THE WORK

The roots of inspiration are unique to each case manager. Although the challenges and obstacles appear endless, the commitment of clinical professionals to excellence in the field of case management knows no bounds and a cause to celebrate the privilege of working in this area can be found in the people, places, and things of day-to-day life. Another open-ended question posed was "What inspires you to continue working in the field of case management?" See Box 3-5 for insights into the mind-set of survey participants.

Case Manager Advice

In the pressure-filled world of health care delivery, case management plays a pivotal role for connecting individuals with services and keeping the wheels of service delivery well-oiled. It is no longer an alternative job for those seeking regular work hours or a less physically demanding job. It is definitely not an option for someone wishing to slow down the pace of work as they head toward retirement. Taking the path toward professional case management requires careful thought and due consideration of many factors, which include preferred care setting and specialty area. Figure 3-1 offers a few thoughts for the health care professional who is interested in becoming a case manager, and Figure 3-2 provides work setting options for consideration.

When asked to share words of advice, interesting thoughts were shared on a number of topics.

On the belief that case management is not for everyone,

- "Not everyone is meant to be a case manager, but for those who are interested in making a difference and are willing to learn how to better interact with patients I will provide encouragement and support."
- "It is not for the 'faint of heart' or if you are looking for better hours. You need to love what you do and be willing to work hard and possibly long hours."

BOX 3-5 Quoted Case Manager Reasons to Continue

Every day is a new adventure. There is no boredom or stagnation in case management as there is constant new learning. There is no better way to serve others than to be a case manager, but not every person has a need to serve. Case management is a vocation as much as it is a job title ... when it is done right!

As a case manager I am better able to assist patients to navigate our very complex health system, provide education and support so that patients can learn to better manage their health, and problem solve, with patients and families, to remove barriers to improved health. Witnessing improvements in self-care, quality of life, and disease burden are what keep me inspired.

The challenge ... each day is unique and each patient brings their individual story. It's the stories that I focus on now. These vignettes are critical in my current role as a TBI Nurse Case Manager with a military treatment facility. At this point in my career, it's not the compensation or the accolades. It's the ability to advocate, comfort, cajole, and motivate that keeps me showing up.

I truly love helping patients and families with their health care needs. I feel that I make an impact on their lives. I also help provide education to case managers, locally and in other areas. I feel it is important to keep yourself up to date with all the changing aspects of healthcare. Things change so fast.

The ever-evolving nature of healthcare, which allows for growth and expansion of the case manager's role. It is an opportunity to help those starting out in case management. The opportunity to be part of a field that positively affects patient outcomes, promotes teamwork among all practitioners, and impacts facility success and growth. CM allows us to be part of the big picture in healthcare, not just isolated in a niche.

It is an excellent use of my skills; I enjoy the challenges. We must be advocates for the profession and we have to embrace the challenges and help to lead them. Now that money is on the table there are other departments are taking over much of the care coordination, which is what we do best. I see myself as a voice for case management and our clients.

The ability to make a difference in the lives of individuals with disabilities.

I love working with patients and teaching them how to negotiate the healthcare system.

There is much in case management as a discipline that overlaps with and resonates with the field of social work: the emphasis on client empowerment and strengths-based practice, the ethical guidelines ... I also particularly like its interdisciplinary focus: a social worker, or a nurse, or an occupational therapist can be a case manager, to name a few. I find the tools of case management practical and easy to apply to myriad situations.

Many days I find case management does not look like it did when we defined it years ago. The complexity, and more time within a computer, not with patients and families, is distressing. However, when I work directly with case management departments to improve efficiencies and bring case managers to the patients and families, I am renewed that it is where the strengths of case management lie. It is where we provide the highest value. When a novice case manager is excited, and something I have done has helped him or her manage a complex patient and they want to share a "success" story ... that is my inspiration!

On the importance of finding a good mentor,

- "Seek out an experienced case manager who can offer insight into the 'real job.' A true mentor is invaluable in offering a true picture."
- "You need to find a good mentor or several!"
- "Find an experienced case manager who can mentor you through the process. I had great mentors and attribute my success to them."

On the value of continuous learning and knowledge,

- "Join local case management association(s) if possible and/or attend continuing education events for case managers to learn how case management integrates with clinical practices, as well as what one needs to learn in order to translate and apply clinical experience in order to transition into case management practice."
- "Jump in. If there are educational opportunities for you to learn case management, take them. Talk to other case managers and find out what works for them. Ingest all you can and be passionate about what you do."
- "Case Management is a true passion. Learn as much as you can. The more education that you have the higher quality of care you can give to your patient's and their families."
- You need to be a lifelong learner, willing to take part in regular continuing education and keep aware of the rapid changes in health care."

On helpful personal characteristics,

- "You need courage, dedication, and a thick skin."
- "I would say to embrace a statement by Winston Churchill, "Never, never, never give up." Tenacity is an essential characteristic for case managers."
- "If you are a person who likes to think out of the box, likes to put puzzles together, is flexible, articulate, and has a tough skin, you may be a good fit for case management. You need to have a strong clinical foundation, and the confidence to lead a care coordination team. It isn't all about clinical knowledge, or fiscal awareness, it is about passion for people, community, and being a champion for those you serve."
- "Be open, flexible, patient, resourceful—the end goal is ensuring your client have all that they need, the basics and beyond. Do not be afraid to ask; the worst answer you will get is, no."

The question of how one becomes a case manager is common. It is not recommended to assume case management (CM) responsibilities without consideration and acquisition of necessary qualifications, skills, and knowledge associated with competent practice. For the health care professional interested in becoming a case manager, the following flow chart provides a process of consideration for gathering information in order to make a knowledge-based decision.

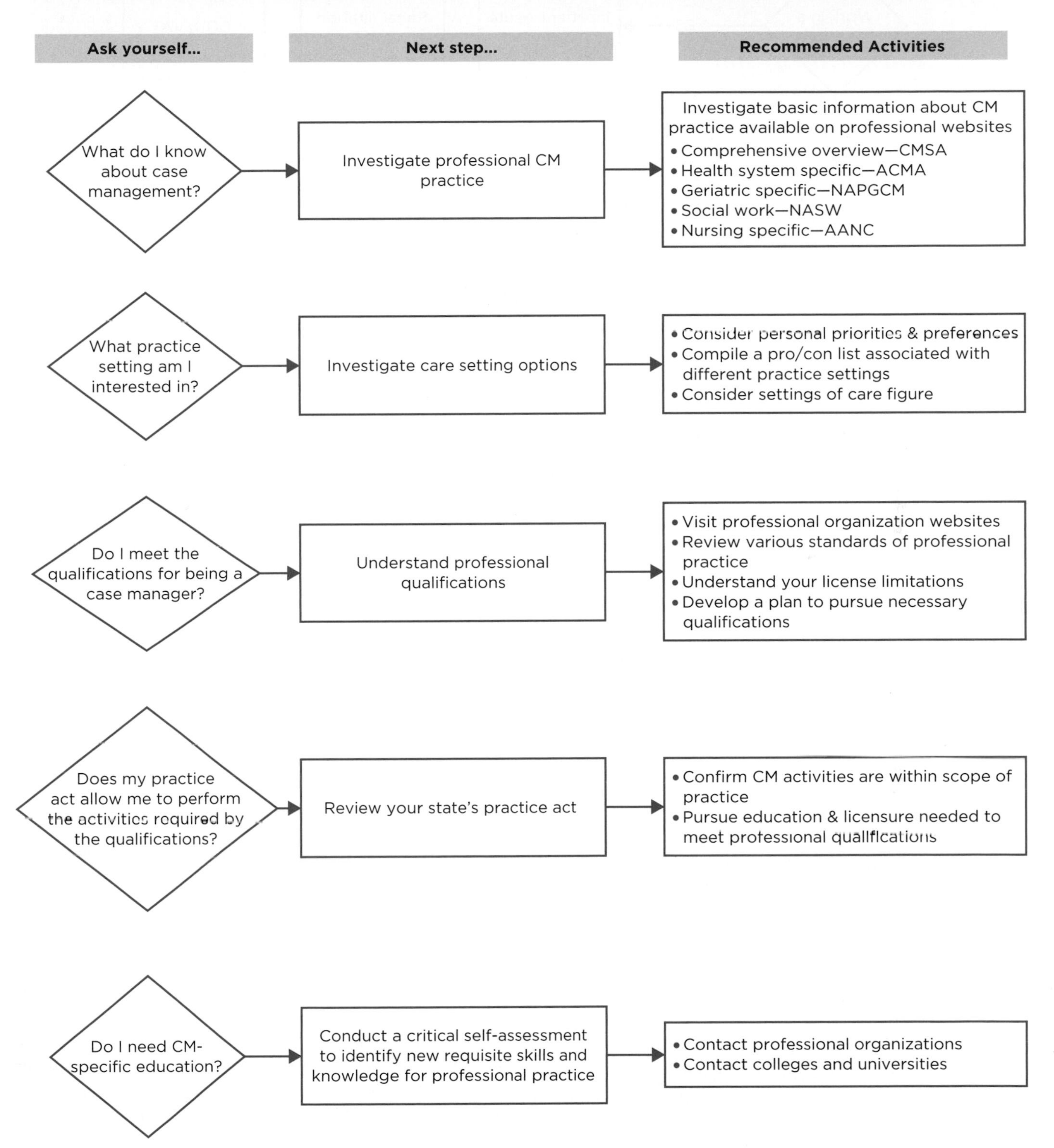

Figure 3-1. Process of consideration for the health care professional interested in becoming a case manager.

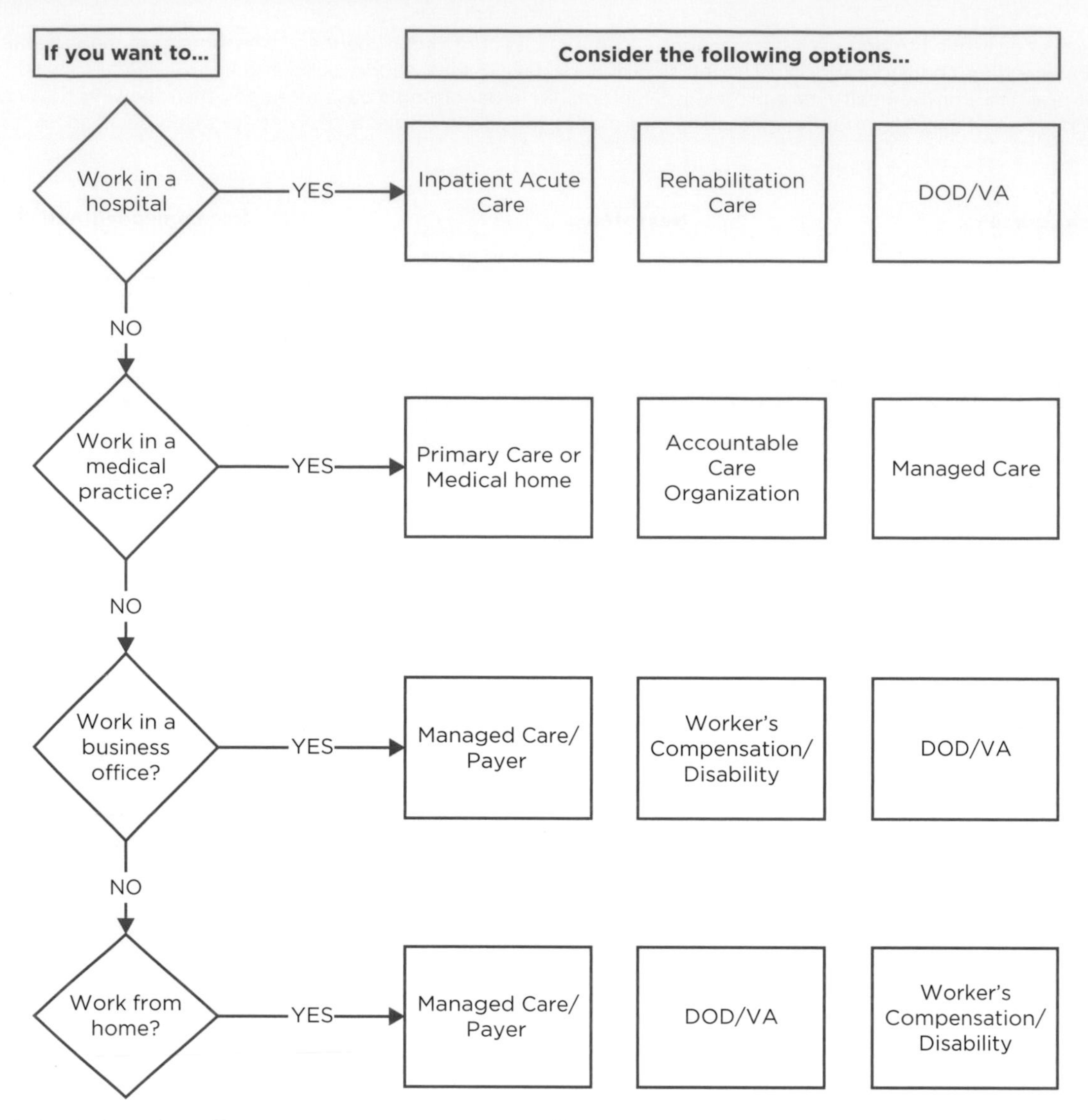

Figure 3-2. Care settings that offer case management opportunities.

On variety of experiences,

- "You will be frustrated, you will be exhilarated, you will be questioned, you will be rewarded, you will be challenged, you will challenge, you will continue to grow, you will find roadblocks, you will succeed. You will never be bored. Buckle up."
- "Case management is a diverse area of practice that allows for new learning every day ... every minute of every day."

On the rewards, both personal and professional,

- "Tough skin is essential, for some days are difficult to navigate with managing a variety of expectations ... it may be the best position that has ever challenged you!"
- "The rewards are many, but it is a challenging profession, make no mistake!

SUMMARY

The multiple paths that lead to case management careers create a valuable diversity of perspectives and knowledge. However, there are issues that detract from the strength and unity of case management practice because of this variety. Industry collaboration relating to common issues such as definition, qualifications, and educational requirements have the potential to bring consistency across the practice. Defining standard expectations, respecting personal strengths, and working for legislation and regulation which identifies the importance of case management in health care delivery is essential for continued growth and enhancement of the practice. As our health care delivery system continues to evolve, so too will expectations on the practitioners who undertake careers in case management. Taking a proactive approach to practice transformation facilitates advancement and recognition across the health care continuum.

References

American Association of Colleges of Nursing. (2014). *Fact sheet: Nursing shortage*. Retrieved from http://www.aacn.nche.edu/media-relations/fact-sheets/nursing-shortage

American Association of Nurse Credentialing. (2012). *Clinical case management practice*. Retrieved from http://www .nursecredentialing.org/Documents/Certification/Review-Manuals/NurseCaseMgmtSampleChap.aspx

American Board of Occupational Health Nurses. (2008). *Case management examination handbook*. Retrieved from http://www.abohn.org/eligibility-cm.cfm

American Case Management Association. (2002). *Case management*. Retrieved from http://acmaweb.org/section.asp?sID=4&mn=mn1&sn=sn1&wpg=mh

American Rehabilitation Counseling Association. (n.d.). *Scope of practice*. Retrieved from http://www.arcaweb.org/?page_id=68

Association of Rehabilitation Nurses. (2010). *The rehabilitation nurse case manager*. Retrieved from http://www.rehabnurse.org/pubs/role/Role-Rehab-Nurse-Case-Manager.html orhttp://www.rehabnurse.org/uploads/files/uploads/File/rdcasemanager10.pdf

Bergen, A. (1992). Case management in community care: Concepts, practices and implications for nursing. *Journal of Advanced Nursing*, *17*, 1106–1113.

Case Management Society of America. (2009). *Case management model act*. Retrieved from http://www.cmsa.org/portals/0/pdf/publicpolicy/cmsa_model_act.pdf

Case Management Society of America. (2010). *CMSA Standards of Practice for case management*. Retrieved from http://www.cmsa.org/portals/0/pdf/memberonly/StandardsOfPractice.pdf

Commission for Case Manager Certification. (n.d.). *Definition and philosophy of case management*. Retrieved from http://ccmcertification.org/about-us/about-case-management/definition-and-philosophy-case-management

Commission on Rehabilitation Counsellor Certification. (n.d.). *CRC/CCRC scope of practice*. Retrieved from http://www.crccertification.com/pages/crc_ccrc_scope_of_practice/56.php

Dierdorff, E. C., & Rubin, R. S. (2007). Carelessness and discriminability in work role requirement judgments: influences of role ambiguity and cognitive complexity. *Personnel Psychology*, *60*, 597–625.

Gray, F. C., & White, A. (2012). Concept analysis: Case management role confusion. *Nursing Forum*, *47*(1), 3–8.

Huber, D., Sarrazin, M., Vaughn, T., & Hall, J. (2003). Evaluating the impact of case management dosage. *Nursing Research*, *52*, 276–288.

Institutes of Medicine (2010). *The future of nursing: Leading change, advancing health*. Washington, DC: National Academies Press.

Lamb, G. (1992). Conceptual and methodological issues in nurse case management research. *Advances in Nursing Science*, *15*(2), 16–24.

Merriam-Webster Dictionary. (2013). *Definition of training*. Retrieved from http://www.merriam-webster.com/dictionary/training

National Association of Professional Geriatric Care Managers. (2013). *What you need to know*. Retrieved from http://www.caremanager.org/why-care-management/what-you-should-know/

O'Donnell, L. (2007a). Ethical dilemmas among nurses as they transition to hospital case management: Implications for organizational ethics, part I. *Professional Case Management*, *12*(3), 160–169.

O'Donnell, L. (2007b). Ethical dilemmas among nurses as they transition to hospital case management: Implications for organizational ethics, part II. *Professional Case Management*, *12*, 219–231.

Park, E., & Huber, D. (2009). Case management workforce in the United States. *Journal of Nursing Scholarship*, *41*, 175–183.

Park, E., Huber, D., & Tahan, H. A., (2009). The evidence base for case management practice. *Western Journal of Nursing Research*, *31*, 693–714.

Pasupuleti, S., Allen, R. I., Lambert, E. G., & Cluse-Tolar, T. (2009). The impact of work stressors on the life satisfaction of social service workers: A preliminary study. *Administration in Social Work*, *33*, 319–339.

Powell, S. (1996). Job stress versus success factors for case management. *Nursing Case Management*, *1*(3), 125–132.

Reimanis, C., Cohen, E., & Redman, R. (2001). Nurse case manager role attributes: Fifteen years of evidence-based literature. *Lippincott's Case Management*, *6*, 230–242.

Schmitt, N. (2005). Role transition from caregiver to case manager, part I. *Lippincott's Case Management*, *10*, 294–302.

Schmitt, N. (2006). Role transition from caregiver to case manager, part II. *Lippincott's Case Management*, *11*(1), 37–46.

Schutt, R., Fawcett, J., Gall, G., Harrow, B., & Woodford, M. (2010). Case manager satisfaction in public health. *Professional Case Management*, *15*(3), 124–134.

Smith, A.C. (2011). Role ambiguity and role conflict in nurse case managers. *Professional Case Management*, *16*(4), 182–196.

Stanton, M. P. (2009). Shortening the case management learning curve: A call to action. *Professional Case Management*, *14*(6), 278–281.

Tahan, H. A. (1999). Clarifying case management: What's in a label? *Nursing Case Management*, *4*(6), 268–278.

Tahan, H. A. & Campagna, V. (2010). Case management roles and functions across various settings and professional disciplines. *Professional Case Management*, *15*, 245–277.

Tahan, H. A. Huber, D. L., & Downey, W. T. (2006). Case managers' roles and functions. *Lippincott's Case Management*, *11*(1), 4–22.

Waterman, H., Waters, K., & Awenat, Y. (1996). The introduction of case management on a rehabilitation floor. *Journal of Advanced Nursing*, *24*, 960–967.

Yun, S., Takeuchi, R., & Lu, W. (2007). Employee self-enhancement motives and job performance behaviors: Investigating the moderating effects of employee role ambiguity and managerial perceptions of employee commitment. *Journal of Applied Psychology*, *92*(3), 745–756.

Zander, K. (1988). Nursing case management: Strategic management of cost and quality outcomes. *Journal of Nursing Administration*, *18*(5), 23–30.

4 CREDENTIALING

OBJECTIVES

After studying this chapter, you will be able to:

1. Explain the concept of credentialing and its components.
2. Understand the scope of authority for credentialing organizations and their hierarchy.
3. Identify the primary functions of credentialing.
4. Discuss the implications of credentialing related to case management.
5. Identify the relationship of credentialing to competency.

KEY TERMS

Accreditation
American Nurses Credentialing Center
Assessment-based certificate programs
Certification
Certificate
Certificant
Commission for Case Manager Certification
Credentialing
Dependent credential
Institute for Credentialing Excellence
Licensure
National Association of Social Workers Credentialing Center
Probation
Professional association
Reprimand
Revocation
State professional boards
Standards
Suspension
Title protection

In recent years, the bar for professional practice has been set at a concerning new level, that of a minimum standard. The quality chasm defined over a decade ago by the Institute of Medicine (IOM, 2001) is now an abyss of epic proportions, spanning between the health care expected and that which is actually rendered. In working to reconcile this issue, an important question beckons: Who has the ultimate responsibility for defining the professional standards which underlie practice for the health care industry? The answer lies with an array of entities that comprise the domain of credentialing.

With organizational credentialing addressed in chapter 2, this chapter's opportunity is to focus on credentialing specific to the diverse professional disciplines that comprise case management. Implications for stakeholders of case management are also addressed.

THE CREDENTIALING CURVE

Credentialing is a term applied to those processes used to designate that an individual, program, institution, or product has met established standards (American Nurses Credentialing Center [ANCC], 2014a). It takes a variety of forms, including licensure, certification, and/or accreditation for both the professionals and the organizations who employ them.

PRIMARY FUNCTIONS

Credentialing's functions are twofold. It provides a mechanism of adherence to professional standards, then assures that those standards protect the public (HRSA, 2011).

Professional Standards

Professional **standards** are traditionally set by an agent (governmental or nongovernmental) that is recognized as qualified to carry out this level of oversight (Styles & Affara, 1997). Examples of agents include state professional boards, professional associations, and accrediting organizations. The standards are clearly framed, authoritative statements which a profession puts forth. These distinguish those members of the profession by describing the unique responsibilities for which its practitioners are accountable. One example is how the CMSA (Case Management Model Act) Standards of Practice (SOPs) (CMSA, 2010) delineate the six components of the case management process, as shown in Table 4-1. Although the CMSA SOPs serve as a prime example of professional industry standards, one must take note that case management continues to be viewed as an advanced practice as opposed to formal profession.

Standards also reflect how exclusive values and priorities of a particular profession are operationalized and understood by mutual stakeholders. It is not uncommon for professional practice values to be included in a distinct ethical code or code of professional conduct as opposed to the overall practice standards. Social workers customarily refer to the National Association of Social Worker (NASW) Code of Ethics to guide their professional endeavors. The values cited are inherent through all professional interactions across the scope of practice and independent of setting, as shown in Table 4-2 (NASW, 2014c). Nurses, in turn, seek guidance with respect to practice values from the nine provisions listed in the ANA (American Nurses Association) Code of Ethics for Nurses (ANA, 2014a), as presented in Table 4-3.

Practice standards may be understood as minimal and mandatory (ANCC, 2014a). For example, an individual who

TABLE 4-1 Components of the Case Management Process

Component	Purpose
Client identification and selection	Focuses on identifying clients who would benefit from case management services. This step may include obtaining consent for case management services, if appropriate.
Assessment and problem/opportunity identification	Begins after the completion of the case selection and intake into case management and occurs intermittently, as needed, throughout the case.
Development of the case management plan	Establishes goals of the intervention and prioritizes the client's needs, as well as determines the type of services and resources that are available in order to address the established goals or desired outcomes.
Implementation and coordination of care activities	Puts the case management plan into action.
Evaluation of the case management plan and follow-up	Involves the evaluation of the client's status and goals and the associated outcomes.
Termination of the case management process	Brings closure to the care and/or episode of illness. The process focuses on discontinuing case management when the client transitions to the highest level of function, the best possible outcome has been attained, or the needs/desires of the client change.

Adapted from Case Management Society of America. (2010). CMSA standards of practice for case management (Rev.). Retrieved December 20, 2012, from http://www.cmsa.org/portals/0/pdf/memberonly/StandardsOfPractice.pdf

TABLE 4-2 NASW Code of Ethics–Values With Operationalized Ethical Principles

Value	Operationalized Ethical Principles
Service	*Social workers' primary goal is to help people in need and to address social problems* Social workers elevate service to others above selfinterest. Social workers draw on their knowledge, values, and skills to help people in need and to address social problems. Social workers are encouraged to volunteer some portion of their professional skills with no expectation of significant financial return (pro bono service).
Social Justice	*Social workers challenge social injustice* Social workers pursue social change, particularly with and on behalf of vulnerable and oppressed individuals and groups of people. Social workers' social change efforts are focused primarily on issues of poverty, unemployment, discrimination, and other forms of social injustice. These activities seek to promote sensitivity to and knowledge about oppression and cultural and ethnic diversity. Social workers strive to ensure access to needed information, services, and resources; equality of opportunity; and meaningful participation in decision making for all people.
Dignity and Worth of the Person	*Social workers respect the inherent dignity and worth of the person* Social workers treat each person in a caring and respectful fashion, mindful of individual differences and cultural and ethnic diversity. Social workers promote clients' socially responsible selfdetermination. Social workers seek to enhance clients' capacity and opportunity to change and to address their own needs. Social workers are cognizant of their dual responsibility to clients and to the broader society. They seek to resolve conflicts between clients' interests and the broader society's interests in a socially responsible manner consistent with the values, ethical principles, and ethical standards of the profession.
Importance of Human Relationships	*Social workers recognize the central importance of human relationships* Social workers understand that relationships between and among people are an important vehicle for change. Social workers engage people as partners in the helping process. Social workers seek to strengthen relationships among people in a purposeful effort to promote, restore, maintain, and enhance the wellbeing of individuals, families, social groups, organizations, and communities.
Integrity	*Social workers behave in a trustworthy manner* Social workers are continually aware of the profession's mission, values, ethical principles, and ethical standards and practice in a manner consistent with them. Social workers act honestly and responsibly and promote ethical practices on the part of the organizations with which they are affiliated.
Competence	*Social workers practice within their areas of competence and develop and enhance their professional expertise* Social workers continually strive to increase their professional knowledge and skills and to apply them in practice. Social workers should aspire to contribute to the knowledge base of the profession.

Adapted from National Association of Social Workers. (2014c). NASW code of ethics (8th ed.). Retrieved April 21, 2014, from https://www.socialworkers.org/pubs/code/code.asp

attains a bachelors' degree in social work (BSW) and the requisite licensure level is expected to have a basic understanding of how to apply knowledge of human behavior in the social environment through a multidimensional perspective. The focus is on understanding and applying theories and knowledge specific to biological, social, cultural, psychological, and spiritual development (CSWE, 2014).

The standards can also be written to reflect practice which is above the minimum expectation and voluntary, such as those individuals who continue on the professional career path. Let us say that the BSW presented in the prior paragraph is now motivated to pursue a master's degree in clinical social work (MSW). This candidate is expected at this level of their education to demonstrate practice competence by integrating the foundational elements of a multidimensional assessment with more advanced concepts, including the behavioral manifestations of clinical psychopathology and psychotherapy interventions.

Protection of the Public

Another primary goal of credentialing is to protect the public (HRSA, 2011). Consumers are provided defined mechanisms to file complaints against those professionals whose actions are not in accordance with established practices and normative guidelines.

Most, if not all, credentialing bodies have administrative rules and governance processes to assess and/or review the

TABLE 4-3 Code of Ethics Provisions

Provision	Explanation
1	The nurse, in all professional relationships, practices with compassion and respect for the inherent dignity, worth, and uniqueness of every individual, unrestricted by considerations of social or economic status, personal attributes, or the nature of health problems.
2	The nurse's primary commitment is to the patient, whether an individual, family, group, or community.
3	The nurse promotes, advocates for, and strives to protect the health, safety, and rights of the patient.
4	The nurse is responsible and accountable for individual nursing practice and determines the appropriate delegation of tasks consistent with the nurse's obligation to provide optimum patient care.
5	The nurse owes the same duties to self as to others, including the responsibility to preserve integrity and safety, to maintain competence, and to continue personal and professional growth.
6	The nurse participates in establishing, maintaining, and improving health care environments and employment conducive to the provision of quality health care and consistent with the values of the profession through individual and collective action.
7	The nurse participates in the advancement of the profession through contributions to practice, education, administration, and knowledge development.
8	The nurse collaborates with other health professionals and the public in promoting community, national, and international efforts to meet health needs.
9	The profession of nursing, as represented by associations and their members, is responsible for articulating nursing values, for maintaining the integrity of the profession and its practice, and for shaping social policy.

Adapted from American Nurses Association. (2014a). Code of ethics for nurses. Retrieved April 21, 2014, from http://www.nursingworld.org/codeofethics

professional conduct of their members. A formal designated committee is traditionally in place, tasked with assessing complaint(s) and defining appropriate action and sanction for the noted violation. While the exact penalties vary across entities, most extend from some type of formal **reprimand** with or without remedial requirements, **probation** for a specified time period, to **suspension** or full **revocation** of the credential. Examples of the most common levels of professional reprimand are culled from credentialing entities across the industry and appear in Box 4-1.

KEY CREDENTIALING TERMS

Credentialing is an umbrella term that refers to concepts inclusive of professional licensure, certification, assessment-based certificate programs, accreditation, and regulation (Institute for Credentialing Excellence [ICE], 2014). The overriding premise of each term is the same; an individual has earned a stamp of quality and achievement which communicates to employers, payers, and consumers what to expect of that particular professional (ANCC, 2014a).

Licensure

Licensure tests an individual's competence and is a mandatory process by which the government grants time-limited permission for that licensed individual to practice his or her profession (ICE, 2014). One is traditionally licensed in the state and/or jurisdiction where their patient population resides. Professionals are beholden to their primary licensure, first and foremost.

Accreditation

Accreditation is the process by which a credentialing or educational program is evaluated against defined standards. When that entity is in compliance with these standards, it is awarded recognition or accreditation by a third party (ICE, 2014). Achieving accreditation speaks volumes to industry stakeholders about an organization's efforts to provide the highest level of quality (The Joint Commission, 2014).

Accreditation is often viewed as a rigorous endeavor, whether faced by the individual or their employer. As readily as health care organizations are subject to strict regulatory oversight through accreditation, professionals face similar analysis when they seek professional certification. Professional certification and assessment-based certificate programs fall under the accreditation realm.

Certification

Certification is a process by which individuals' preacquired knowledge, skills, or competencies are evaluated against

BOX 4-1 Levels of Professional Reprimand

Censure
This is the least restrictive discipline. The imposition of censure acts as a public reprimand that is permanently kept in the licensee's file.

Probation
Probation places terms and conditions on the licensee's license. The licensee must comply with the terms and conditions throughout the probationary period, which may extend for several years.

Suspension
Suspension requires that the licensee cease practicing for a period of time.

Revocation
This is the most restrictive discipline. It mandates that the licensee immediately loses his or her license and may no longer practice. Once a license is revoked, the individual may not apply for relicensure for a defined period of time starting from the date of revocation. Upon application, the individual may be relicensed at the discretion of the Board after compliance with all the requirements relative to a new applicant, including, but not limited to, retaking the licensure examination.

Missouri Division of Professional Registration, 2014

Limited Licensure
A practitioner's professional activities can be restricted to only those areas allowed by the board. In such cases, the practitioner is permitted to practice, albeit within a limited scope

Reprimand
This is a more formal censure or statement of wrongdoing on the part of the practitioner. It is generally used where a board believes that a formal notice of wrongdoing is necessary but without the removal of licensure or removal of the individual from practice.

Fines
Boards may be empowered to issue fines up to certain statutory limits against individuals found to have violated the practice act. These are generally penal in nature and subject the individual to payment of a monetary amount to the general funds of the jurisdiction.

Assessment of Costs
Boards should be empowered to assess costs upon individuals for the investigations, prosecutions, and adjudications of administrative matters where individuals are found guilty of violating the practice act.

The assessment of these costs should include all costs associated with the administrative prosecution including attorney's fees.

Use of Examinations
The successful completion of the initial licensure examination may be required as part of the disciplinary process, sanction, and subsequent reinstatement of licensure.

Mandatory Continuing Education
Successful completion of certain continuing education courses may be part of the disciplinary process. Continuing education courses may be specific to certain subject matter (i.e., ethics) or may be general in scope.

ASWB, 2011

predetermined standards. The focus is on an assessment that is independent of a specific class, course, or another education or training program. Those individuals who demonstrate that they can meet the standards by successfully completing the assessment process are granted the certification. Traditionally, this process is by an examination. A specific acronym or letters are awarded to the person to signify they have obtained and maintained the credential. While professional certification is viewed as a voluntary process, it can also be a requirement for employment or practice (ICE, 2014).

From case management's vantage, certification is viewed as confirming that someone has met a certain set of predetermined criteria by the certifying body. It is recognized as an acceptable standard of practice by general consent of the population it certifies (CMSA, 2014). Those who hold a particular certification are traditionally referred to as **certificants**. Other terms commonly used are *certified* and *board certified*.

There are an expanding number of certifications across health care. Some are aligned with a particular professional discipline or background, and are offered through professional associations. The **National Association of Social Workers Credentialing Center** has been providing specialty certifications to social workers for over 50 years. There are currently 20 distinct credentials available to those who meet defined eligibility (NASW, 2014).

In comparison, the **American Nurses Credentialing Center**, a subsidiary of the ANA, offers board certifications which extend across roles of nurse practitioner and clinical nurse specialist. They extend over 25 defined specialty areas, with 12 in advanced practice (ANCC, 2014b).

The scope of certifications for both NASW and ANCC encompasses the full span of patient populations and continues to evolve. Each credential denotes that a practitioner has demonstrated expertise through fulfilling defined requirements. A listing of the certifications from both entities is shown in Table 4-4.

Despite the evident merit of demonstrating excellence in one's profession through specialty certification, there is a caution that exists. How do stakeholders of the industry understand the unique differences of each certification, whether patients, practitioners, providers, or payers? It has been suggested that the emergence of new certifications with each new practice trend, such as those newly developed for health information technology and informatics, only dilutes the value of the concept of certification itself. More may not necessarily be better in this instance.

TABLE 4-4 NASW and ANCC Certifications

<table>
<tr><th>NASW</th><th>ANCC</th></tr>
<tr><td>Leadership
• Academy of Certified Social Workers (ACSW)
• Diplomate in Clinical Social Work (DCSW)</td><td>Nurse Practitioner
• Acute Care
• Acute
• Adult—Gerontology Acute Care
• Adult—Gerontology Primary Care
• Adult Psychiatric Mental Health
• Family
• Gerontological
• Pediatric Primary Care
• Psychiatric-Mental Health
• School</td></tr>
<tr><td>Advanced Practice Specialty Credentials
Military
• Military Service Members, Veterans, and Their Families—Social Worker
• Military Service Members, Veterans, and Their Families—Advanced Social Worker
• Military Service Members, Veterans, and Their Families—Clinical Social Worker

Clinical
• Qualified Clinical Social Worker

Gerontology
• Clinical Social Worker in Gerontology
• Qualified Social Worker in Gerontology
• Advanced Social Worker in Gerontology

Hospice and Palliative Care
• Advanced Certified Hospice and Palliative Social Worker
• Certified Hospice and Palliative Care Social Worker

Youth and Family
• Certified Advanced Children, Youth, and Family Social Worker
• Certified Children, Youth, and Family Social Worker

Addictions
• Certified Clinical Alcohol, Tobacco, and Other Drugs Social Worker

Health Care
• Certified Social Worker in Health Care

Case Management
• Certified Advanced Social Work Case Manager
• Certified Social Work Case Manager

Schools
• Certified School Social Work Specialist</td><td>Clinical Nurse Specialist Certifications
• Adult Health
• Adult-Gerontology
• Adult Psychiatric-Mental Health
• Child/Adolescent Psychiatric-Mental Health
• Gerontological
• Home Health
• Pediatric
• Public/Community Health

Specialty Certifications
• Ambulatory Care
• Cardiac Rehabilitation
• Cardiac-Vascular
• Certified Vascular
• College Health
• Community Health
• Diabetes Management—Advanced
• Faith Community
• Forensic Nursing—Advanced
• General Nursing Practice
• Gerontological Nursing
• High-Risk Nursing
• Informatics Nursing
• Medical-Surgical Nursing
• Nurse Executive
• Nurse Executive Advanced
• Nursing Case Management
• Nursing Professional Development
• Pain Management Nursing
• Pediatric Nursing
• Perinatal Nursing
• Psychiatric-Mental Health Nursing
• Public Health Nursing
• School Nursing

Assessment-Based Certificates
• Guided Care Nursing
• Fundamentals of Magnet</td></tr>
</table>

Adapted from National Association of Social Workers. (2014b). NASW professional social work credentials and advanced practice specialty credentials. Retrieved April 16, 2014, from http://www.socialworkers.org/credentials/list.asp; American Nurses Credentialing Center. (2014b). ANCC certification center. Retrieved April 16, 2014, from http://www.nursecredentialing.org/Certification

Assessment-Based Certificate Programs

Assessment-based certificate programs are educational or training programs used to teach learning objectives and assess whether the student has achieved those objectives. **Certificates** are awarded only to those individuals who meet the performance, proficiency, or passing standard for the assessment(s). No acronyms or letters are awarded for use after a person's name on the completion of the certificate (ICE, 2014).

A new generation of certificate programs in case management have emerged over the past decade. These programs, offered through community colleges and institutions of higher learning, appeal to health care professionals interested in advancing their careers and joining what has been identified as the fastest growing segment of the healthcare industry (UCSD, 2014). Course work is offered through a range of modalities, including distance education, intensives which occur over a day or weekend, and/or traditional in-person classes. These programs offer a certificate for the completion of required and clearly designated coursework and/or fulfilling a defined number of continuing education units. However, this endeavor should not be viewed as a substitute for formal certification, such as those provided through official credentialing bodies as the **Commission for Case Management Certification (CCMC)** or ANCC. Box 4-2 provides a glimpse of the course requirements for several case management certificate programs.

It should be noted that admission requirements are defined by the program sponsor and may not necessarily be consistent with established industry qualification standards. A solid example includes those established guidelines defined by the Qualification Standard for CMSA's Standards of Practice. This standard states the need for "case managers to maintain competence in their area(s) of practice by having a current, active, and unrestricted licensure or certification in a health or human services discipline that allows the professional to conduct an assessment independently as permitted within the scope of practice of the discipline, or baccalaureate or graduate degree in social work, or another health or human services field" (CMSA, 2010). The sponsoring programs may indicate that a college degree is not a requirement to enroll in the certificate programs, though may set other stipulations to take individual courses or certificate completion (UCSD, 2014). This presents as a contradiction between the industry's best practice' guidelines for case management practice and the expectations for those who may obtain these certificates.

CREDENTIALING OVERSIGHT

The daunting responsibility for the credentialing of professionals across health care's vast transitions of care is shared among a series of entities. This accountability spans regulatory bodies, including state professional boards, plus professional associations, accreditation and certification organizations.

BOX 4-2 Examples of Case Management Certificate Programs

Rutgers University
School of Social Work (2014)

Five Required Workshops
- Building the Helping Relationship: 5 CE hours
- Comprehensive Assessment and Care Planning: 10 CE hours
- Advocacy and Collaborating Skills in Case Management: 5 CE hours
- Improving Networking Skills and Enhancing Interagency Relationships: 5 CE hours
- Handling Crisis in Case Management: 5 CE hours

Two Elective Workshops
- Disaster-Planning for Service-Providing Agencies
- Case Plan Essentials
- Case Documentation in Social Work Practice
- The Role of the Case Manager in Working with Child Abuse and Neglect
- Working with Children and Families in Crisis

Program length, 8 days

University of Southern Maine
Professional Development (2014)

All content required:

Day 1: Case Management—Basic Elements
- History and role of the case manager
- Multidisciplinary collaborative practice
- The physician as advocate
- Length of stay and extended stay management
- A career in case management

Day 2: Outcomes Management—Critical Thinking and Critical Pathway Development
- Critical thinking concepts for everyday practice
- Description, development, and critical pathway implementation strategies
- Variance/exception analysis
- Alternatives to using a critical pathway

Day 3: Discharge Planning: Role and Departmental Integration
- Integration and other models
- Levels of care
- Referral service
- Process of discharge
- Outcomes

Day 4: Utilization Management
- Payers
- Reimbursement systems
- Utilization process
- Building relationships with payers
- Working toward zero denial rate

Program length, 4 days
Continuing education credit, 24 contact hours/2.4 CEUs

State Professional Boards

State professional boards of nursing, social work, and/or behavioral health are examples of those administrative bodies tasked with the regulatory oversight of professional licensure. A number of states also offer certifications. Although the individual roles of state boards vary, it is understood that most are tasked with protecting the public by ensuring that standards of practice are met and the requisite professionals are competent in their practice (ANA, 2014b). Examples of the roles for state boards in both nursing and social work appear in Box 4-3.

Professionals are beholden primarily to the professional licensure of the state(s) and jurisdictions in which they practice. Although this was referred to earlier in the chapter, it is a point which bears reminding amid the quagmire of credentials available across the workforce. Case management certification and other specialty certifications are often referred to as **dependent credentials**. In this instance the individual's eligibility is dependent on that person holding another credential such as a professional license or certification (CCMC, 2014).

BOX 4-3 Typical Duties of State Boards

- Interpreting and enforcing the state nurse practice act
- Administering nurse licensure by overseeing examinations to grant licenses and taking action against licenses of nurses who have exhibited unsafe nursing practice
- Accrediting or approving nurse education programs
- Developing nursing practice standards from the regulatory standpoint
- Developing policies, administrative rules, and regulations

The board investigates complaints concerning nurses' compliant with the nurse practice act law in each state, holds hearings for license holders, and determines and administers disciplinary actions based on evidence of violations of the law.

ANA, 2014b

- Establish the rules and regulations of the profession and the standards for licensure
- Issue licenses to those social workers who have met these professional standards
- Require that social workers complete continuing education in order to maintain their licensed status in good standing
- Investigate complaints and, when necessary, decide whether a social worker continues to deserve a license

In short, the mission of these regulatory bodies is the protection of the public and that public includes anyone who is the recipient of social work services.

ASWB, 2014

Certification/Accreditation Organizations

Institute for Credentialing Excellence

The **Institute for Credentialing Excellence (ICE)** is a professional membership association for accreditation and certification programs. It is tasked with setting the standards for these entities, though does not offer certification directly to professionals.

As a developer of standards for both certification and certificate programs, ICE serves as a provider of and a clearinghouse for information on trends in certification, test development and delivery, assessment-based certificate programs, and other information relevant to the credentialing community. They offer accreditation to professional certification programs through the National Commission for Certifying Agencies (NCCA) (ICE, 2014). This includes the case management credentials of the CCM and ACM, which are offered through the CCMC and American Case Management Association (ACMA), respectively. ICE also provides education, networking, and resources for organizations and individuals who work in and serve the credentialing industry (ICE, 2014).

PROFESSIONAL ASSOCIATIONS

A **professional association** is a body of persons engaged in the same profession, formed with the intent to control entry into the profession, maintain standards, and represent the profession in discussion with other bodies (*Collins English Dictionary*, 2014). CMSA, NASW, and ANA are those which case managers traditionally join.

Several professional associations have created formal credentialing divisions which provide oversight for voluntary certifications. NASW and ANA are included in this effort through the NASW Credentialing Center and ANCC. Particularly with huge variation in the definitions and scope of licensure from state to state, these specialty designations certify an individual's knowledge and experience meets or exceeds excellence at a national level (NASW, 2014a). The certifications that are relative to case management are listed in Table 4-5.

CASE MANAGEMENT'S CREDENTIALING CHASM

Case Management's Identity Disorder

Case management certification is on the rise, reflecting the expanding role that case managers play in team-based delivery models (Tahan & Campagna, 2010). The evolving opportunities through health care reform, as those provided by Accountable Care Organizations (ACOs), have only amplified the number of career options.

Over the past 20 years, the health care industry has exploded with more case management associated titles, roles, functions,

TABLE 4-5 Case Management-Related Certifications

Certification	Sponsoring Organization	Nursing	Transdisciplinary	Social Work
ACM	American Case Management Association		X	
ABDA	American Board of Disability Analysts		X	
ABQAURP	American Board of Quality Assurance Utilization Review Physicians		X	
C-ACSWCM C-SWCM	National Association of Social Workers			X
NACCM	National Academy of Certified Case Managers		X	
CMAC	Center for Case Management		X	
CCM	Commission for Case Manager Certification		X	
CDMS	Certified Disability Management Specialists		X	
CMCN	American Board of Managed Care Nursing		X	
COHN-CM	American Board for Occupational Health Nurses	X		
CPDM	Insurance Educational Association		X	
CPHQ	National Association for Healthcare Quality		X	
CPUR	McKesson		X	
CRC	Commission on Rehabilitation Counselor Certification		X	
CRRN CRRN-A	Rehabilitation Nursing Certification Board	X		
PAHM FAHM	Academy for Healthcare Management/American Health Insurance Professionals		X	
RN-BC	American Nurses Credentialing Center	X		

and job descriptions than one could have ever foretold. These framings span business models, practice settings, professional disciplines, and across the transitions of care. Some experts might challenge this expansion has contributed to a paradoxical effect on case management's identity to become the profession it strives to become (Treiger and Fink-Samnick, 2013).

Does the vast range of certifications lead to quality or confusion? Amid a lack of industry consensus on how certification is defined across the industry (Lundmark et al., 2012), how can the expanding number of certifications be compared to each other?

As presented in this chapter, certifications are administered through state professional boards, professional associations, and accreditation entities. Some certifications are voluntary, while others mandatory. Who administers the certification can serve to leverage or devalue it, simply based on their position in the regulatory and/or administrative hierarchy of sponsoring organizations. Which of these credentials holds greater employer significance: the CCM administered by the CCMC or the C-ASWCM administered by the National Association of Social Workers (NASW)? Both are understood as case management certifications and respected by the certificants who possess them. The answer to which is the more valuable certification varies, for it is dependent on an array of factors from the potential employer and their target population, to the individual's other credentials, experience, education, and/or training.

The lack of a consistent definition for certification also contributes to a challenge in identifying a meaningful, as well as causal relationship between the value of certification and patient outcomes (Lundmark et al., 2012). There have been efforts to link case management certification itself to enhanced patient care. It has been claimed that case management certification is aligned with competency, with competent case management professionals having an impact on the success and outcomes of care coordination programs (Tahan & Campagna, 2010). Others content that certification sends an important message to health care stakeholders and acknowledges that case managers possess a unique body of knowledge that is testable (Tahan, 2005). However, these affirmations are far different from a direct cause and effect relationship between certification itself and positive outcomes which reflect quality patient care.

Professional Fragmentation

Case management's diffusion is evidenced through the number of emerging case management professional associations, each with unique practice standards that are aligned, though still distinct. Several associations have developed their own specialty credential(s). At the time of this writing, there are over 21 unique certifications and six distinct organizational accreditations for case management (CMSA, 2014).

One has to wonder what value this vast array of professional distinctions serve to the consumers and/or populations served by case management. Although competition can result in a better quality and wider variety of product offerings, it should always be undertaken in the spirit of raising the bar for the entire practice rather than to create market confusion for the case management consumer (Treiger & Fink-Samnick, 2013).

A question for consideration beckons: Who gains the greatest benefit from case management certification? Is it the professional, their employer, the patient, the industry, or another entity? Given the wide berth of case management-related certifications alone, one could debate this translates as a credential available for everyone; expanded options yield opportunity. Some experts equate the earning of multiple credentials as a means of simply seeking more letters after their name, at times going the fastest and easiest route (Mullahy, 2014).

A growing trend involves a flow of case management certifications offered through professional associations and other organizations, as those listed in the NASW and ANCC Comparison. Many have a population-specific focus, as those geared to the military or a specific disease state. Others are defined by the professional discipline or background of the individual, such as those which denote social work or nursing case management. It is with respect to this latter group that one should wonder, do theses certifications dilute the value of larger and more overriding certifications?

A majority of case management certifications include the mandate for an individual to hold appropriate licensure in the health and human services area as part of the eligibility criteria, as the CCM and ACM. In the hierarchy of credentialing, one is first beholden to his or her professional licensure and the administrative laws which underlie it. This translates to the case management certification being viewed as a dependent credential—one which is dependent on licensure.

One would think that the majority of licensed professionals fully comprehend the scope of practice of their primary license, whether nurse, social worker, or other member of the allied health workforce. How would they understand this scope any better with a dependent credential which is qualified by their professional discipline of origin as opposed to certification reflecting global case management practice? The CMSA (2009) speaks to case management and case managers throughout the document, as opposed to nursing or social work case management.

How much does this fragmentation interfere with case management maturing from its current status of advanced practice to full-fledged profession? A model grounded primarily in case management–specific competencies would be an asset to this end. Why should the expertise defined by and demonstrated through case management certification be diluted by adding a professional discipline as a qualifier?

The Certificate Conundrum

At a time when the race is on to demonstrate competency and excellence in a chosen field, professionals are eager to obtain specialty certifications, particularly in case management. Many are obtained through formal professional boards as state boards of nursing, social work, and/or behavioral health. Others originate with formal accreditation entities as CCMC or CRCC, as have been discussed.

However, a false notion exists about the value of those certificates obtained from continuing education programs, conferences, and/or other educational trainings: that they are somehow equal to formal case management certification. These certificates do validate an individual's attendance at a conference, training, and/or fulfillment of continuing education hours. They are not, however, substitutes for passing an examination of evidence-based knowledge, theories, and skills.

TITLE PROTECTION

Title Protection refers to the legal designation that it is unlawful for an individual to call himself or herself by a specific professional title without the requisite education and training for that title, plus potentially the minimal level of licensure. Although the efforts and language of the laws in each jurisdiction vary, the theme is similar.

The movement has been occurring within a number of health professions across the globe for the past several decades. Title protection has been motivated by one of the primary roles of credentialing, that of consumer protection (Powell, 2011).

Social Work

Social work has been instrumental in leading the Title Protection movement. This action was motivated by assorted factors from consumer protection to recognition of social work as a specialized profession and not just a job title.

In the year 2000, the United Kingdom passed Title Protection under its Care Standards Act of that year. Per section Chapter 14 (Part 1V) Section 61, "no one can describe herself or himself as a social worker unless he or she is registered in the Social Care Registry maintained by the General Social Care Council" (Murray and Hendricks, 2011).

The National Association of Social Workers (NASW) and its individual chapters have worked diligently to move Title Protection forward. Almost every state with social work licensure has a licensure law and/or regulation that protects the use of the title "social worker" by use from anyone who is not a social worker (Social Work Examination Services, 2014). Virginia's law HB 2037, enacted July 2013, extends to it being unlawful for any person not licensed by the Board of Social Work to use the title "social worker" in both writing or in advertising in connection with his practice unless he simultaneously uses the clarifying initials signifying a degree in social work (Legislative Information System, 2014). Box 4-4 provides a view of title protection language comparisons across several states.

One of title protection's challenges for social workers lies in the fact that not every state legislates licensure for all social work roles, such as those hired by public institutions plus several other settings as discussed in chapter 2. This has led to public protection challenges for consumers as they work to reconcile the difference between social workers who have formal education from an accredited school of social work at the bachelor's and potentially master's level of practice, as well as the requisite level of licensure and those who do not. The case scenario in Box 4-5 illustrates an example of why title protection is aligned with one of the prime reasons cited for credentialing at the start of this chapter, that of protecting the public.

Nursing

Thirty-nine states currently include language to reflect title protection in their Nurse Practice Act. Some states, such

BOX 4-4 Title Protection Legislation Wording Comparison—Social Work

HB 2037: Social work: unlawful for person not licensed by Board of Social Work to use title social worker

Social work; title protection. Provides that it shall be unlawful for any person not licensed by the Board of Social Work to use the title "Social Worker" in writing or in advertising in connection with his practice unless he simultaneously uses the clarifying initials signifying a degree in social work. The bill provides exceptions for federally required and defined social workers in nursing homes and hospices and has a delayed effective date of July 1, 2013.

Legislative Tracking System, 2014

North Carolina Code: Chapter 90B Social Worker Certification and Licensure Act § 90B-16. Title protection

Except as provided in G.S. 90B-10, an individual who (i) is not certified, licensed, or associate licensed by this Chapter as a social worker, (ii) does not hold a bachelor's or master's degree in social work from a college or university having a social work program accredited or admitted to candidacy for accreditation by the Council on Social Work Education, or (iii) has not received a doctorate in social work shall not use the title 'Social Worker' or any variation of the title.

NCSW Board, 2014

BOX 4-5 Title Protection Case Scenario

Mrs. Kelly is a resident of Glen Ray Nursing Home. Her family is visiting and has requested to meet with the social worker. Mrs. Kelly has a history of colon cancer, which is now metastasized to the bone. Prior to her admission, Mrs. Kelly was clear with her family, "There will be no prolonging of my time on earth to fight this illness. My doctors have been clear about my lousy prognosis and when I say I'm done, I'm done. I've had all the pain I can handle and want as much control over my death as I can. You will call hospice when I say so."

James is employed as the social worker at Glen Ray. He appears in Mrs. Kelly's room. Before Mrs. Kelly or her family can speak, James verbalizes strong disapproval of this plan to the family. There is a loud, verbal altercation between James and the resident, with the family shocked at what they are experiencing.

The family contacts the State Board of Social Work for their jurisdiction to file a complaint against James for what they feel is blatant unprofessionalism. However, the family is first asked, "Is the social worker licensed?" The family thinks, "How can a social worker NOT be licensed?" The state board informs the family that in this particular state, social workers who are employed in nursing homes are exempt from licensure. The family decides to call the nursing home to find out more about James and his credentials.

The family contacts Glen Ray and is directed to the administrator. They become appalled when they are informed that James does not hold a degree in social work. He also holds no licensure as a social worker.

The family is informed that there is no regulatory oversight for the "social worker's" actions. They contact NASW's Legal Department and are provided information concurrent with what they have already heard from both the State Board of Social Work and Glen Ray's administrator. NASW tells them they can file a complaint with the local ombudsman, or perhaps explore civil suit with a private attorney against the social worker. They advise the family to also contact the NASW chapter for their state since they happen to be currently advocating for Title Protection legislation in the state.

as Arkansas, Pennsylvania, and Washington State, have explicit language to restrict use of the title "nurse" to only those who are licensed. Others such as Arizona, Mississippi, and Nebraska use more implicit language to restrict use of any words implying the individual is a licensed nurse (ANA, 2014d). Similar to social work, both the wording and implications for nursing practice vary across the states, though the intent of title protection legislation is the same; to restrict use of the title "nurse" to only those individuals who have fulfilled the requirements for licensure as outlined in each state's nurse practice act is a protection for the public against unethical, unscrupulous, and incompetent practitioners (ANA, 2014e). Box 4-6 provides a comparison of how vastly different title protection language for nursing can manifest across the states.

BOX 4-6 Title Protection Legislation Wording Comparison—Nursing

Kansas 65-1115

(d) Title and abbreviation. Any person who holds a license to practice as a registered professional nurse in this state shall have the right to use the title, "registered nurse" and the abbreviation "RN." No other person shall assume the title or use the abbreviation or any other words, letters, signs, or figures to indicate that the person is a registered professional nurse.

Pennsylvania (2012) P.L.317, No.69

Section 3 Registered Nurse, Clinical Nurse Specialist, Use of Title and Abbreviation "RN" or "CNS"; Credentials; Fraud— (a) Any person who holds a license to practice professional nursing in this Commonwealth, or who is maintained on inactive status in accordance with section 11 of this act, shall have the right to use the [title] titles "nurse" and "registered nurse" and the abbreviation "RN." No other person shall engage in the practice of professional nursing or use the [title] titles "nurse" or "registered nurse" or the abbreviation "RN" to indicate that the person using the same is a registered nurse[.], except that the title "nurse" also may be used by a person licensed under the provisions of the act of March 2, 1956 (1955 P.L.1211, No.376), known as the "Practical Nurse Law." No person shall sell or fraudulently obtain or fraudulently furnish any nursing diploma, license, record, or registration or aid or abet therein. (b) An individual who holds a license to practice professional nursing in this Commonwealth who meets the requirements under sections 6.2 and 8.5 of this act to be a clinical nurse specialist shall have the right to use the title "clinical nurse specialist" and the abbreviation "CNS." No other person shall have that right. c) Notwithstanding subsection A, this section shall not prohibit the use by a person if a descriptive title for nurse assistive personnel. For the purposes of this subsection, the term "nurse assistive personnel" shall mean an individual providing health services under the supervision of a professional or practical nurse.

P.L.423, No.110, Section 14. Violations— Except (A) EXCEPT as otherwise herein provided, it shall be unlawful for any person, association, partnership, corporation, or institution, after the effective date of this act, to (1) Furnish, sell or obtain by fraud or misrepresentation a record of any qualification required for a license, or aid or abet therein; (2) Use in connection with his or her name the words nurse, practical nurse, licensed practical nurse, or the letters "PN," or "LPN," or any designation tending to imply that he or she is a practical nurse, or licensed practical nurse, unless he or she is duly licensed to so practice under the provisions of this act, except that the title "nurse" also may be used by a person registered under the provisions of the act of May 22, 1951 (P.L.317, No.69), known as "The Professional Nursing Law "; (3) Practice practical nursing during the time his or her license issued under the provisions of this act is suspended or revoked; (4) Practice practical nursing without a valid current license; (5) To transfer, offer to transfer, or permit the use by another of any license issued under this act; (6) To aid or abet any person to violate any provision of this act; (7) Otherwise violate any of the provisions of this act. (B) Notwithstanding subsection A, this section shall not prohibit the use by a person if a descriptive title for nurse assistive personnel. For the purposes of this subsection, the term "nurse assistive personnel" shall mean an individual providing health services under the supervision of a professional or practical nurse.

ANCC, 2014d

Case Management

Title Protection has also been broached as a means to professionalize case management (Powell, 2011). The last several decades have witnessed strong efforts to ground and formalize case management, including the development of model acts to establish templates for professional practice through legislation. The Case Management Model Act proposed standards for case management services with key provisions identified to encompass staff qualifications, case management functions, scope and payment of services, training requirements, quality management programs, and antifraud and consumer protections. The Act has strong potential to serve as a template for title protection legislation at the federal, local, or regulatory levels (CMSA, 2009). Consider case scenarios in Box 4-7 reflecting the implications of title protection for case management.

In this patient-centric health care environment, the following question is posed: Shouldn't consumers receiving intervention from health care professionals, especially case managers, be assured that this intervention is rendered by competent, licensed professionals who have received the requisite education and training? (Treiger & Fink-Samnick, 2013)

BOX 4-7 Title Protection Case Scenarios

Scenario 1

Janine has been employed for the past 10 years by Soho Insurance, a large national managed care organization. She loves her job in the Claims Department and a Senior Claims Analyst. Janine's role is focused on assuring that all the explanation of benefits (EOB) documentation is coded accurately. Janine then mails the EOBs out to Soho's customers. She is also responsible for tracking and resolving any appeals to the codes by customers, whether patients or their providers. Courtesy of a recent reorganization at Soho, the Claims Department now reports to the Director of Clinical Operations, It has been decided that because of the strong financial implications of Janine's role, her job title will be changed. Effective immediately, all Senior Claims Analysts will be known as Claims Case Managers. Janine has an associates' degree in human services from a local community college.

Scenario 2

Andrew has been working in utilization management at Masters Community Hospital (MCH) for the past 5 years. His job title is case manager. His responsibilities include medical necessity review of all new admissions, application of appropriateness criteria, communication with payer source, and communication with his colleague Carter, whose focus is discharge planning. A major focus for Carter is to coordinate transitions by communicating requests for evaluations to post-acute care settings and overseeing efficient patient transfers. His job title is case manager. Both Andrew and Carter work with various payer's clinical coordination departments obtaining authorizations for admissions and other services. During these interactions, they come in contact with many individuals who review incoming information and make determinations based on evidence-based criteria. Many of these contacts work under the job title of case manager. Although all of these individuals have either social work or nursing degrees, each attends to a small part of overall care, many do not conduct comprehensive patient assessments, and few are responsible for development or execution of a case management plan.

SUMMARY

This chapter has delivered a comprehensive view of credentialing as it impacts case management professionals. Credentialing provides the mechanism to assure adherence to professional standards, then mandates those standards protect health care's consumers. This is equally integral to how stakeholders understand the delivery of quality case management intervention.

Moving forward, one must consider that if credentialing assures standards of practice are adhered to by professionals, what provides those qualifiers by which to judge and validate that the practice standards have actually been met? Therein lies the function of competencies.

The question of how a competent case manager is defined has been a source of great debate. Although a number of indicators have been suggested, a clearly defined answer continues to warrant attention. Is the reply based on those minimum standards defined by the assorted credentialing entities, as presented in this chapter? Do the tools which measure the quantity of a case manager's intervention shed light on a response, such as caseload calculators, or outcomes to define return on investment?

The answer to how a competent case manager can be found among those entities that share accountability for educational, professional, organizational, and institutional oversight. We invite you to enter the realm of competency's history, scope, value, and innovation—the focus of chapter 5.

References

American Nurses Association. (1979). *The study of credentialing in nursing: A new approach.* Kansas City, MO: American Nurses Association.

American Nurses Association. (2014a). *Code of ethics for nurses.* Retrieved April 21, 2014, from http://www.nursingworld.org/codeofethics

American Nurses Association. (2014b). *FAQs: Roles of state boards of nursing: licensure, regulation, and complaint investigation.* Retrieved April 21, 2014, from http://www.nursingworld.org/mainmenucategories/tools/state-boards-of-nursing-faq.pdf

American Nurses Credentialing Center. (2014a). *Credentialing definitions.* Retrieved April 9, 2014, from http://www.nursecredentialing.org/Functional Category/ANCC-Awards/Grants/Credentialing-Definitions.html

American Nurses Credentialing Center. (2014b). *ANCC certification center.* Retrieved April 16, 2014, from http://www.nursecredentialing.org/Certification

American Nurses Credentialing Center. (2014c). *Adult psychiatric-mental health clinical nurse specialist certification eligibility criteria.* Retrieved April 18, 2014, from http://www.nursecredentialing.org/AdultPsychCNS-Eligibility.aspx

American Nurses Credentialing Center. (2014d). *Title protection.* Retrieved April 20, 2014, from http://www.nursingworld.org/MainMenu Categories/Policy-Advocacy/State/Legislative-Agenda-Reports/State-TitleNurse

American Nurses Credentialing Center. (2104e). *Summary of title protection language by state.* Retrieved April 20, 2014, from http://www.nursingworld.org/MainMenuCategories/Policy-Advocacy/State/Legislative-Agenda-Reports/State-TitleNurse/Title-Nurse-Summary-Language.html

Association of Social Work Boards. (2011). *Disciplinary guidebook.* Retrieved April 22, 2014, from http://www.aswb.org/wpcontent/uploads/2013/10/ASWBDisciplinaryGuidebook.pdf

Case Management Society of America. (2009). *Case Management Model Act.* Retrieved April 18, 2014, from http://www.cmsa.org/portals/0/pdf/publicpolicy/cmsa_model_act.pdf

Case Management Society of America. (2010). *CMSA standards of practice for case management* (Rev.). Retrieved December 20, 2012, from http://www.cmsa.org/portals/0/pdf/memberonly/StandardsOfPractice.pdf

Case Management Society of America. (2014). *Accreditation and certification resources.* Retrieved April 9, 2014, from http://www.cmsa.org/Individual/Education/AccreditationCertification/Certification/tabid/261/Default.aspx

Commission for Case Manager Certification. (2014). *Certification and renewal.* Retrieved April 21, 2014, from http://ccmcertification.org/node/428

Council on Social Work Education. (2008). *Education policy and accreditation standards (EPAS) implementation.* Retrieved from http://www.cswe.org/Accreditation/EPASImplementation.aspx

Institute of Credentialing Excellence. (2014). *About us.* Retrieved April 9, 2014, from http://www.credentialingexcellence.org/p/cm/ld/fid=32

Institute of Medicine. (2001). *Crossing the quality chasm: A new health system for the 21st century.* Washington, DC: The National Academies Press.

Legislative Tracking System. (2014). *HB 2037.* Retrieved April 11, 2014, from https://lis.virginia.gov/cgi-bin/legp604.exe?111+sum+HB2037

Lundmark, V., Hickey, J., Haller, K., Hughes, R., Johantgen, M., Koithan, M., ... Unruh, L. (2012). *A national agenda for credentialing research in nursing (ANCC Credentialing Research Report).* Silver Spring, MD: American Nurses Credentialing Center.

Missouri Division of Professional Regulation. (2014). *Board of nursing discipline.* Retrieved December 11, 2014 from http://pr.mo.gov/nursing-discipline.asp

Mullahy, C (2014). *The Case Manager's Handbook* (5th ed.). Burlington, MA: Jones and Bartlett Learning.

Murray D., & Hendricks G. (2011). *A collaborative project to achieve title protection in North Carolina.* The New Social Worker. Retrieved December 25, 2012, from http://www.socialworker.com/home/Feature_Articles/General/A_Collaborative_Project_to_Achieve_Title_Protection_in_NC/

National Association of Social Workers. (2014a). *Credentialing center.* Retrieved April 16, 2014, from http://www.socialworkers.org/credentials/default.asp

National Association of Social Workers. (2014b). *NASW professional social work credentials and advanced practice specialty credentials.* Retrieved April 16, 2014, from http://www.socialworkers.org/credentials/list.asp

National Association of Social Workers. (2014c). *NASW code of ethics* (8th ed.). Retrieved April 21, 2014, from https://www.socialworkers.org/pubs/code/code.asp

North Carolina Social Work Board. (NSCW). (2014). *Statute chapter 90B-16, title protection,* Retrieved April 22, 2014, from http://www.ncswboard.org/page/statute1#b16

Powell, S. (2011). The gestalt of case management. *Professional Case Management, 16*(5), 227–228.

Professional Association. (n.d.). *Collins english dictionary—Complete & unabridged* (10th ed.). Retrieved April 22, 2014, from http://dictionary.reference.com/browse/professional association

Rutgers School of Social Work. (2014). *Certificate program in case management.* Retrieved April 22, 2014, from http://socialwork.rutgers.edu/continuingeducation/ce/certificateprograms/certcasemanagement.aspx

Social Work Examination Services. (2014). *Regulatory Issues.* Retrieved December 11, 2014, from http://www.swes.net/licensing/reg_issues.html

Styles, M. M., & Affara, F. A. (1997). *ICN on regulation: Toward 21st-century models.* Geneva: International Council of Nurses. Retrieved April 16, 2014, from http://www.icn.ch/publications/regulation/

Tahan, H. (2005). Clarifying certification and its value for case managers. *Professional Case Management, 10*(1), 14–21.

Tahan, H., & Campagna, V. (2010). Case management roles and functions across various settings. *Professional Case Management, 15*(5), 245–277.

Treiger, T., & Fink-Samnick, E. (2013). Collaborate: A universal competency-based paradigm for professional case management, part 1: Introduction, historical validation and competency presentation. *Professional Case Management, 18*(3), 122–135.

University of California San Diego Extension. (2014). *Case management certificate.* Retrieved April 22, 2014, from http://extension.ucsd.edu/programs/index.cfm?vAction=certDetail&vCertificateID=13

University of Southern Maine, Professional Development Programs. (2104). *Certificate program in case management.* Retrieved April 22, 2014, from https://usm.maine.edu/pdp/certificate-program-case-management#Details

U.S. Department of Health and Human Services, Health Resources and Services. (2010). *Health licensing board, report to congress administration.* Retrieved April 9, 2014, from http://www.hrsa.gov/ruralhealth/about/telehealth/licenserpt10.pdf

5 COMPETENCY-BASED APPROACHES

OBJECTIVES

After studying this chapter, you will be able to:

1. Discuss the historical constructs of how competency is understood and applied across the health care industry.
2. Define the various contexts of competency applicable to case management.
3. Explain the importance of competency-based job descriptions.
4. Describe the evolution of competency-based oversight for higher education, health care organizations, and the workforce.
5. Identify the primary organizational influencers of competency-based models for health care.
6. Discuss interprofessional competencies and their decisive role in the provision of quality health care.
7. Identify barriers specific to interprofessional education and practice.
8. Identify the impetus for competency-based exit examinations in higher education and their significance for hiring.

KEY TERMS

Accreditation
Autonomy
College Learning Assessment+
College Work Readiness Assessment+
Competency
Competent
Common competency
Core competency
Five core competencies
Hard competency
Interprofessional competency
Interprofessional Education Collaborative (IPEC)
Institute of Medicine (IOM)
Professional competency
Soft competency
The National Quality Aims
The Canadian Interprofessional Health Collaborative

Competencies are a vital factor of the quality health care equation. They set the tone for academic and professional **accreditation** by defining educational program priorities and required coursework. Job descriptions are now guided by the inclusion of competency-based skills and practice behaviors. Amid the fluid nature of the industry, competencies are that constant by which organizational return on investment is measured and validated.

This chapter provides a comprehensive view of the evolution and significance of competencies across health care. It will extend from basic definitions and utilization across practice contexts to the recent cultural transformation for competencies, one that reflects a new generation of interprofessional approaches which generate unique synergy to leverage quality-driven care coordination. A timeline is shown in Figure 5-1.

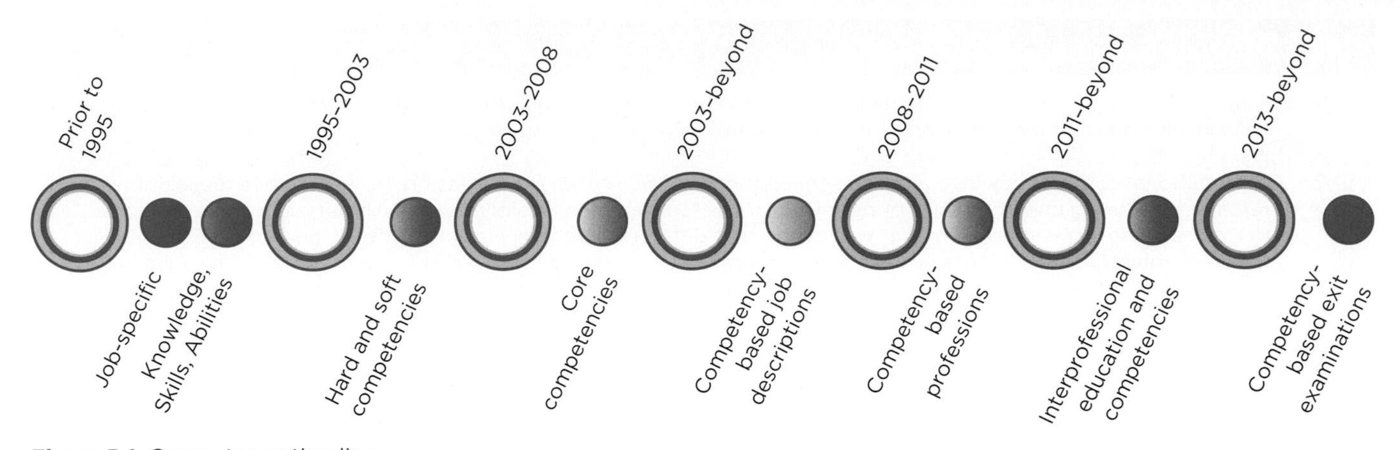

Figure 5-1. Competency timeline.

TOWARD A COMPETENCY CULTURE

Definitions and Contexts

The term **competency** has a complex heritage with extremely broad use across all industries, including health care. Although some experts suggest there is little consensus in how the term is understood by professionals (Welie & Welie, 2001), there are widely accepted definitions to frame application. These extend across the myriad of contexts where competencies have strong potential to drive the patient care process.

The Patient

A person thought to have the necessary ability or skills, or is able to do something well enough to meet a standard is viewed as **competent** (Merriam-Webster Online, 2014a). This is a general framing with application across society. For example, an event planner and a patisserie chef are each viewed as competent when they complete their assigned tasks to meet the benchmark, whether facilitation of a successful party or preparation of a flaky croissant.

Case managers may have their initial introduction to the term *competence* through the context of a patient assessment. In this situation, a case manager may have to determine whether a patient is able to understand informed consent specific to particular treatment options and/or the consequences of his or her decisions. In these types of situations, there can easily be confusion between patient **autonomy** and competence (Welie & Welie, 2001). The respect for autonomy is a basic patient right that is understood as an individual's ability to be free, independent, and self-directing (Merriam-Webster Online, 2014b). However, some professionals might suggest that a patient who can self-direct his or her care is competent, implying a direct relationship between the two terms. As a result, the question beckons: Is an autonomous patient who can complete an informed consent, or for that matter refuse the care presented by that informed consent, always competent?

The need to define patient *competency* is often viewed as a formal legal process to determine the capability of that individual to act on his or her own behalf (McGraw Hill Concise Dictionary of Modern Medicine, 2014). A psychiatrist or other mental health professional may be consulted to provide an assessment of a patient's *competence*, but the court will render the ultimate decision. It is for this reason that many professionals subscribe to a definition for *competency* used in the law. In this scope, the patient is required to have the mental capacities to reason and deliberate, hold appropriate values and goals, appreciate his or her circumstances, understand information given, and communicate a choice (Buchanan, 2004). This is a far more complex concept than that which underlies patient autonomy.

The Workforce

The application of competency to the workforce evolved over time. In this context, competence was first viewed as an organism's ability to interact effectively and purposefully with the environment. This biological perspective provided a sound view of human nature that resonated with many. Yet it became equally powerful to ground competence through a range of psychological theories, including, but not limited to, psychoanalysis (Freud), cognitive development (Piaget), and attachment (Harlow). Each theory equated the direct impact of one's instincts and behaviors on the immediate environment. This presented as a natural leap to relate motivation and purposeful behavioral intent to each person's unique level of competency (White, 1959). White's work ultimately aligned competency with workplace performance, a concept that reverberated with great force across human resource professionals. By the 1960s, competencies took root as the means to assess an employee's workplace performance.

From the 1970s to 1990s, a series of new definitions for competency continued to appear. Each one of these empowered human resource departments to both define and operationalize workplace competency. The focus evolved from defining competence for business (Lundberg, 1972) to distinguishing it from intelligence (McClelland, 1973), establishing

TABLE 5-1 New Definitions of Competency

<table>
<tr><td>1972</td><td>Competence is a set of defined behaviors that provide a structured guide enabling the identification, evaluation, and development of the behaviors in individual employees. (Lundberg)</td></tr>
<tr><td>1973</td><td>Occupational competency leveraged the concept of specific self-image, values, traits, and motive dispositions (i.e., relatively enduring characteristics of people) that are found to consistently distinguish outstanding from typical performance in a given job or role. It was posed that different competencies predict outstanding performance in different roles, and that there are a limited number of competencies that predict outstanding performance in any given job or role. As a result, a trait that is a "competency" for one job might not predict outstanding performance in a different role. (McClelland)</td></tr>
<tr><td>1980</td><td>Stages of Competency Development
<table>
<tr><td>Novice</td><td>Rule-based behavior, strongly limited, and inflexible</td></tr>
<tr><td>Experienced beginner</td><td>Incorporates aspects of the situation</td></tr>
<tr><td>Practitioner</td><td>Acting consciously from long-term goals and plans</td></tr>
<tr><td>Knowledgeable practitioner</td><td>Sees the situation as a whole and acts from personal conviction</td></tr>
<tr><td>Expert</td><td>Has an intuitive understanding of the situation and zooms in on the central aspects</td></tr>
</table>
(Dreyfus & Dreyfus)</td></tr>
<tr><td>1990</td><td>Core competency is a specific factor that a business sees as central to the way the company or its employees work. It fulfills three key criteria:
1. It is not easy for competitors to imitate.
2. It can be reused widely for many products or markets.
3. It must contribute to the end consumer's experienced benefits and the value of the product or service to its customers.
(Prahalad & Hamel)</td></tr>
</table>

stages for development (Dreyfus & Dreyfus), and ultimately drilling down to **core competencies** (Prahalad & Hamel, 1990). These framings presented across management development circles, with the main concepts shown in Table 5-1.

Meanwhile, health care's culture began to transition and reflect a more economically motivated industry, one especially associated with business acumen. The introduction of diagnostic-related groups and an expanding managed care presence contributed to an increased focus on the financial drivers of quality, including reimbursement, utilization of services, and efficiency and effectiveness of care (Fink-Samnick, 2008). Competition and expansion in health care now paralleled the business sector. The race was on for health care providers to offer trendsetting interventions and customer-focused environments. Employment growth was staggering, increasing over 292%, with more than 10% of the workforce employed in the health care sector (Sultz & Young, 1999).

Health care employers became increasingly attentive to the importance of defining and assessing workplace performance by more consistent means. Knowledge, skills, and one's ability to perform core job functions were among the key areas of appraisal (Alspach, 1992). In this way performance could ultimately be measured by those primary job functions, core skills, and behaviors specific to the responsibilities of a position. Organizations began to align job titles, roles, and functions with related professional standards. However, industry concern prevailed on whether competencies were still the best means to measure an individual's overall expertise.

HARD PLUS SOFT COMPETENCIES SET THE STANDARD

The specific job-related tasks and responsibilities are known as **hard competencies** (Parsons & Capka, 1997). Examples might include a nurse's ability to administer different types of medications (e.g., intravenous injections) or a social worker's expertise to engage and establish rapport with diverse patient populations.

In 1995, the Joint Commission on Hospital Accreditation began to require that hospitals assess, prove, track, and improve the competence of all employees. This new direction proved as daunting as one might expect any shift in organizational culture would be. Competency became viewed as the determination of an individual's capacity to perform his or her job functions up to defined expectations (The Joint Commission, 2000). This proved to be a shift in mind-set, as a professional's commitment to complete a task became as integral a component as the demonstrated proficiency of that task itself.

As health care's workforce approached the 20th century, the competency focus experienced yet another shift in how it was operationalized. An innovative concept, **soft competencies**, infused its way into both the job market and the employee assessment models. Defined as the traits to reflect individual personality and unique style, soft competencies became quickly viewed as a determining factor when evaluating for successful performance mastery in the new outcomes-focused practice culture (Parsons & Capka, 1997).

The times were ripe for these soft competencies, also referred to as "soft" business skills. Health care's new business culture framing, discussed earlier, continued to drive competition and expansion across all sectors. This was fueled in part by expansion of medical knowledge from biomedical research and manifesting technology, yielding expanded care options and longer lives for health care consumers (Fink-Samnick, 2008). This atmosphere set the stage for a full-on business perspective, one that emphasized the value of these interpersonal and participative competencies to the optimal candidate. Soft competencies were identified to have the right prescriptions for leadership success moving forward (Wilson & O'Grady, 1999).

COMPETENCY-BASED JOB DESCRIPTIONS

The practice bar was raised with a new course defined on health care's horizon, one directed toward competency-based practice. A steady stream of new competency programs across the industry was viewed as not only mandated for the Joint Commission adherence but also served:

1. To help facility leaders stay focused on their primary objective: the facility's mission statement
2. To assist in matching applicants to open positions
3. To ensure ongoing assessment of staff competency from system entry through the remainder of the person's association with the organization (Summers & Woods, 2008)

Despite the popularity of the hot and soft competencies model, not all were fans. Many viewed soft competencies as too subjective a means by which to assess an individual's appropriateness for a particular job. Although human resource experts viewed the merging of soft with hot competencies as the right ticket for organizational success, this combined effort had other pitfalls. Too large and exhaustive a list of competencies had the potential to evoke confusion among academicians and the next generation of health care leaders. Questions emerged regarding how educational priorities would be established. Of equal concern was the best means to appraise work performance. Others wrestled with how to define hiring priorities. Although those in leadership positions sought to define the fundamental value of workforce competencies, there was little professional consensus. Optimal utilization remained an overwhelming task in health care's increasingly complex world (Parsons & Capka, 1997).

During this time it was not uncommon for organizations to develop job descriptions with included focused competencies as opposed to the more traditional format of roles and/or functions. This contributed to supporting organizational expectations for high-quality services (Summers & Woods, 2008). Those in the industry at this time might recall both their surprise amid elation when seeing their job description decrease dramatically in size, along with the removal of that language, "other duties as assigned." However, this was driven by another powerful force: a grander focus on providing health care consumers with care reflective of their needs rendered by quality professionals.

COMPETENCY-BASED OVERSIGHT ACROSS THE INDUSTRY

The Institute of Medicine's Pathway

The National Quality Aims

As noted in chapter 2, the **Institute of Medicine (IOM)** had become a respected voice for the health care industry. They had published a series of reports since the 1970s that closely examined the overall quality of care, as displayed in Table 5-2.

Tens of thousands of Americans were dying annually from errors in their care, with additional numbers suffering or barely escaping from nonfatal injuries that a truly high-quality care system would largely present (IOM, 2003). There was consensus and evidence that the American health care delivery system was in need of monumental change.

Quality issues presented across all transitions of care which was concerning in and unto itself. Yet, new evidence yielded just how many of the quality issues occurred at the hands of those health care professionals entrusted to render that care. Although it was identified that these professionals were most likely committed to do the best job possible, they were equally forced to work within a system that failed to prepare and/or support them once they were in practice to achieve the best for their patients (IOM, 2003). This was surprising and alarming to all stakeholders.

The IOM's profound words still resonate for many: "The nation's current healthcare system often lacks the environment, the processes and the capabilities needs to ensure that services are safe, effective, patient-centered, timely, efficient and equitable" (IOM, 2001). The manifesting call for action involved an ambitious redesign of the broken health care system involving what became known as the National Quality Aims, which are highlighted in Table 5-3.

The Core Competencies

The Aims were geared to enhance the quality processes underlying health care delivery, quite the massive undertaking. However, a grander vision accompanied this project: serving as the precursor for competency-based oversight of the overall industry.

The expectation for this endeavor was that the Aims' agenda could be aligned with the current array of

TABLE 5-2 IOM Foundational Reports

Title	Publication Date	Context
To Err Is Human: Building a Safer Healthcare System	1999	• Lays out a comprehensive strategy by which government, health care providers, industry, and consumers can reduce preventable medical errors. • Concluding that the know-how exists to prevent many of these mistakes, the report sets as a minimum goal a 50% reduction in errors over the next 5 years. • Recommendations strike a balance between regulatory and market-based initiatives, and between the roles of professionals and organizations.
Crossing the Quality Chasm: A New Health System for the 21st Century	2001	• Identified that tens of thousands of Americans were dying annually from errors in their care, with additional numbers suffering or barely escaping from nonfatal injuries that a truly high-quality care system would largely present.

A Bridge to Quality	2003	• Identifies how doctors, nurses, pharmacists, and other health professionals are not being adequately prepared to provide the highest quality and safest medical care possible, and there is insufficient assessment of their ongoing proficiency.
		• Educators and accreditation, licensing, and certification organizations should ensure that students and working professionals develop and maintain proficiency in five core competency areas:
		  • Delivering patient-centered care,
		  • Working as part of interdisciplinary teams,
		  • Practicing evidence-based medicine,
		  • Focusing on quality improvement, and
		  • Using information technology.

professional competencies in place for the requisite accrediting bodies. Since these competencies were used toward obtaining and maintaining continued licensure, linkage to quality-based initiatives was logical. This information would further be used toward determining plus fine-tuning the competencies clinicians needed to fulfill it (the agenda). Ultimately, there would be further implications for study, including means to better understand how the workforce could be educated for practice, deployed, and ultimately held accountable (IOM, 2003).

TABLE 5-3 IOM National Quality Aims

Aim	Operationalized
Safety	Patients should not be harmed by care that is intended to help them, nor should harm come to those who work in health care.
Effectiveness	Care that is based on the use of systematically acquired evidence to determine whether an intervention, such as a preventive service, diagnostic test, or therapy, produces better outcomes than alternatives ... including the alternative of doing nothing.
Patient-centeredness	Focuses on the patient's experience of illness and health care and the systems that work to fail or work to meet individual patient's needs. Encompasses qualities of compassion, empathy, and responsiveness to the needs, values, and expressed preferences of the individual patient.
Timeliness	A valued commodity for all patients and stakeholders. Delays can pose physical harm and/or emotional distress and signal a lack of attention to flow and lack of respect for the patient. It suggests care has not been designed with the welfare of the patient at the center.
Efficiency	Resources are used to obtain the best value for the money spent through reducing quality waste and administrative or production costs.
Equity	This involves securing health care benefits which reduce the burden of illness, injury, and disability, and improve the health and functioning for all at the levels of the population and individual.

TABLE 5-4 IOM Core Competencies

Competency	Explanation
Provide patient-centered care	Identify, respect, and care about patient's differences, values, preferences, and expressed needs. Relieve pain and suffering, coordinate continuous care; listen to, clearly inform, communicate with, and educate patients. Share decision making and management. Continuously advocate disease prevention, wellness, and promotion of healthy lifestyles, including a focus on population health.
Work in interprofessional teams	Cooperate, collaborate, communicate, and integrate care in teams to ensure that care is continuous and reliable.
Employ evidenced-based practice	Integrate best research with clinical expertise and patient values for optimum care, and participate in learning and research activities to the extent feasible.
Apply quality improvement	Identify errors and hazards in care. Understand and implement basic safety and design principles, such as standardization and simplification. Continually understand and measure quality of care in terms of structure, process, and outcomes in relation to patient and community needs. Design and test interventions to change processes and systems of care, with the objective of improving quality.
Utilize informatics	Communicate, manage knowledge, mitigate error, and support decision making using information technology.

Adapted from Institutes of Medicine. (2003). Health professions' education: A bridge to quality. The quality chasm series. Washington, DC: The National Academies Press.

A multidisciplinary summit was convened across the accreditation, licensing, and credentialing organizations spanning the spectrum of all health professions. The **five core competencies** were developed using a rigorous approach (see Table 5-4) and spanned the practice realm and its workforce. It was evident these could not serve as an exhaustive list, particularly amid an industry where change was the only constant. It was expected that discipline-specific additions would be mandated as practice evolved. Further competencies might also be created to reflect the maturation of professionals through their career, from novice to advanced (IOM, 2003)

There was applause for the IOM vision by many across the health care continuum. However there was one major pitfall noted. The Core Competencies like the Six Aims that preceded them were recommendations only. As a result it was understood that they would yield limited influence on their own to effect the change required throughout the industry. To evoke the level of global system transformation deemed necessary by the IOM and other industry stakeholders, there would need to be involvement by other tiers of the professional institutional hierarchy.

ACCREDITATION AND COMPETENCY-BASED PROFESSIONAL MODELS IN EDUCATION

As the IOM considered how to evolve their competency-based vision toward the achievement of higher standards of care, the urgency to ground core competencies was being acknowledged by another sector of the professional spectrum. Efforts were underway to dramatically transform the focus of higher education.

To heed the IOM vision for care, students required a revised understanding of their professional practice paradigms. To render a patient-centered approach which reflected quality standards, students needed a more focused preparation. They required an enhanced understanding of their individual practice discipline that practice of their health care colleagues. The boundaries defined by each professional practice scope were valuable, but at times could silo the practitioner within his or her own realm. This action had potential to limit needed expertise by other team members. A new framing would promote increased communication, interaction, and collaboration.

TABLE 5-5 Accreditation Competencies

QSEN	CSWE	AACN Synergy
1. Quality improvement 2. Safety 3. Teamwork and collaboration 4. Patient-centered care 5. Evidenced-based practice 6. Informatics (QSEN, 2014)	1. Identify as a professional social worker and conduct oneself accordingly. 2. Apply critical thinking to inform and communicate professional judgments. 3. Advance human rights, and social and economic justice 4. Apply knowledge of human behavior and the social environment. 5. Engage in research-informed practice and practice-informed research. 6. Apply social work ethical principles. 7. Engage diversity and difference in practice. 8. Engage in policy practice to advance social and economic well-being. 9. Respond to contexts that shape practice. 10. Engage, assess, intervene, and evaluate with individuals, families, groups, organizations, and communities. (CSWE, 2014)	1. Clinical judgment 2. Advocacy and moral agency 3. Caring practices 4. Collaboration 5. Systems thinking 6. Response to diversity 7. Facilitation of learning 8. Clinical inquiry (innovator/ evaluator) (AACN, 2014a)

Accreditation

Higher education had long been viewed as the established gateway for budding professionals entering the workforce. As discussed in chapter 2, the accreditation entities have the rigorous job of developing professional standards to assure practice quality for specific disciplines. They play a valuable role in academia by ensuring the education provided by colleges and universities meets specific measures of quality (ACE, 2014).

With this strong emphasis placed on the quality of education and training, it stands to reason each accreditation entity could serve a valuable role in developing the needed professional competencies to leverage quality-driven care. Growing recognition had already emerged for the power of competency-based assessments and learning across health care (Baker, 2003). It was now time to connect the dots between the discipline-specific competencies and the practice behaviors expected of graduates once they entered the workplace.

Academic accreditation entities began to revise their approach to learning and how they framed professional practice within their unique disciplines. Leaders within nursing drew from the IOM framework of the five core competencies to craft prelicensure and graduate-level competency statements geared toward quality and safety outcomes, which became operationalized through the Quality and Safety Education for Nurses Institute (QSEN) (2014). Beginning in 2008, the American Association of Colleges of Nursing (AACN) developed behavioral expectations for bachelor's, master's, and doctoral education for advanced practice (IPEC, 2011). In the Synergy Model developed in this timeframe, AACN posed that the needs or characteristics of patients and families influence and drive the characteristics and competencies of nurses. This solidified the perspective that synergy results when the needs and characteristics of a patient, clinical unit, or system are matched with a nurse's competencies (AACN, 2014).

The Council on Social Work Education (CSWE) developed 10 core competencies which were common to all social work practice. The Educational Policy and Accreditation Standards (EPAS) released in 2008 outlined each of the competencies. EPAS is used to accredit baccalaureate- and master's-level social work programs plus support academic excellence by establishing thresholds for professional competence (CSWE, 2014). Advanced practice for social work incorporates the entire core competencies augmented by knowledge and practice behaviors specific to the practice concentration, such as clinical practice or that for social change. EPAS is amid a current revision scheduled for release in 2015. The EPAS competencies plus those for AACN and QSEN are shown in Table 5-5.

INTERPROFESSIONAL EDUCATION

Meanwhile, a parallel movement took root which recognized academia as that ideal entry portal for education of health care professionals. Since health professional schools bore the primary responsibility for developing core competencies, logic had it that a competency-based model implemented at this juncture could have the greatest potential to influence professional practice across the industry (IPEC, 2011).

Professional practice was already undergoing an evolution across practice settings. New roles emerged across the industry, with a vast change in the balance of power between patients and practitioners. The team-based approach to care begged for an interactive dialogue among members of the process. It was established that only when individual professions learned to appreciate their distinctive qualities, could they call upon each other intelligently and respond more fully to the needs of patients. A collaborative approach to educating students needed to mirror the new collaborative practice environment they would enter upon graduation (Barr, 1998).

The Canadian Interprofessional Health Collaborative

In 2007, a team of representatives from health organizations, health educators, researchers, professionals, and students from the health care sector was convened in Canada. The goal of this **Canadian Interprofessional Health Collaborative (CIHC)** was to identify and share best practices plus its extensive and growing knowledge in interprofessional education (IPE) and collaborative practice.

The CIHC knew exactly where to begin this journey. The members identified a gross lack of clarity surrounding the terms used to denote this continually advancing concept of team practice. Multidisciplinary, interdisciplinary, and team approaches were cited interchangeably. Communication among those involved on these teams occurred both within and/or across the involved disciplines (CIHC, 2007). There was little to any consistency in how these teams and their practices were framed particularly in the context of IPE.

The CIHC worked to compare and contrast the vast body of information that would ultimately serve as the foundational work for their seminal report, Interprofessional Education & Core Competencies: A Literature Review. Paramount to this study was the way in which CIHC specifically noted how the shared accountability to accomplish competency mastery belonged to all professional stakeholders: educators, learners, and practitioners. Verma's quote rang true: "Competencies in education create an environment that fosters empowerment, accountability, and performance evaluation which is consistent and equitable. The acquisition of competencies can be through talent, experience, or training" (Verma, Paterson, & Medves, 2006). They culled the research to compile an exhaustive listing of the benefits of IPE, which are noted in Box 5-1.

The report went on to identify core competencies implemented across several organizations globally. Among those included were:

- The Pew Health Professions Commission
- The American Council on Pharmaceutical Education
- The Accreditation Council for Graduate Medical Education
- The Interprofessional Education Consortium

An exciting array of tables was developed. One framed two prominent universities, University of Toronto and where core competencies were implemented. Another table compared and contrasted the unique competencies that had been developed across accrediting bodies. A final table listed the most commonly used or core competencies and viewed which manifested across the literature. This latter list included:

- Problem solving
- Decision making
- Respect
- Communication
- Shared knowledge and skills
- Patient-centered practice
- Collaborative work (or teamwork)

Although it was no doubt empowering to view these concepts aligned, looks were deceiving. An overriding concern emerged, in that there were far more differences than similarities among the competencies. This was identified to be due mainly to the unique perspectives of discipline-specific goals and variations in terminology (CIHC, 2007).

Barriers to appropriate IPE were identified, such as lack of uniformity with varying definitions of IPE around the world. There were an expanding number of definitions of IPE in the health care field, and although they all may describe similar goals, no common set of goals was present for all disciplines to adhere. The second challenge involved how the industry had differing interpretations of what IPE is. In order to develop effective education strategies, there must be agreed-upon goals that educators, learners, and professionals understand.

While the report acknowledged that clearly defined competencies existed across IPE and the involved professions, they were bound by disciplines, geography, and varying interpretations. The conclusion was clear: that it was best intent of those disciplines within the health care system to take the initiative in developing and implementing core competencies, yet the efforts fell short (CIHC, 2007). There were miles to go before any of IPE's vested stakeholders could sleep.

BOX 5-1 Benefits of Interprofessional Education

The benefits of interprofessional education are:

- Describe one's roles and responsibilities clearly to other professions.
- Recognize and observe the constraints of one's role, responsibilities, and competence, yet perceive needs in a wider framework.
- Recognize and respect the roles, responsibilities, and competence of other professions in relation to one's own.
- Work with other professions to effect change and resolve conflict in the provision of care and treatment.
- Work with others to assess, plan, provide, and review care for individual patients.
- Tolerate differences, misunderstandings, and shortcomings in other professions.
- Facilitate interprofessional case conferences, team meetings, etc.
- Enter into interdependent relations with other professions.

Canadian Interprofessional Health Collaborative, 2007

The Interprofessional Education Collaborative

The World Health Organization (2010) had identified the power of what was now being framed as IPE; when students from two or more professions learn about, from and with each other to enable effective collaboration and improve health outcomes. Leveraging this concept plus recognizing the IOM recommendations, a group of six distinct accreditation entities aligned. Each had already integrated competency-based models to guide their respective professional education and training programs:

- American Association of Colleges of Nursing
- American Association of Colleges of Osteopathic Medicine
- American Association of Colleges of Pharmacy
- American Dental Education Association
- Association of American Medical Colleges
- Association of Schools of Public Health

Each accrediting body was at a different phase of its own competency journey, though they shared a common vision. As a group they believe strongly in the value of an IPE approach toward creating a culture of outcome-based competency expectations for the industry. Ultimately they joined forces to form the **Interprofessional Education Collaborative (IPEC)**.

IPEC set the goal to prepare health professions students for deliberatively working together, with the common aim of building a safer and better patient-centered and a population-oriented U.S. health care system. This was an ambitious one considering the recent publication of CIHC and its concluding barriers to the concept. However, the CIHC report also set a strong precedent of commitment to the IPE cause and was fuel to IPEC's fire.

PROFESSIONAL AND INTERPROFESSIONAL COMPETENCIES

In 2011, IPEC published Core Competencies for Interprofessional Collaborative Practice: Report of an Expert Panel (IPEC, 2011). In moving forward, IPEC not only framed an innovative rationale for IPE but also went on to develop key definitions, including those to distinguish between professional and **interprofessional competencies**. These set the tone for the next phase of needed work and an innovative framing of IPE, presented in Table 5-6.

IPEC took a similar position to the IOM, in that the competency domains and specific core competencies should be general in nature and function as guidelines only. They believed this would promote a sense of needed industry cohesion among all involved disciplines. IPEC also believed this approach would equally allow for some flexibility with respect to interpretation of the competencies within each profession along with at the institutional level. Educators and organizational leaders would be able to access, share, and build on IPEC's overall guidelines in order to develop future programs of study for their requisite disciplines or institution. These programs would be aligned with more general interprofessional competency statements but contextualized to individual professional, clinical, or institutional circumstances (IPEC, 2011). Refer to these rationales, domains, and principles in Box 5-2.

The IPEC document not only leveraged the work of the IOM and academic accreditation entities, but also served to reinforce a powerful message. Health care quality was now viewed as a comprehensive and consolidated team effort. It was intended to be interprofessional and thus transdisciplinary in scope (IPEC, 2011). With integral role competencies positioned to ground accreditation and institutional and organizational approaches, it was expected that their popularity in defining and framing a profession's perspective would be equally valuable (Treiger & Fink-Samnick, 2013).

Interprofessional collaboration's long-term acceptance across the health care industry remains to be seen. Despite the initial excitement surrounding the concept, sustainability will ultimately be driven by how the industry and its unique stakeholders interpret and operationalize the term, interprofessional, as a construct.

How the next generation of discipline-specific competencies-based models will be aligned with the still present "siloed" approaches to care continues to be a point of concern. As industry leaders wrestle to manage the strong fiscal influences on their organizational bottom line, one overriding question for consideration remains: Will competition ultimately supersede quality-driven competency-based collaboration?

THE VALUE OF COMPETENCY-BASED EDUCATION

An equally compelling value of competency-based models speaks to their connection with experiential learning. The education process comes alive through this approach as budding professionals engage with their chosen career paths through an intricate weave of theory, knowledge, and practical application. Competency-based degree programs merge reality with practicality.

TABLE 5-6 Professional and Interprofessional Competency Definition Comparison

Professional Competencies	Interprofessional Competencies
Integrated enactment of knowledge, skills, and values/attitudes that define the domains of work of a particular health profession applied in specific care contexts.	Integrated enactment of knowledge, skills, and values/attitudes that define working together across the professions, with other health care workers, and with patients, along with families and communities, as appropriate to improve health outcomes in specific care context.

Adapted from Interprofessional Education Collaborative. (2011). Core competencies for interprofessional collaborative practice: Report of an expert panel. Washington, DC. Retrieved from http://www.aacn.nche.edu/news/articles/2011/ipec

BOX 5-2 IPEC Rationales, Domains, and Principles

Rationales	Domains	Principles
Create a coordinated effort across the health professions to embed essential content in all health professions education curricula. Guide professional and institutional curricular development of learning approaches and assessment strategies to achieve productive outcomes. Provide the foundation for a learning continuum in interprofessional competency development across the professions and the lifelong learning trajectory. Acknowledge that evaluation and research work will strengthen the scholarship in this area. Prompt dialogue to evaluate the "fit" between educationally identified core competencies for interprofessional collaborative practice and practice needs/demands. Find opportunities to integrate essential IPE content consistent with current accreditation expectations for each health professions education program. Offer information to accreditors of educational programs across the health professions that they can use to set common accreditation standards for IPE, and to know where to look in institutional settings for examples of implementation of those. Inform professional licensing and credentialing bodies in defining potential testing content for interprofessional collaborative practice.	Values/Ethics for interprofessional practice roles/responsibilities Interprofessional communication teams and teamwork	Patient/family-centered (hereafter termed "patient-centered") Community/population-oriented relationship focused Process-oriented Linked to learning activities, educational strategies, and behavioral assessments developmentally appropriate for the learner Able to be integrated across the learning continuum Sensitive to the systems context/applicable across practice settings Applicable across professions Stated in language common and meaningful across the professions Outcome drive

Adapted from Interprofessional Education Collaborative. (2011). Core competencies for interprofessional collaborative practice: Report of an expert panel. Washington, DC. Retrieved from http://www.aacn.nche.edu/news/articles/2011/ipec

These innovative degree programs have become an attractive option for the rising number of students who seek value plus immediately applicable and industry-relevant skills (Shapiro, 2014). Many schools also offer credit for past experience, which provides further incentive to students to apply since they can complete their degree faster as result.

Over the past several years a number of competency-based degree options have appeared at the University of Wisconsin, Western Governors University, and Excelsior College, to name a few locations (Waters, 2013). Although these programs have a prevailing number of strengths, there are concerns voiced by experts. One pivotal area for consideration is how the success of these programs will be measured. As one expert notes, "Great education isn't just about content. It challenges students to consider others' viewpoints, provides conflicting information, and forces students to reconcile, set priorities, and choose. In the best cases, it engenders a growth of intellect and curiosity that is not easily definable" (Shapiro, 2014).

Competency-based methodologies and models will continue to appear throughout higher education and the health care industry. It is expected they will evolve to meet the new programs and professions that are manifesting courtesy of health care reform, such as ACOs.

COMPETENCY-BASED EXIT EXAMINATIONS

A grand challenge exists at the exit door of the academic gateway: assessing the relevance of theoretical content taught to the job a graduate walks into. Potential employers echo this concern with one survey from Hart Research Associates providing compelling validation. Ninety-three percent of the employers surveyed identified that a candidate's ability to demonstrate the capacity to think critically, communicate clearly, and solve complex problems was far more important than what their undergraduate major may have been. Seventy-five percent indicated colleges should place increased emphasis on competencies that reflect critical thinking, complex problem solving, written and oral communications, and applied knowledge in real-world settings (Tempera, 2013).

As discussed previously, one challenge of competency-based degree programs involves the most accurate means to assure them. It presents there is a resolution to this dilemma. A series of new and innovative examinations claim to help new graduates, independent of major, demonstrate to potential employers that they have mastered the aforementioned coveted competencies. The primary goal of these examinations is to assess the outcome(s) of academia's competency-based approach.

The Council for Aid to Education

Driving the train for competency-based examinations for higher learning is the Council for Aid to Education (CAE). CAE is a national nonprofit established in 1952 to conduct policy research on and promote corporate support of education. Their primary focus is to help educational institutions measure and improve learning outcomes for their students (CAE, 2014a).

CAE has developed two examinations to test the critical thinking ability of graduates: the **College Work Readiness Assessment+** (CWRA+) and the **College Learning Assessment+** (CLA+). Experts profess both examinations support the value of competency-based learning as the new standard of academic practice (Tempera, 2013).

The CWRA+ is given to graduating high school seniors while the CLA+ to college students. Both examinations provide employers tangible means to demonstrate evidence of a candidate's work readiness skills. The foci identified for both examinations include

- critical thinking,
- problem solving,
- scientific and quantitative reasoning,
- writing, and
- the ability to critique and make arguments.

For the CLA+, digital badges are provided which note advanced mastery of skills. These are specifically designed to be loaded to professional networking sites as a way to note proficiency. The examination has been administered to over 700 institutions across the United States and internationally (CAE, 2014b).

This competency-based organizational culture change is in sync with the domains identified by IPEC, plus validates the important work which propelled this concept forward (Treiger and Fink-Samnick, 2014). Experts hope the examination scores serve as evidence to support expansion of this unique approach to validate competency exit examinations. However, given the slower pace at which higher education tends to function, it may be some time before there is full acceptance of this examination across the education arena.

SUMMARY

Competency-based approaches have matured through a series of developmental life stages. This chapter has provided a glimpse into their evolution, from the earliest definitions through professional, interprofessional, and workplace models and their implementation. A new generation of educational degree programs and exit examinations is poised to further propel competencies to another dimension of application; one to more purposefully link higher education with occupation. This latter element is especially crucial to workplace performance measurement, which will be discussed in section 3 of this book.

At this juncture it is fair to wonder exactly how competency-based approaches will be implemented to reflect industry best practice standards, particularly for case management. Some experts have suggested that established practice standards and codes of ethics serve as driving forces for best practice in case management (Henning & Cohen, 2008). These documents serve a persuasive role in framing certain aspects of industry best practice such as qualifications and ethical and legal parameters. However, in order for case management to attain its long-awaited position as a profession of and unto itself, another critical element is mandated—a defined paradigm of practice competencies specific to professional case management itself. Herein lies the opportunity for case management to define a unique competency-based approach of its own, which is the focus of section 2.

References

Alspach, J. G. (1992). Concern and confusion over competencies. *Critical Care Nurse*, *12*(4), 9–11.

American Association of Colleges of Nursing. (2014). *AACN synergy model of patient care*. Retrieved from http://www.aacn.org/wd/certifications/content/synmodel.pcms?menu=certification#Basic

American Council of Education. (2014). *Accreditation and standards page*. Retrieved from http://www.acenet.edu/advocacy-news/Pages/Accreditation-and-Standards.aspx

Association of Social Work Boards. (2013). *Exam content outline*. Retrieved, http://www.aswb.org/exam-candidates/about-the-exams/exam-content-outlines/

Barr, H. (1998). Competent to collaborate: Towards a competency-based model for interprofessional education. *Journal of Interprofessional Care* *12*(2), 181.

Buchanan, A. (2004). Mental capacity, legal competence and consent to treatment. *Journal of the Royal Society of Medicine*, *97*(9), 415–420. Retrieved from http://www.ncbi.nlm.nih.gov/pmc/articles/PMC1079581/

Canadian Interprofessional Health Collaborative. (2007). *A national interprofessional competency framework*. Retrieved from http://www. cihc.ca/resources/publications

Council for Aid to Education. (2014a). *Home page*. Retrieved from http://cae.org/about/category/home/

Council for Aid to Education. (2014b). *Collegiate learning assessment + overview*. Retrieved from http://cae.org/performance-assessment/category/cla-overview/

Council on Social Work Education. *Education policy and accreditation standards (EPAS) implementation*, Retrieved from http://www.cswe.org/Accreditation/EPASImplementation.aspx

Dreyfus, S., & Dreyfus, H. (1980). *A five-stage model of the mental activities involved in directed skill acquisition*. Washington, DC: Storming Media.

Fink-Samnick, E. (2008). Developing a resilience accountability continuum: Workplace resilience, part 2. *Professional Case Management*, *13*(6), 338–343.

Henning, S., & Cohen, E. (2008). The competency continuum: Expanding the case manager's skill set. *Professional Case Management*, *13*(3), 127–148.

Institute of Medicine. (1999). *To err is human: Building a safer healthcare system*. Washington, DC: National Academies Press.

Institute of Medicine. (2001). *Crossing the quality chasm: A new health system for the 21st century*. Washington, DC: National Academies Press.

Institute of Medicine. (2003). *Health professions' education: A bridge to quality. The quality chasm series*. Washington, DC: The National Academies Press.

Interprofessional Education Collaborative. (2011). *Core competencies for interprofessional collaborative practice: Report of an expert panel*. Washington, DC. Retrieved from http://www.aacn.nche.edu/news/articles/2011/ipec

The Joint Commission on Accreditation of Healthcare Organizations. (2000). *Hospital accreditation standards* (vols. 261–263, pp. 219–225, 319). Oakbrook Terrace, IL: Author.

Lundberg, C. C. (1972, Fall). Planning the executive development program. *California Management Review*, *15*(1), 10–15.

McClelland, D. (1973, January). Testing for competence rather than intelligence. *American Psychologist*, *28*(1), 1–14.

McGraw Hill Concise Dictionary of Modern Medicine. (2014). *Competence*. Retrieved from http://medical-dictionary.thefreedictionary.com/competence

Merriam-Webster Online. (2014a). *Competency*. Retrieved http://www.merriam-webster.com/dictionary/competent

Merriam-Webster Online. (2014b). Retrieved from http://www.merriam-webster.com/dictionary/autonomy

National Council of State Boards of Nursing. (2013). *Exam FAQs*. Retrieved from https://www.ncsbn.org/1201.htm

Parsons, E. C., & Capka, M. B. (1997). Building a successful risk-based. *Competency Assessment Model*, *66*(6), 1065–1068.

Prahalad, C. K., & Hamel, G. (1990). The core competence of corporation. *Harvard Business Review*, *68*(3), 79–91.

Quality and Safety Education for Nurses Institute (QSEN). (2014). *Quality and safety education for nurses competencies*. Retrieved from http://qsen.org/competencies/

Shapiro, J. (2014). *Competency-based degrees: Coming soon to a campus near you, the chronicle for higher education*. Retrieved http://m.chronicle.com/article/Competency-Based-Degrees-/144769/?cid=wb&utm_source=wb&utm_medium=en

Sultz, H. A., & Young, K. A. (1999). *Health care USA: Understanding its organization and delivery* (2nd ed.). Gaithersburg, MD: Aspen Press.

Summers, B. G., & Woods, W. S. (2008). *Competency-based assessment: A practical guide to the joint commission standards* (3rd ed., p. 4). Danvers, MA: HCPro, Inc.

Tempera, J. (2013). Post-College Exam seeks to determine employability. *USA Today*. Retrieved from http://www.usatoday.com/story/news/nation/2013/08/29/learning-assessment-plus-test-colleges-employers/2726031

Treiger, T. M., & Fink-Samnick, E. (2013). COLLABORATE©: A universal, competency-based paradigm for professional case management practice, part I. *Professional Case Management*, *18*(3), 122–135.

Treiger, T.M., & Fink-Samnick, E. (2014). COLLABORATE©: A universal, competency-based paradigm for professional case management practice, part III. *Professional Case Management*, *19*(1), 4–15.

Verma, S., Paterson, M., & Medves, J. (2006). Core competencies for health care professionals: What medicine, nursing, occupational therapy, and physiotherapy share. *Journal of Allied Health*, *35*(2), 109–116.

Waters, J. K. (2013). *Inside competency-based degrees, inside campus technology*. Retrieved, http://campustechnology.com/articles/2013/12/18/inside-competency-based-degrees.aspx

Welie, J. V., & Welie, S. (2001). Patient decision making competence: Outlines of a conceptual analysis. *Medicine, Health Care and Philosophy*, *4*(2), 127–138.

White, R. W (1959). Motivation reconsidered-the concept of competence. *Psychological Review*, *66*(5) 297–333.

Wilson, C. K., & O'Grady, T. P. (1999). *Leading the revolution in health care: Advancing systems, igniting performance* (2nd ed.). Grand Rapids, MI: Aspen Publishing.

SECTION 2

Clarifying the Paradigm

6 CREATING COMPETENCY EXCELLENCE

OBJECTIVES

After studying this chapter, you will be able to:

1. Identify five approaches to case management process.
2. Describe how CMSA Standards of case management practice align with Institute of Medicine Aims for health care.
3. Consider how patient centered care and engaged care are aligned and how they differ.
4. Consider how communication style impacts patient engagement.
5. Align the COLLABORATE competencies with the case management process.

The case manager collaborates with all members of the care team across all settings of the care continuum. Health care professionals working as case managers must learn flexibility and accommodation skills to address evolving client priorities quickly. However, the talent required to adapt-on-the-fly to the wide variety of circumstances in the day-to-day lives of clients also proves to be problematic in that it carries a risk of variation in practice approach based on each situation.

In order for case management (CM) practice to progress beyond its present-day status, it is imperative that thought leaders generate theoretical doctrine and practical solutions to address the challenges of health care delivery, including definition of best practice, terminology (e.g., common language), dedication of resources (e.g., dosage), expected outcomes (e.g., outcomes), and qualifications for practice (e.g., education, experience, credentials). Case managers must begin to speak the same language across ranks. COLLABORATE is positioned to be a part of the knowledge progression regarding what constitutes professional, high-quality CM practice.

This introduction to section 2 provides an overview of CM process, practice standards, and their relationship to the COLLABORATE practice paradigm.

CONSIDERATIONS ASSOCIATED WITH THE CM PROCESS

The process of CM practice provides a consistent approach to working with individuals. According to Powell and Tahan (2008), the components of the contemporary CM process, applicable in all settings of practice (Figure 6-1), are:

- Client identification and selection,
- Assessment and problem/opportunity identification,
- Development of the CM plan,
- Implementation and coordination of care activities,
- Evaluation of the CM plan and follow-up, and
- Termination of the CM Process.

It is necessary to recognize the relative importance and the level of effort spent on each phase of the process, and in how it varies according to one's practice setting. For example, in managed care the identification of individuals

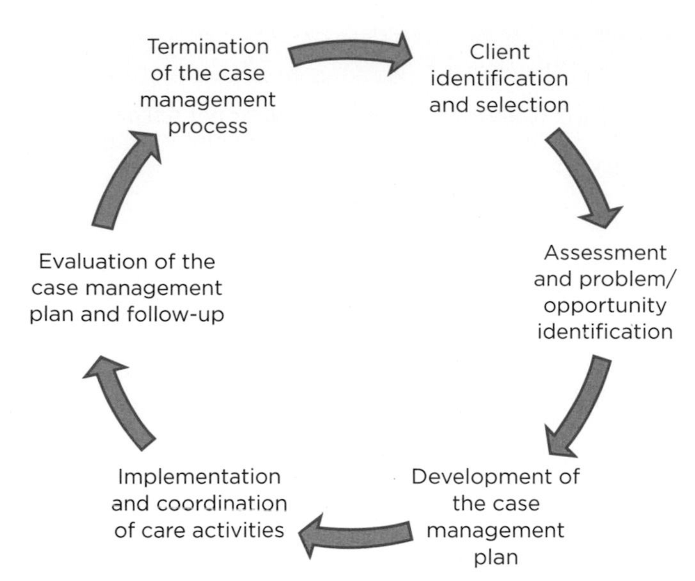

Figure 6-1. CM process. (Adapted from Case Management Society of America. (2010). *CMSA standards of practice for case management* (Rev.). Retrieved from http://www.cmsa.org/portals/0/pdf/memberonly/StandardsOfPractice.pdf)

appropriate for CM intervention often relies on automated screening mechanisms that mine claims history data (e.g., predictive algorithms, risk analysis). In worker's compensation, CM intervention is triggered by a work-related illness or injury, often coupled with the complexity and/or the projected length of the resulting lost work period. These examples highlight an identification process facilitated by a trigger event or analysis of utilization history rather than the manual effort of a case manager. However, subsequent to the identification of individuals who may benefit from CM intervention is the screening process, which involves the direct attention of a case manager. A consistent screening process narrows the eligibility pool to individuals falling within the scope of the CM program, highlights the potential impact that CM may have, and includes obtaining individual consent to participate in CM, especially in situations where program type, regulation, or law does not mandate participation.

THE CM PROCESS

CM process steps have been identified as part of various practice models. In 1985, Weil, Karls, and Associates, identified client identification and outreach, individual assessment and diagnosis, service planning and resource identification with client and members of the service network, linking client to needed services, service implementation and coordination, monitoring service delivery, advocacy for and with client in service network, and evaluation of service delivery and CM (may result in continued service with same or revised service plan, termination, or basic follow-up). Cesta and Tahan (2003) proposed assessment, diagnosis, planning, implementation, and evaluation. Powell and Tahan (2008) identified stages as case selection, assessment/problem identification, development and coordination of the case plan, implementation of the plan, evaluation and follow-up, continuous monitoring, reassessing, and reevaluating, and case closure and termination of CM services. The Case Management Society of America integrates a CM process in their Standards of Practice (2010) as client identification and selection, assessment and problem/opportunity identification, development of the CM plan, implementation and coordination of care activities, evaluation of the CM plan and follow-up, and termination of the CM process. The National Association of Social Workers (NASW) provides core functions of social work, which relate to process stages as engagement, assessment, planning, implementation/coordination, advocacy, reassessment/evaluation, and disengagement (2013). Table 6-1 displays the various process models. Although there are differences in the terminologies used across each of the noted models of CM process, it is important to note that the components follow similar cycles which include identification, investigation, planning, implementation, and appraisal activities.

OVERVIEW OF THE CM PROCESS PHASES

The process of CM recognizes functional phases or components. For the purpose of this text, the process as described in the CMSA Standards of Practice for Case Management (2010) demonstrates a consistent approach to which case managers should adhere, regardless of practice setting, population served, educational preparation, or certification status. For one to appreciate the process, it is essential to understand frequently used terminology such as:

- A role is a conceptual or abstract term referring to a set of behaviors associated with a position within a structure and identified with a title or job name (Tahan, Huber, & Downey, 2006). Examples of roles include care coordinator and case manager.
- A function is a derivation of a role, referring to groupings of activities specific to the role. These activities are interrelated and share common goal. Functions are the activities performed to accomplish tasks required for a particular outcome (Tahan, Huber, & Downey, 2006). An example of a function is care coordination, which is comprised (in part) of assessing, analyzing, and prioritizing.
- An activity, as distinguished from a function, is a discrete action, task, or behavior undertaken by an individual within a role in order to meet the desired goals of said role (Tahan, Huber, & Downey, 2006). An example of an activity is documenting a CM plan.

Another important context, which requires clarity, is the vision of CM process. CM is not a linear progression of activities, but rather it is iterative. What is the reason for this approach? Individuals enrolled in CM are inherently complex in terms of the fluid, multifactorial bio-psycho-social-spiritual challenges of their health status. As a result, a rigid and linear work process does not work. Clearly, there is a distinct starting point (e.g., identification) and it is reasonable

TABLE 6-1 CM Process Comparison

Weil and Karls (1985)	Cesta and Tahan (2003)	Powell and Tahan (2008)	Case Management Society of America (2010)	National Association of Social Workers (2013)
Client identification and outreach	Assessment	Case selection	Client identification and selection	Engagement
Individual assessment and diagnosis	Diagnosis	Assessment/problem identification	Assessment and problem/opportunity identification	Assessment
Service planning and resource identification with client and members of the service network	Planning	Development and coordination of the case plan	Development of the CM plan	Planning
Linking client to needed services	Implementation	Implementation of the plan	Implementation and coordination of care activities	Implementation/coordination
Service implementation and coordination	Evaluation	Evaluation and follow-up	Evaluation of the CM plan and follow-up	Advocacy
Monitoring service delivery		Continuous monitoring, reassessing, and reevaluating	Termination of the CM process	Reassessment/evaluation
Advocacy for and with client in service network		Case closure and termination of CM services		Disengagement
Evaluation of service delivery and CM				

to expect that one phase will routinely precede another (e.g., assessment before planning). It is recognized that the approach to CM is repetitive and cyclical in order to reach the desired outcome (Weil, Karls, & Associates, 1985; Powell & Tahan, 2000; Powell, 2000; Case Management Society of America, 2010; Kathol, Perez, & Cohen, 2010).

A demonstration of this iterative process is the manner in which a case manager continuously assesses a client's situation. A comprehensive assessment occurs at the beginning of the CM engagement in order to become acquainted with the individual, gain an understanding of barriers and needs, and prioritize needs to ensure the most urgent issues are addressed early in the CM plan. When a serious health event takes place subsequent to the initial assessment, the case manager reassesses the client to determine if the event had an impact on previously identified priorities and desired outcomes. When necessary, adjustments in the CM plan serve to mitigate new risks and may modify the desired goals to optimize achievement. This cycle runs continuously during the course of an engagement (Figure 6-2).

CONSIDERATIONS ASSOCIATED WITH CM PRACTICE STANDARDS

As discussed in section 1, the importance of CM practice standards cannot be overemphasized, especially in light of its practice being secondary to an individual's baseline educational preparation. In June 1998, the Institutes of Medicine (IOM) formed the Quality of Health Care in America Committee, charging it to develop a blueprint for improvement in the delivery of quality health care. To Err Is Human: Building a Safer Heath System (1999) set the stage for addressing the systemic quality shortcomings outlined in the subsequent report *Crossing the Quality Chasm: A New Health System for the 21st Century*, released in 2001. In light of these milestone reports, health care professionals need practice standards toward which to aim in order to deliver quality care, goods, and services.

When considering practice standards, it is important to identify with those that have the tenure to apply across practice settings and populations served. The Case Management Society of America's Standards of Practice for Case Management were first published in 1995 and subsequently updated in 2002 and 2010. The process followed for each update included using a cross continuum representation of individuals on a core task force, as well as having a reference group, industry experts from various accreditation and certification organizations, academic institutions, a wide variety of practice settings, and working case managers. The process also featured public comment periods.

The transparency with which the CMSA practice standards were developed ensures objectivity and as global a practice perspective as was possible. It is because of the thorough

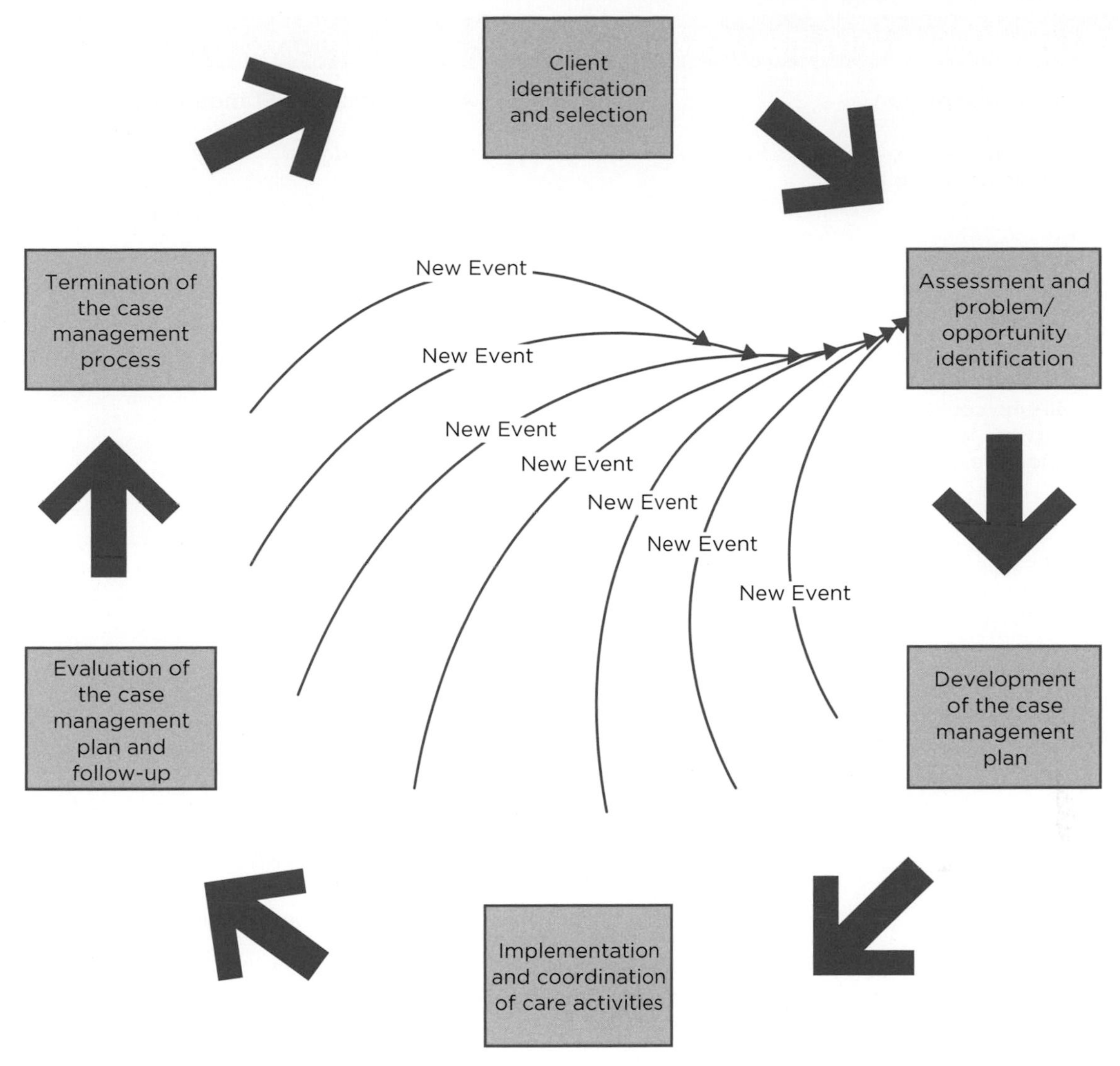

Figure 6-2. The iterative CM process.

effort and attention to detail given to these standards that they are so widely adopted across practice settings by both individual and institutional practitioners. Highly regarded, these standards are incorporated into accreditation and organization documentation across the continuum of care as voluntary guidance for the practice of high-quality CM.

The CMSA practice standards reflect a broad spectrum of practice. Although important to practitioners in specialty areas, subset or specialty standards may also serve as sources of confusion to the noncase manager. When introducing one's self as a case manager, the person to whom one is speaking is generally not asking about the nuances of practice setting or specialty. To those outside the CM industry, a case manager is a case manager and the demand is for high-quality care and excellent client service.

When one considers how each of the CMSA standards for professional CM practice aligns with the IOM's vision for health care, it is evident that both individually and collectively the Standards of Practice support activities and behaviors contributing to the achievement of the IOM's aims (Table 6-2). This is especially important to acknowledge because of the multidisciplinary nature of both health care and CM.

The CMSA case manager qualification standard points to an individual's practice act as a foundation with the overlay of CM standards. Practice within one's licensure is of tantamount importance. However, CM requires that individuals have the ability to conduct a comprehensive assessment, "Current, active, and unrestricted licensure or certification in a health or human services discipline that allows the professional to conduct an assessment independently as permitted within the scope of practice of the discipline" (CMSA, 2011). In the exceptional situation when an individual comes from a state that does not require licensure or certification, the standard contains additional qualifying language. There are other practice standards associated with care/CM in particular practice settings or populations that do not articulate levels of qualification. As a result, it is difficult for those outside of CM to discern the value proposition presented through the delivery of authentic CM provided by qualified practitioners versus performance of discreet tasks by lesser educated/

TABLE 6-2 CM Standards of Practice Aligned with IOM Aims

Aim	IOM Description	Aligned Practice Standards
Safe	Avoiding injuries to patients from the care that is intended to help them.	Client Assessment Problem/Opportunity Identification Monitoring Qualifications for Case Managers
Effective	Providing services based on scientific knowledge to all who could benefit and refraining from providing services to those not likely to benefit (avoiding underuse and overuse, respectively).	Client Assessment Problem/Opportunity Identification Planning Outcomes Termination of CM Services
		Legal Ethics Advocacy Resource Management and Stewardship Research and Research Utilization
Patient-centered	Providing care that is respectful of and responsive to individual patient preferences, needs, and values and ensuring that patient values guide all clinical decisions.	Client Assessment Problem/Opportunity Identification Planning Monitoring Facilitation, Coordination, and Collaboration Ethics Advocacy Cultural Competency
Timely	Reducing waits and sometimes harmful delays for both those who receive and those who give care.	Planning Monitoring Outcomes Facilitation, Coordination, and Collaboration Advocacy Resource Management and Stewardship

Aim	IOM Description	Aligned Practice Standards
Efficient	Avoiding waste, including waste of equipment, supplies, ideas, and energy.	Client Selection Process for CM Client Assessment Planning Outcomes Termination of CM Services Facilitation, Coordination, and Collaboration Advocacy Cultural Competency Resource Management and Stewardship
Equitable	Providing care that does not vary in quality because of personal characteristics such as gender, ethnicity, geographic location, and socioeconomic status.	Problem Opportunity Identification Planning Facilitation, Coordination, and Collaboration Ethics Advocacy Cultural Competency Resource Management and Stewardship

Adapted from Institutes of Medicine. (2001). Crossing the quality chasm: A new health system for the 21st century. Washington, DC: National Academies Press; Case Management Society of America. (2010). CMSA standards of practice for case management (Rev.). Retrieved from http://www.cmsa.org/portals/0/pdf/memberonly/StandardsOfPractice.pdf

trained individuals devoted to coordinating administrative aspects of care or applying predetermined criteria in an authorization process. Although there is a certain amount of administrative work associated with CM, it should not be the predominating aspect of the work.

The issues relating to the applicability of CM practice standards in a legal context need to be recognized. The first thing to acknowledge is that the CMSA practice standards are voluntary, which means there is no legal requirement to adopt or uphold them in practice. In a situation where a registered nurse case manager is involved in a civil action, the plaintiff attorney looks to the registered nurse practice act of the state in which the nurse is licensed and practicing. A knowledgeable attorney may also look to the American Nurses Association Standards of Practice for additional information. When one's practice is CM, it is essential that a registered nurse case manager involved in a lawsuit (or criminal prosecution) educates their attorney as to the existence and applicability of the CM standards of practice as well as how that standard applies more directly to the nurse-specific practice act. If the same case manager also happens to be certified, the additional code of conduct or practice standard should be brought forward for consideration.

DISTINGUISHING THE COLLABORATE PRACTICE PARADIGM

The COLLABORATE paradigm distinguishes itself through emphasis of its interrelationships, both within the work process and across the care team. Past and current models of practice were (and continue to be) critically important to the advancement of CM. However, if the CM process is to stay ahead of health care trends, it must continue to define itself with careful consideration paid to the essential aspects of practice, qualification requirements, and educational prerequisites. In other words, the stakeholders of CM must avoid the tail wagging the dog and remain relevant to the ideal health care approach—patient-centered and engaged care.

Patient-Centered Care

Patient-centered care was among the aims outlined by the IOM (2001) as a beacon toward which 21st century health care should strive. This concept, defined as "providing care that is respectful of and responsive to individual patient preferences, needs, and values and ensuring that patient values guide all clinical decisions." Although the term is bandied about, it is not so easy to nail down in terms of consistent practice because of the issues attached to health and health care. However, coalescing around a definition and articulating the concept are clearly a starting point.

Copious words have been written about patient-/client-centered care. Various practice standards include discussion regarding the role of the patient in the decision-making process in terms of self-determination. The philosophical underpinning of CM describes holistic and client-centered care that is an integral part of achieving the highest possible level of health and wellness (CMSA, 2010). Delivering this level of service requires guiding principles that include respect, collaboration, advocacy, shared decision making, cultural competence, evidence-based, knowledge, and safety (CMSA, 2010; NAPGCM, 2013).

The IOM's definition stands as a touchstone for those seeking to establish professional practice excellence. Consider the impact of these words and think about how authentic CM practice embodies patient-centered care. Leveraging a process originally presented by American Geriatrics Society Expert Panel on the Care of Older Adults with Multimorbidity (2012), initiating a more patient-centered approach to CM encounters becomes easier to understand (Figure 6-3).

Engaged Care

For health care professionals, patient engagement is the holy grail of health care. It is the key to patient adherence – a prerequisite to achieving better outcomes, fewer ER visits and hospitalizations and more satisfied patients. It is easy

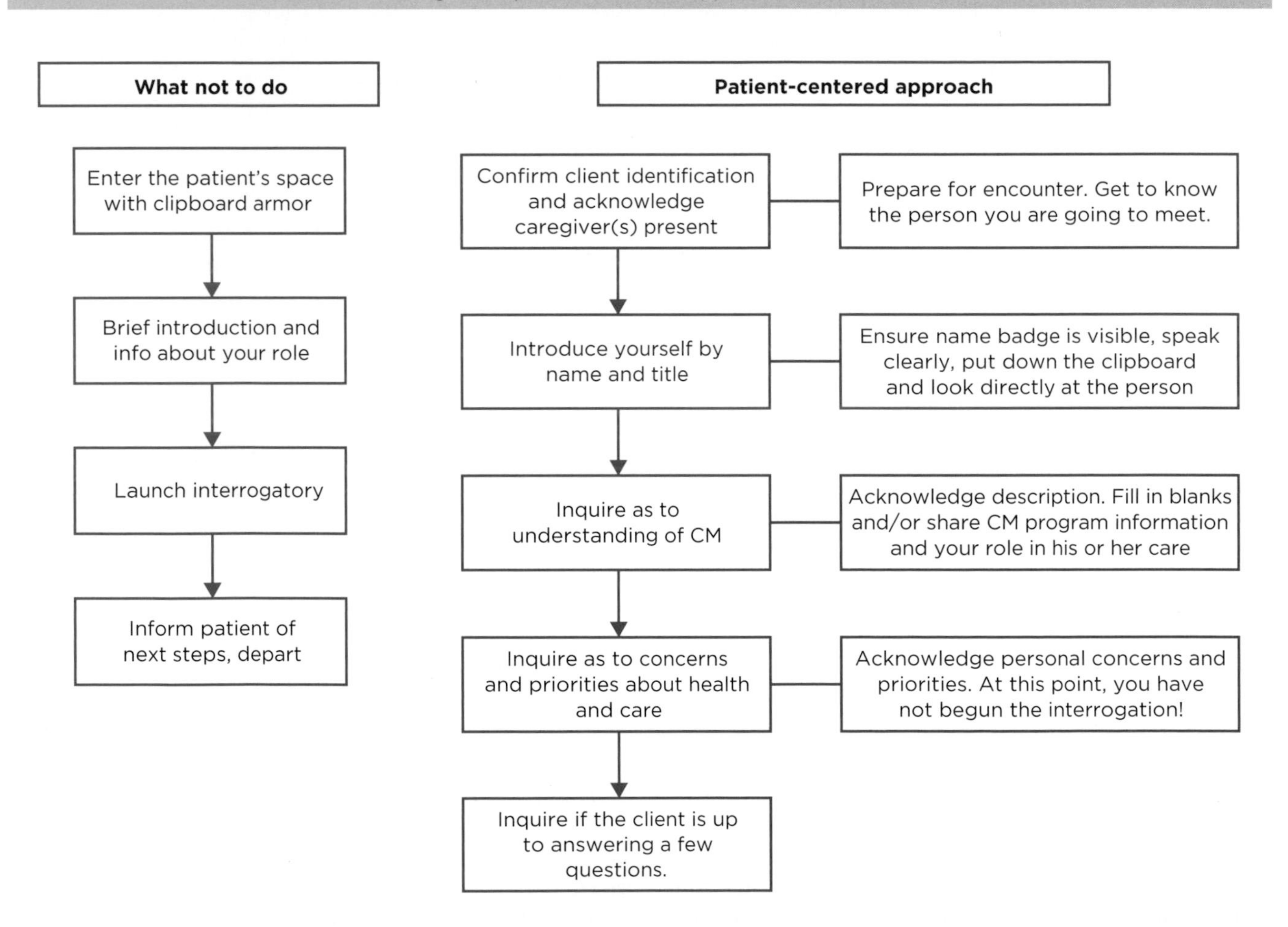

Figure 6-3. The patient-centered approach to the initial CM encounter.

> to recognize an engaged patient – they do what their health care providers recommends ... what their health care team knows what is right for them.
>
> *S. Wilkins, 2012*

Individuals engage in their health and care management to varying degrees; not all of these efforts are recognized as "patient engagement." Engagement has been the source of numerous articles and whole conferences have been devoted to the topic, yet it still seems subjective and arbitrary with regard to the overall health care system. Although system-wide engagement is too broad a topic to delve into here, engagement in the CM process is extremely relevant.

Consider Mary, a 45-year-old relatively healthy woman who eats a well-balanced diet and exercises regularly, sharing her meal choices and jogging distances with her social network. From time to time, Mary forgets to take a medication. Recently she put off undergoing a recommended procedure because of the financial burden of her plan's required coinsurance and co-payment. So what does Mary's primary care provider label her? At a recent appointment, her primary care provider documented that she was noncompliant to prescribed treatment. She was lectured for most of her 10-minute visit about what she had not done instead of acknowledging the fact that she had shed 20 pounds since her appointment last year and had made lasting changes in her diet and exercise. Put yourself in Mary's shoes for a moment. Would this appointment interaction result in you being more engaged?

Perhaps, it is time to consider that it may not be patients who need to engage in the health care system, but rather it is the system that needs to engage with the individual at a point at which they are most comfortable and productive. It is time to acknowledge that it takes two (or more) parties to make an engagement. Mary's commitment to herself carries the utmost impact. However, what she needs is someone else to invest in her efforts in order to be in an engagement in the health care system. In situations where a case manager is involved, this is where she or he demonstrates tremendous value in the equation of health.

Bodenheimer, Lorig, Holman, and Grumbach (2002) identified an important point, which remains relevant as a significant influencer of patient interactions today. People are socialized in a paternalistic medical model that fosters dependence on the health care professionals rather than creates a partnership model between the health care provider and the individual. There is little evidence to suggest that the health care industry (on the whole) has made significant progress beyond this approach; few recommendations are made as to transformation methodology. Although there are a number of tools to identify readiness to change (Miller & Rollnick, 1991; Prochaska, DiClemente, & Norcross, 1992), activation and confidence level (Hibbard, Stockard, Mahoney, & Tusler, 2004), readiness and motivation (Zimmerman, Olsen, & Bosworth, 2000), support system adequacy and ability (Broadhead, Gehlbach, de Gruy, & Kaplan, 1988; Coleman & Williams, 2007), and other variables which affect individual self-management, these remain actions which are done to, rather than with, the patient. Case managers have a tremendous potential to bridge the gap from the medical model paradigm, as discussed by Bodenheimer, to the engaged care model, as is at the foundation of the COLLABORATE model. Figure 6-4 provides a further look at Mary, who engages in taking care of her health, as well as two different approaches to working with Mary. In which of the scenarios presented is the case manager positively engaged with Mary?

BRIDGING CM PROCESS TO THE COLLABORATE PARADIGM

As the line goes, if it were that easy, everyone would be doing it! The competencies of professional CM practice may sound easy to find (or develop) in health care professionals, but they are not. The combination of knowledge, experience, skills, and behaviors are not present in nonclinical or undereducated administrative staff. This general knowledge gap across health care industry is cause for concern. There is a critical need to build a bridge of understanding for both business executives and clinical professionals since the passage of the Affordable Care Act. Care coordination efforts have flourished in association with numerous pilot and demonstration projects. Unfortunately, so have jobs with underpowered education, qualifications, and skill requirements. These so-called CM and care coordination positions are essential in order to bring projects to life, but in the end, less-than-anticipated outcomes reflect badly on the name of CM because that is the job title that has been most frequently used. However, the question that must be considered is, were these jobs truly authentic CM positions in the first place?

Enter the COLLABORATE model. The model serves to build and maintain competent professional practice through essential skills, behaviors, and characteristics. Because it is a characteristic-based model, the paradigm integrates into existing CM process and programs without major systems retooling. The keys to success are in hiring the appropriate candidates into authentic CM staff and managerial positions, providing an objective career progression process, creating measurable performance goals, and continuing to support professional growth through educational opportunities (e.g., professional conferences, certifications, advanced degrees).

The characteristics and performance indicators associated with CM processes are found in both qualitative and quantifiable expressions within the competencies. However, it is essential to state that unrealistic performance expectations should not anticipate finding salvation in a professional practice paradigm. In situations where management-determined production levels outpace the limits of human capacity, the system will ultimately experience staff resignation and overall failure. The momentary push of higher quantitative output succumbs to the need for quality in the form of well-reasoned decisions and appropriate application of evidence-based guidance.

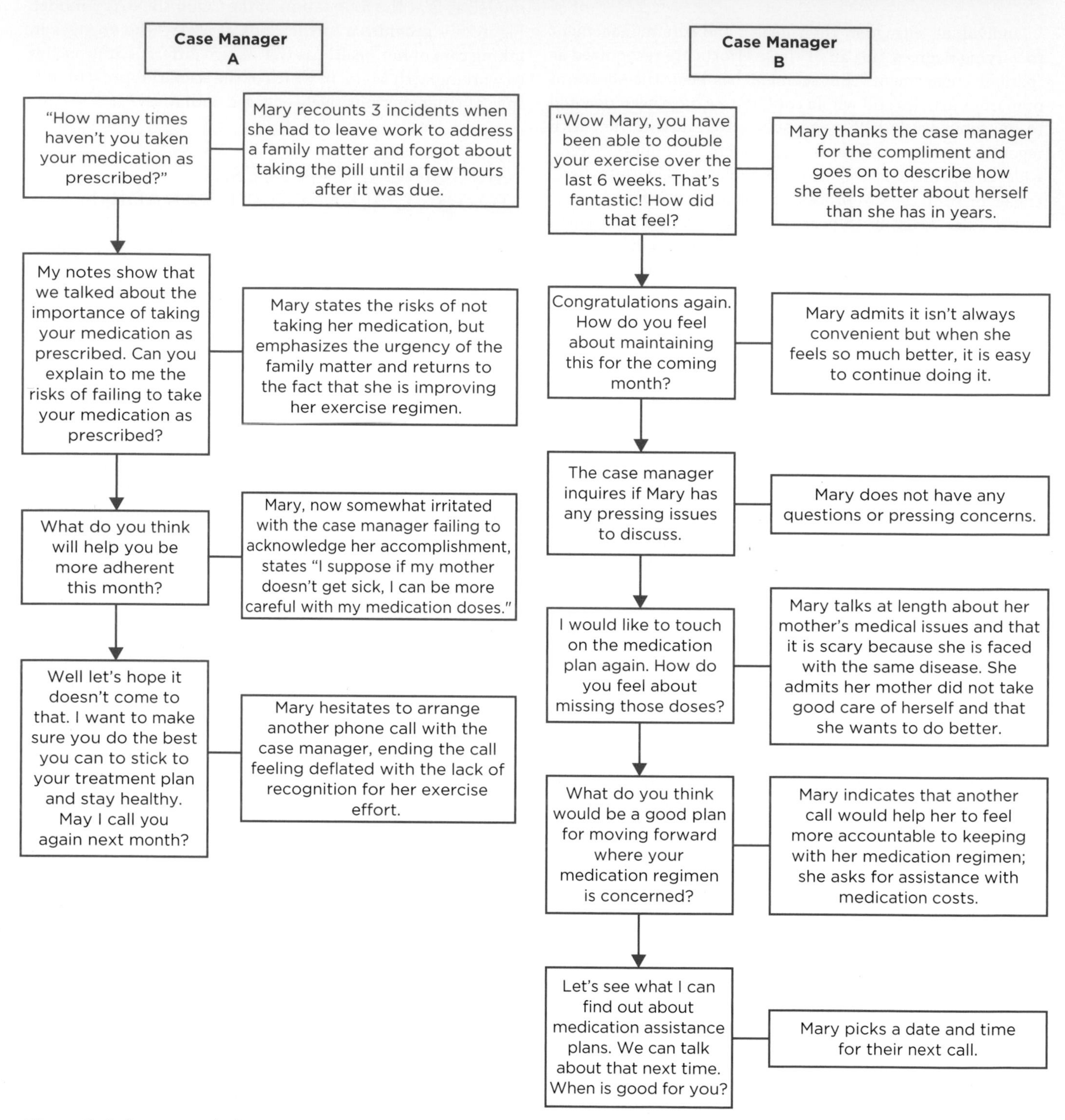

Figure 6-4. An engaged client in CM.

A basic failure in organizational CM programs is the lack of care taken in using the case manager title. Applying the job title to every position in the care coordination department is a mistake. The process and practice of CM requires adherence to professional practice standards, which serve the full spectrum of the health care continuum, not just a specific care setting or population subset. The industry must embrace standards of practice as an expectation for quality care, not out of convenience or simply because it is fashionable or politically correct to do so. The failure to select the appropriate positions for CM job classification sets the entire concept of professional CM practice on its edge. The critical distinguishers are, not every clinical position in a care coordination department performs authentic CM and simply performing some of the practice standards does not equate to one being a case manager. Hence, attempting to measure the processes of CM against a performance management description for a job that is not actually CM will result in dismal outcomes.

The essential ingredient of COLLABORATE is the action-oriented and engaged approach to all activities associated with the CM cycle. A professional case manager cannot be passive in any aspect of practice. CM adds value, not layers of complexity, to the health care team. In Treiger's words, "Case management is a bridge, not a crutch" (Miller, 2012).

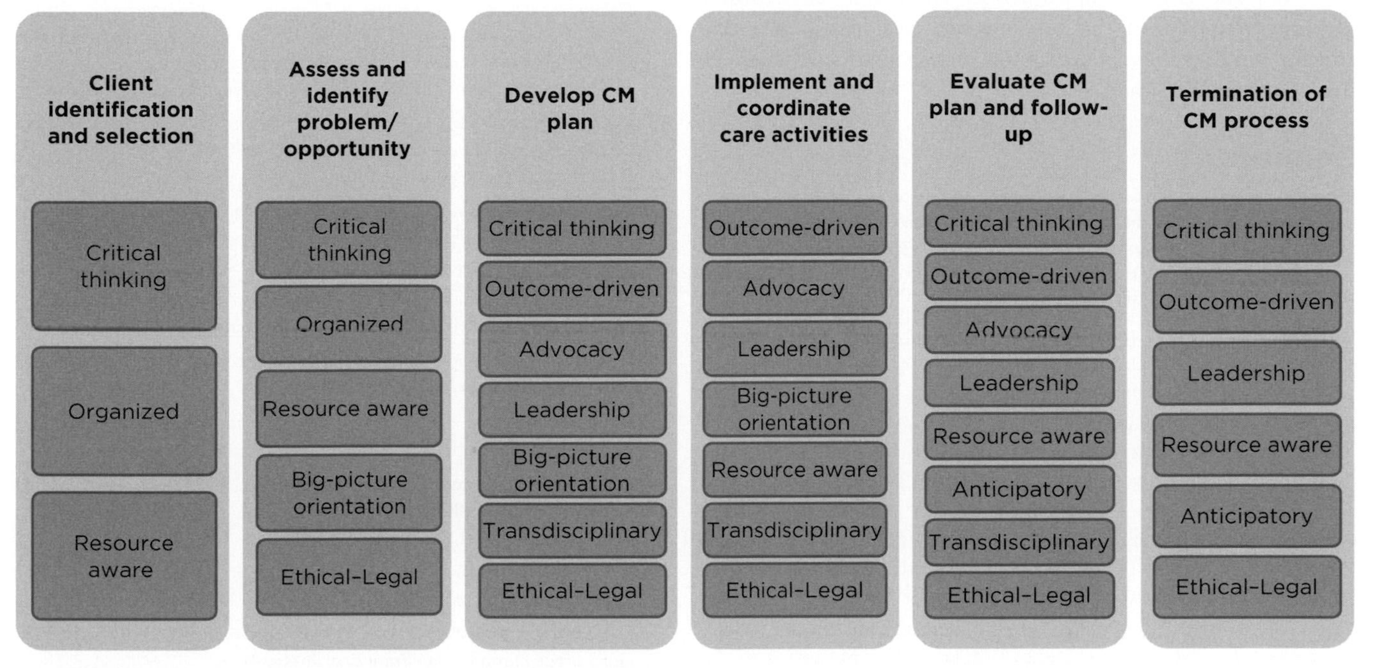

Figure 6-5. COLLABORATE competencies integration to CM process.

TABLE 6-3 An Activated and Engaged Take on CM Process

Client Identification and Selection	Assessment and Problem/ Opportunity Identification	Development of the CM Plan	Implementation and Coordination of Care Activities	Evaluation of the CM Plan and Follow-up	Termination of the CM Process
Identify, select, and engage	Assess, agree, and prioritize	Plan development and consensus-building	Activation of the collaborative CM plan	Evaluation and realignment of interventions	Disengagement from active CM
Taking an organized and methodical approach	Maintaining focus on big-picture implications	Creating achievable plan interventions and goals	Addressing barriers to goal achievement	Remaining aware of resource limitations	Preparing client for positive disengagement from active CM
Critically analyzing pros and cons of CM intervention prior to offering CM	Mindful consideration of ethical and legal ramifications	Leading efforts to secure necessary products and services	Building client satisfaction and enthusiasm through regular check-ins	Building anticipation toward client independence	Anticipating and addressing risks to backsliding after disengagement
Engaging individual in visualizing his or her contribution to CM efforts	Recognizing resource supply and demand	Calling for multidisciplinary care team meetings to discuss progress and barriers	Acknowledging all wins, big and small	Addressing ethical or legal situations directly to maintain knowledge of current situation and risks	
			Creative pursuit of needed resources leveraging client strengths		

SUMMARY

The COLLABORATE competencies, embedded throughout the CM process cycle, foster professional practice and set the tone for a patient's positive health care experience. Figure 6-5 provides a depiction of action-oriented, competence-based CM process. Table 6-3 provides basic expansions on common activated and engaged approaches. The intent of section 2 is to amplify each of the 11 competencies with descriptive content, evidence, and means to incorporate each element into professional practice.

References

American Geriatrics Society. (2012). American geriatrics society expert panel on the care of older adults with multimorbidity. *Journal of the American Geriatrics Society*. Retrieved from http://www.americangeriatrics.org/files/documents/MCC.principles.pdf. doi:10.1111/j.1532-5415.2012.04188.x

Bodenheimer, T., Lorig, K., Holman, H., & Grumbach, K. (2002). Patient self-management of chronic disease in primary care. *Journal of the American Medical Association*, *288*(19), 2469–2475.

Broadhead, W. E., Gehlbach, S. H., de Gruy, F. V., & Kaplan, B. H. (1988). The Duke-UNC functional social support questionnaire. Measurement of social support in family medicine patients. *Medical Care*, *26*(7):709–723.

Case Management Society of America. (2010). *CMSA standards of practice for case management* (Rev.). Retrieved from http://www.cmsa.org/portals/0/pdf/memberonly/StandardsOfPractice.pdf

Cesta, T. G., & Tahan, H. A. (2003). *The case manager's survival guide: Winning strategies for clinical practice* (2nd ed.). St. Louis, MO: Mosby.

Coleman E. A., & Williams, M. V. (2007). Executing high quality care transitions: A call to do it right. *Journal of Hospital Medicine*, *2*(5), 287–290.

Hibbard, J. H., Stockard, J., Mahoney, E. R., & Tusler, M. (2004). Development of the Patient Activation Measure (PAM): Conceptualizing and measuring activation in patients and consumers. *Health Services Research*, *39*(4, Pt. I), 1005–1026.

Institutes of Medicine. (2001). *Crossing the quality chasm: A new health system for the 21st century*. Washington, DC: National Academies Press.

Kathol, R. G., Perez, R., & Cohen, J. (2010). *The integrated case management manual: assisting complex patients regain physical and mental health*. New York, NY: Springer.

Miller, C. (2012). *Meet healthcare case management manager Teresa Treiger: Helping clients bridge gaps to self-advocacy, self-management*. [Interview]. Health Intelligence Network. Retrieved from http://hin.com/blog/2012/09/14/meet-healthcare-case-management-manager-teresa-treiger-helping-clients-bridge-gaps-to-self-advocacy-self-management

Miller, W. R., & Rollnick, S. (1991). *Motivational interviewing: preparing people to change addictive behavior*. New York: Guilford.

National Association of Professional Geriatric Care Managers. (2013). *NAPGCM standards of practice*. Retreived from http://www.caremanager.org/about/standards-of-practice

National Association of Social Workers. (2013). *NASW standards for social work case management*. Retrieved from http://www.socialworkers.org/practice/naswstandards/CaseManagementStandards2013.pdf

Powell, S. (2000). *Advanced case management: Outcomes and beyond*. Philadelphia, PA: Lippincott Williams & Wilkins.

Powell, S., & Tahan, H. (2008). *CMSA core curriculum for case management*. Philadelphia, PA: Lippincott Williams & Wilkins.

Prochaska, J. O., DiClemente, C. C., Norcross, J. C. (1992). In search of how people change. Applications to addictive behaviors. *The American Psychologist 47*, 1102–1104.

Tahan, H. A., Huber, D. L., & Downey, W. T. (2006). Case Managers' Roles and Functions. *Lippincott's Case Management*, *11*(1), 4–22.

Weil, M., Karls J. M., & Associates. (1985). *Case management in human service practice* (1st ed.). San Francisco: Jossey-Bass.

Zimmerman, G. L., Olsen, C. G., & Bosworth, M. F. (2000). A stages of change approach to helping patients change behavior. *American Family Physician*, *61*(5), 1409–1416. Retrieved from http://www.aafp.org/afp/2000/0301/p1409.html

7 COLLABORATE MODEL OVERVIEW

OBJECTIVES

After studying this chapter, you will be able to:

1. Identify each model competency and respective key elements.
2. Prepare for study of subsequent chapter content.
3. Describe the significance of the Venn diagram in the context of the COLLABORATE practice model.

KEY TERMS

Advocacy
Anticipatory
Big-picture orientation
Critical thinking
Ethical–Legal
Leadership
Lifelong learning
Organized
Outcome-driven
Resource awareness
Transdisciplinary
Venn diagram

Independent of health care's ongoing challenges, case managers must be sufficiently agile to frame (and reframe) professional practice in order to facilitate the client's best outcomes. This is why defining a competency-based case management model, which is sufficiently fluid to fit into any setting of care and apply to all populations, is essential (Treiger & Fink-Samnick, 2013). Ultimately, a competency-based model elevates the quality of practice and contributes to optimal case management and health care outcomes. The purpose of section 2 is to define and explore each competency (see Table 7-1) associated with the COLLABORATE model.

FRAMING THE PARADIGM

While seeking balance and consistency between work process and scope of responsibility, the case manager must embrace flexibility and practice with professionalism in the face of competing priorities. To accomplish this, the case manager must methodically assess, plan, facilitate, coordinate, evaluate, and advocate for the client whose needs are best addressed comprehensively through clear communication and by utilizing available resources in the promotion of quality cost-effective outcomes (CMSA, 2010).

TABLE 7-1 COLLABORATE Competencies

Acronym	Competency	Key Elements
C	Critical thinking	Out-of-the-box creativity Analytical Methodical approach
O	Outcome-driven	Patient outcomes Strategic goal setting Evidence-based practice
L	Lifelong learning	Valuing: • Academia & advanced degrees • Professional development • Evolution of knowledge requirements for new & emerging trends (e.g., technology, innovation, reimbursement) • Practicing at top of licensure and/or certificationAcknowledging that no one case manager can and does know all
L	Leadership	Professional identity Self-awareness Professional communication: verbal/nonverbal Team coordinator: a unifier rather than a divider
A	Advocacy	Patient Family Professional
B	Big-picture orientation	Bio-psycho-social-spiritual assessment Macro (policy) impact on micro (individual) intervention
O	Organized	Efficient Effective
R	Resource awareness	Utilization management Condition/Population-specific Management of expectations per setting
A	Anticipatory	Forward thinking Proactive vs. reactive practice Self-directed
T	Transdisciplinary	Transcending • Professional disciplines • Across teams • Across the continuum
E	Ethical-Legal	Licensure Certification Administrative standards Organizational policies and procedures Ethical codes of conduct

©Treiger, T. M., & Fink-Samnick, E. (2013). COLLABORATE©: A universal, competency-based paradigm for professional case management practice, part I. Professional Case Management, 18(3), 122–135..

How does one illustrate this construct visually? The development of a graphical depiction of the COLLABORATE model proved challenging. It was essential for the paradigm to align the tenets defined by various standards of professional practice with those of case management. The dynamic influences of industry, organization, and institution trends add layers of additional considerations, which are essential to consider when implementing a foundational change. Add to this the importance of best practice at a specific point in time; the resulting image was rather chaotic.

Stepping back to examine the big picture (which most case managers do quite well) enabled deconstruction of the complex to an elegantly simple concept captured by a **Venn diagram** (Figure 7-1). Through its overlapping circles the

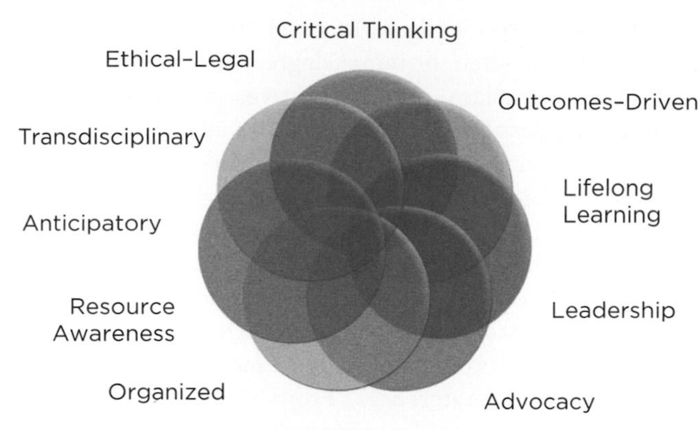

Figure 7-1. The COLLABORATE paradigm. (© Treiger, T. M., & Fink-Samnick, E. (2013). COLLABORATE©: A universal, competency-based paradigm for professional case management practice, part I. *Professional Case Management, 18*(3), 122–135.)

classic Venn diagram reveals logical relationships that exist across a multitude of considerations. This symbol highlights the interrelatedness of the professional competencies associated with case management's roles and responsibilities. It is this depiction which provides for the flexibility of one's individual circumstance (e.g., licensure, practice setting) as well as promotes professional case management practice.

THE COLLABORATE MODEL COMPETENCIES

Although discussed comprehensively in subsequent chapters, the following briefly introduces each competency.

Critical Thinking

The key elements of the **Critical Thinking** (CT) competency include:

- Out-of-the-box creativity;
- Analytical; and
- Methodical approach.

Out-of-the-Box Creativity

Simpson and Courtney (2002) explore the fundamental grounding of the dimensions of CT and distinctions as opposed to more traditional problem solving, clinical decision making. They set the foundation for CT as a process, which fuels a more ingenious effort, a blending of knowledge and creativity. "Creative thinkers employ an attitude of interest in everything, continuously exploring for new ideas, options, alternatives and approaches" (Simpson and Courtney, 2002).

Herein lies the alignment with professional case management practice: "In order to step outside the everyday reasoning and approaches to problem solving, a person needs to develop an imagination of the possibilities and potentials inherent in a particular circumstance. This often demands a creative leap of faith and a willingness to be 'playful' with future possibilities" (Simpson & Courtney, 2002).

Analytical

While CT is integral to evidence-based practice (EBP), it allows one to accurately describe the extent to which the related underlying research can rigorously test established practice (Gambrill, 2012). One might emphasize that CT strives to go beyond the black and white of prevailing research, to address that which is gray. Many interpretations of how professional case managers work within the gray are manifested across practice settings, diverse job roles, and associated functions.

Methodical Approach

The goal of CT by its very premise is to approach decision making from a strategic perspective toward the purpose of well-reasoned decisions (Gambrill, 2012). Although there is great variation and perspective in the implementation of this approach, there is consensus on both the merits of templates to this end across health care professional disciplines and of CT's vital role for the industry. Whichever model a case manager utilizes, utilization of a formal framework is vital to assure a proactive, logical, and purposeful action.

Chapter 8 expands on the significance of CT to the model. Included are relevant frameworks as emotional intelligence, new modes of engaging CT plus expansion of Gambrill's list to depict the balance involved in the case managers' CT Gray Zone.

Outcome-Driven

The key elements of the **Outcome-Driven** competency include:

- Client;
- Strategic goal setting; and
- Evidence-based practice.

Client

The COLLABORATE perspective focuses on client outcomes and the case manager's strength in identifying client needs and strengths associated with producing positive outcomes. The case manager focuses on maximizing his or her client's health, wellness, as well as other considerations involving caregivers, providers, and payers. This approach is at the heart of the case management philosophy. The underlying premise is that when an individual reaches an optimum level of wellness and functional capability, everyone benefits (CMSA, 2010). Outcomes is a practice standard demonstrating the value of case management intervention in terms of plan of care goal attainment, use of evidence-based criteria and guidelines, and measures of client satisfaction (CMSA, 2010). To the case manager, it is not only about what barriers and needs a client faces, but also incorporates the client's strengths and abilities in planning and executing the agreed-upon management plan.

Strategic Goal Setting

Goals, which are unattainable, are frustrating. Regardless of whether the goals are set for a client (as part of a case management plan), for a case manager (as part of performance management), or for a case management department, goals must be well considered and reasonably attainable.

Poorly designed case management plan goals are the cause of many intervention failures. Therefore, goal setting must be strategic in terms of taking into account client variables (e.g., readiness, willingness to participate), achievability of the desired outcome, and the anticipated length of the case management engagement. The utilization of short, intermediate, and long-term goals provides a platform for ongoing client engagement in the case management plan. This approach also alleviates possible discouragement when a client feels as though he or she is not making progress.

Where management or participation in a team setting applies, the case manager must take the same well-considered approach to goal setting and achievement. In addition, supervisory staff must incorporate appropriate goal-setting strategies into performance management programs so that case management staff goals align with team, department, and organizational targets.

Evidence-Based Practice

COLLABORATE takes the perspective that the outcomes-driven case manager should understand the essentials of EBP. The case manager utilizes evidence-based findings as rationale for his or her activities such as care planning, authorization requests, and health education efforts. EBP contributes toward overall effectiveness and efficiency of the case management intervention.

Chapter 9 discusses the importance of outcomes at various levels of case management (e.g., process, practice) as well as outcomes of research and impact on current practice.

Lifelong Learning

The key elements of the **Lifelong Learning** competency value:

- Academia and advanced degrees;
- Professional development;
- Evolution of knowledge requirements for new and emerging trends (e.g., technology, innovation, reimbursement);
- Practicing at the top of licensure and/or certification; and
- Acknowledging that no one case manager can and does know all.

Education and learning are cardinal values instilled during the formative years of many. These experiences, plus how each individual reflects on them, shape how professional case managers engage in their continued educational endeavors. Few would argue the vast amount there is to constantly learn in the health care industry. An abundance of evolving societal trends mandates that professional case managers commit to traveling the highway of lifelong learning.

Academia and Advanced Degrees

Knowledge is power, especially for today's case manager. It is not surprising how many professionals pride themselves on being avid learners. There is increased motivation and incentive for case managers to excel through formal education and seek their terminal degree. In the competitive health care workplace, grand incentives motivate many to attain the highest level of education possible, including promotional and/or expanded job opportunities

Professional Development

Expanding numbers of credentialed case managers, as discussed in chapter 4, equals increased demand for innovative and empowering continuing education. The options are massive and present through a variety of modes, based on each person's learning preferences. From traditional in-person conferences, to distance learning webinars, the professional development realm is the case manager's oyster.

Evolution of Knowledge Requirements for New and Emerging Trends

Addressing new trends comes with a professional case manager's territory. Many have embraced technology proficiency, though far from all.. Most case managers use some element of technology daily. The workday can involve entering or reviewing documentation in an electronic health record, or contacting a colleague via a mobile device.

Case managers continue to grasp the full scope of the Health Insurance Portability and Accountability-Health Information Technology for Economic and Clinical Health Act (HIPAA HITECH) 1, 2, and 3. Recent studies validate that innovation is here to stay, and will continue to dominate the energies, if not budgets, of most health care organizations. The global telemedicine market went is expected to hit $27.3 billion by 2016. About 2.8 million patients are being remotely monitored (Lewis, 2012), with this number expected to climb. Sixty percent of the 8,745 persons surveyed move between anywhere from one to three mobile devices each day to access health information (Manhattan Research, 2012). It is not uncommon for case managers to discuss the technology evolution as a precipitator for early retirement.

Practicing at the Top of Licensure and/or Certification

Professional case managers are motivated to practice at the pinnacle of their expertise and education. However, more urgently, achieving the highest level of licensure and certification is becoming an industry expectation. New job opportunities and competition for those roles, are prompting an increased demand for case managers already holding certification, which was touched on in chapter 4.

There is a renewed focus on case manager's adherence to the established professional standards and codes of conduct, which guide practice. CMSA Standards of Research and Research Utilization present the responsibility of each case manager to maintain familiarity with current research findings and the ability to apply research to practice, as appropriate (CMSA, 2010). This also relates to CCMC's Code of Professional Conduct, which speaks to certificants maintaining their competency at a level to ensure each client receives the benefit of services appropriate and consistent for their conditions and circumstances (CCMC, 2009). Both NASW's Code of Ethics and the administrative regulations that underlie social work clinical licensure mandate one advance their knowledge base, develop and enhance professional expertise, and continually strive to increase professional knowledge and skills to apply them in practice (NASW, 2008).

Acknowledging That No One Case Manager Can and Does Know All

Whatever the source of knowledge, the goal should be to learn daily from each interaction and experience, whether that experience is with a client or another professional. With professional case managers at the core of care coordination, experiences and interactions across industry stakeholders abound. Each one of these experiences provides additional data for that lessons-learned file each individual should possess.

Chapter 10 expands on the emphasis of lifelong learning for professional case managers. Particular focus is on the practical implications of continued education as a means to demonstrate competence to industry stakeholders and assure professional sustainability.

Leadership

The key elements of the **Leadership** competency include:

- Professional identity;
- Self-awareness;
- Professional communication (verbal/nonverbal); and
- Team coordinator (a unifier rather than a divider).

Professional Identity

COLLABORATE fixes a spotlight on the professional case manager who leverages the tools and resources at their disposal to provide thoughtful case management interventions that add value, rather than layers, to the delivery of health care services (Treiger, 2008). The professional case manager applies knowledge and experience in the form of clinical judgment, ensuring optimal, cost-effective quality care and leads by facilitating the care delivery process.

It is by weaving professional identity through every COLLABORATE competency and key element that we create a fabric of sufficient strength to bind seemingly disparate (and occasionally competing) agendas into a cohesive synergy.

Self-Awareness

Self-awareness is the ability to engage in reflective awareness and is associated with executive processes essential to self-regulation. The self-aware individual is controlled and intentional in his or her actions (Hull, 2007). In the context of case management, the individual is mindful that every interaction leaves a lasting impression both of him or her and of what case management is (or is not). It is essential to understand that how one conducts him or herself as important as the result.

Leadership is also inclusive of the self-regulation concept. By definition, self-regulation means that society confers a group with the mandate to police itself. Because case management requires specialized knowledge to effectively practice, it follows that case managers are in the best position to accomplish this oversight responsibility. However, accountability accompanies this privilege. Case management, as an overarching whole, must assume responsibility to continuously monitor practice patterns, acknowledge and learn from deviations from standard practice, and continuously seek information to build and advance our collective competence.

Professional Communication

A leader respects cross-continuum care team partners by working toward a goal, using mindful and evocative communication techniques. This approach is a hallmark of the case management philosophy. The case manager leader considers the tone, appearance, and impact of verbal, nonverbal, and written communication and uses a clear and concise approach in the course of conducting business.

Team Coordinator

A case manager does not make assumptions about which solution may work best, but instead seeks to gain consensus across the care team. As a high-functioning team member, the case manager strives to work effectively with other team members. As a coordinator of care, the case manager facilitates the completion of tasks, consistently encouraging other care team members, especially the client/caregiver to take action rather than personally performing every intervention.

Chapter 11 provides discussion of various ways in which formal and informal leadership impact care coordination.

Advocacy

The key elements of the **Advocacy** competency pertain to:

- Patient and family/support system and
- Professional (individual and the profession).

Patient and Family/Support System

A majority of case managers have an easier time advocating for their patients and families than they do for themselves. It is an occupational hazard for health and human service professionals to prioritize the needs of others in lieu of their own (Fink-Samnick, 2007).

Most professional case managers know how to advocate for those whom they intervene on behalf of and aspire to do so. However, a lengthy list of impeding priorities affects the ability to fulfill this goal. Amid time management demands and responsibilities of various tasks, the extra time and energy needed to advocate for others evade us. One may contend that a case manager's adherence to advocacy as a competency enhanced through a commitment to achieve balance between occupational stressors and life challenges while fostering professional values and career sustainability (Fink-Samnick, 2009).

Professional

This element cuts to the core of a case manager's professional identity. It involves how to put that professional foot forward, occurring at levels to address the needs of the client as well as the case management profession itself.

The Individual

This competency pertains to a case manager's awareness of how to present with a professional presence and involves implementation of solid and eloquent communication, whether written, verbal, or even nonverbal messaging. This extends to those skills and strategies used to effectively manage and lead a **transdisciplinary** team. Case managers are team leaders and expected to facilitate the care coordination process. This involves the skillful art of negotiation to obtain authorization for extended days, treatments, or other identified resources for clients. How a case manager connotes unique expertise is critical to the success of his or her individual professional effort.

The Profession

Case managers advocate for the profession in a variety of ways. Examples include engagement in a professional association, working on a public policy committee, supporting title protection activity, and facilitating interstate license portability.

Through the lens of COLLABORATE the case manager believes strongly in the value of case management, addresses devaluation of practice with colleagues, and utilizes best practice information to demonstrate to his or her employing organization in order to raise awareness and improve working conditions. Chapter 12 explores various aspects of advocacy that are necessary for effective practice as well as discusses the danger of advocacy becoming inappropriately demanding or negatively controlling over a care team activity or client desire and self-determination.

Big-Picture Orientation

The key elements of the **Big-Picture Orientation** competency include:

- Bio-psycho-social-spiritual assessment and
- Macro interventions on micro practice.

Bio-Psycho-Social-Spiritual Assessment

Case managers possess expanded power by assessing clients through the largest lens possible. Generations of social work professionals have had their practice grounded by learning how to assess the human behavior of clients through a bio-psycho-social-spiritual framing. Viewed collectively, the distinct realms of the biophysical, psychological, sociological, and spiritual dimensions provide a fundamental template to assure a thorough and comprehensive evaluation of vital patient clinical pathophysiology and psychopathology. Ashford and Lecroy (2013) state, "Practitioners must be clear about how they will systematically assess, measure, or describe the characteristics of their clients and their various life troubles in the changing social and physical contexts."

Macro Impact on Micro Interventions

Macro impact signifies those larger scale policy implications, also known as the *view from 30,000 feet*. This pertains to all aspects of a case manager's role and associated functions, from quality of and access to appropriate patient care, to assessing and intervening with patients across state lines, to lack of ability to obtain authorization for behavioral health care despite the presence of a benefit for it. It behooves each case manager to maintain awareness of policy initiatives which impact their practice and potentially their patient population.

In this COLLABORATE, the case manager engages in several efforts across personal and professional realms to assure their awareness to and education about the current regulations which impact their licensure and their case management certification.

Organized

The key elements of the **Organized** competency include:

- Efficiency and
- Effectiveness

Efficiency

An organized case manager balances practice standards, regulatory changes, legal mandates, and organization-specific administrative constructs in order to provide services in a manner where effort expended results in optimal outcomes without unnecessary waste (e.g., expense, resource, time).

COLLABORATE focuses on the development of meaningful case management metrics that contribute toward efficient achievement of performance and strategic goals. How meaningful metrics are incorporated into a wide variety of documentation (e.g., job description, performance management program, department goals) impacts the realization of real efficiency.

Effectiveness

An effective case manager leverages evidence to improve the effectiveness of interventions and tools. For instance, an effective case manager is knowledgeable of best practices and utilizes interventions that demonstrate positive results. Effectiveness also points to the habit of knowledge sharing in order to improve consistency across the case management department and ultimately deepen program impact. COLLABORATE encourages use of evidence-based guidelines to develop measurable and meaningful case management interventions and improve consistency of team-wide service delivery and outcomes (e.g., adherence rate, biometric measures, utilization).

Chapter 14 delves into various models of efficiency as well as using process improvement to gain efficiency and best practice research and outcomes, which may be applicable across settings of case management practice.

Resource Awareness

The key elements of the **Resource Awareness** competency include:

- Utilization management;
- Condition/population-specific; and
- Management of expectations per setting.

Utilization Management

The term utilization management seems to have gotten itself a black eye as a result of indiscriminate application of rules designed to restrict access to service or dollars spent. Recognizing that all resources are eventually finite, the resource-aware case manager considers multiple aspects of a situation and various options for utilization of available resources by consulting with the patient–client and relevant care team members and by understanding the benefits and risks associated with each option as a part of proposing case management plan interventions. Mindfulness of available resources and advocating for their appropriate use focus on what is best to address the needs of each client.

Using the COLLABORATE approach, the case manager proposes a phased approach for the transition plan, beginning with an admission to a skilled nursing facility. The proposal includes milestone goals that trigger level of care reevaluation and possible transfer to an acute rehabilitation facility.

Condition/Population Specificity

The resource-aware case manager maintains current knowledge of health conditions, insurance coverage, community resources, and care criteria sets in order to prepare realistic and responsible case management plan to meet each client's individual needs.

Management of Expectations

The resource-aware case manager understands that setting and managing client expectations from the point of initial contact facilitates subsequent interactions and contributes to building a trust-based relationship. Failing to manage expectations risks a suboptimal outcome, including, but not limited to, low client satisfaction and care delays.

COLLABORATE encourages the case manager to work with the client and caregiver to clearly communicate the facts and likely process steps. The case manager takes a thoughtful approach to explaining issues (e.g., insurance coverage, level of care determinations). Chapter 15 explores aspects of utilization management in the context of finite benefits and strategies for managing client and family expectations.

Anticipatory

The key elements of the **Anticipatory** competency include:

- Forward thinking;
- Proactive vs. reactive practice; and
- Self-directed.

To anticipate means that one takes measures to prevent, mitigate, or otherwise nullify the possible harms of a predictable outcome in order to realize a more positive result. This does not mean to imply that one jumps into the middle of a situation and takes control, but rather takes a circumspect approach to considering and offering educated, evidence-based, and well-informed recommendations to optimize a positive result or minimize a downside impact or outcome. In case management, the desired goal is to use education, experience, CT, and clinical judgment to assess a client's status and weigh the risks for experiencing untoward outcomes. Based on that analysis, the case manager is able to work with the client or caregiver and care team to activate measures aimed to avoid, or appreciably reduce, those negative consequences.

Forward Thinking

The forward thinking case manager takes into consideration immediate, as well as future, implications of his or her actions and interventions. For instance, a forward thinking case manager actively engages on a public policy committee in order to advocate for multistate licensure policy. This individual realizes that his contribution is essential to advancing case management through reduction of artificial barriers to practice.

Proactive

The professional case manager embodies proactivity by developing and implementing client-centered interventions that address existing barriers to care and includes risk mitigation strategies that stem the tide on reasonably foreseeable challenges. The COLLABORATE paradigm highlights the proactive attitude as a hallmark of a professional case manager, focusing on prevention and mitigation strategies that highlight their value to the health care team.

Self-Directed

COLLABORATE defines self-directed practice in terms of functional autonomy to practice independently within the scope of one's professional practice act and/or other accepted limits (e.g., legislation, regulation, certification, organization). The self-directed case manager maintains a collaborative yet independent approach to practice. This is evidenced in the performance of responsibilities without the necessity of prompting by another care team member.

The issue of professional autonomy extends well beyond the scope of a particular practice model to address, let alone to resolve. Due to the issues that need to be incorporated in any productive discussion, as well as inclusion of consumer confidence and protection, the COLLABORATE model heartily encourages key case management stakeholders to undertake an organized and unified approach to developing consensus as to the definition and intent of professional autonomy where case management is concerned.

Chapter 16 explores the necessity of case managers being able to anticipate care needs of the client in order to contribute to care planning and team discussions. The concept of practice independence versus interdependence is also covered.

Transdisciplinary

The key elements of the Transdisciplinary competency transcend:

- Professional disciplines;
- Across teams; and
- Across the continuum.

Transdisciplinary expertise within teams presents as the optimal means to address the scope of obstacles that have emerged on health care's horizon. The increased number of facilities seeking Magnet accreditation is cited as a key motivator for evidence-based transdisciplinary team expertise (Satterfield et al., 2009).

The point loudly resonates through the emergence of accountable care organizations, mandating the collaboration of a group of providers and suppliers of services including the hospitals, physicians, and others involved to coordinate care for the clients they serve with original Medicare. They are to be true partners in care decisions (Healthcare.gov., 2013).

Professional Disciplines

Chapter 5 discusses the importance of the competencies underlying the professional practice within and across health care disciplines. These competencies set the cornerstones for individual and collective practice, reinforced through education, training, licensure, and/or other regulatory and organizational constructs. Health care quality is a comprehensive and consolidated team effort, which is interprofessional, and thus transdisciplinary in scope (Treiger & Fink-Samnick, 2013).

Across Teams

The increased cost of health care continues as a fiscal priority for all stakeholders, begs for transdisciplinary team involvement. Health expenditures in the United States alone neared $2.6 trillion in 2010, over 10 times the $256 billion spent in 1980. About 75% of these national health expenditures alone have been related to chronic disease treatment. (KaiserEDU, 2013). This adds additional fuel to the fire to optimize health care processes, treatments, and accompanying interventions.

Across the Continuum

Communication challenges across the continuum of care are a compelling motivator speaking to transdisciplinary teams. Poor communication processes manifesting across care settings with their often fragmented and siloed approaches to care have a negative impact on the quality of care (Treiger & Lattimer, 2011). Focus on the nature, quality, and frequency of team communication has become even more heightened in our global society. Clients now access care across settings regionally, nationally, and internationally.

Chapter 17 provides expansion of how the transdisciplinary competency is operationalized across the transitions of care. Information about fresh perspectives, including the application of interprofessional teams, will be provided.

Ethical–Legal

Key elements include:

- Licensure;
- Certification;
- Administrative and professional standards;
- Organizational policies and procedures; and
- Ethical codes of conduct.

Ethical and legal realms have a synergistic relationship, both with tremendous potential to impact a professional case manager's interventions. One hears the term legal and their brain embarks on a lengthy journey from malpractice to adherence of laws and regulations specific to their employer, a client, or potentially the scope of their professional practice. Ethics focuses on the analysis of principles, rules, or language that characterize an action or judgment bearing on human welfare as right, good, or beneficial or wrong, harmful, evil, burdensome, etc. (Beauchamp & Childress in Powell & Tahan, 2008).

The more philosophical and subjective interpretation of ethical practice mandates it be viewed in tandem with its objectively defined and rigid legal partner. In the litigious society in which case managers work, concerns exist with an ethical–legal conflict in which case managers strive to provide quality intervention, obey the laws, and yet still act as an advocate for their patients (Muller, Powell, & Tahan, 2008). The COLLABORATE perspective unites the integral ethics and legal foci to assure a comprehensive and realistic means to guide case management.

Licensure

Case managers are prone to prioritize legal over ethical concerns, yet each deserves its due attention. For example, the laws related to practicing outside of the scope of a license pose equally dramatic ethical implications. A case manager who potentially misrepresents him or herself via fraudulent credentials and/or fails to advocate appropriately for a client is subject to potentially both ethical and legal sanctions. There are disciplinary consequences from both legal and ethical lens, ranging from rendering an informal warning to the revoking of that individual's professional license. With respect to licensure, the ethical and legal intersection is evident.

Certification

A growing number of certification entities provide advisory opinions to address the burgeoning ethical and legal concerns of professionals. While professional case managers are bound to comply primarily with their professional licensure, legal and ethical connections manifest when case managers instead defer primarily to the scope of their certification. Especially with expanding parameters for case management intervention including increased frequency of practice across state lines and cyberspace, challenges abound reconciling both legal and ethical implications for professional practice.

Administrative and Professional Standards

It is not uncommon for a case manager to analyze the legal implications of his or her practice and ignore the ethics and vice versa. Particularly in our litigious society, case managers are concerned with ethical–legal conflict in which they want to provide quality case management services (Muller, Powell, & Tahan, 2008).

Space does not permit for the full list of all individual ethical and legal professional standards and codes, particularly in light of the exhaustive number of case management–related credentials. However, most, if not all, professional associations include related content encompassing legal and ethical standards for practice. Each one of these is specific in framing the parameters for ethical and legal adherence with respect to one's professional discipline of origin (e.g., nursing, social work, medicine).

Organizational Policies and Procedures

Ethical and legal issues are tangled and quite intertwined. It becomes tough to see where one ends and the other begins. Professional ethics encompass personal and corporate standards of behavior expected (Chadwick, 1998). Case managers may identify these as autonomy, nonmaleficence, beneficence, and justice (Powell & Tahan, 2008). There is a daily juggling act of ethical and legal stakeholder balls, manifesting through privacy and confidentiality of protected electronic health information, adherence to informed consent, and the extent one can appeal the decision of a managed care organization related to known client care needs.

Bioethics involves the philosophical implications of certain biological and medical procedures, technologies, and treatments as organ transplants, genetic engineering, and care of the terminally ill (Bioethics, 2012). Case managers walk an especially lengthy and convoluted ethical and legal tightrope when these situations emerge, one which extends from assuring personal values align with professional ethics and in turn comply with laws, regulations, and related organizational policies and procedures.

Ethical Codes of Conduct

Ethical codes of conduct are consistent in their language that case managers are beholden to behave and practice ethically, adhering to the tenets of the code of ethics that underlies the individual case manager's professional credential. These tenets are beneficence, nonmalfeasance, autonomy, justice, and fidelity (CMSA, 2010).

The five ethical tenets of case management are a constant amid rapid industry change. Ethical–legal convergence emerges as case managers wrestle with the decision of whether to practice as guided by their ethical codes or by their employer. Consistent challenges greet case managers as they struggle to ascertain if telehealth intervention is "coaching or assessing." Case managers ponder the limits of privacy and confidentiality in the age of the internet. As a result, one must wonder why ethical codes are not viewed simultaneously from a legal context, particularly given the fact that their basic objective is to protect the public interest (CCMC, 2009). CCMC's code, like a majority of others, speaks as well to the certificants obeying all applicable laws and regulations governing their scope of practice (2009).

Chapter 18 probes the **ethical–legal** competency justification, relevance, and paramount importance to case managers, both individually and collectively. Application of the creative synergy of these concepts is demonstrated.

SUMMARY

This chapter introduces each of the COLLABORATE competencies. Chapters 8 to 18 expand on these simplifications in order to illustrate the depth, meaning, and impact on professional case management practice.

References

Ashford, J. B., & Lecroy, C. W. (2013). *Human behavior in the social environment: A multi-dimensional perspective* (5th ed.). Belmont, CA: Brooks/Cole, Cengage Learning.

Beauchamp, T., & Childress, J. (2008). Ethical issues in case management practice. In S. K. Powell & H. A. Tahan (Eds.), *CMSA core curriculum for case management* (2nd ed., chap. 27). Philadelphia, PA: Lippincott Williams & Wilkins.

Bioethics. (2012). *Dictionary.com Unabridged.* Random House, Inc. Retrieved April 30, 2012, from http://dictionary.reference.com/browse/bioethics

Case Management Society of America. (2010). *CMSA standards of practice for case management* (Rev.). Retrieved April 25, 2013, from http://www.cmsa.org/portals/0/pdf/memberonly/StandardsOfPractice.pdf

Chadwick, R. (1998). *Routledge encyclopedia of philosophy, professional ethics.* Retrieved April 30, 2013, from http://www.rep.routledge.com/article/L077

Code of Ethics of the National Association of Social Workers. (2008). *NASW Press.* Retrieved April 28, 2013, from http://www.naswdc.org/pubs/code/code.asp

Commission for Case Manager Certification. (2009). *Code of professional conduct for case managers.* Retrieved April 26, 2013, from http://ccmcertification.org/content/ccm-exam-portal/code-professional-conduct-case-managers

Fink-Samnick, E. (2007). Fostering a sense of professional resilience: Six simple strategies. *The New Social Worker Magazine, 14*(3), 24–25.

Fink-Samnick, E. (2009). The professional resilience paradigm: Defining the next generation of professional self-care. *Professional Case Management, 14*(6), 330–332.

Fink-Samnick, E. (2013, March 9). *The global assessment lens©, managing the client village: The ethical tango.* PowerPoint presentation. DFW CMSA Annual Conference, Irving, TX

Gambrill, E. (2012). *Critical thinking in clinical practice: Improving the quality of judgments and decisions* (3rd ed.). Hoboken, NJ: Wiley and Sons.

Healthcare.gov. (2013). *Accountable care organization fact sheet.* Retrieved April 28, 2013, from http://www.healthcare.gov/news/factsheets/2011/03/accountablecare03312011a.html

Hull, J. (2007). Self-awareness. In R. Baumeister, & K. Vohs (Eds.), *Encyclopedia of social psychology.* Thousand Oaks, CA: SAGE. doi:10.4135/9781412956253.n473, p. 791-793

KaiserEDU.org: Health Policy Explained. (2013). *U.S. Healthcare costs: Issues, modules, background brief.* Retrieved April 28, 2013 from http://www.kaiseredu.org/issue-modules/us-health-care-costs/background-brief.aspx

Lewis, N. (2012). *Global telemedicine market headed for 27 billion.* Retrieved, April 28, 2013 from http://www.informationweek.com/healthcare/mobile-wireless/global-telemedicine-market-headed-for-27/232602930

Manhattan Research. (2012). *Multiscreen health activity on the rise.* Retrieved April 28, 2012 from http://manhattanresearch.com/News-and-Events/Press-Releases/multiscreen-health-activity

Muller, L. S. (2008). Legal issues in case management practice. In S. K. Powell & H. A. Tahan (Eds.), *CMSA core curriculum for case management* (2nd ed., chap. 26). Philadelphia, PA: Lippincott Williams & Wilkins.

National Association of Social Workers. (2008). Code of ethics of the national association of social workers. *NASW Press.* Retrieved April 28, 2013, from http://www.naswdc.org/pubs/code/code.asp

Powell, S. K., & Tahan, H. A. (Eds.). (2008). *CMSA core curriculum for case management* (2nd ed.). Philadelphia, PA: Lippincott Williams & Wilkins.

Satterfield, J. M., Spring, B., Brownson, R. C., Mullen, E. J., Newhouse, R. P., Walker, B. B. & Whitlock, E. P. (2009). Toward a Transdisciplinary model of evidence-based practice. *Milbank Quarterly*, *87*(2), 368–390.

Simpson, E., & Courtney, M. (2002). Critical thinking in nursing education: A literature review. *International Journal of Nursing Practice*, *8*(2), 89–98.

Treiger, T. M. (2008). *Business communication* [Electronic mail message to C. Gehrke]. Broomfield, CO: McKesson Corporation.

Treiger, T. M., & Fink-Samnick, E. (2013). COLLABORATE©: A universal, competency-based paradigm for professional case management practice, part I. *Professional Case Management*, *18*(3), 122–135.

Treiger, T. M., & Lattimer, C. (2011). The interdisciplinary team and transitions of care. In P. Dilworth-Anderson & M. H. Palmer (Eds.), *Annual review of gerontology and geriatrics* (chap. 9). New York, NY: Springer.

8 CRITICAL THINKING

OBJECTIVE

After studying this chapter, you will be able to:

1. Define critical thinking.
2. Understand the historical context and evolution of critical thinking.
3. Describe the stages of critical thinking relevant to case management.
4. Identify how the key elements of critical thinking enhance professional case management.
5. Describe how critical thinking supports the case management process.

KEY TERMS

Analytic thinking
Case Manager's Critical Thinking Gray Zone
Competency Outcomes Performance Assessment (COPA) Model
Critical thinking
Stage Theory
Emotional intelligence
Evidence-based
Habit
Judgment
Objective
Reflective thinking
Socratic questioning
Subjective
TACTICS
The 3E Model

The concept of **critical-thinking** (CT) has experienced a vast evolution over the years. What appeared centuries ago as a means by which to assess whether the ideas and beliefs of those in authority were sound or rational (The Foundation for Critical Thinking, 2014a), now has far grander significance. The U.S. Department of Labor has labeled CT as the foundation for key personal and workplace skills such as problem solving, decision making, creativity, and strategic planning (Ward, 2012).

CT serves a pivotal role for health care's interprofessional workforce. It is a formally recognized and frequently identified mandatory professional competency that presents across academic accreditation entities and regulatory bodies. CT is prominently identified as the number one workplace competency executives seek in employees (Ward, 2012).

It is imperative to note at the start of this chapter that CT's positioning as COLLABORATE's initial competency is deliberate. As the hallmark for professional decision making, CT serves dual duty for the COLLABORATE paradigm, as a competency in and unto itself plus one integral to each of those (competencies) which follow it in the model. When CT is actively engaged, it supports and advances all the components comprising the case management process (Powell & Tahan, 2008) presented in chapter 2. Consider the decision making required to identify those patients who would benefit from case management intervention. How does a case manager strategize with team members, as well as those in the C-suite, to implement care coordination plans? What skills of analysis are needed for case managers to evaluate patient goals toward return on investment initiatives and/or outcomes measurement? CT's influence serves a vital role in each of these endeavors.

It is not an overexaggeration to state that most, if not all, case managers engage in some type of thinking to guide their actions. This includes the way individual work functions are organized, as an example. Is each (function) evaluated in a strategic and proactive manner, or is it more haphazard and reactive to emotion, whether self-induced stress or that of the environment within which one works? Organized chaos and baptism by fire strategies work for most only for the short term. There are clear benefits of a more intentional thinking process, where emotion is kept at bay. Thinking on its own has the potential to be biased, distorted, partial, and/or uninformed (The Foundation for Critical Thinking, 2014b). CT's inclusion augments the quality of how a case manager actively participates in the thinking process. As eloquently stated by author Christopher Hitchens, "the essence of the independent mind lies in not what it thinks but in how it thinks" (Hitchens, 2005).

DEFINITIONS

CT's diverse definitions span education, medicine, nursing, philosophy, social work,etc. However, one foundational common thread weaves together the unique renderings of CT. Decision making is at the heart of clinical practice and CT involves how to think critically about decisions (Gambrill, 2012).

Over the years, there have been assorted definitions for CT, with those most integral to health care provided in this chapter. There have equally been a series of concepts closely aligned with CT. These concepts validate the importance of more intuitive modes of thinking, plus offer a unique twist on CT. This chapter provides a comprehensive retrospective of those most pertinent to the health care industry, and case management specifically. The definitions and models included in this chapter each advances the messaging that CT involves what can feel like an unconventional yet necessary approach to decision making.

IN THE BEGINNING: SOCRATIC QUESTIONING

CT has a rich and lengthy history that some challenge began several centuries ago with Socrates and his method of **Socratic Questioning**. These probing or reflective questions were deemed necessary by society to assess whether the beliefs of those in leadership positions could be taken at face value, or required further evidence or proof. Socrates established the importance of carefully distinguishing beliefs that are reasonable and logical from those which lack evidence or rational foundation to warrant one's beliefs (The Foundation for Critical Thinking, 2014a). This concept sets the tone for CT's maturation through the ages, one which took a dramatic turn in the early 20th century.

DEWEY DEVELOPS REFLECTIVE THINKING

If Socratic questioning begins the ancestral lineage of CT, **reflective thinking** (RT) is its modern grandparent. Developed by John Dewey in the early 1900s, RT is defined as thought based on reflection, related to beliefs, purposeful, and involving outcomes (Zori & Morrison, 2009). Dewey was a philosopher, psychologist, and educational reformer who believed in advocacy of democracy. He brought these concepts into academia, where he felt strongly that a curriculum aimed at building thinking skills had a more universal function. It would benefit not only the individual learner, but in turn their community and entire democracy.

Not only did RT pose that a natural leap was involved in all thinking, but it forced individual members of society to accept accountability for their thinking process. Dewey asked that they contemplate the true depth and scope of their own thinking process. He invited individuals to suspend **judgment**, maintain a healthy skepticism, and exercise an open mind. These were to be accompanied by active, persistent, and careful consideration of any concept in light of the ground that supports it (Dewey, 1910). Imagine the cultural shift for the population. This was an innovative concept for the times; thinking about one's thinking was not the norm.

Although Dewey framed how facts are a critical component of any thinking process, he was adamant they are not the sole motivator of it. Dewey's analysis of the stages of RT placed emphasis on the significance that an individual's frame of reference has on the outcome of efforts where thinking plays a role. His five-step RT process served as a template to guide this novel model and is shown in Figure 8-1 (Dewey, 1910).

Dewey (1910) is also acknowledged for his perspective on the way influences can ultimately dictate the course of any thinking process. A broad range of contributing influences were identified, ranging from experience to self-interest, personal norms and/or biases, plus expectations, to name only a few. Dewey felt strongly about the likelihood of influencers to alter the outcome of any situation.

Consider how influencers have the potential to impact a case manager's thinking process. Imagine two patients who appear at first glance as similar in the context of their clinical presentation, diagnosis, or even the treatment protocols used in the respective level of care (e.g., ambulatory, acute) where intervention is being rendered. The prognosis can be profoundly altered when the influencers of each covering case manager's education, training, and/or experience meet the unique organizational priorities such as length of stay or even treatment biases of the physicians and team members.

Dewey's work brought more-complex thinking practices out of the shadows and into a more global consciousness. Getting students to process didactic knowledge with their

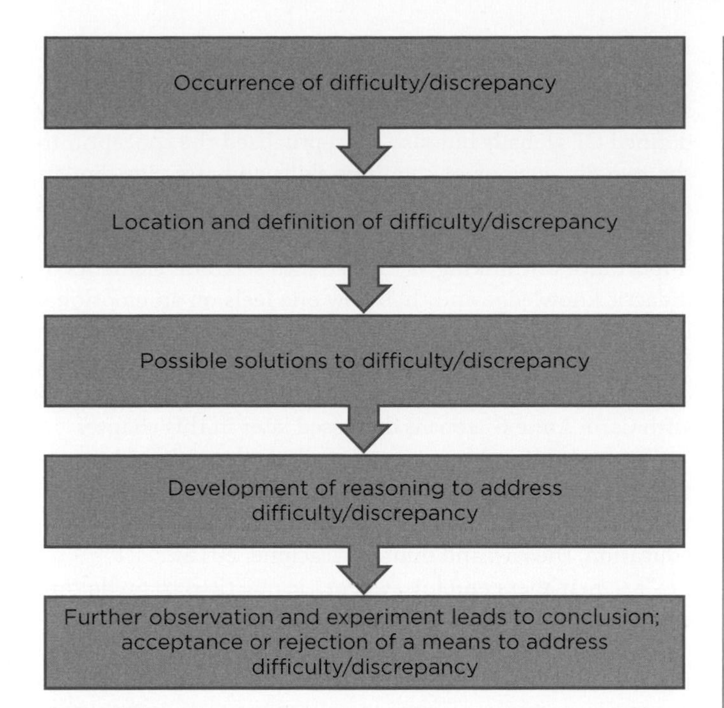

Figure 8-1. John Dewey's five steps of reflective thinking. (Adapted from Dewey, J. (1910). *How we think*. Lexington, MA: D.C. Health.)

related emotions became a powerful means to enhance learning, and serves equal benefit to other professionals.

CRITICAL THINKING COMES OF AGE

As the 20th century advanced, a wide range of professionals contributed definitions to the CT evolution. From the research of Glaser to Paul and Elder's development of the Foundation for Critical Thinking, CT's maturation continued full throttle, primarily in realm of higher education. CT is a focus of educators at every level of education (Walker, 2003).

Each of the experts discussed in this section played pivotal roles in the CT movement. Their contributions and the definitions developed by each are presented in Box 8-1, Contemporary Definitions for Critical Thinking.

BOX 8-1 Contemporary Definitions of Critical Thinking

The ability to think critically . . . involves three things:

1. An attitude of being disposed to consider in a thoughtful way the problems and subjects that come within the range of one's experiences,
2. Knowledge of the methods of logical inquiry and reasoning, and
3. Some skill in applying those methods.

Glaser, 1941

We understand critical thinking to be purposeful, self-regulatory judgment which results in interpretation, analysis, evaluation, and inference, as well as explanation of the evidential, conceptual, methodological, criteriological, or contextual considerations upon which that judgment is based. Critical Thinking is essential as a tool of inquiry.

American Philosophical Association, 1990

Critical thinking is purposeful, reflective judgment that manifests itself in giving reasoned and fair-minded consideration to evidence, conceptualizations, methods, contexts, and standards in order to decide what to believe or what to do.

Facione, 2013

Critical thinking (in nursing) is an essential component of professional accountability and quality nursing care. Critical thinkers in nursing exhibit these habits of the mind: confidence, contextual perspective, creativity, flexibility, inquisitiveness, intellectual integrity, intuition, open-mindedness, perseverance, and reflection. Critical thinkers (in nursing) practice the cognitive skills of analyzing, applying standards, discriminating, information seeking, logical reasoning, predicting and transforming knowledge.

Scheffer and Rubenfeld, 2000

To engage in processes of reflection, judgment, evaluation, and criticism that leads to decisiveness, so vital to the achievement of intentioned outcomes.

Zori and Morrison, 2009

Critical Thinking is thinking about your thinking while you're thinking in order to make your thinking better. Two things are crucial:

1. Critical thinking is not just thinking but thinking which entails self-improvement, and
2. This Improvement comes from skill in using standards by which one appropriately assesses thinking.

Paul, 1992

Self-guided, self-disciplined thinking which attempts to reason at the highest level of quality in a fair-minded way.

Elder and Paul, 2012

A purposeful endeavor with enhanced emphasis on having defined standards of clarity and fairness, along with careful attention to beliefs and actions.

Gambrill, 2012

Edward M. Glaser

Glaser (1941) was emphatic that those who engage in CT stand out among the rest of the population. He is known for being one of a small group of educators who called for a change from the didactic paradigm of knowledge and learning to a Socratic, critically reflective one (Paul, 1992). Glaser's solo and duo contributions support and guide how educational programs develop CT in children and adult learners, through individual and group problem solving and decision making. Glaser's work is referred to as the cornerstone for the CT movement (Paul, 1992).

While a student at Columbia Teachers College in the 1920s, Glaser worked with his professor, Goodwin Watson, to develop the Watson test of fair-mindedness. This was ultimately revised in 1941 as the Watson–Glaser Test of Critical Thinking (Think Watson, 2014), and then again in the 1990s with Richard Paul (Paul, 1992). This psychometric test is administered globally and viewed as the gold standard to measure CT ability. It is also used by employers, recruiters, and institutions of higher education for both academic evaluations of CT plus job selection and talent management (TestPrep-Online, 2014).

Facione Sets a Standard for Higher Education

Facione's work on CT toward the end of the 20th century serves as one of the main resources on the topic for students and faculty in higher education. Many of Facione's articles are integrated into syllabi as course-required reading.

During his time with the American Philosophical Association, Facione spearheaded the study to develop an international expert consensus of CT and its core cognitive skills, shown in Table 8-1. The summation of this work became known as the Delphi Report. The report not only defined CT globally but also conceptualized the concept into the two dimensions of cognitive skills and affective dimensions (Insight Assessment, 2014). This validated the focus of previous CT visionaries such as Dewey who touted the importance of thinking as divided into separate elements of didactic knowledge and then how one feels on an emotional level about that knowledge. Facione continues committed to CT as best practice, engaged in research and the developing of tools to assess reasoning. The IDEAS Process he co-wrote with Carol Anne Gittens is discussed later in this chapter.

Facione's efforts bring a unique lens through which professionals across numerous business sectors are influenced to take charge of a situation, including those in health care, education, the law, and military (Facione, 2015).

Case managers employ systematic practices to guide care coordination's diverse and associated components to fruition. It is in these situations where CT thrives for it provides the rich opportunity to individualize and objectively analyze a variety of situations. CT is especially meaningful for case managers who often find themselves in situations which can

TABLE 8-1 The Delphi Report: Core Cognitive Skills

Core CT Skills	Definition	Subskills
Interpretation	To comprehend and express the meaning or significance of a wide variety of experiences, situations, data, events, judgments, conventions, beliefs, rules, procedures, or criteria.	1.1 Categorization 1.2 Decoding Significance 1.3 Clarifying Meaning
Analysis	To identify the intended and actual inferential relationships among statements, questions, concepts, descriptions, or other forms of representation intended to express beliefs, judgments, experiences, reasons, information, or opinions.	2.1 Examining Ideas 2.2 Detecting Arguments 2.3 Analyzing Arguments
Evaluation	To assess the credibility of statements or other representations which are accounts or descriptions of a person's perception, experience, situation, judgment, belief, or opinion; and to assess the logical strength of the actual or intended inferential relationships among statements, descriptions, questions or other forms of representation.	3.1 Assessing Claims 3.2 Assessing Arguments
Inference	To identify and secure elements needed to draw reasonable conclusions; to form conjectures and hypotheses; to consider relevant information; and to educe the consequences flowing from data, statements, principles, evidence, judgments, beliefs, opinions, concepts, descriptions, questions, or other forms of representation.	4.1 Querying Evidence 4.2 Conjecturing Alternatives 4.3 Drawing Conclusions
Explanation	To state the results of one's reasoning; to justify that reasoning in terms of the evidential, conceptual, methodological, criteriological, and contextual considerations upon which one's results were based; and to present one's reasoning in the form of cogent arguments.	5.1 Stating Results 5.2 Justifying Procedures 5.3 Presenting Arguments
Self-regulation	Self-consciously to monitor one's cognitive activities, the elements used in those activities, and the results educed, particularly by applying skills in analysis and evaluation to one's own inferential judgments with a view toward questioning, confirming, validating, or correcting either one's reasoning or one's results.	6.1 Self-Examination 6.2 Self-Correction

From The American Philosophical Association (1990). Critical thinking: A statement of expert consensus for purposes of educational assessment and instruction. The Delphi Report, Committee on Pre-College Philosophy.

play out in any number of ways. In fact, if one were to ask 10 different case managers how each would address a particular patient situation, there would most likely be 10 different assessments and plans.

Consider how the slightest change in a patient's condition often translates to major adjustments in the treatment plan. These situations usually occur without warning, with the case manager having little or no time to consider how best to validate the rationale of this new treatment course. This new treatment direction usually warrants additional authorization for approved days and/or services. This important task often falls to the case manager who must strategically evaluate and reflect on each component of the treatment plan. There is little margin for error in these circumstances. When CT is engaged toward this purpose, it fuels each case manager's ability to transition what can feel like a disorganized effort akin to herding cats to one far smoother, and for that matter more tactical.

Paul and the Foundation for Critical Thinking

Another renowned philosopher, Richard Paul, is viewed as a major leader and founder of the modern CT movement. His vast contributions to the education sector are now mainstreamed across business and other segments of society. Paul, in both solo and shared efforts with Elder and Glaser to name a few, has influenced the way the world understands CT.

Paul's commitment to CT led him to work toward the development of the Center for Critical Thinking, an educational nonprofit organization whose mission is to promote essential change in education and society through the cultivation of fair-minded CT (The Foundation for Critical Thinking, 2014d). The Center works under the auspices of the Foundation for Critical Thinking created in 1990. Its goal is to integrate the Center's research and theoretical developments, and to create events and resources designed to help educators improve their instruction. The Foundation is also instrumental in working with institutions to design their own CT professional development programs.

Gambrill Distinguishes Between CT and Evidence-Based Practice

Eileen Gambrill's perspective draws on her background as an educator in social work research and practice. Like those previously mentioned, Gambrill (2012) views CT as a purposeful action. Emphasis is placed by clinical practitioners and helping professionals on thinking in accordance with defined standards of clarity and fairness. In addition, Gambrill (2012) notes there must be equal awareness and processing of distinct beliefs and actions. It is through this powerful combination that each practitioner is able to arrive at well-reasoned decisions.

Consider the endurance and commitment required to get all treatment team members on the proverbial same page of a treatment plan. There are multiple professionals of diverse backgrounds, each with unique standards of practice and ethical codes, not to mention personal and professional beliefs, values, and biases. When there is greater awareness of these factors, plus a mutual starting point of understanding and expectation, the outcomes and the effort will usually be far more favorable.

Gambrill also noted the importance of skepticism to the CT effort. A thoughtful approach to decision making requires a skeptical attitude. Yet how skeptical is too skeptical, and when might it impede solid clinical judgment? Gambrill's (2012) message to the professional community is clear: clinicians should be able to offer cogent reasons for decisions they make regarding choice of assessment, intervention, and evaluation methods. She adds, "We should be as skeptical as we need to be to avoid influence by propaganda in the helping professions, which is rife."

CT can be synonymous with thinking and/or decision making which is **evidence-based**, and Gambrill (2012) notes the distinction between these concepts. CT's purpose is to arrive at well-reasoned decisions. To the contrary, evidence-based practice (EBP) describes a distinct process to facilitate this aim, one which incorporates the effective use of professional judgment in integrating information regarding each client's unique characteristics, circumstances, preferences and actions, and external research findings (Gambrill, 2012). EBP describes a process which is designed to help practitioners link evidence, ethics, and application of concepts to purposeful interventions.

Scheffer and Rubenfeld Strive for CT Consistency

The expansion and increased utilization of CT over the last decade of the 20th century yielded a paradoxical response, one of confusion in terms of application in the nursing profession especially. Despite formal acknowledgment by a number of entities, including the U.S. Department of Education, the National League for Nursing, and American Association of Colleges of Nursing (AACN), there was little consensus on the meaning and application of CT in nursing (Scheffer & Rubenfeld, 2000).

Scheffer and Rubenfeld (2000) engaged in an international effort to achieve professional agreement through an international panel of nursing experts in education, practice, and research. Their seminal work included an exhaustive historical retrospective of CT from across the nursing profession. Five rounds of expert panel interviews, research, and analysis were conducted which yielded a strong consensus statement as to the nature of CT in nursing and how it could be defined.

Standardized language for CT in nursing has particular benefits in the education realm in standardizing learning activities and assessments of students, self-evaluation by students of their own abilities, and in addressing professional accreditation criteria (Scheffer & Rubenfeld, 2000).

There were equally a list of questions which emerged for further study, including querying the relationships among CT and the associated skills of diagnostic reasoning, clinical judgment, problem solving, and the nursing process. This query continues to this day across the literature spanning professional disciplines. Many strive to weave what presents as subtle differences among a number of terms associated with CT, such as clinical reasoning, clinical judgment, and analytical thinking (Victor-Chmil, 2013; Elder & Paul, 2012).

Zori and Morrison Align CT With Nursing Management

In their retrospective article on CT, Zori and Morrison (2009) worked to create a comprehensive definition of CT applicable to nursing management. What evolved has considerably strong application to case management as well—to engage in processes of reflection, judgment, evaluation, and criticism that lead to decisiveness, so vital to the achievement of intentioned outcomes. This promotes the ability to challenge assumptions and work past them to a more thorough comprehension of causes and implications of problems. Ultimately more creative solutions are attained (Zori & Morrison, 2009).

The concepts framed by Zori and Morrison are in alignment with a professional case manager's standard of practice. Consider the case manager, or any health care professional who is unable to engage in critical thinking. The individual's efforts will result in a more reactive if not emotional response. This response will be **subjective**, based on feelings or opinions rather than on facts (Merriam-Webster Online, 2014a). Subjective, emotionally laden responses will do little to enhance an individual case manager's professional presentation.

This is in opposition to what supports case management intervention, a response that is **objective**. This is information based on facts rather than feelings or opinions (Merriam-Webster Online, 2014b). An objective response is more conducive to the proactive practices, which are essential to case management success.

Amid the confluence of definitions which exist for CT, prevailing common denominators exist. CT takes the stance that for thinking to be critical it cannot be accepted at face value. Instead there must be allowance for analysis and assessment of its clarity, accuracy, depth, breadth, and logicalness plus interpretation through a variety of frames of reference (The Foundation for Critical Thinking, 2014b).

PAST AND CURRENT THINKING

Over the years, CT has been the focus of and/or incorporated as a component of an exhaustive number of influential models, enough to fill many books on the topic. This list has recently expanded to include several models where CT is identified as a core competency. These models transverse the health care industry from those developed for discipline-specific interventions, to those applied across the business, education, and health care sectors, including case management. Those that have been chosen serve to provide readers with a diverse yet comprehensive foundation of models to include CT as opposed to an all-inclusive listing.

Before moving forward, one major point beckons amid the many CT models for consideration. Health care professionals, especially those in case management, can feel pressured to align with a particular model, whether recommended by new organizational leadership or presented at a recently attended conference. The decision to implement any single model can be related more to industry popularity or "the greatest thing since sliced bread" syndrome as opposed to a more formal and strategic means for application (e.g., evidenced-based or SWOT analysis).

Picking from the assortment of CT perspectives that appear in the literature does not make a professional case manager competent in CT. This would be akin to calling oneself a case manager without the requisite education, training, and credentialing. Instead, case managers must pledge to put energy and emphasis on what is commonly referred to as **habit**, the intellectual commitment to use those CT skills as a means to guide their behavior (The Foundation for Critical Thinking, 2014b). Simply stated, a case manager's overall acknowledgment to accept and embrace a new CT state of mind is as important as defining which CT model to implement. The concept of habit and its importance to professional case management practice is further addressed in chapter 14, Organized.

NURSING

An essential component of nursing practice, CT forms the foundation of many nursing specialties, including infection control and case management (American Sentinel, 2012). The promoting of CT competence is an important way to improve problem-solving and decision-making competence to further improve quality of care (Feng et al., 2010). Quality is integral to nursing practice and thus no surprise that nursing includes a number of theories and models that align with and/or include CT as a core component.

The Competency Outcomes Performance Assessment Model

As discussed in chapter 5, competency-based approaches entered the health care industry in the final decade of the 20th century. Education of the industry's next generation of practitioner equally transitioned to a competency-based approach in response to an array of individuals, initiatives, and organizations who became committed to heed the competency charge (Barr, 1998; CIHC, 2007; IOM, 2003; IPEC, 2011). The strong focus on both quality and patient safety (IOM, 1999) translated to a need to train more competent nurses. Nurse leaders, educators, and students were caught in the struggle of shifting from past practices to contemporary requirements of unlearning and relearning, of shifting from a past-to-present dimension to an informed present-to-future practice (Lenburg, Klein, Abdur-Rahman, Spencer, & Boyer, 2009).

In direct response to the industry's need to reframe the professional training of its next generation of nurses, Lenburg's **Competency Outcomes Performance Assessment (COPA) Model** was developed. It was designed and structured as a theoretical curriculum framework to promote competence for practice Lenburg et al. (2009). Considered a holistic yet focus-based model, the COPA required the integration of practice-based outcomes, interactive learning methods, and performance assessment of competencies. In essence, the models merged the significance of theory, with the expectations of professional practice and the reality of workplace expectations. These areas were organized around four conceptual pillars (Lenburg et al., 2009):

1. The specification of essential core practice competencies
2. End result competency outcomes
3. Practice-driven interactive learning strategies
4. Objective competency performance examinations

CT is identified in the second pillar as one of eight core practice competency categories. In the context of the COPA, CT is defined as using evidence for practice, integrating theory for practice, problem solving, decision making, and scientific inquiry (Lenburg et al., 2009).

The COPA has been applied to case management for its focus on the broad array of skills along a continuum. This includes basic problem solving and analysis to more complex and higher-level reflective judgment, scientific inquiry, and research-based knowledge development (Lenberg, in Cohen & Henning, 2005).

AACN's Synergy Model

CT is included by AACN in the Synergy Model (2014) under clinical judgment and shown in detail in Table 8-2. The model was triggered by industry curiosity around defining a better way to dialogue about patients and nurses' relationships with them. Increasing attention was focused on delineating what nurses tangibly add to this relationship that improved patient outcomes (Edwards, 1999).

Developed to link clinical practice with patient outcomes, the core concept of the Synergy Model is that the needs or characteristics of patients and families influence and drive the characteristics or competencies of nurses. Synergy results when the needs and characteristics of a patient, clinical unit, or system are matched with a nurse's competencies (AACN, 2014).

Paul's Eight Elements of Thought

Richard Paul noted that if all thinking is purposeful, it includes eight elements of thought. He identified that for nurses especially the thinking process could easily become flawed or limited by the lack of understanding a specific problem (Paul, in The Foundation for Critical Thinking, 2014). For example, consider how important it is for a case manager to fully understand each of the unique components of a patient's history and physical. Think how vital it becomes to fully ascertain information ranging from the patient's allergies to spiritual beliefs and end-of-life choices, and how these details impact the comprehensive treatment plan.

Paul applied his Elements of Thought model toward enhancing a nurse's ability to sort out difficult questions and critically monitor thinking. By moving through the eight distinct elements, nurses could assure that they engaged in a thorough and comprehensive thought process, one which meets the standards for level of intellectual thought expected. This model finds particular application in the health care industry, especially in these times where there is a strong focus on assuring professional standards of practice are met. The Elements of Thought are displayed in Figure 8-2 (Paul, in The Foundation for Critical Thinking, 2014).

TACTICS Achieve the IOM Competencies

Rubenfeld and Sheffer (2015) viewed health care delivery and nursing, in particular, in need of critical thinkers. Their commitment to this concept culminated in providing a

TABLE 8-2 AACN Clinical Judgment Competency, Synergy Model-Presentation

Clinical Judgment	Clinical reasoning, which includes clinical decision making, critical thinking, and a global grasp of the situation, coupled with nursing skills acquired through a process of integrating formal and informal experiential knowledge and evidence-based guidelines.
Level 1	Collects basic-level data; follows algorithms, decision trees, and protocols with all populations and is uncomfortable deviating from them; matches formal knowledge with clinical events to make decisions; questions the limits of one's ability to make clinical decisions and delegates the decision making to other clinicians; includes extraneous detail.
Level 3	Collects and interprets complex patient data; makes clinical judgments based on an immediate grasp of the whole picture for common or routine patient populations; recognizes patterns and trends that may predict the direction of illness; recognizes limits and seeks appropriate help; focuses on key elements of case while sorting out extraneous details.
Level 5	Synthesizes and interprets multiple, sometimes conflicting, sources of data; makes judgment based on an immediate grasp of the whole picture, unless working with new patient populations; uses past experiences to anticipate problems; helps patient and family see the "big picture"; recognizes the limits of clinical judgment and seeks multidisciplinary collaboration and consultation with comfort; recognizes and responds to the dynamic situation.

Adapted from the American Association of Critical-Care Nurses. (2014). The AACN synergy model for patient care. Retrieved July 23, 2014, from http://www.aacn.org/wd/certifications/content/synmodel.pcms?menu=

1. The problem, question, concern, or issue being discussed or thought about by the thinker
   - What the thinker is attempting to figure out
2. The purpose or the goal of thinking
   - Why are we attempting to figure something out and to what end?
   - What do we hope to accomplish?
3. The frame of reference, points of view, or even world view that we hold about the issue or problem
   - How might this invoke bias in our thinking?
4. The assumptions that we hold to be true about the issue on which we base our claims or beliefs?
   - How do our values, norms, morals, and ethics impact our thinking?
5. The central concepts, ideas, principles, and theories that we use in reasoning about the problem
   - What didactic knowledge, theories, and interventions drive our thought process?
6. The evidence, data, or information provided to support the claims we make about the issue or problem
   - How do we incorporate evidenced-based decision making?
7. The interpretations, inferences, reasoning, and lines of formulated thought that lead to our conclusions
   - Can I identify how I used the evidence to validate my conclusions?
8. The implications and consequences that follow from the positions we hold on the issue or problem
   - How does this process contribute to new and or different thinking?

Figure 8-2. The Elements of Thought. (Adapted from Paul in The Foundation for Critical Thinking. (2014e). *Analyzing and assessing.* Retrieved, December 12, 2014, from http://www.criticalthinking.org/pages/analyzing-and-assessing-thinking-/783)

robust model for educators and practitioners that resonated with the real world of practice.

Their **TACTICS** model addresses the CT required by a health care professional to achieve the IOM's five core competencies, which were presented in chapter 5. There is innovative energy from the direct application of CT strategies with those valued competencies of quality improvement and safety, patient-centered care, interdisciplinary teams, EBP, and informatics. Health care professionals live these competencies daily, independent of practice setting. They must equally engage CT to address, evaluate, revise, and develop care that reflects the ever-evolving definition of best practice. In these rapidly changing times best practice is only good for a specific moment, for it becomes obsolete within minutes when replaced by a newer best practice model. The acronym and the scope of the model's individual elements are presented in Table 8-3.

SOCIAL WORK

The competency-based models discussed in chapter 5 place heightened focus on operationalizing CT at the gateway of professional learning, with several accreditation entities

TABLE 8-3 TACTICS

CT Activities	Scope
Tracking	Following thinking paths, making them visible and open for study and enhancement
Assessing	Discerning the quality of thinking
Cultivating Thinking	Implies a growth-enhancing process
Improve	Promote better CT
Competency-based	Derived from the IOM core competencies, this relates to performance of CT in the real world as opposed to an academic checklist.
Strategies	Means by which CT is practiced and enhanced so that health care quality may be enhanced.

From Rubenfeld, M. G., & Scheffer, B. (2015). Critical thinking TACTICS for nurses: Achieving the IOM competencies (3rd ed.). Burlington, MA: Jones and Bartlett.

highlighting CT as a distinct competency (AACN, 2014; CSWE, 2008). In doing so, the expectation for knowledge acquisition and professional attainment is clearly noted.

The Council on Social Work Education

The Council on Social Work Education (CSWE) defined the Educational Policy and Accreditation Standards (EPAS) to accredit programs at the baccalaureate and master's level social work programs, plus establish thresholds for professional competence. Toward this end, they developed explicit curriculum criteria that are to be accomplished through the mastery of core competencies, 10 in total for social work. Each distinct competency also includes a description of the knowledge, values, skills, and practice behaviors that may be used to operationalize the curriculum and assessment methods. Individual educational programs have permission of CSWE to add competencies, which reflect their respective missions and goals (CSWE, 2008).

Box 8-2 provides the CSWE Education Policy 2.1.3, which addresses how social workers are expected to "apply critical thinking to inform and communicate professional judgments" (2008). The psychosocial stressors of poverty, family violence, child abuse and exploitation, and severe mental illness evoke strong feelings within social workers, as well as society. Those real and often raw feelings must be placed in a proverbial box while social workers intervene with each individual patient and/or family situation. This can be a tough lesson to reconcile for new practitioners.

The use of CT as a competency in this context assures social work students truly understand the importance of separating their presumed bias from each unique patient situation. They must be able to assess and identify what biological, psychological, and sociocultural factors impact each specific event. In this way there can be individualized attention to assuring the manifesting treatment plan is developed with consummate attention to the reality of the situation, reflecting patient self-determination and need, as opposed to being influenced by personal feelings.

A revised edition of the EPAS is currently under development and scheduled for release in 2015 (CSWE, 2014). The competencies and their practice behaviors have become a highly valued and respected resource across the social work professional domain.

BOX 8-2 CSWE CT Competency-Presentation

Educational Policy 2.1.3: Apply critical thinking to inform and communicate professional judgments.

Social workers are knowledgeable about the principles of logic, scientific inquiry, and reasoned discernment. They use critical thinking augmented by creativity and curiosity. Critical thinking also requires the synthesis and communication of relevant information. Social workers:

- Distinguish, appraise, and integrate multiple sources of knowledge, including research-based knowledge, and practice wisdom,
- Analyze models of assessment, prevention, intervention and evaluation, and
- Demonstrate effective oral and written communication in working with individuals, families, groups, organizations, communities and colleagues.

CSWE, 2008

CASE MANAGEMENT

The diverse professional landscape of case management's workforce contributes to difficulty in establishing substantive and clearly defined competencies. Contributing factors include the diverse skills, knowledge, and abilities, plus unique facility's hiring criteria and range of experiences for the workforce (Henning & Cohen, 2008).

All readers are reminded at this point that case management is not identified as a full-fledged profession. With the CMSA Standards of Practice (2010) for qualification being explicit for case managers to have current, active, and unrestricted licensure or certification in a health and human services discipline, it is a fair presumption that case managers will identify primarily with those competencies which underlie their unique professions, whether for nursing, social work, or others (ASWB, 2014; CSWE, 2008; QSEN, 2014).

Although a number of authors have cited CT as a principal skill of case management practice (Cohen, 2005; Cunningham & Cesta, 2009; Daniels & Ramey, 2005; Kelley, 2003; Powell & Tahan, 2008), there are a limited number of formal models written for case management specifically that include CT as a distinct competency. This continues to be surprising in light of the important role that CT serves to support the case management process. Table 8-4 includes each CT competency and how it is demonstrated within the models below.

The Competency Continuum

The competency continuum developed by Henning and Cohen (2008) draws from competencies grounded in the professional case management standards of practice of the time. The fluid nature of standards can be an issue to reconcile with respect to their long-range utilization. Ten competencies are included, with CT as a distinct competency. The others being screening, utilization management, assessment-care management, planning, care coordination and intervention, discharge planning, evaluation, advocacy, and professional practice.

A Competency Model for Lead Case Managers in Integrated Case Management

In 1995, the Children's Cabinet was established in Maine to address identified problems with the fragmented delivery of

TABLE 8-4 Case Management Competency Comparison: Critical Thinking

Model	The Clinical Competency Assessment Form (Henning and Cohen, 2008)	A Competency Model for Lead Case Managers in Integrated Case Management (Bernotavicz and Spence, 2000)	CMSA Competency Map (CMSA, 2014)
Competency	Critical Thinking	Critical Thinking	Analytical and Critical Thinking
Explanation	1. Demonstrates critical thinking skills in modifying plan of care to meet changing needs 2. Assesses overall status of patient and identifies changes including failure to achieve interim outcome goals 3. Collaboratively determines whether goals have been met for discharge form care management	Uses knowledge of the system to identify opportunities and problems; demonstrates the ability to think critically and strategically	Demonstrates defined expertise across roles levels designated 1–6 (CM Assistant-Executive)

services to the state's children and families. Recognizing the complex challenges faced by this population when attempting to access identified social services, the Children's Cabinet of Maine established the Integrated Case Management (ICM) initiative in 1997. The project's goal was to develop improved outcomes for children and families (especially in instances of child abuse and neglect, complicated by substance abuse, mental illness, and domestic violence) through interdisciplinary case management and integrated service delivery. The ICM recognized the importance of integrating case management business practices across departmental lines to create a fully coordinated and seamless delivery system (Bernotavicz & Spence, 2000).

The competency-based case management model and interdisciplinary training program were developed through a grant from the U.S. Department of Health and Human Services, Administration for Children, Youth and Families, and by the Institute for Public Sector Innovation at the University of Southern Maine's Edmund S. Muskie School of Public Service, in collaboration with the Maine Children's Cabinet (Bernotavicz & Spence, 2000). A component of this endeavor involved the development and publication of the competency model specific to the roles of lead or primary case managers, one that laid the foundation for those from a range of disciplines to enhance their professional case management and group facilitation skills (Bernotavicz & Spence, 2000).

The ICM model drew from the works of Covey (1989) and a range of other experts across case management, education, and child welfare. It details a complex and exhaustive list of lead case manager competencies organized into five primary domains, each with a series of subcompetencies. Critical thinking appears under the Work Management primary domain, within the subcompetency breakdown of Team Leadership. The other primary domains include Interpersonal Knowledge, Conceptual Knowledge, Self-Management, and Case Management Technical Knowledge (Bernotavicz & Spence, 2000).

CMSA's Competency Map

CMSA debuted their Competency Map in June 2014, seeking preliminary industry public comment. At present Analytical and CT are combined. When evidence is examined and organized into the competencies, there may be significant workforce impact. Preliminary information on the CMSA CT competency is included. However, the final product and research supporting the Competency Map were not available for critical review at the time this text was prepared.

GENERAL PERSPECTIVES

A number of models in the literature introduce CT to more global audiences. Several were written for education and business sectors, though all have application for those who acknowledge the commitment to engage in the CT habit.

IDEAS

IDEAS—a five-step critical thinking problem-solving process—was developed by Peter Facione and Carol Anne Gittens. The model seeks to engage individuals in solving their own problems. Through their experiential and evidence-based approach, Facione and Gittens created a CT model that can be engaged in by educators and college students as easily as professionals in health care, legal analysis, arbitration, and negotiation, and across the business sector.

Popularity of the IDEAS process lies in how it also has application to real-life situations, including, but not limited to, buying a car, dealing with a difficult boss or coworker, career changes, relationship challenges, to name a few (Facione & Gittens, 2013). IDEAS is shown in Figure 8-3.

Stage Theory

Linda Elder and Richard Paul believed that for students to develop as thinkers, they must pass through several key stages

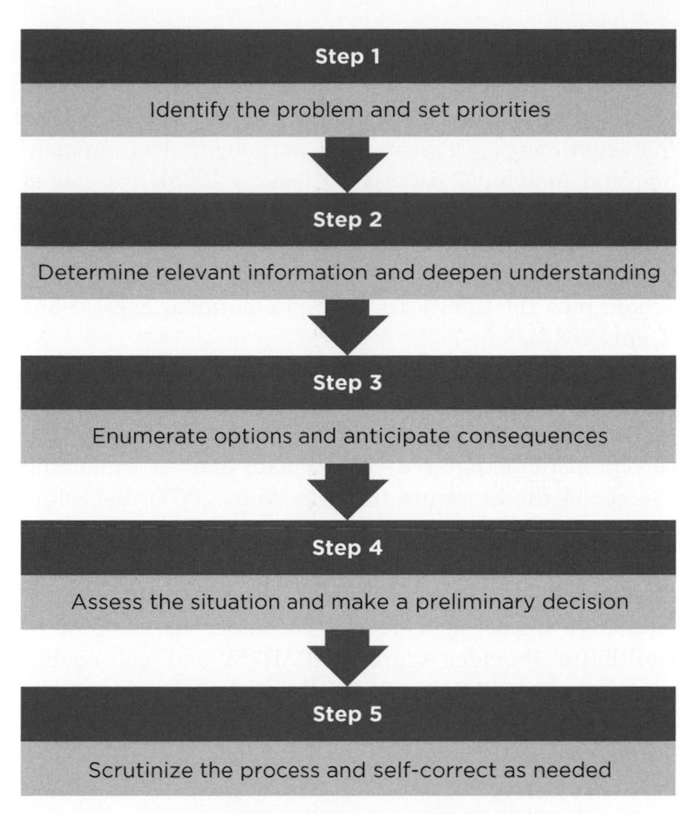

Figure 8-3. The IDEAS model. (Adapted from Facione, P. A. (2015). *Critical thinking: What it is and why it counts*. Retrieved August 21, 2014, from www.insightassessment.com)

of development in CT. However, they were clear that few educators were aware of these levels of intellectual development, a needed area of change. Through their **Stage Theory** Model, Elder and Paul reinforced the message that learning is a reciprocal process, one where cognizance by educators of defined stages of CT development enhances the student's overall intellectual quality. It also fosters the full maturity of CT (The Foundation for Critical Thinking, 2014c).

In developing the six stages of the Stage Theory, Elder and Paul made four assumptions:

1. There are predictable stages through which every person who develops as a critical thinker passes.
2. Passage from one stage to the next is dependent on a necessary level of commitment on the part of an individual to develop as a critical thinker, and is not automatic.
3. Success in instruction is deeply connected to the intellectual quality of student learning, and
4. Regression is possible in development.

The stages are presented in Figure 8-4.

The 3E Model

The 3E model includes three simple yet comprehensive steps: examine, explore, and evaluate, which are shown in Figure 8-5. Each of the steps is deliberate, focused, and action-oriented, strategies which speak to the core of a case manager's practice.

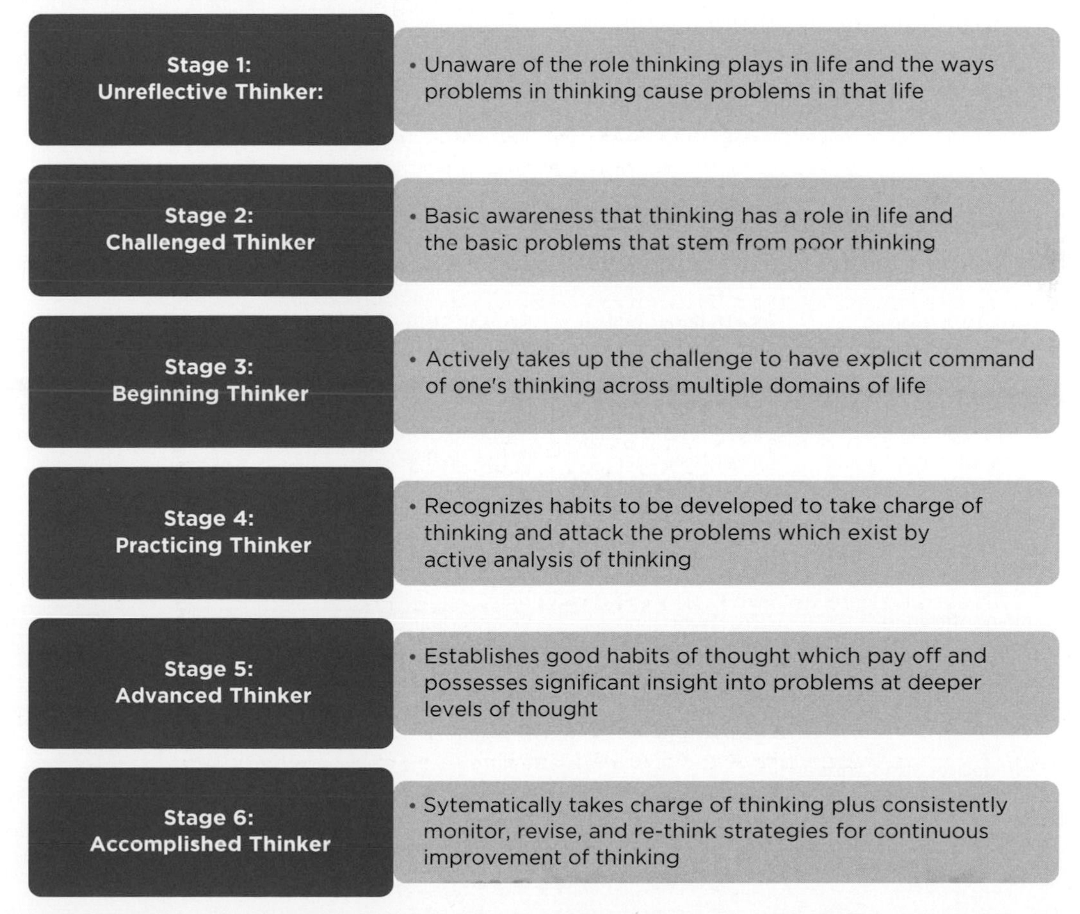

Figure 8-4. Critical thinking development: A stage theory. (Adapted from The Foundation for Critical Thinking. (2014d). *The mission*. Retrieved August 22, 2014, from http://www.criticalthinking.org/pages/our-mission/599)

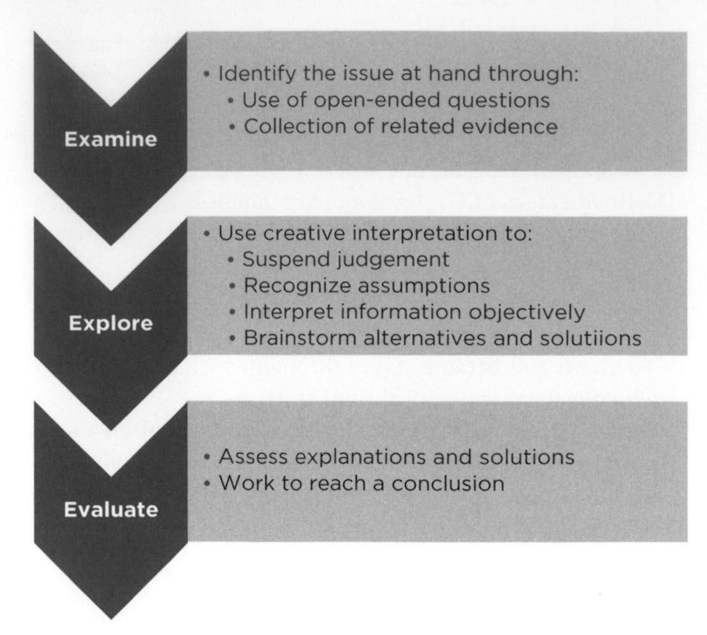

Figure 8-5. The 3E model. (Adapted from Ward, K. (2012). *Critical thinking: How to improve your decision-making skills*. King of Prussia, PA: HRDQ.)

People who excel at CT are better able to comprehend the issues at hand, evaluate evidence, make rational decisions, and work efficiently with others (Ward, 2012). These are skills that are especially applicable for case managers who live each of these concepts daily through their interventions with patients, family members, treatment teams, and other providers engaged in care coordination.

Emotional Intelligence

It could be argued that **Emotional Intelligence** (EI) is a cousin of CT, or certainly a distant relative. The concept that emotions play a greater role in thought, decision making, and individual success (Goleman, 2005) has gained appeal across business sections since it was introduced in 1995. High EI has been positively correlated with job performance and satisfaction, stress management, social interaction, plus the ability to identify emotional expressions (Dunn, 2013).

It has also been suggested that professionals with a mastery of EI can more effectively connect and communicate successfully with patients. This is especially vital in the current patient-centered care climate and an expanding concept in the literature (Birks & Watt, 2007). Behaviors of professionals and patients, plus outcomes affect a hospital's bottom line. When the providers have poor EI, it can negatively impact patient satisfaction and quality scores, ultimately impacting Hospital Consumer Assessment of Healthcare Provider scores (HCAHPS) and subsequent reimbursement (Gamble, 2013).

Table 8-5 frames the five essential elements of EI and includes a case scenario to reflect each (element).

Competency-Based Exit Examinations

CT is now considered a gauge of learning for education's continuum from high school to higher education. It is equally viewed as an indicator of each individual graduate's readiness to engage in the professional workforce

TABLE 8-5 Emotional Intelligence

Emotional Intelligence: The Ability to Identify, Assess, and Control Emotions of Oneself, Others, and Groups					
	Self-Awareness	**Self-Regulation**	**Social Skill**	**Empathy**	**Motivation**
Definition	Know emotions, strengths, weaknesses, drives, values, and goals, plus recognize their impact on others while using gut feelings to guide decisions.	Control or redirect disruptive emotions & impulses, then adapt to changing circumstances.	Manage relationships to move others in the desired direction.	Consider feelings of others in decision making.	Driven to achieve for the sake of achievement.
Hallmarks	Self-confidence Realistic self-assessment Self-deprecating sense of humor	Trustworthiness and integrity Comfort with ambiguity Openness to change	Strong desire to achieve Optimism in the face of failure Organizational commitment	Expertise in building and retaining talent Cross-cultural sensitivity Service to clients and customers	Effectiveness in leading change Persuasiveness Expertise in building and leading teams

Emotional Intelligence: The Ability to Identify, Assess, and Control Emotions of Oneself, Others, and Groups					
	Self-Awareness	**Self-Regulation**	**Social Skill**	**Empathy**	**Motivation**
CM Application	Sam is offered a new case management supervisor position (CM) at Gambosh Hospital (GH). He transitioned roles from bedside nursing, postcompletion of a degree program in CM from Nightingale Nursing School. Most of the CM's are new hires. Sam is totally overwhelmed! He seeks to discuss the offer with Mindy, his long-time mentor.	Sam enters the CM department to find it in a state of flux. The director who hired him has been fired. Toxic talk surrounds him whenever he is in the office. A consultant is hired to reorganize the department. Sam thinks what Mindy would say. "Focus, remember your strengths, and show 'em what you can do."	Sam strives to keep his colleagues focused on the work. He seeks to shift the toxic talk, to engage them in purposeful dialogues that will assure their ongoing employment. Sam has engaged the other CM's in efforts to demonstrate successful department outcomes.	Sam attends his first team conference. He heard the team has members who vie for leadership. On this day, team consensus is needed to extend Mr. James' stay beyond the current approval. Sam presents the challenge as a team effort. He engages each member to provide input. Sam submits the review to his MCO counterpart, Jyneal. Jyneal applauds the organized review focused on Mr. James: Current status Realistic objectives and goals Assures team input and consensus Approval is granted for 5 more days	The interim consultant, Sandy, is impressed with what Sam and his colleagues have accomplished during her 6-month tenure. They have successfully implemented: Interprofessional team conferences Population-based outcomes Expanded CM to the new ambulatory care unit Obtained CM certification Sandy agrees to stay on at GH to mentor Sam as the new department director.

Adapted from Goleman, D. (2004). What makes a leader. Harvard Business Review, Retrieved April 20, 2013, from http://hbr.org/2004/01/what-makes-a-leader

(Tempera, 2013). The new generation of competency-based examinations, discussed in chapter 5, are especially focused on how well students demonstrate CT. This is assessed through questions highlighting problem-solving and scientific quantitative reasoning skills. The popularity and frequency of those examinations administered by the Council for Aid to Education (2014) is evolving to be the industry norm.

CONTEXT FOR COLLABORATE CRITICAL THINKING

Case managers are positioned smack in the middle of care coordination efforts. As a result, there is engagement in a variety of interactions and situations in the workplace that can and will evoke intense emotional responses. These can easily bubble up to the surface such as confrontations with team members and intense discussions with patients and their families. Strong feelings can be triggered and the first impulse will be to lash out or project the frustrations at whoever is perceived as the source. Objectivity is replaced by subjective and emotional reactivity, far from the standard of professionalism expected by any case manager.

Key Elements of the Critical Thinking Competency

The key elements of the critical thinking competency include:

- Out-of-the-box creativity
- Analytical
- Methodical

Out-of-the-Box Creativity

Simpson and Courtney (2002), in their article, CT in Nursing Education, explore the fundamental grounding of the dimensions of CT and distinctions as opposed to more traditional problem solving, clinical decision making. The foundation is framed for CT as a process that fuels a more ingenious effort, a blending of knowledge and creativity which by its very nature is endemic to case management. The individuality of a patient's condition and life circumstance can evoke the need for a case manager to recommend plans that are beyond the traditional. Consider the situation in Box 8-3, one of many opportunities whereby case managers are able to engage this high level of innovative thinking to assure safe and quality-driven patient-centered care.

When creativity intersects with thinking, a renewed and fresh sense of purpose influences a case manager's actions. Interest in everything prevails with motivation to continuously explore new ideas, options, alternatives, and approaches (Simpson & Courtney, 2002).

Herein lies the alignment with professional case management practice:

> In order to step outside the everyday reasoning and approaches to problem solving, a person needs to develop an imagination of the possibilities and potentials inherent in a particular circumstance. This often demands a creative leap of faith and a willingness to be 'playful' with future possibilities.
>
> *Simpson and Courtney, 2002*

Individual case managers may feel challenged to allow their "creativity" to flow, especially in light of health information technology's influence. Some may view this type of creativity as counter to the latest generation of tools and templates which have emerged, particularly with increased electronic health records. When a machine defines, facilitates, and completes an assessment, cues documentation needs, and identifies medication reconciliation, what is the value of case management qualifications that speak to eligibility guidelines, such as those across several credentialing organizations which require a professional to be licensed at a level which allows for independent practice?

BOX 8-3 Out-of-the-Box Creativity Case Scenario

Jason is a strapping 25-year-old man admitted to the hospital following the sudden onset of nausea and fever, with a painful and swollen ankle. He is diagnosed with osteomyelitis and needs 4 to 6 weeks of intravenous antibiotics. The plan is for Jason to be discharged home from the hospital. However, Lydia, who is Jason's case manager, gets an earful from the treatment team when they find out that home is a trailer in the rural part of the state. Dr. Jones tells Lydia, "This is far from an optimal location for the patient to recuperate. He will land right back in here. Or worse than that, the osteo will invade his system and kill him. Nobody will ever find him out there. This guy has to go to a nursing home, so just set it up."

Lydia talks to Jason, who tells her, "No way am I going to a nursing home. I'm going home to my trailer and that's it." Lydia understands the trailer is home to the patient and the only discharge plan up for consideration. She knows her colleagues would tell her to set up a nursing and tell Jason this is the only safe option. Besides, she has other patients to see and can't take the time for complicated discharge arrangements. However, Lydia knows patient competence and self-determination trump a very well-intended physician and team members. 'There has to be another safe option," Lydia thinks to herself.

Jason has a case manager through his health insurance, a large managed care organization (MCO) for the state. Lydia explores the resources in the community, then calls Marco, the case manager at the MCO.

Lydia is able to arrange IV medication management through a clinic down the road from Jason's trailer, including medications and supplies. The clinic has a registered nurse onsite and a separate community-based program to complete needed home visits, referrals, and care coordination with Dr. Jones. Although the clinic is out of network for the MCO, Marco is able to provide approval under the circumstances. He is also able to continue to case manage Jason with the clinic and assure ongoing intervention.

Dr. Jones is thrilled about the plan and tells Lydia, "If this is what case management can do for patients, I'm convinced of its success."

An overreliance on technology also has gross potential to negatively impact a case manager's ability to engage in a meaningful critical thinking process. For example, consider the art of unique patient assessment. Perhaps, the greatest variance of a clinical pathway should be the ability of a case manager to trigger put on his or her CT switch, and then assess the uniqueness of the patient's situation. In this way, individual patient need becomes factored into the process as opposed to allowing autopilot to take charge. Why devalue the unique practitioner CT process, such as how one completes a biopsychosocial–spiritual assessment for a distinct patient and family system? This concept will be further addressed in chapter 13, Big-Picture Orientation.

Analytical

The COLLABORATE approach engages a unique CT model which aligns the pivotal analysis and decision-making elements of professional practice with fundamental action-oriented phases (Treiger & Fink-Samnick, 2013).

CT is integral to EBP, for it allows one to accurately describe to what extent the related underlying research can rigorously test established practice (Gambrill, 2012). Some view CT on par with analytical or **analytic thinking**, though the two have different definitions. Analytic thinking is defined as the abstract separation of a whole into its constituent parts in order to study those parts and their relations (The Free Dictionary by Farlex, 2014). Analytic thinking is involved in many CT models, in that several provide a process for an individual to actually break down complex information or a particular problem, then assess it step by step. This is far more reflective of true CT, which strives to go beyond the black and white of a situation to address the complexity of the gray.

The complexity of CT for case managers is operationalized in Figure 8-6, the **Case Manager's Critical Thinking Gray Zone**. This model draws from Paul's work (cited in Gambrill, 2012), in which he created a list of opposite cognitive forces, which accompany most, if not all, CT efforts experienced by professionals. A high likelihood exists that the list and graphic representation will resonate with every case manager.

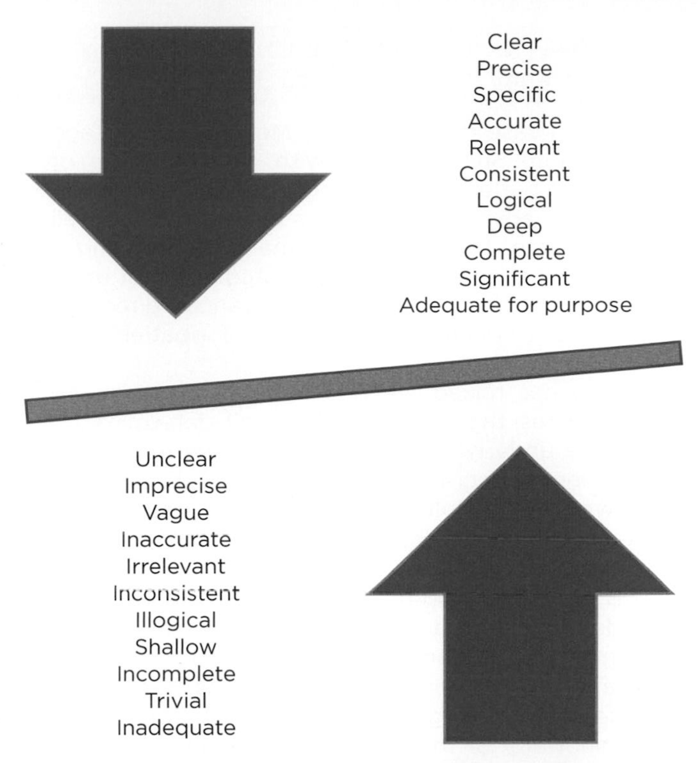

Figure 8-6. A professional case manager's critical thinking gray zone. (Adapted from Paul in Gambrill, E. (2012). *Critical thinking in clinical practice: Improving the quality of judgments and decisions* (3rd ed.). Hoboken, NJ: John Wiley and Sons.)

Methodical

The goal of CT is to approach decision making from a strategic perspective toward the purpose of well-reasoned decisions (Gambrill, 2012). Although there is great variation and perspective in how this approach is implemented, there is consensus on both the merit of templates to this end across health care professional disciplines and on CT's vital role for the industry.

When case managers take the helm with the COLLABORATE approach and CT competency, they gain confidence in having done due diligence with what can present as a complex and overwhelming problem-solving effort. The model in Figure 8-7 operationalizes CT specific to COLLABORATE. A case scenario is provided in Box 8-4 to apply this unique CT

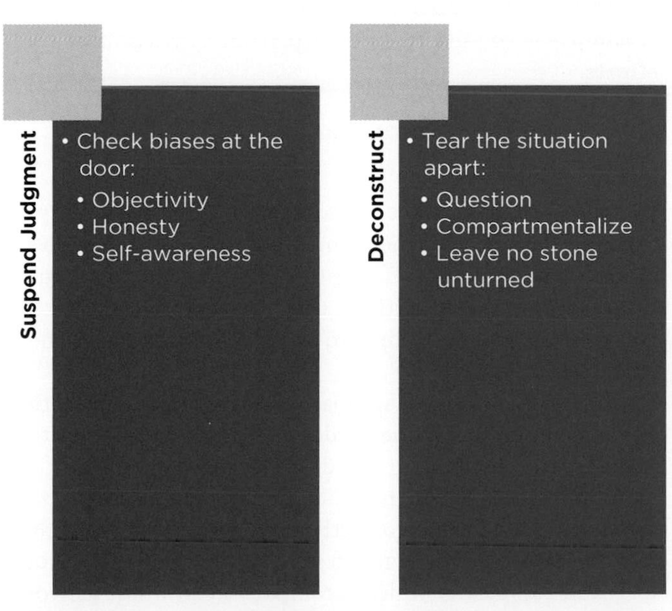

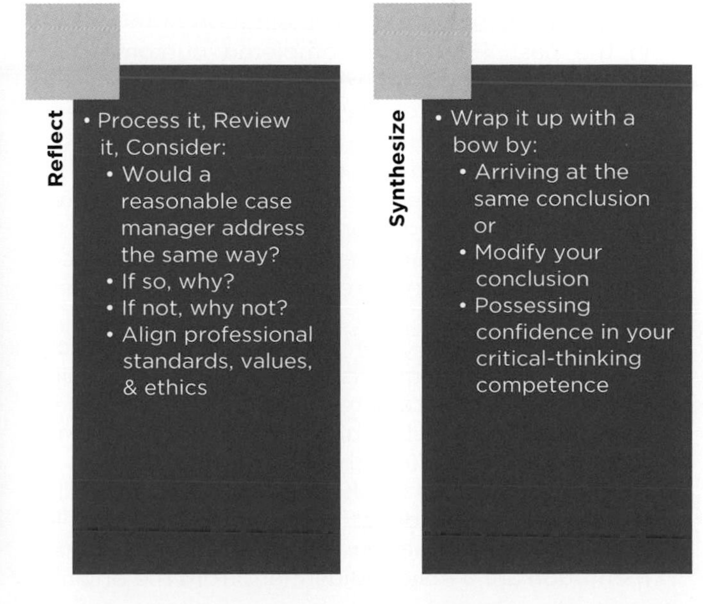

Figure 8-7. Critical thinking for professional case managers.

BOX 8-4 COLLABORATE Critical Thinking Competency in Action: Case Scenario

Julia is a case manager for a Medicare advantage population. She is faced with the challenge of engaging patients in meaningful dialogues to verify that their advanced directives are in place as well as complete. This issue has remained an organizational objective due to Julia's outcomes that demonstrated that the presence of advanced directives translates to decreased utilization of inpatient hospital days.

Julia has mixed feelings about this topic. She appreciates the importance of self-determination and the underlying professional values to support a patient's decision making. However, she also knows how difficult it can be for case managers to broach this topic with some patients and their family members.

The medical director, Dr. Liberio, has asked Julia to develop a proactive plan to assure high compliance with advanced directives. The plan is to expand this program to all populations across clinical resource management department. Considering the enormity of this project, Julia uses a CT template to move forward this process.

Step 1: Suspend judgment—Julia dialogues with her mentor, Miriam, about her personal and professional biases surrounding this topic. Julia verbalizes her frustration that not all her colleagues are as patient as they can be with family members. As tough as this honesty may be, it is essential to assure viewing this situation and the assignment through the most objective framing. A high level of self-awareness is an asset with this step. With a plan in mind, Julia wonders how her bias about the topic itself impacts her intended approach. The importance of the project translates to knowing that a personal perspective is not a welcome visitor to this process.

Step 2: Deconstruct—Julia identifies what challenges have impacted implementation of this effort in the past. Previously completed outcomes are available and reviewed extensively. A questionnaire is then developed to survey her case management colleagues engaged with this population based on the obstacles noted in the outcomes, as well as to obtain their interpretations of the data. A comprehensive and strategic presentation is defined to address vital areas of the project focus, historical challenges, new survey results, and the implementation plan.

Step 3: Reflect—Julia reviews her presentation and plan with Miriam. It is recommended that Julia insert established case management standards as referencing. This will assure professional grounding for her colleagues. Together they revise the plan.

Step 4: Synthesize—Julia is confident due diligence has been done in devising a workable solution to the situation. The timelines for implementation are a major adjustment from the original version though she now feels the preliminary version was related to subjective bias on her part. With this issue, plus other issues fully discussed, Julia is ready to engage purposefully and confidently with this effort.

model. Consider whether or not you would reach the same conclusion as Julia. If you have, then contemplate why this is so. You may come to a different conclusion and should that be the case, make sure to reflect on both why this occurred and exactly what would be done differently.

Whether a case manager utilizes a defined CT model to facilitate his or her thought process such as the one presented, it affords the utilization of a formal framework. This is vital to ensure case managers are proactive, logical, and purposeful in considering the multifaceted and difficult challenges they face in the workplace.

Implication for Practice

CT is core to the case management process. It is aligned in action with evidence-based knowledge and conducted within the ethical and legal realm of a case manager's scope of practice (CMSA, 2010). It has been included as a core competency for implementation (Daniels & Ramey, 2005; Henning & Cohen, 2008). When case managers take the helm with CT, it provides the opportunity to gain confidence in having done due diligence with the full scope of the problem-solving effort.

Skepticism over how to facilitate any component of the case management process accompanies the decision-making process of any professional. A cognitive wrestling match occurs within each case manager's brain as the objective facts of patient's situation come face to face with a subjective emotion being experienced in response. This is where CT achieves it consummate victory as it strategically guides a professional case manager from the fog of the moment to crystal clear conditions and purposeful conviction of their efforts.

SUMMARY

CT serves an integral role as a competency that advances professional case management interventions across the entire practice landscape, including the full scope of roles, functions, and workplace settings. CT is the switch to trigger the mental calisthenics required to engage the case management process.

The COLLABORATE approach calls for CT to be a tactical action. It follows a defined order of cognitive processes that mandate the suspending of judgment, deconstructing of the situation, reflecting on individual actions, then synthesizing thoughts. When done correctly, these processes contribute to propelling case managers from that gray zone of discomfort, and complexity which accompany most if not all workplace situations, to confidence in their CT competence.

References

American Association of Critical-Care Nurses. (2014). *The AACN synergy model for patient care*. Retrieved July 23, 2014, from http://www.aacn.org/wd/certifications/content/synmodel.pcms?menu=

American Sentinel. (2012). Critical nursing can make or break a nursing career. *NurseTogether.com*. Retrieved July 22, 2014, from http://nursetogether.com/critical-thinking-can-make-or-break-a-nursing-career#.UL1i-4ZAOSo

Association of Social Work Boards. (2014). *Exam content outlines*. Retrieved July 25, 2014, from http://www.aswb.org/exam-candidates/about-the-exams/exam-content-outlines/

Barr, H. (1998). Competent to collaborate: Towards a competency-based model for interprofessional education. *Journal of Interprofessional Care, 12*(2), 181–187.

Bernotavicz, F., & Spence, R. (2000). *Report: A competency model for lead case managers integrated case management*. National Child Welfare Resource Center for Organizational Development, Administration for Children, Youth and Families, U.S. Department of Health and Human Services (Grant #90-CT-0001).

Birks, Y. F., & Watt, I. S. (2007). Emotional intelligence and patient-centered care. *Journal of the Royal Society of America, 100*(8), 368–374.

Canadian Interprofessional Health Collaborative. (2007). *A national interprofessional competency framework*. Retrieved June 10, 2014, from http://www. cihc.ca/resources/publications

Case Management Society of America. (2010). *CMSA standards of practice for case management* (Rev.). Retrieved April 10, 2014, from http://www.cmsa.org/portals/0/pdf/memberonly/StandardsOfPractice.pdf

Cohen, E. (2005). *Nursing case management: From essentials to advanced practice applications*. St Louis, MO: Elsevier Health Sciences.

Council for Aid to Education. (2014). *Home page*. Retrieved April 22, 2014, from http://cae.org/about/category/home/

Council on Social Work Education. (2008). *Education policy and accreditation standards (EPAS) implementation*. Retrieved July 20, 2014, from http://www.cswe.org/Accreditation/EPASImplementation.aspx

Council on Social Work Education. (2014). *EPAS revision*. Retrieved August 21, 2014, from http://www.cswe.org/Accreditation/EPASRevision.aspx

Covey, S. (1989). *The seven habits of highly effective people*. New York: Simon & Shuster.

Cunningham, B., & Cesta, T. (2009). *Core skills for hospital case managers: A training toolkit for effective outcomes*. Marblehead, MA: HCPro.

Daniels, S., & Ramey, M. (2005). *The leaders guide to hospital case management*. Sudbury, MA: Jones and Bartlett.

Dewey, J. (1910). *How we think*. Lexington, MA: D.C. Health.

Dunn, L. (2013). Developing healthcare workers' emotional intelligence: Q&A with emotional intelligence coach Harvey Deutschendorf. *Becker's Hospital Review*. Retrieved August 18, 2014, from http://www.beckershospitalreview.com/workforce-labor-management/developing-healthcare-workers-emotional-intelligence-qaa-with-emotional-intelligence-coach-harvey-deutschendorf.html

Edwards, D. F. (1999). The synergy model: Linking patient needs to nurse competencies. *Critical Care Nursing, 19*(1), Retrieved July 29, 2014, from http://www.aacn.org/wd/certifications/content/synpract2.pcms?menu=certification

Elder, L., & Paul, R. (2013). *The thinker's guide to analytical thinking*. Tomales, CA: The Foundation for Critical Thinking.

Facione, P. A. (2015). *Critical thinking: What it is and why it counts*. Retrieved August 21, 2014, from www.insightassessment.com

Facione, P., & Gittens, M. A. (2013). *Think critically* (2nd ed.). Saddle River, NJ: Pearson Education.

Feng, R. C., Chen, M. J., Chen, M. C., & Pai, Y. C. (2010). Critical thinking competence and disposition of clinical nurses in a medical center. *The Journal of Nursing Research, 18*(10), 77–87.

The Foundation for Critical Thinking. (2014a). *A brief history of critical thinking*. Retrieved June 9, 2014, from http://www.criticalthinking.org/pages/a-brief-history-of-the-idea-of-critical-thinking/408

The Foundation for Critical Thinking. (2014b). *Defining critical thinking*. Retrieved May 29, 2014, from http://www.criticalthinking.org/pages/defining-critical-thinking/766

The Foundation for Critical Thinking. (2014c). *Critical thinking development: A stage theory*. Retrieved June 9, 2014, from http://www.criticalthinking.org/pages/critical-thinking-development-a-stage-theory/483

The Foundation for Critical Thinking. (2014d). *The mission*. Retrieved August 22, 2014, from http://www.criticalthinking.org/pages/our-mission/599

The Free Dictionary by Farlex. (2014). *Analytic thinking*. Retrieved August 20, 2014, from http://www.thefreedictionary.com/analytic+thinking

Gamble, M. (2013). How and why emotional intelligence is affecting hospitals' bottom lines. *Becker's Hospital Review*. Retrieved August 18, 2014, from http://www.beckershospitalreview.com/hospital-management-administration/how-and-why-emotional-intelligence-is-affecting-hospitals-bottom-lines.html

Gambrill, E. (2012). *Critical thinking in clinical practice: Improving the quality of judgments and decisions* (3rd ed.). Hoboken, NJ: John Wiley and Sons.

Glaser, E. (1941). *An experiment in the development of critical thinking*. Retrieved July 29, 2014, from https://www.criticalthinking.org/pages/defining-critical-thinking/766

Goleman, D. (2005). *Emotional intelligence: Why it can matter more than IQ* (10th Anniversary ed.). New York, NY: Bantam Books.

Henning, S., & Cohen, E. (2008). The competency continuum: Expanding the case manager's skill set. *Professional Case Management, 13*(3), 127–148.

Hitchens, C. (2005). *Letters to a young contrarian*. Cambridge, MA: Basic Books, Perseus Book Group.

Insight Assessment. (2014). *Expert consensus on critical thinking*. Retrieved August 22, 2014, from http://www.insightassessment.com/CT-Resources/Expert-Consensus-on-Critical-Thinking

Institutes of Medicine. (1999). *To err is human: Building a safer healthcare system*. Washington, DC: National Academies Press.

Institutes of Medicine. (2003). *Health professions' education: A bridge to quality* (The Quality Chasm Series). Washington, DC: National Academies Press.

Interprofessional Education Collaborative. (2011). *Core competencies for interprofessional collaborative practice: Report of an expert panel*. Washington, DC. Retrieved April 30, 2014, from http://www.aacn.nche.edu/news/articles/2011/ipec

Kelley, T. (2003). Critical Thinking and Case Management. *The Case Manager (TCM), 14*(3), 70–72.

Lenburg, C. B. (2005). Nursing case management: From essentials to advanced practice applications. In E. Cohen & T. Cesta. *The competency outcomes and performance assessment model* (chap. 25). St. Louis, MO: Elsevier.

Lenburg, C. B., Klein, C., Abdur-Rahman, V., Spencer, T., & Boyer, S. (2009, September/October). The COPA model: A comprehensive framework designed to promote quality care and competence for patient safety. *Nursing Education Perspectives, 30*(5), 312–317.

Merriam-Webster Online. (2014a). *Subjective*. Retrieved June 3, 2014, from, http://www.merriam-webster.com/dictionary/subjective

Merriam-Webster Online. (2014b). *Objective*. Retrieved June 3, 2014, from, http://www.merriam-webster.com/dictionary/objective

Paul, R. (1992). *Critical thinking: What every person needs to survive in a rapidly changing world* (rev. 2nd ed.). San Rosa, CA: Foundation for Critical Thinking.

Paul, in The Foundation for Critical Thinking (2014). *Critical thinking and nursing*. Retrieved July 23, 2014, from http://www.criticalthinking.org/pages/critical-thinking-and-nursing/834

Powell, S. K., & Tahan, H. A. (2008). *Case management society of America (CMSA) core curriculum for case management* (2nd ed.). Philadelphia: Lippincott Williams & Wilkins.

Rubenfeld, M. G., & Scheffer, B. (2015). *Critical thinking TACTICS for nurses: Achieving the IOM competencies* (3rd ed.). Burlington, MA: Jones and Bartlett.

Scheffer, B. K., & Rubenfeld, M. G. (2000). A consensus statement of critical thinking in nursing. *Journal of Nursing Education*, *39*(8), 352–359.

Simpson, E., & Courtney, M. (2002). Critical thinking in nursing education: A literature review. *International Journal of Nursing Practice*, *8*(2), 89–98.

Tempera, J. (2013). Post-college exam seeks to determine employability. *USA Today*. Retrieved May 30, 2014, from http://www.usatoday.com/story/news/nation/2013/08/29/learning-assessment-plus-test-colleges-employers/2726031

TestPrep-Online. (2014). *Watson-Glaser critical thinking appraisal:How to prepare?* Retrieved August 20, 2014, from http://www.testprep-online.com/watson-glaser-test.aspx

Think Watson. (2014). *The gold standard critical thinking test*. Retrieved August 20, 2014, from http://www.thinkwatson.com/assessments/watson-glaser

Treiger, T., & Fink-Samnick, E. (2013). COLLABORATE©: A universal competency-based paradigm for professional case management, part II: Competency clarification. *Professional Case Management*, *18*(5), 219–243.

Victor-Chmil, J. (2013). Clinical thinking versus clinical reasoning versus clinical judgment. *Nurse Educator*, *38*(1), 34–36.

Walker, S. (2003). Active learning strategies to promote critical thinking. *Journal of Athletic Training*, *38*(3) 263–267.

Ward, K. (2012). *Critical thinking: How to improve your decision-making skills*. King of Prussia, PA: HRDQ.

Zori, S., & Morrison, B. (2009). Critical thinking in nurse managers. *Nursing Economics*, *27*(2). Retrieved on June 2, 2014, from http://www.medscape.com/viewarticle/707855_3

9 OUTCOMES-DRIVEN

OBJECTIVES

After studying this chapter, you will be able to:

1. Define basic terminology and concepts relating to outcomes-driven case management practice.
2. Outline the important aspects that need to be taken into consideration when evaluating case management-related research and evidence.
3. Define the steps associated with critical appraisal and apply to case management research.
4. Provide historical and environmental factors that influence the development of consistent case management performance outcomes.
5. Describe the domains and attributes associated with case management outcomes.
6. Discuss the importance of using a SMART approach to patient goal setting.
7. Demonstrate how practice and accreditation standards influence outcomes-driven case management.

KEY TERMS

Baseline
Benchmarking
Council for Case Management Accountability
Critical appraisal
Evidence-based practice
Metric
Outcome
Outcomes management
Research
SMART
Target

The case manager's ability to affect client health in measurable ways has been a topic of debate. Practitioners see the impact on their client's lives on a daily basis. However, the translation from frontline effort to bottom-line results has been difficult to capture, in part due to the misapplication of the job title to include positions that are heavily weighted with utilization review responsibilities combined with a lack of clear industry-wide definition as to consistent case management accountability and outcomes measurement.

A case manager's value to a client, as well as to an organization, is as meaningful as the measuring stick used. If one uses a ruler rather than a yardstick to measure cloth, there is a great risk of inaccuracy if having to measure out many yards of fabric. Along the same line, using ill-suited means to quantify and/or qualify case management value all but assures erroneous results. Application of the wrong metrics may mislead attention from the actual derived benefits to less meaningful statistics (e.g., case closure counts) which do not reflect case complexity, level of effort, impact on client condition, or improved quality of life.

Having an outcome-orientation evidences itself differently at various levels of health care bureaucracy. At the client level, it influences individualized assessment and goal planning. Case management performance expectations affect and results influence compensation and professional growth. A department's outcomes dictate regulatory compliance and accreditation status. At the systems level, research and research utilization are considered so important that they stand as a practice standard (Case Management Society of America [CMSA], 2010). However, a practice standard is not a performance mandate unless it comes with the force of legal ramifications. Unfortunately, no formal agreement exists amongst case management stakeholders as to best practice for measuring outcomes and utilization of research findings is ill-defined.

It is incumbent on every professional case manager to understand how outcomes relate to and demonstrate case management's overall contribution to the equation of health care delivery (e.g., client health, organizational viability, health care quality). From an organizational chart perspective, case management placement is frequently consumed under the umbrella of medical management programs. This is one point at which differentiation can be clearly illustrated. As previously noted by Fetterolf (2010), case management programs are materially different from standard medical management or disease management programs in a number of ways. The patients have complex medical conditions, combined with many other variables, that tend to increase their costs and patterns of utilization. Because of the wide-ranging clinical and cost variation of individuals participating in case management programs across the continuum of care, there are clear challenges as to a standard return on investment methodology (Fetterolf, 2010).

The case manager collaborates with the health care team to incorporate best practices; assesses outcomes at the level of the individual and the point of service; and designs, monitors, evaluates, and manages aggregate outcomes at the macrosystems level, as a case management administrator. The skills set for different case management roles must be cultivated through formal education and ongoing professional development (Stanton & Packa, 2010). This chapter delves into this topic to highlight the importance of possessing outcomes-driven competence.

DEFINITION

Before going further, it is important to provide the definitions of frequently used terminology pertaining to this case management model to ensure clarity and maximize understanding. As pointed out in chapter 3, the lack of consistent definition results in confusion and misapplication of terms and their use. Consequently, outcomes that do not clearly articulate the use of terminology should be suspect as to their implications to practice. Case management means different things to different audiences. At this time, because of the absence of industry agreement as to a unified definition, every mention of the term *case management* should include a defining statement as to the author(s) use of the term. That backdrop raises the importance to be clear as to the intent of terms in this text.

Outcome

The Agency for Healthcare Research and Quality (2014) defines an **outcome** as the result of health care practices. Outcomes demonstrate the effectiveness of an intervention (or lack thereof) and may indicate the need for change. The value-add of an entity (or intervention) arises from a collection of outcomes, not from activities and processes (Chatterjee, 1998). Outcome measurements include, but are not limited to, principles of continuous quality/performance improvement, use of benchmarks, analysis of trends, incorporation of evidence-based practice, processes that promote the understanding of current condition, outcomes, and the examination of return on investment related to a specific intervention (Zander, 2008).

The outcomes movement draws from four techniques: a greater reliance on standards and guidelines; the routine and systematic interval measures of patient function and well-being, associated with disease-specific clinical outcomes; pooled clinical and outcome data; and appropriate results from the database analyzed and disseminated in order to meet each decision maker's needs (American College of Emergency Physicians, 2013).

As pertains to case management, an outcome is the measurable result of an intervention or action taken in the accomplishment of a task or goal relating to the case management plan. The array of outcomes include, but are not limited to, access, experience, knowledge, adherence, functional ability, and customer satisfaction (CMSA, 2010). An outcome may be the result or consequence of the care received or that which was not received (Powell & Tahan, 2008).

Metric

A **metric** is a gauge to measure things such as efficiency, performance, progress, quality, or process (The Business Dictionary.com, 2014). Metrics relate to, but are not the same as, objectives. An objective is a target, whereas a metric is the indicator of whether we are achieving the objective (Okes, 2013). Reliable metrics are required to examine whether targets are met and to assess impact on the provision of services (Stevens, Stokes, & O'Mahony, 2006). In the business world, sustained success of a company depends on executing a superior strategy within an organization. This and overall objectives are achieved through constant monitoring, evaluating, and modification (Askar, Iman, & Prabhaker, 2009). Along this theme of continuous evolution, business priorities continue to shape health care to more refined and accountable care models; however, not all of health care moves at the same speed of change. In many instances, institutions with larger bandwidth for managing change take the lead, while smaller provider practices implement less costly, and at times less impactful, models of care.

On point with distinguishing the difference in terms, it is important to note the differentiation of a metric from a measure. This is not to say that the same definitions apply to the use of this terminology. This point becomes clear in some of the referenced works within this text. A measure is how we use some standard way or tool to determine a value. For instance, we use a thermometer to measure temperature. A metric is a calculated value in which a formula combines numbers to create it. The heat index is a metric, which takes into account factors such as heat, humidity, and wind (Lee, 2013).

Metrics provide tangible value with significance at different organizational levels. A strategic metric looks at overall company performance (e.g., market share, sales, new product launches). An operational-level metric demonstrates achievement of objectives of importance to the frontline (e.g., error rates, cycle time). The impact of a metric may have meaning internally and/or externally to the organization (e.g., consumer, staff member, stockholder). Sharing significance of effort through metrics connects those associated with the product/process with a common element, the desire to improve and be successful.

There are various types of metrics, and the terminology used to describe them is helpful to understand. Okes's (2013) similar but different pairings (Table 9-1) distinguish these intricacies. The bottom line is that an organization, department, or individual shall understand their core business and responsibilities in order to identify the metrics that are most useful to demonstrating that efforts are paying off.

To that point, a common problem is the selection of metrics that are easier to calculate, rather than those that are strategically useful or demonstrative of real value (Okes, 2013). Another pitfall is having too many metrics; more is not necessarily better, nor are a multitude of metrics reflective of better business practice. In some instances, redundancy causes confusion and forces those on the receiving end of reports to create their own interpretations as to meaning and business performance (Lee, 2013). One must consider the paradoxical effect of too much information. If the continuous stream of numbers and graphical representations become more of a nuisance than a benefit, the risk of shutting down the inflow increases. End users will simply shut off the source. On the other hand, there is a risk associated with having too few metrics. The company monitoring too few metrics is like a boat in the middle of the ocean, minus navigating instruments (Lee, 2013).

In case management, the number of closed cases per case manager is an easy metric to collect, but it does little to give the organization an understanding of the level of effort required or of consumer satisfaction with the outcome. If a key metric within an organization is the case closure rate, one must consider the internal definition of the term *case* and *case management* as well as the service being performed. Is the work performed actually more of a utilization management–focused function? If it is bona fide case management, what useful snapshot does case closure rate portray in terms of the value of the intervention, and are there other measures which provide a balanced perspective as to case management's overall effort and/or value?

There are different levels of metrics. A metric may be primary or advanced. Primary metrics address the results you intend to produce and the value provided to others, and support alignment of effort, accountability, monitoring, and reporting. Within this category fall customer service, productivity, and cost savings. Advanced metrics highlight work processes and capabilities of an organization. These metrics support efficiency and future planning. Cycle time, defect reduction, productivity, and organizational agility are examples of advanced metrics (Frost, 2000).

Transparency in the collection and reporting of metrics promotes accountability in care access, quality, and cost. However, if a metric is ill-suited to be a gauge of demonstrating success associated with stated objectives, then transparency becomes moot. The shared results are ultimately irrelevant to that which the audience seeks to understand.

Baseline

A **baseline** is the measurement that establishes current or existing performance (Spitzer, 2007). Baseline data are necessary in order to understand what is currently taking place in an organization. Examination of baseline data contributes to the decision-making process as to what, if any, change is necessary to improve (e.g., productivity, quality). When considering a new metric, it is customary to collect baseline data in order to establish a starting point prior to instituting a change in process. The case example (Box 9-1) amplifies on the use of baselines in case management.

TABLE 9-1 Okes's Similar but Different Terminology of Metrics

External: Evaluates trends/environmental feedback	Internal: How well an organization uses its resources
Effectiveness: How well an organization satisfies stakeholders	Efficiency: How well an organization uses its resources
Leading: Predicts future outcomes	Lagging: Measures past activity outcomes
Outcomes: Focuses on end-of-process results	Controls: Used to adjust or stabilize performance of the process itself
Monitoring: Long-term measures associated with performance management	Diagnostic (ad hoc): Short-term measures used to assess/solve specific problem(s)
Objective: Easily quantified items	Subjective: Less quantifiable measures (e.g., customer satisfaction)

Adapted from Okes, D. (2013). Performance metrics—The levers for process management. Milwaukee, WI: Quality Press.

BOX 9-1 Baseline and the New System Implementation

In order to evaluate the successful installation and use of the information system software, the case management department manager decides to collect user and usage data. Productivity reports within the previous system were limited; however, information regarding user output and use is available. Prior to system installation, all users receive training appropriate to their role. In addition, a vendor representative remains onsite following implementation to conduct refresher training, provided one-on-one guidance, and troubleshoot end-user issues.

The 3-month period following installation is defined the "introductory phase." During this time, staff acclimates to the new system and associated processes. Although a few reports are generated and progress is observed, it is recognized that there is a learning curve during which users develop system fluency. Following this period, a 2-week period is designated as a data collection interval. During this interval, users are assessed for baseline operator proficiency. This sets each user's baseline as to system proficiency and productivity. This represents the first evaluation as to the extent that anticipated gains from the previous to the new information system were realized. Subsequent data collection intervals tracked additional gains in efficiency as measured against an agreed-upon acceptable range. Evaluation of the information produced during these measurement periods produces metrics that are used to demonstrate user and department performance.

With regard to client goals, having a baseline provides a starting point from which an individual's progress may be measured. For example, Donald is a newly discharged person diagnosed with chronic obstructive pulmonary disease. Barriers to Donald's self-care include dyspnea and shortness of breath on exertion. The case manager requests that spirometry testing be performed at his first follow-up office appointment in order to objectively measure pulmonary function. This test shall be repeated intermittently to gauge Donald's pulmonary status.

Target

Simply put, a **target** is a desired level of performance as defined by an organization or individual. Examples of targets include specifications, control limits, and organizational process objectives (Okes, 2013). An important consideration in target setting is that it be reasonably attainable. Setting a target that is impossible to achieve may look impressive at face value, but setting an individual or department up for failure is both demoralizing and demotivating.

For the case manager, a target (or goal) may come into play when working with an individual on a recovery path. Generally, a target sets interim and/or end-result expectations toward which to strive. The key is that the target is clear, specific, reasonably achievable for the given situation, and agreed upon by the client and care team. For example, Bob Jones is on a return-to-work trajectory. He must achieve specific functional targets in order to resume his regular work. In conjunction with his health care provider, the worker's compensation case manager coordinates therapy and other care to facilitate resuming regular work duties. Sadie Simpler is recovering from a sports-related knee injury. Her health plan case manager evaluates her progress in functional ability against targets to evaluate progress. Based on measurable improvement, the case manager approves continued outpatient physical therapy visits.

A target may be set as part of a quality improvement initiative (e.g., gain in productivity, error reduction rate). For example, the case management director at a small health plan recently instituted a new after-hours workflow. A spike in emergency department (ED) usage triggered a process review. The investigation revealed some individuals had self-referred to the ED after a failed attempt to call the after-hours program. In tracing the problem backwards, it was learned that calls were being forwarded to a nonworking telephone number. A contributing factor to ED misuse was an incorrect number programmed into the telecommunication system. This resulted in member frustration, unnecessary emergency room visits, and at least one hospital admission. The contact number was correctly programmed. Upon activation of the new workflow, a target set was for no ED self-referrals for individuals calling the after-hours program. In subsequent data collection, performance met the target.

Benchmarking

Benchmarking is a performance improvement method involving measurement of an organization's internal processes followed by identifying, understanding, and adapting outstanding practices from other organizations considered to be best-in-class (The Benchmarking Exchange, 2013). It is the comparison of an organization's practices and performance against those of other companies. A benchmark seeks to identify standards, or "best practices," to apply in measuring and improving performance (Management Analysis and Budget, 2014). It is a search for the best practices that lead to performance improvement. It is a way to establish operating targets based on constantly reviewed and updated best practices (Camp, 1989). To muddy the water a bit, a benchmark may also be used as a target if it is determined that the performance level is a desirable goal to set for performance improvement.

Research

The dictionary definition of **research** is a careful study that is done to find and report new knowledge about something (Merriam-Webster, 2014). Camwell (2014) describes research as a systematic, planned, investigation of a specified problem, with a predetermined outcome, which will contribute to our understanding of the phenomena in question. As pertains to outcomes, research examines the goals of health care itself (e.g., improved functional status, quality of life) by examination of patient-level care and system-level environment as influences on the endpoint(s) (Huber, 2010). Outcomes research aims to understand the results of health care practices and interventions.

The CMSA's (2010) final practice standard is research and research utilization. It is stated that the case manager maintains familiarity with current research findings and be able to apply them, as appropriate, in his or her practice as evidenced by familiarity with current literature, compliance with legitimate and relevant research efforts, incorporation of meaningful research into individual practice, and identification of practical best practices. A review of case/care management practice standards of the American Case Management Association (2013) or the National Association of Professional Geriatric Care Managers (2013) did not reveal research-specific guidance. However, the National Association of Social Workers' (2013) Standards for Social Work Case Management highlight practice evaluation and improvement as the expectation that the social work case manager participates in ongoing, formal evaluation of her or his practice to maximize client well-being, assess appropriateness and effectiveness of services, ensure competence, and improve practice (2013).

Case managers have an opportunity to use and change practice, based on research-generated evidence in current literature. Often case managers are working with population aggregates, disease management groups, or cohorts of patients who can benefit immensely by using best evidence or practices in terms of care coordination (Stanton & MacRobert, 2007).

Evidence

As Winston Churchill said, "However beautiful the strategy, you should occasionally look at the results." Evidence is proof of success (or failure) related to an intervention or action. Where current case management is concerned, organizations look to evidence (also known as results) to justify investment in case management resources (e.g., staff, information systems). As has been acknowledged, some measurements may not indicate the actual impact of case management intervention, so it behooves leadership to step back from the "plan" and consider if actions demonstrate the intended result. Taking time to evaluate results at regular intervals ensures the right interventions have the intended impact at regular intervals and to that action be taken to adjust one's approach if that is not the case.

One such use of evidence requires keeping abreast of research. For instance, a comparative effectiveness report published by the AHRQ, Outpatient Case Management for Adults with Medical Illness and Complex Care Needs provides evidence, which may be useful to reshaping case management definition where research and evidence-based practice is concerned. The report focuses on this single segment of practice and specific questions pertaining to case management as an intervention strategy for chronic illness outpatient management. In their findings, it is clearly noted that there was a wide diversity in the included study populations, interventions, and outcomes. That notwithstanding, the overall conclusion was case management demonstrated limited impact on patient-centered outcomes, quality of care, and resource utilization among patients with chronic medical illness (Hickam et al., 2013). A use of these findings to identify and implement program modifications is one way in which research-generated evidence may influence practice.

Regardless of application, a point to keep in mind is that past performance does not assure future success (or failure). Evidence must be applied judiciously while taking into consideration forward-looking and continuously changing variables, such as environmental changes, program scope, and other important influences, in order to duplicate results and maximize benefit.

PAST AND CURRENT THINKING

Historically, outcomes were considered a patient-centric measure of case management intervention. In 2000, Powell pointed out that case managers were just beginning to add an outcomes manager role to their scope of practice. Today, the expectation of having an outcomes-driven orientation is noted by the increasing inclusion of the expectation in case management job descriptions and as an integral part of performance management expectations. Case managers are accountable for case management outcomes and case management interventions drive outcomes.

The historic perspective on case management outcomes pointed toward volume-related statistics including, but not limited to, cases opened or closed, cost–benefit derivation, and return-to-work rate. Other measures that attached themselves to proving the value of case management included length of stay, emergency room usage, and cost of care. Many of these measures were a result of utilization management efforts more so than case management intervention. The misapplication of the case manager job title contributed to blurring the attribution of the results to activities not solely specific to case management.

While qualitative measures serve as part of care plan implementation and monitoring tools, objective measures (e.g., functional ability) were not routinely integrated into case management plans as a means to assess the impact of case management involvement in patient care. This may be related to the reality that there are numerous influences relating to improvement or decline in any given measure. It is important to recognize that any measure selected as a scale for monitoring progress be based on that which is within the case manager's scope of responsibility to impact. The degree to which case management should be held accountable for any measure should be tempered by their relative impact of their interventions. Would functional ability be a fair assessment of case management value? Perhaps this is specific to

TABLE 9-2 Case Management-Influenced Outcomes

Quality	Access to Care	Safety	Cost
Case managers have the capacity to balance quality and cost in many health care settings, and particularly in the case management of patients with chronic health problems near the end of life. (Stanton & Packa, 2010)	... there is ample evidence of the need for professional case managers to undertake a care coordination role to improve delivery of health services to patients. (Consornery-Fairnot & Serbin, 2012)	Case management administrators at this level perform root cause analysis to protect patient safety and deal with medical issues and provide the performance indicators or "dashboard" for monitoring at the point of service or care. (Smith, 2008)	Outcomes at the organizational level include: aggregate clinical; functional; and quality outcomes; as well as costs of care; lengths of stay; re-hospitalizations; use of acute services; cost benefit; return on investment; and satisfaction rates for different patient populations. (Lehrman, Gimbel, Freedman, Savicki, & Tackley, 2002)

the setting of care and relationship of the case manager to the client. Table 9-2 provides examples of case management's influence over outcomes. These, and similar, may be considered as a means for demonstrating case management impact. However, quantifying case management's influence of measures, such as mentioned above, requires additional study.

Satisfaction scales for assessing case management services, similar to Likert, have been employed sporadically. These tools have shortcomings, including, but not limited to, specificity to the sponsoring organization, inconsistent administration techniques, and inclusion of generic queries not specific to case management. Due to the design of these tools, as well as the lack of uniform case management practice, it has been impossible to generalize the results. This continues to be an evidence gap, for demonstrating case management value.

Case Management Outcomes Accountability

There was a promising initiative in the area of case management outcomes, the **Council for Case Management Accountability** (CCMA). Organized around 1996, CCMA recognized the importance of establishing evidence-based measures consistent with the CMSA Standards of Case Management Practice. The purpose of CCMA was to establish a framework for case management accountability on which case managers and clients could agree. The framework would establish mutually agreed-upon expectations relating to case management achievement as well as how it would be demonstrated. CCMA held promise as a means to facilitate consumer-informed decision making regarding purchasing and utilization of case management services (Hamilton, 1999; Braeden, 2002). Its goals were to provide a framework for measuring accountability by providing the methodology for data collection and documentation of results, and thus demonstrating value to establish a standard for assessing the value of case management, and finally to provide the information necessary to identify best practice and thereby improve the delivery of case management services (CCMA, 1999).

Due to a lack of accessible documentation and continuing activity, researching the work of CCMA proves difficult. However, three State of the Science (SoS) documents were published on the topics of patient adherence, involvement/participation, empowerment, and knowledge, and finally care coordination. Within these documents, one finds an addendum which provides a high-level overview of the Council's intended work. Unfortunately, following the publication of the SoS documents, there was apparently no substantive work published by the Council.

The Triple Aim

The focus on outcomes raises the urgency on having knowledge and ability to apply an outcomes-driven mentality to case management intervention in a consistent manner. Understanding the basics of outcomes and quality management guides both operational and patient-specific case management efforts. The overarching principles for high-quality care are relatable to the Triple Aim.

Developed at the Institute for Healthcare Improvement (IHI), the Triple Aim is a framework describing an approach to optimize health system performance. Key to this framework is the belief that improvements in health care design must address three important dimensions of care delivery. As identified by Berwick et al. (2008), these dimensions of care—quality, access, and cost—make up the Triple Aim of:

- Improving the patient experience of care (including quality and satisfaction);
- Improving the health of populations; and
- Reducing the per capita cost of health care.

To understand the genesis for the Triple Aim, it is important to place context as to how it came about. Efforts to define shortcomings in the U.S. health care system coalesced in the landmark publication of *To Err Is Human: Building a Better Healthcare System* in 2000 (Institute of Medicine, 2000) and *Crossing the Quality Chasm: A New Health System for the 21st Century* in 2001 (Institute of Medicine, 2001).

The former defined the safety and quality crisis within the U.S. health care system, and the latter provided a means for addressing its dangerous shortcomings.

Achieving the Triple Aim requires simultaneous pursuit of improving the experience of care delivery, improving the health of aggregate populations, and reducing the cost of care. This aligns with the foci of 21st century care outlined by the Institutes of Medicine (2001) as key dimensions defining that health care should be safe, effective, patient-centered, timely, efficient, and equitable (Box 9-2). Movement to a more quality-driven system continues through public quality reporting (e.g., Hospital Compare), demonstration projects (e.g., Premier Hospital Quality Incentive Demonstration), and incentive programs (e.g., Medicare and Medicaid Electronic Health Records (EHR) Incentive Programs).

However, the task of improving individuals' care remains incomplete. In addition to the previously acknowledged barriers to achieving truly safe and effective care, there is a tenuous relationship existing between the politics and philosophical underpinnings of health care. As was pointedly identified, "The remaining barriers to integrated care are not technical; they are political" (Berwick et al., 2008). One only need look at the partisanship demonstrated during the passage and implementation of the Patient Protection and Affordable Care Act (PPACA), also referred to as the Affordable Care Act (ACA) or Obamacare, to observe the political divide over health care in the United States.

The goals of the ACA are to provide consumer protections, improve quality and affordability of care, increase access to affordable care options, and increase insurer accountability. Its passage is an historic landmark when one considers the successive federal administrations, starting with Truman, who failed to pass comprehensive health care reforms (Sultz & Young, 2014). The ACA is also historic, in that it succeeded in addressing the three most problematic areas—quality, access, and cost—which the health care industry has been unable, or unwilling, to manage.

BOX 9-2 Institute of Medicine Health Care Dimensions

Safe

Avoiding injuries to patients from the care that is intended to help them

Effective

Providing services based on scientific knowledge to all who could benefit and refraining from providing services to those not likely to benefit (avoiding underuse and overuse, respectively)

Patient-Centered

Providing care that is respectful of and responsive to individual patient preferences, needs, and values and ensuring that patient values guide all clinical decisions

Timely

Reducing waits and sometimes harmful delays for both those who receive and those who give care

Efficient

Avoiding waste, including waste of equipment, supplies, ideas, and energy

Equitable

Providing care that does not vary in quality because of personal characteristics such as gender, ethnicity, geographic location, and socioeconomic status

Adapted from Institute of Medicine. (2001). Crossing the quality chasm: A new health system for the 21st century. Washington, DC: National Academy Press.

Outcomes Management

Ellwood (1988) initially offered the concept of **outcomes management**. In setting the tone of his proposal, Ellwood (1988) stated that health care was an organism guided by misguided choices relating to the divergent and conflicting perspectives of stakeholders each holding that their primary concern was for the patient. He goes on to define outcomes management as "a technology of patient experience, designed to help patients, payers, and providers make rational, medical care-related choices based on better insight into the effect of these choices on the patient's life."

As pertains to case management, Wojner's (2001) perspective is applicable to nursing when providing the following case management definition parameters:

- A process of sophisticated outcomes management and measurement
- Interdisciplinary primary nursing care
- A technology of patient experience designed to help patients, payers, and providers make rational care-related choices
- A nursing process supported by the principles of autonomy, accountability, authority, and financial advocacy

Subsequently, Wojner defined outcomes management with the following parameters:

- Synonymous with nursing case management
- A research-based process that complements and drives a grass-roots case management initiative
- A mechanism to support payer-driven health care systems
- A second-generation primary nursing

Although this text does not use the above definition of case management, the detail is intended to provide perspective as to the development of outcomes management theory. The value of outcomes management is that providers may bring best practice to life through provision of care that has been validated through research, which contributes to reduction of health care cost (Wojner, 2001).

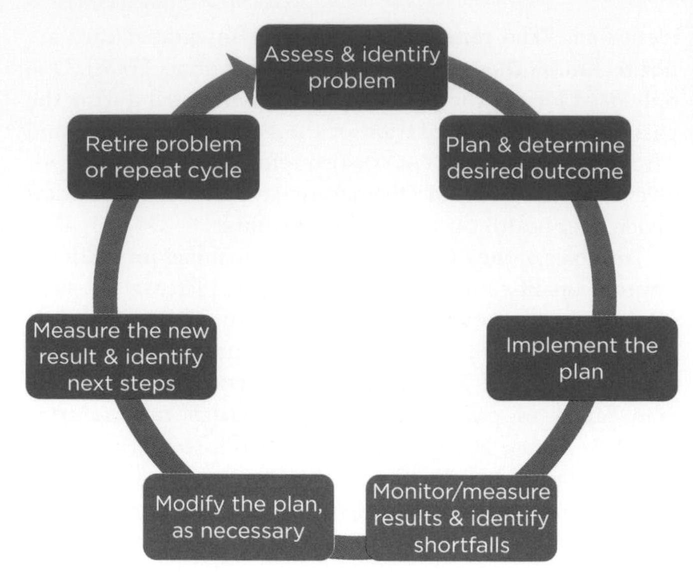

Figure 9-1. Outcomes management in action.

Another perspective of outcomes management relates that there is one reason for measuring and monitoring client outcomes and that is to use the feedback to modify intervention plan as it unfolds, thereby improving the quality of the plan, as well as the impact/outcome for the client (Orme & Combs-Orme, 2012). Rather than setting a specific course, implementing interventions, and waiting to see what transpires, outcomes management dictates that modifications to the original plan should be made that will ultimately bring about a better outcome than would have been observed had no adjustment been implemented. This approach allows for a more effective and efficient case management intervention as demonstrated in Figure 9-1.

The Conundrum of Capturing Case Management Value

How might case management's value best be assessed and demonstrated? There has been no clear case management industry consensus as to case management's definition, value, or standardized ways to measure value. As was previously noted, the AHRQ evidence review of outpatient case management impact clearly stated that case management demonstrated limited impact, which was related to the wide variances in the application of terms.

Indicators have been applied as a means of providing medical management outcomes. Powell (2000) provided case management outcome domains (Boxes 9-3 through 9-5). Howe and Greenberg (2005) outlined a knowledge attribute framework (Boxes 9-6 through 9-10) for various case management functional domains. Fetterolf (2010) recognized that case management programs are materially different from standard medical management or disease management programs including condition complexity, program specialization, and relatively small targeted population (1%–5% of membership). However, he identified major categories that although used to evaluate medical management programs, were more focused on case management cost drivers fall into categories of activity/operational, clinical quality indicators, clinical utilization, financial, and other metrics (e.g., quality-of-life improvement, patient satisfaction).

BOX 9-3 Powell's Case Management Clinical and Financial Economic Outcomes Domains

Clinical

(CM facilitated appropriate clinical outcomes in collaboration with multidisciplnary team)

- Management of the therapeutic regimen
- Appropriateness of clinical care
- Necessity of ED visit
- Disease-specific complications, exacerbations, and comorbidities
- Adverse drug reactions
- Infection rate
- Unscheduled return to the ED within 72 hours
- Delay in diagnosing condition
- Readmission
- Complication of procedure/therapy
- Disease condition present in acute care or skilled nursing care

Financial/Economic

(CM facilitated appropriate resource utilization and management)

- Length of stay
- Facilitated change in level of care
- Facilitated change to contracted provider/facility
- Facilitated appropriate number of days (acute, postacute, skilled, home care)
- Facilitated productivity
- Facilitated reduction of disease exacerbation
- Facilitated adherence to therapeutic regimen
- Negotiated rates of service/equipment
- Negotiated intensity of service/equipment
- Negotiated frequency/duration of service/equipment
- Provided assessment of equipment "rent vs. buy"
- Avoided inappropriate/ineffective services
- Avoided insurance denial

Adapted from Powell, S. K. (2000). Advanced case management: outcomes and beyond. Baltimore, MD: Lippincott, Williams & Wilkins.

DISCUSSION OF KEY ELEMENTS

Key elements of the outcomes-driven competency include:

- Client
- Strategic goal setting
- Evidence-based practice

BOX 9-4 Powell's Case Management Humanistic and Quality Outcomes Domains

Humanistic

- Facilitated recovery of functional status
- Facilitated improved patient comfort through effective pain/symptom management
- Facilitated improved quality of life for the patient as evidenced by satisfaction with CM services
- Facilitated caregiver well-being
- Facilitated improved level of physical independence
- Facilitated improved cognitive performance
- Facilitated employability
- Facilitated psychosocial adjustment/coping with life changes
- Facilitated patient/family satisfaction
- Facilitated provider satisfaction
- Facilitated payer satisfaction
- CM satisfaction
  - Job
  - Roles
  - Case load
  - Autonomy
  - Ethical dilemmas
  - Challenging cases
  - Adequate training

Quality Outcomes

- Facilitated access to health care/avoidance of delay in services
- Facilitated reduced mortality and morbidity
- Facilitated prevention of adverse occurrences
- Facilitated improved compliance with organizational standards/guidelines
- Facilitated decreased fragmentation of care/services
- Recognized important psychosocial need/risk
- Recognized important clinical need/risk
- Facilitated health-seeking behavior
- Facilitated compliance issues (patient and provider)
- Facilitated patient self-care

Adapted from Powell, S. K. (2000). Advanced case management: outcomes and beyond. Baltimore, MD: Lippincott, Williams & Wilkins.

BOX 9-5 Powell's Case Management Organizational/Administrative/Systems Outcomes Domain

- Facilitated assessment of patient/family support/financial/psychosocial/insurance benefits
- Facilitated coordination and development of case management plans and services
- Facilitated education of patient/significant other/family
- Facilitated appropriate monitoring, reassessment, and reevaluation of cases
- Facilitated appropriate discharge planning/changing levels of care
- Facilitated appropriate utilization management/resource management
- Facilitated appropriate clinical activities for each patient
- Facilitated improved organizational communication on outcomes data, plans for improvement
- Facilitated appropriate use of on-site vs. telephonic case management services
- Facilitated the reconsideration process when necessary
- Facilitated expedited appeals process when necessary
- Facilitated standard appeals process when necessary
- Facilitated appropriate referrals to hospice, SNF, rehabilitation, home health
- Facilitated increased health plan membership retention rate (relatable to customer satisfaction)
- Facilitated member satisfaction with networks provided
- Facilitated patient access to providers/services
- CM records are accurate and complete
- Facilitated appropriate length of case management services
- Facilitated high confidentiality standards
- Facilitated appropriate CM problem identification
- Provided appropriate CM educational material/instruction
- Facilitated availability of inpatient and outpatient services (rehabilitation)
- Reduced delay in diagnosis condition
- Facilitated timeliness of CM intervention
- Facilitated appropriate use of "reasons for case closure"
- Facilitated appropriateness of discharges or referrals
- Facilitated beneficiary retention

Adapted from Powell, S. K. (2000). Advanced case management: outcomes and beyond. Baltimore, MD: Lippincott, Williams & Wilkins.

Client

The COLLABORATE perspective focuses on client outcomes. The outcomes-driven case manager contributes interventions which aim to maximize client health, function, and wellness. This approach is at the heart of the case management philosophy. When an individual reaches an optimum level of wellness and functional capability, everyone benefits (CMSA, 2010). As pertains to the practice standard,

BOX 9-6 Howe and Greenberg's Case Management Attributes in the Assessment Domain

- Know a particular disease/clinical expertise
- Accurately assess patient status and functioning
- Possess clinically relevant technical skills
- Collect, analyze, and synthesize data
- Develop specific markers to track patient progress
- Act as a change agent by assessing relevant systems and organizations
- Continuously monitor the quality of care and make appropriate adjustment to the care plan
- Monitor the delivery of services to patient
- Identify patient needs and issues
- Assess clinical, social, or other patient needs
- Assess caregiver or family needs
- Determine the type and level of cultural influences on client
- Identify and acknowledge the client's belief or value system
- Identify potential barriers to client goals or treatment plan
- Reassess plan of care
- Maintain accurate and detailed records

Adapted from Howe, R., & Greenberg, L. (2005). Performance management for case management: principles and objectives for developing standard measures. Case Manager, 16, 52–56.

BOX 9-7 Howe and Greenberg's Case Management Attributes in the Planning Domain

- Educate patient, family, and other providers
- Provide consultation to patients
- Utilize creativity in finding new or unique solutions
- Act as a coach or a guide to patient
- Assist patient in setting appropriate goals (individual or long-term)
- Discuss the potential pros and cons of various treatment options with patient and family
- Develop an appropriate plan of care to reach clinical goals
- Develop contingency plans care

Adapted from Howe, R., & Greenberg, L. (2005). Performance management for case management: principles and objectives for developing standard measures. Case Manager, 16, 52–56.

BOX 9-8 Howe and Greenberg's Case Management Attributes in the Facilitation Domain

- Collaborate with various agencies and types of people
- Facilitate, coordinate, and maintain continuity of care
- Possess general problem-solving ability, written communication skills (email, letters, etc.), verbal communication skills (telephone call, in person, etc.)
- Successfully link patient to needed services
- Locate needed services or community resources for patients
- Successfully implement and coordinate patient services
- Know health plan benefits and services
- Facilitate access to providers and services, as needed
- Maintain continuity of care by coordinating all services seamlessly

Adapted from Howe, R., & Greenberg, L. (2005). Performance management for case management: principles and objectives for developing standard measures. Case Manager, 16, 52–56.

outcomes seek to demonstrate case management value in terms of client-centered goal achievement, which leverage evidence-based criteria and guidelines (CMSA, 2010). However, client outcomes may be adversely affected if not undertaken concurrently with measures of client satisfaction as an integral part of the process.

Consider Maureen who suffers from debilitating rheumatoid arthritis. Following a recent flare-up, Maureen's strongest desire is to return to work as soon as possible. Her practice-based case manager focuses on getting Maureen into outpatient therapy and scheduling follow-up medical appointments. She also works on simplifying Maureen's

BOX 9-9 Howe and Greenberg's Case Management Attributes in the Advocacy Domain

- Negotiate on behalf of others.
- Recognize and identify the potential for ethical dilemmas.
- Openly address and discuss potential ethical dilemmas with patient, family, or caregiver.
- Act as patient advocate with physicians or various organizations.

Adapted from Howe, R., & Greenberg, L. (2005). Performance management for case management: principles and objectives for developing standard measures. Case Manager, 16, 52–56.

BOX 9-10 Howe and Greenberg's Case Management Attributes in the Performance Domain

Display a high amount of integrity or values in interactions with others.
Build and maintain trust.
Acquire flexibility and ability to quickly adapt to changing situations.
Work independently and set deadlines.
Maintain a professional and a well-polished image/appearance to others
Possess solid interpersonal (relational), computer, active listening skills.
Promote client/family autonomy.

Adapted from Howe, R., & Greenberg, L. (2005). Performance management for case management: principles and objectives for developing standard measures. Case Manager, 16, 52–56.

medication schedule. All of this activity leads in the direction of returning to work. Unfortunately, the ultimate context of Maureen's desire to return to work gets lost in the myriad of follow-up appointments and check-in telephone calls. Identifying and leveraging Maureen's abilities and strengths as well as communicating with Maureen's employer from the outset could have reduced her out-of-work time. Instead, the bulk of time was devoted to activities that, although valuable, misused precious time as pertains to Maureen's priorities. The interventions were driven by a system-generated care plan without due consideration of Maureen's personal goal.

As pointed out by Rikkert (2012), understanding patient-centered care involves asking the patients to rate or judge their own care. Although health care providers like to think they know the patient and his or her needs, it is not appropriate to base this opinion on a gut feeling. To truly understand patient needs and determine if health care intervention is meeting it, one must ask the patient. Case managers must transform their interactions from barriers-based, what-is-your-problem interrogations to strengths-centric, what-is-most-important-to-you conversations. In making this paradigm shift, case managers begin to integrate and build on client strengths rather than their barriers, weaknesses, and needs.

Client-Centered Goal Development

An essential yet often overlooked aspect of the case management planning process is that of goal setting. Although overarching quality and health outcomes reporting are a staple of health care delivery, accreditation, and reimbursement schema, they have failed to incorporate patient-centeredness into the equation, assuming there is a universally agreed-upon definition of patient-centered.

The case management assessment produces information, which is intended to be considered when developing a case management plan. However, the plan is simply a proposal until the client, caregiver, and care team members reach consensus as to its feasibility and likelihood for producing desired results. A truly client-centered assessment provides insight to the entire care team into those things held most important by the individual. Failing to incorporate assessment findings into care planning and goal setting, not only slights the care team's ability to interact on a personalized level but also short-circuits the individual's contribution to supposed patient-centered care.

It is essential that the case manager understand the multifaceted issues faced by the client in order to develop a strategy, which takes the individual's strengths, weaknesses, and available resources into consideration. The client's desires, revealed during the examination of identified opportunities for case management intervention, are to be considered through the lens of what the client believes to be a success.

Outcomes must be addressed within time periods, such as short-, intermediate-, and long-term horizons. Providing the distinctions of periods supports fulfillment of accreditation requirements, such as are found in URAC Case Management Accreditation Standards (2011), version 4.1—CM10 Case Review and Evaluation of Goals, CM 24 Case Management Plan, and CM 25 Case Management Goals.

The professional case manager presents both plan and goals to the care team, client, and caregiver. Feedback received is incorporated into the plan and supports consensus building, ultimately contributing to ongoing collaboration, motivation, and goal achievement. Once activated, the professional case manager methodically monitors and evaluates intervention effectiveness, documenting the progress made toward goals. Updates, shared with all care team members, invite stakeholders to identify different approaches toward success.

Although goal setting and outcome achievement are essential to case management success, it is just as important for the case manager to recognize the necessity of case management plan modification, involving desired outcomes and periods, which may change based on the client's health condition or other circumstances. This flexibility supports the use of the SMART approach to setting goals.

SMART Thinking

Organizations often provide a format for writing case management goals or prepare goal statements within their respective information system software. Unfortunately, the way in which goals are conceived or formulated is not always clearly articulated. Goals written in a manner that are too vague or are unachievable are defeating to the client's sense of accomplishment. The use of the **SMART** methodology provides a consistent and organized framework in which to write goal statements. To be effective, goal statements must reflect the following parameters: Specific, Measurable, Attainable, Realistic, and Tangible (Doran, 1981; Morrison, 2010). Box 9-11 provides further explanation of each SMART goal component, and Box 9-12 provides a case example of how SMART thinking influences case management plan formulation.

BOX 9-11 Tenets of SMART Goal Formulation

Specific

The expectation is specific if it is clearly written so that it is easily understood by the patient and care team.

The statement defines that which needs to be accomplished including a rationale or benefit related to the desired outcome or goal

Measurable

Desired outcome and monitoring of progress toward achievement must include at least one measure associated with an objective yardstick (e.g., quality, volume, time, cost).

A measurement is provided (e.g., unit, degree) which it must be met.

Individual accountability for determining success is defined.

Attainable

Written in context with the level of each patient's ability and knowledge

Culturally and linguistically appropriate

Realistic

Goals encourage an individual to reach for success but not to such a degree that they defeat the patient's capacity.

Tangible

The goal includes a time parameter by which it may be accomplished.

The goal is objectively trackable, which enables interval determinations of success and reformulation, if necessary.

BOX 9-12 SMART Thinking Case Example

Case Facts

Donald O. Masters is a 66-year-old man recently discharged from the hospital for a severe chronic obstructive pulmonary disease (COPD) exacerbation. Until recently, he had quit smoking for 3 years (self-reported). He began to smoke again following a family visit, within a few weeks returning to his previous pack-a-day habit. Donald's comorbidity profile includes COPD (emphysema with past respiratory failure), congestive heart failure, severe depression, substance misuse (alcohol), and a history of gastrointestinal hemorrhage.

He has a history of aggressive behavior toward family and staff and multiple arrests for domestic violence and assault and battery. This is the main reason that his wife sought separation 5 years ago and moved about 40 miles away. Although she remains in contact with Donald, she recently moved forward with divorce proceedings. His siblings (two brothers and a sister) live in the same small town but have no contact with him. Both parents are deceased.

Donald is an expert carpenter. Due to his recent hospitalization, he is unable to work away from home this year and is upset about this due to the loss of income as well as not being able to get out of the cold weather.

He feels tired all the time, does not eat regularly, and "nods off" just sitting in his easy chair a lot more. He began limiting his physical activity, including hygiene efforts, in order to avoid getting short of breath and having "coughing jags." He wants to quit smoking again but feels it will take too long to regain his energy and head out of state to find work saying "all the good jobs will be filled so what's the use."

When asked, Donald denies having a primary care provider and cannot name any of the medications prescribed to him at the time of discharge. He adds that he filled them initially but has to watch his pennies now that he is not going back to work any time soon. Donald does not articulate an understanding of how smoking affects his breathing and activity tolerance, but acknowledges that he felt much better when he did not smoke. He denies ever having been for admitted for pulmonary rehabilitation.

He lives alone in a single-story home, which he owns outright. However, on returning home from the hospital, he discovered a utility notice that his electric service was scheduled to be terminated unless he paid his outstanding bill. He has a limited support system which consists of the spouse from whom he is separated and one adult child, both of whom work full-time.

During his home visit, the following areas of concern are identified:

- Does not have a primary care provider
- Uses the ED for routine health care services
- Does not take medications as prescribed
- Does not reliably fill medication prescriptions
- Does not understand COPD pathology or the progressive nature of the disease
- Does not understand the connection between smoking and COPD
- Short of breath with activity and tires very easily
- Does not eat regular or nutritious meals
- Does not have a lot of food in the home
- Has a very limited support system
- Received service cutoff notices from the electric company
- Potential loss of health benefits (due to impending divorce)

Donald's barriers to care are extensive; however, his strengths should also be taken into consideration in crafting opportunity statements and goals. His strengths include willingness to make necessary changes in his lifestyle, receptivity to health education, and a strong motivation to return to work.

Application of SMART Thinking

Donald's current problem list is worded in the traditional barrier-specific manner. By applying SMART thinking, two related problems are recognized in a single statement: "Lack of primary care provider contributing to misuse of emergency department (ED) resources." Two desired outcomes of case management intervention are for Donald to engage with a primary care provider as a consistent first-line source of health care services and a reduction in ED utilization. SMART thinking provides a framework for constructing an opportunity and goal dyad through the identification of critical elements.

S	Select and engage a primary care provider as a trusted source of health care. • This expectation is specific and expresses what needs to be accomplished.
M	Identify and complete tasks relating to provider selection. • The tasks are identifiable and completion is easily determined.
A	Willing and able to make necessary telephone calls and attend appointments. • The individual voices willingness and desire to change and engage in case management activities.
R	Acknowledges his need to have a primary care provider and having the physical and intellectual ability to find someone. • The goal is realistic and well within the individual's physical and intellectual abilities and resources within the given time frame.
T	Selection of primary care provider will take place within 2 weeks of case management engagement. An appointment will be scheduled within 3- weeks of case management engagement. • The time frame is specific and achievable.

The agreed-upon opportunity and desired outcome statement appears in Donald's case management plan as:

Opportunity: Requires a primary care provider

Desired outcome: Donald selects a primary care provider, schedules an initial appointment, and the appointment within the first 30 days of case management engagement.

Time frame for completion:

Provider selection takes place within 2 weeks of case management engagement.

Initial appointment occurs within 3 weeks of case management engagement.

Strategic Goal Setting

The use of the term *strategic* is often applied to executive level function and output. However, for the purpose of this competency, the term is used in a much broader sense. The discussion of outcome-driven competence pertains to all levels of organization as well as goal setting and outcomes achievement. As Senge (2006) points out, a shared vision is just one component of guiding organizational aspirations. The quadrangle of vision, values, purpose/mission, and goals are the underpinning of what guides and shapes the destiny of an organization or department. A standalone case management company has the ability to define these four legs of its strategic table. However, within larger organizations case management departments take their cue for tactical and operational goals from that which is defined by higher levels of management.

Department Goal Setting

Case management department leadership must determine what it wants to accomplish by taking actions to understand its business, knowing what it wants to accomplish, and defining itself in the form of a goal(s) (Powell, 2000). Regardless of its position in an organizational hierarchy, goal setting should be factor in the various forces exerting themselves on the case management operation (e.g., competition, workforce, program scope).

Assessing the competitive market in which an organization functions requires leadership to look inward and, perhaps more importantly, to scan the business horizon external to itself. Use of benchmarking as an element in the process of goal setting can prove valuable if undertaken in an organized and informed manner. The spirit that underlies any benchmarking initiative is the desire to learn from and overcome the competition. Benchmarking is about comparing, learning from the outcomes of such comparison, and consequently learning how to do the job better (Anderson-Miles, 1994). As health care organizations compete for market share, the edge of competition sharpens so that the desire to outperform becomes the norm. Benchmarking may precede goal setting as it can lead to a clearer perspective of environmental demands and reasonableness of staff expectations.

The basic approach to the benchmarking process includes the following oversimplified steps: operational understanding, industry knowledge, incorporation of others' successes, and continue to gain and grow (Camp, 1989). Camp's process for benchmarking is adapted and displayed in Figure 9-2. Benchmarks may be internal or external to an organization. External benchmarking requires significant advance work but can yield good ideas and processes for an organization to emulate. However, finding suitable and willing partners with applicable ideas from other industries can be time consuming and costly. Bad benchmarking is about as valuable as no benchmarking at all. Box 9-13 reveals a story relating a failed benchmarking.

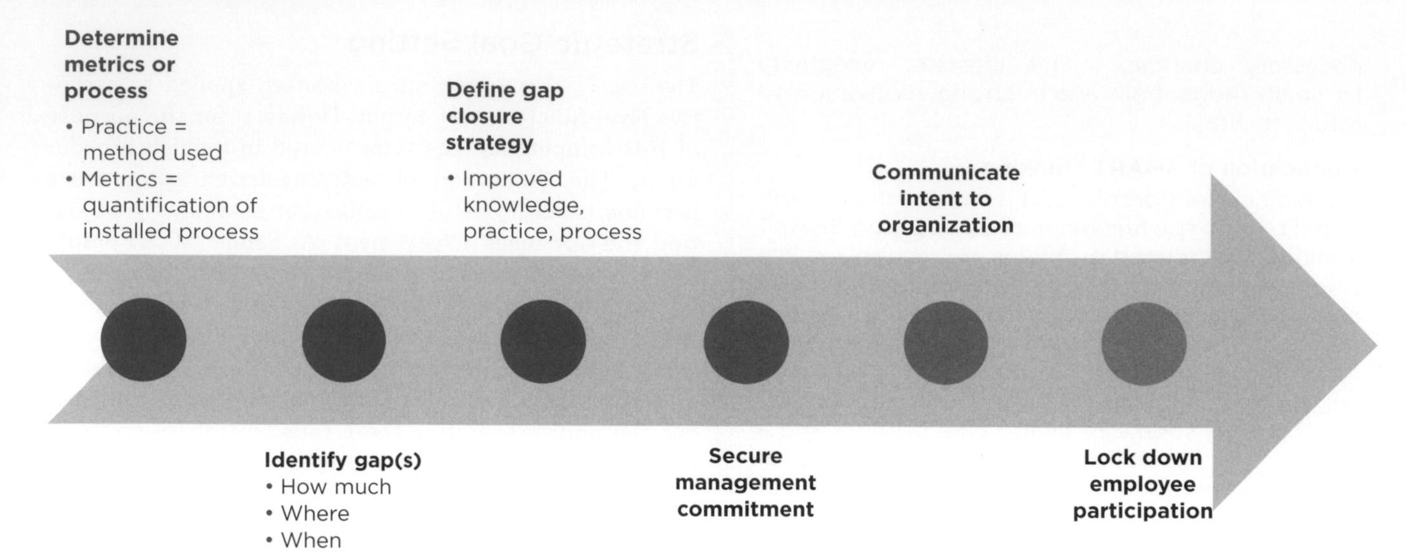

Figure 9-2. Basic benchmark process. (Adapted from Camp, R. C. (1989). *Benchmarking: The search for industry best practices that lead to superior performance.* Milwaukee, WI: ASQC Quality Press.)

BOX 9-13 The Tale of Bad Benchmarking

Many years ago, a case manager worked for a large managed care and health insurance company as a special project liaison. During medical management department reorganization, her background and organizational talent placed her on the radar as an asset. She was asked to step in as the manager of a large utilization review (UR) team with the understanding that additional supervisory staff would be put into place as part of the transition. She accepted the temporary transition. An initial assessment of the team uncovered a range of performance abilities and production levels. Staff ranged from highly motivated and positive to outright obstructionist and passive-aggressive personalities. It was fairly clear why previous supervisory staff had difficulty managing the team. Based on an evaluation of routine tasks and responsibilities, a proposal to reorganize the team and designate new roles was submitted and accepted. The transition began.

Within a couple months, the vacant position of department director was filled by a rather abrasive individual who shall be referred to as Suzie. Once in place, Suzie nullified all previous agreements for the UR area reorganization. She also diverted financial resources from the frontline staff to hiring senior managers to report directly to her. When it came to the UR area, open full-time slots were eliminated. Concurrently, incoming volume increased as a result of the expanding number of covered lives. Review backlog continued to rise; temporary help band-aided the problems. Experienced team resource staff were tasked with full caseload responsibilities and denied anticipated promotions. The department's general tone was negative and fearful. It was fairly clear to see that Suzie was intent on achieving the level of vice president at all costs.

Change was taking place everywhere in the medical management department. Suzie thought that it would be a good idea to do some benchmarking, so she tasked all managers in the department to identify organizations with "best practice" reputations and inquire as to their willingness to serve as benchmarkers. That was it. She left everyone to figure out what she wanted. There was no clear articulation as to what the department's vision and goals were in order to identify the best organizations to approach. When results summaries were submitted, Suzie threw them back at some of the managers complaining that it was not what she wanted. The benchmarking failure was not due to a lack of managerial effort, which took hours away from their core responsibilities, but rather it was because Suzie refused to provide both necessary instructions to managers as to what she wanted benchmarked as well as any leadership or oversight to ensure a successful outcome.

Applying the Balanced Scorecard Approach to Case Management

In business, many organizations undertake a "balanced scorecard" approach to strategic metrics and subsequent goal setting. The scorecard framework emphasizes provision of financial and nonfinancial measures throughout an organization for assisting employees at every level of an organization to understand the impact of individual actions and decisions—from frontline staff to senior executives (Kaplan & Norton, 1996). The four major components of a balanced scorecard approach are financial, customer, business process, and learning/growth. This approach focuses a top-down process driven by organizational mission and strategic vision, yet it also translates to the business unit and department level, assuming it is a framework adopted

BOX 9-14 Critical Inquiry for Balanced Scorecard Implementation

1. Did your organization have a well-defined vision, mission, and strategy before utilizing the balanced scorecard?
2. What motivated your organization to adopt the balanced scorecard?
3. How did the balanced scorecard differ from other measurement systems?
4. What process was followed to develop and implement the balanced scorecard?
5. What major challenges and barriers arose during the balanced scorecard development and implementation?
6. What benefits did your organization receive?

Adapted from Noorein, I., Kaplan, R. S., & Reynolds, K. (2002). Applying the balanced scorecard in healthcare provider organizations. Journal of Healthcare Management, 47(3), 179–196.

throughout the entire organization. The balance struck between external measures of importance to stockholders and board members and internal measures of business process. It is also a balance between past performance outcomes measures and future performance indicators. Finally, it is a balance between objective, quantifiable measures, and more subjective performance measures (Kaplan & Norton, 1996).

In terms of health care, the benefits that may be derived when applied throughout organizations include alignment, facilitation, communication, accountability, and continual feedback (Noorein, Kaplan, & Reynolds, 2002). However, an innovation of this nature should not be undertaken without clear organizational buy-in and advanced planning. To that point, examination of department considerations requires a methodical implementation approach in the form of critical inquiry. Questions, which may be helpful to the discovery and implementation process, include those utilized by Noorein in research into application of balanced scorecard in health care organizations (Box 9-14). Table 9-3 provides description of these benefits as well as how case management departments may apply them within a balanced scorecard environment.

Evidence-Based Practice

Where case management practice is concerned, **evidence-based practice** is important for reasons including, but not limited to, quality, access to care, safety, and cost. There are many kinds of evidence, and rating conventions vary according to the review source. Although evidence-based practice is an essential skill for case managers to possess, few have the time or resources to complete the extensive literature reviews and analyses required to determine what is applicable to individual practice in order to base every function of work on solid evidence (Throckmorton & Windle, 2009).

More commonly, case managers rely on evidence-based tools such as health condition guidelines and decision-support criteria on which to base authorization decisions, develop case management plan interventions, and anticipate future client needs. These serve as that valued resource allowing the case manager to be proactive in planning, educating the patient and the multidisciplinary team, as well as anticipate transition needs and scheduling. Utilizing these tools assists the case manager in facilitating quality-focused and timely medical services for the consumer (Powell & Commander, 2007).

COLLABORATE takes the perspective that an outcomes-driven case manager understands the essentials of judging evidence and applying reliable evidence to practice. It is also important to understand the value associated with basing care interventions on reliable, objectively proven information. The case manager utilizes evidence-based findings as rationale for his or her activities, such as care planning, authorization requests, and health education efforts. Using strong and reliable evidence contributes to development of effective and efficient interventions. The skill of identifying what qualifies as a strong and reliable source is an essential aspect of the outcomes-driven approach to case management.

TABLE 9-3 Balanced Scorecard Philosophy Applied to Case Management

Alignment	Facilitation	Communication	Accountability	Feedback
Moves the organization/department to a market-driven, customer-focused operational approach	Monitors and assesses implementation of strategy	Opens collaborative opportunities	Assigns responsibility across all organizational levels	Promotes continual adjustment to dynamic environmental factors
Use of highly rated patient preference for customizing portal layout for monitoring case management plan progress	Identification of authorization process delay relating to telecomm program error in new submission portal	Development of intranet tools enabling project management deliverables tracking during conversion of case management software	Development of tool requiring source to provide plain-English interpretation of case management outcome reports	Providing bidirectional care team communication tool to expedite transition planning

Adapted from Noorein, I., Kaplan, R. S., & Reynolds, K. (2002). Applying the balanced scorecard in healthcare provider organizations. Journal of Healthcare Management, 47(3), 179–196.

Critical Appraisal

Critical appraisal is a process of careful and systematic examination of research in order to judge its trustworthiness, value, and relevance in a particular context (Burls, 2009). The outcomes-driven case manager must develop a critical appraisal mentality in order to evaluate and correctly apply health care research. This is especially true when evaluating case management research because of the previous issues identified with wide variation in practice and application of the job title to work that is substantively utilization review in nature. Possessing critical appraisal skills allows for the efficient discovery and application of research evidence.

When evaluating research, Delfini (2013) recommends evaluating multiple aspects of the work in question, starting with a look at the study's date, purpose/aim, type, and sponsorship/funding source, which are simple, yet essential, details useful to validate the applicability of the study and possible bias. Next, look at study design to determine if it was appropriate to the research question posed and that the research question was useful and clinically significant. Other things to examine are the research questions, population, and outcomes predefined and appropriate.

The next step in critical appraisal has to do with assessing the validity of the work. The purpose of this is to determine if the study results can be attributed to bias, confounding, or chance rather than a product of the research itself. Figure 9-3 illustrates the four areas of assessing research validity. There are additional consideration and usefulness factors to evaluate. Delfini (2013) provides a framework for these issues in its Short Critical Appraisal Checklist that includes meaningful clinical benefit, external validity, patient perspective, and provider perspective.

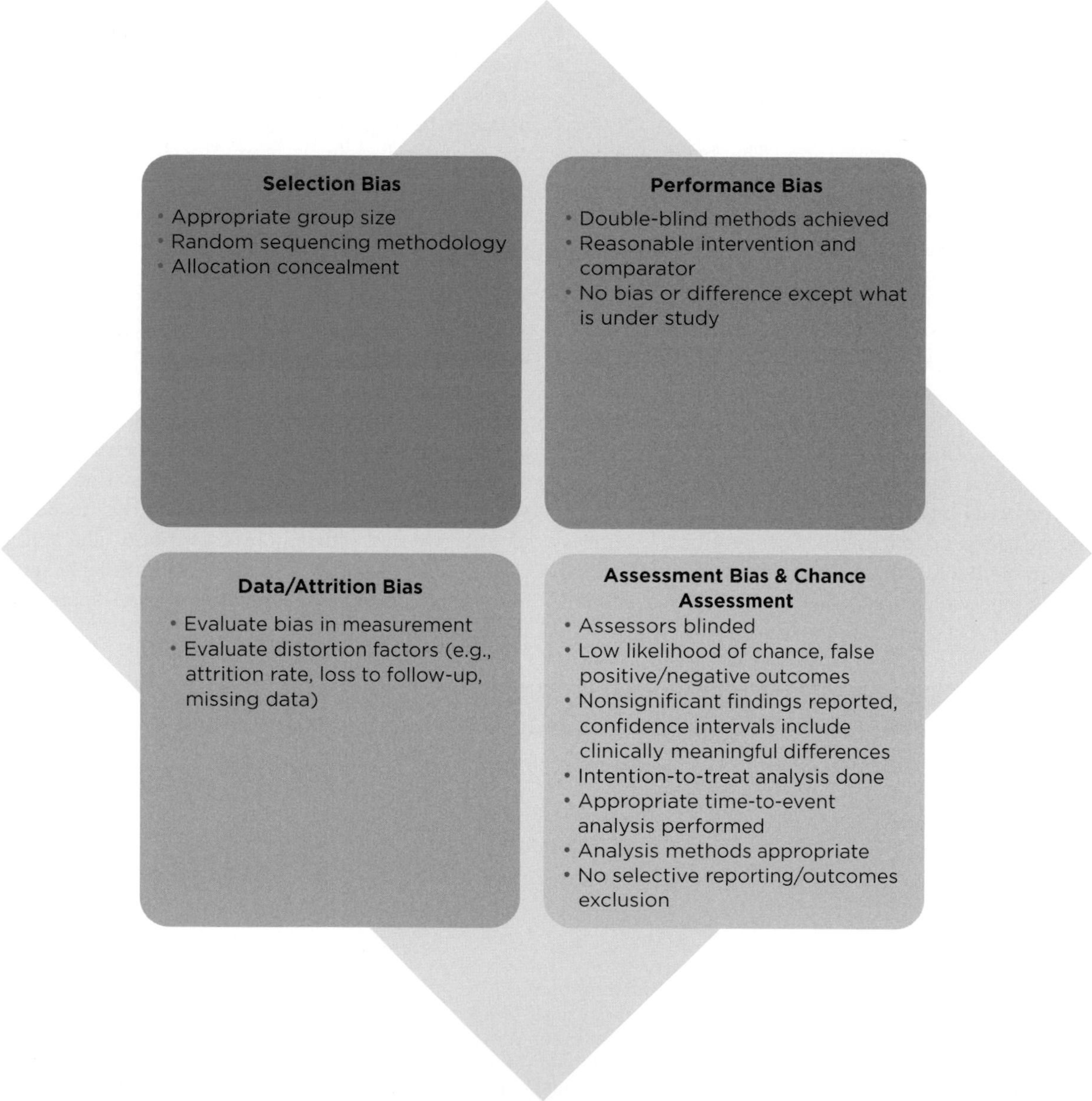

Selection Bias

- Appropriate group size
- Random sequencing methodology
- Allocation concealment

Performance Bias

- Double-blind methods achieved
- Reasonable intervention and comparator
- No bias or difference except what is under study

Data/Attrition Bias

- Evaluate bias in measurement
- Evaluate distortion factors (e.g., attrition rate, loss to follow-up, missing data)

Assessment Bias & Chance Assessment

- Assessors blinded
- Low likelihood of chance, false positive/negative outcomes
- Nonsignificant findings reported, confidence intervals include clinically meaningful differences
- Intention-to-treat analysis done
- Appropriate time-to-event analysis performed
- Analysis methods appropriate
- No selective reporting/outcomes exclusion

Figure 9-3. Internal validity assessment. (Adapted from Delfini Evidence Tool Kit. (2013). *Short critical appraisal checklist: Interventions for prevention, screening & therapy*. Retrieved June 16, 2014, from http://www.delfini.org)

Finally, it is important to maintain consistency in critical appraisal review process regardless of the methodology used. Organizations need to identify a common approach and evidence rating in order for there to be consistency in critical appraisal practice across multiple disciplines. Failure in doing this risks creation of additional imbalance in attribution and application of research findings.

Implication for Practice

The implication of adopting an outcomes-driven perspective is transformative for case management practice in that it shifts the client approach from a gut-reaction, formulaic, and barrier-centric "what-is-your-problem" interrogation to a strengths-centric, evidence-based, and outcome-informed "what-is-most-important-to-you" conversation. In making this paradigm shift, the case manager seeks out and integrates formal education, experience, and skills to build strengths in support of professional practice. This swings the perception of case management away from that of serving as a crutch and elevates the practice to being understood as a bridge to improved self-management and wellness (Treiger, 2013). This fulfills the philosophical promise of case management and furthers recognition of case management as a truly professional practice applicable across the continuum of care.

SUMMARY

This chapter explores the outcomes-driven competence for professional case management practice. At any level of an organization, the case manager's ability to impact health (e.g., quality, access, cost) in measurable ways is essential to the long-term success of the health care industry. One's position in case management's hierarchy also affects the need for and application of outcomes and research findings. Measuring value becomes an essential activity requiring mastery for case management practice. Continuing to apply inappropriate measures will not make the case for case management value. Application of the wrong metrics misdirects attention from the real derived benefits of the intervention and focuses on less meaningful statistics, which do not reflect case complexity, level of effort, or impact on client condition.

Identifying how case management quantifies its value contribution is important to the overall practice and to health care industry stakeholders (e.g., purchasers, patients, providers, insurance companies). Three key reasons why capturing consistent case management performance measures remains critical are as follows (Howe & Greenberg, 2005):

- Providing information to drive quality improvement,
- Allowing the CM provider to compare performance to benchmarks or competitors, and
- Allowing purchasers and consumers to differentiate CM providers based on quality.

Understanding as well as leveraging performance outcomes for improved case management practice is an essential competency for the professional case manager. This translates into design of meaningful goals at client, individual, and organizational levels. It influences human resource performance management, exerting increased influence over compensation and job security. At the department and organization level, performance expectations and outcome thresholds must align with an organization's mission, vision, and value in order to optimize their contribution to projected operational and strategic outcomes. At the systems level, research outcomes advance case management practice so much so that research and its utilization stand as a practice standard, according to the CMSA (2010). Thus, it is incumbent on every case manager to understand how outcomes relate to and demonstrate case management's contribution to health care delivery, more effective case management interventions, and ultimately to better client outcomes.

References

Agency for Healthcare Research and Quality. (2014). *Definition of outcomes*. Retrieved April 25, 2013, from http://www.ahrq.gov/health-care-information/topics/topic-outcomes.html

American Case Management Association. (2013). *Standards of practice and scope of services for healthcare delivery system case management and transition of care professionals*. Retrieved April 25, 2013, from www.acmaweb.org/Standards

American College of Emergency Physicians. (2013). *Quality of care and the outcomes management movement* Retrieved June 13, 2014, from http://www.acep.org/content.aspx?id=30166

Anderson-Miles, E. (1994). *Benchmarking in healthcare organizations: An introduction*. Healthcare Financial Management. Retrieved May 3, 2014, from http://www.allbusiness.com/management/benchmarking/467664-1.html

Askar, M., Iman, S., & Prabhaker, P. R., (2009). Business metrics: A key to competitive advantage. *Advances in Competitiveness Research*, *17*(1,2), 91–109.

The Benchmarking Exchange. (2013). *What is benchmarking?* Retrieved May 30, 2014, from http://www.benchnet.com/wib.htm

Berwick, D. M., Nolan, T. W., & Whittington, J. (2008). The triple aim: Care, health, and cost. *Health Affairs*, *27*(3), 759–769. doi:10.1377/hlthaff.27.3.759. Retrieved June 14, 2014, from http://content.healthaffairs.org/content/27/3/759.full

Braeden, C. J. (2002). *Involvement/participation, empowerment and knowledge outcomes indicators of case management* [State of the Science Paper 2/3]. Little Rock, AR: CMSA.

Burls, A. (2009). *What is critical appraisal?* London: Hayward Medical Communication. Retrieved June 13, 2014, from www.whatisseries.co.uk

The Business Dictionary. (n.d.). *Definition of metric*. Retrieved May 15, 2014, from http://www.businessdictionary.com/definition/metrics.html#ixzz32wXVay8M

Camp, R. C. (1989). *Benchmarking: The search for industry best practices that lead to superior performance*. Milwaukee, WI: ASQC Quality Press.

Camwell, R. (2014). Essential differences between research and evidence-based practice. *Nurse researcher*, *8*(2), 55–68. Retrieved May 31, 2014, from http://rcnpublishing.com/doi/pdfplus/10.7748/nr2001.01.8.2.55.c6150

Case Management Society of America. (2010). *CMSA standards of practice for case management* (Rev.). Retrieved April 25, 2013, from http://www.cmsa.org/portals/0/pdf/memberonly/StandardsOfPractice.pdf

Chatterjee, S. (1998). Delivering desired outcomes efficiently: the creative key to competitive strategy. *California Management Review*, *40*(2), 78–95.

Consornery-Fairnot, D., & Serbin, K. M. (2012, May 1). *Tracking case management outcomes: New thinking for existing measures*. Retrieved July 4, 2013, from http://www.dorlandhealth.com/case_management/best_practice/Tracking-Case-Management-Outcomes-New-Thinking-for-Existing-Measures_2238.html

Council for Case Management Accountability. (1999). *A framework for case management accountability* [Addendum to CCMA State of the Science Paper #1 (5/99)]. Little Rock, AR: CMSA.

Delfini Evidence Tool Kit. (2013). *Short Critical Appraisal Checklist: Interventions for Prevention, Screening & Therapy*. Retrieved June 16, 2014 from http://www.delfini.org.

Doran, G. T. (1981). There's a S.M.A.R.T. way to write management's goals and objectives. *Management Review, 70*(11) (AMA Forum), 35–36.

Ellwood, P. M. (1988). Outcomes management: a technology of patient experience. *New England Journal of Medicine, 318*(23), 1549–1556.

Fetterolf, D. (2010). Estimating clinical and economic impact in case management programs. *Population Health Management, 13*(2), 73–82. doi:10.1089pop.2009.0032.

Frost, B. (2000). *Measuring performance*. Dallas, TX: Measurement International.

Hamilton, G. A. (1999). *Patient adherence outcome indicators & measurement in case management healthcare* [State of the Science Paper 1/3]. Little Rock, AR: CMSA.

Hickam, D. H., Weiss, J. W., Guise, J-M., Buckley, D., Motu'apuaka, M., Graham, E., ... Saha, S. (January 2013). Outpatient case management for adults with medical illness and complex care needs. *Comparative Effectiveness Review, 99*. (Prepared by the Oregon Evidence based Practice Center under Contract No. 290-2007-10057-I.) AHRQ Publication No.13-EHC031-EF. Rockville, MD: Agency for Healthcare Research and Quality. www.effectivehealthcare.ahrq.gov/reports/final.cfm

Howe, R., & Greenberg, L. (2005). Performance management for case management: principles and objectives for developing standard measures. *Case Manager, 16*, 52–56.

Huber, D. (2010). *Leadership and nursing care management* (4th ed.). Maryland Heights, MO: Saunders Elsevier.

Kaplan, R. S., & Norton, D. P. (1996). *The balanced scorecard*. Boston, MA: Harvard Business Review Press.

Institute of Medicine. (2000). *To err is human: Building a safer health system*. In L. T. Kohn, J. M. Corrigan & M. S. Donaldson (Eds.), Washington, DC: National Academy Press.

Institute of Medicine. (2001). *Crossing the Quality Chasm: A New Health System for the 21st Century*. Washington, D.C: National Academy Press.

Lee, R. T. (2013, May/June). Managing with metrics. *Industrial Management 55*(3), 16–21.

Lehrman, S., Gimbel. R., Freedman, J., Savicki, K., & Tackley, L. (2002). Development and implementation of an HIV/AIDS case management outcomes assessment programme. *AIDS Care, 14*(6), 751–761.

Management Analysis and Budget. (2014). *What is benchmarking?* Retrieved May 30, 2014, from http://www.mad.state.mn.us/benchmarking

Merriam-Webster. (2014). *In Merriam-Webster.com*. Retrieved June 16, 2014, from http://www.merriam-webster.com/dictionary/research

Morrison, M. (2010). *History of SMART objectives*. Retrieved June 10, 2014, from http://rapidbi.com/history-of-smart-objectives

National Association of Professional Geriatric Care Managers. (2013). *Standards of practice*. Retrieved April 29, 2013, from www.caremanager.org/about/standards-of-practice

National Association of Social Workers. (2013). *NASW standards for social work case management*. Retrieved April 25, 2013, from http://www.socialworkers.org/practice/naswstandards/CaseManagementStandards2013.pdf

Noorein, I., Kaplan, R. S., & Reynolds, K. (2002). Applying the balanced scorecard in healthcare provider organizations. *Journal of Healthcare Management, 47*(3), 179–196.

Okes, D. (2013). *Performance metrics—The levers for process management*. Milwaukee, WI: Quality Press.

Orme, J. G., & Combs-Orme, T. (2012). *Outcome-informed evidence-based practice*. Upper Saddle River, NJ: Pearson.

Powell, S. K. (2000). *Advanced case management: outcomes and beyond*. Baltimore, MD: Lippincott, Williams & Wilkins.

Powell, S.K., & Commander, C. (2007). A tale of two initiatives case management and evidence-based practice. *Professional Case Management, 2*(1), 1–2.

Powell, S. K., & Tahan, H. A. (Eds.). (2008). *CMSA core curriculum for case management* (2nd ed.). Philadelphia, PA: Lippincott Williams & Wilkins.

Rikkert, J. (2012). Patient-centered care: what it means and how to get there. *Health Affairs* [web blog]. Retrieved June 10, 2014, from http://healthaffairs.org/blog/2012/01/24/patient-centered-care-what-it-means-and-how-to-get-there

Senge, P. M. (2006). *The fifth discipline: the art and practice of the learning organization*. (2nd ed.). New York: NY: Currency.

Smith S. (2008). *Cultivating a culture of safety in healthcare: A systematic approach to root cause analysis*. Cullman: QIG Publishing.

Spitzer, D. R. (2007). *Transforming perforance measurement: Rethinking the way we measure and drive organizational success*. New York, NH: Amacom.

Stanton, M. P., & Packa, D. (2010). Outcomes analysis-the role of case management. *Journal of Healthcare Leadership, 2*, 25–30. doi:10.2147/JHL.S7844.

Stanton, M. P., & MacRobert, M. (2007). Putting the "easy" into evidence-based practice. *Professional Case Management, 12*(1), 5–13.

Stevens, P., Stokes, L., & O'Mahony, M. (2006). Metrics, targets and performance. *National Institute Economic Review, 197*(80), 80–92. doi:0.1177/002795010619700103.

Sultz, H. A., & Young, K. M. (2014). *Health care USA: understanding its organization and delivery* (8th ed.). Burlington, MA: Jones & Bartlett Learning.

Throckmorton, T., & Windle, P. E. (2009). Evidence-based case management practice—part II: meta-analysis. *Professional Case Management, 14*(5), 226–232.

Treiger, T. M. (2013). *The role of case managers in emerging care delivery models* [interview and webinar] Health Intelligence Network. Retrieved June 16, 2014, from http://www.hin.com/soundclips/Treiger_role_case_managers_full0213.mp3

URAC. (2011). *Case management accreditation standards, version 4.1*. Retrieved June 19, 2014, from https://www.urac.org/resource-center/standards-interpretations

Wojner, A. W. (2001). *Outcomes management: Applications to clinical practice*. St. Louis, MO: Mosby.

Zander, K. (2008). *Hospital case management models: Evidence for connecting the boardroom to the bedside*. Marblehead, MA: HCPro.

10 LIFELONG LEARNING

OBJECTIVES

After studying this chapter, you will be able to:

1. Define various terms associated with education of professional case managers.
2. Describe the distinctions between experiential and didactic learning.
3. Identify Knowles's Six Characteristics of Adult Learners.
4. Discuss Gardner's Multiple Intelligences.
5. Present the four priority areas needed to transform nursing education.
6. Relate the GO FAR Framework to case management practice.
7. Discuss the key elements of the Lifelong Learning competency.

KEY TERMS

Andragogy
Continuing education units
Contact hours
Didactic learning
Digital omnivores
Education
Evidence-based
Experiential learning
Intelligence
Learning
Logic
Mentoring
Professional development
Reason
Seven intelligences

Learning is a lifelong process of keeping abreast of change (Drucker, 2003). Most professionals strive to live by this mantra though for case managers it is especially vital. Health care has transformed in the blink of an eye, as the influencers of technology and the Patient Protection and Affordable Care Act (PPACA) alone have altered how the industry and its stakeholders experience patient care. Although case managers should assure a proactive versus reactive stance to that constant of industry change, the grand question beckons: How does a case manager stay abreast of change when he feels like the learning curve is now an endless road?

It was not long ago that the mailman would deliver an abundance of monthly and/or quarterly professional journal(s). A stack would gradually grow on a desk or night table, one created in earnest with the dog-eared pages of articles and highlighted titles in the table of contents that you pledged to make time to get to though never did. With any luck, your employer offered on-site trainings, or even reimbursement for attending relevant courses, trainings or conferences that provided those coveted continuing education units (CEUs).

The current generation of professionals access learning through an array of diverse genres, both the traditional aforementioned modes and those which now appear as if by magic at our fingertips online. Digital versions of professional and **evidence-based** journals and e-books can be delivered to any one of several mobile devices. Continuing education portals, webinars, and conferences are attended from the comfort of a case manager's favorite chair or coffee shop at any hour of the day. Even academia's continuum of vast degrees is now accessible through distance education programming. Multimodal platforms allow for resource provision and sharing of knowledge across cyberspace through professional online groups and list serves.

There are extensive means and modes by which case managers can now advance and achieve a lifelong learning (LLL) attitude. These extend across workplace settings, the organizational hierarchy of those settings, and the overall case management profession. Chapter 10 provides a manageable context for this competency's enormous scope, one that transforms LLL from (what can present as) a burdensome task to a more normalized essential process that raises the overall bar on professional case management practice to a maximum standard.

DEFINITIONS

Grounding Terms

An important initial point of distinction in the literature emerges with the definition of learning as opposed to education. **Education** is an activity undertaken or initiated by one or more agents that is designed to effect changes in the knowledge, skill, and attitudes of individuals, groups, or communities (Knowles et al., 2012). The term emphasizes the role of the educator, who is viewed as the agent of change. That person is responsible for how to present appropriate stimuli and reinforcement for learning. It is essential that activities be designed to induce change. The power of the education process and comprehension of the content can easily lie with how the content is delivered (Knowles et al., 2012).

It is common for students and professionals alike to dialogue with each other about the quality of a particular conference or course. Perhaps, there were positive evaluations because of the educator's use of related real-life experiences, humorous anecdotes, or a creative interactive breakout discussion. To the contrary, maybe the educator read the content on the slides verbatim and spoke in a monotone manner, or did little to engage those attending in the information. As a result boredom ensues and potentially those present are not motivated to engage in the content being taught.

The word **learning** emphasizes the person in whom the change occurs or is expected to occur (Knowles et al., 2012). Merriam-Webster (2014a) defines learning as the activity or process of gaining knowledge or skill by studying, practicing, being taught, or experiencing something. There are a several types of learning that one may hear referenced, such as didactic in contrast to **experiential learning**. **Didactic learning** involves lecture or textbook instruction as opposed to demonstration (Merriam-Webster, 2014b). This also involves the array of theories, tools, professional jargon, and other established resources (e.g., codes of ethics, professional standards of practice, competencies) that are specific to that profession. For example, a case manager who educates herself or himself on new outcomes measurement tools by reading a recently published article or new research in an evidence-based practice journal is engaging in didactic learning.

Experiential learning is that learning which occurs through an individual's reflection on doing. Learning is the process whereby knowledge is created through the transformation of experience (Kolb, 1983). It requires self-initiative, an intention to learn, and an active phase of learning (Moon, 2004). When that same case manager enhances her comprehension of an outcomes measurement tool through its direct application to a targeted patient population through a pilot project, she is engaging in experiential learning. Several experiential models further operationalized the learning by doing premise and are presented in further detail later in this chapter.

Logic is another term that weaves its way into understanding LLL. It is a proper or reasonable way of thinking about or understanding something (Merriam-Webster, 2014c). Perhaps a rehabilitation hospital case manager (RCM) is requesting additional inpatient days for an adolescent female patient status-post a motor vehicle accident. Admitted with multiple fractures, and a mild traumatic brain injury, the RCM does not understand the logic used by her MCO case manager (CM) counterpart has just issued a denial for the request, instead requesting the patient be discharged to a subacute rehabilitation program for the next week. The MCO CM sees no logic in why a treatment team would want to advocate so strongly, using their valuable time expertise on a patient who has met the original treatment goals and can be transferred to another level of care. In their dialogues with each other, the two CMs use **reason** to work through the disparity in their perspectives and achieve an agreeable patient plan. Reason is a statement or fact that explains why a situation is the way it is, why someone does, thinks or says something, or why someone behaves a certain way (Merriam-Webster, 2014d).

The RCM meets with the treatment team to strategize on obtaining further facts to answer the 64-thousand-dollar question asked by her MCO counterpart: How will the additional requested days, services and/or treatments change the patient's outcome? In partnership, the RCM and treatment team develop finite goals to be accomplished in the requested timeframe to enable a safe transition home. The two CMs discuss the fiscal incentives of keeping the patient one more week, as the MCO CM is reminded of the potential to lose valuable treatment time as the patient transfers between facilities and adjusts to the new treatment environment and team.

Measuring Professional Learning

Within our case management world, learning occurs across a multitude of mediums, often identified as **professional development** or continuing education opportunities, with the terms used interchangeably across the industry. Both refer to the advancement of skills or expertise to succeed in a particular profession, especially through continued education (Dictionary.com., 2014a). Examples include workshops, seminars, conferences, study groups, teleconferences, online programs, self-guided study, academic coursework, and even manuals.

Contact hours (CEs or CHs) are provided for attending the event. This term refers to a 50- or 60-minute hour of organized didactic or clinical learning, which is used as the standard measurement of time for continuing education programs (Dictionary.com., 2014b). **Continuing education units** are the defined credits that are awarded to an individual case manager by a professional organization, for having attended the education program (Dictionary.com., 2014c). Case managers often experience confusion around the distinction between the two terms, CEs and CEUs. Although they are often viewed as interchangeable, in reality they are not. Traditionally, one CEU equals 10 CEs.

Most, if not all, state boards require that those whom they license and/or certify obtain a specific number of CEUs over each designated renewal period in order to be eligible for relicensure. This is the same for a majority of the certification and accrediting bodies (e.g., CCMC, ACMA, ANCC). One of the many requirements for case managers to maintain their state licensure and certification involves fulfilling the defined continuing education requirements and attaining the necessary CEs. Given the variation in requirements across states, professional disciplines, and accrediting organizations, case managers are strongly encouraged to verify the exact number of CEUs and/or CEs mandated with respect to ongoing eligibility for each credential they possess.

PAST AND CURRENT THINKING

An immense number of theories and frameworks exist for understanding how individuals learn. These span the biological, psychological, sociological, and educational dimensions. For the purposes of this chapter, a limited selection of perspectives have been chosen to enhance how a case manager understands and embraces the LLL competency.

PSYCHOLOGY

John B. Watson and Classical Conditioning

John B. Watson was a psychologist who is viewed as the father of behaviorism, a learning theory based on observable behavior. He believed that individual development depends on learning. Watson was emphatic that all individuals are born as blank slates. With the opportunity to engage in a range of life experiences, when given the proper experiences, learning will proceed (Ashford & LeCroy, 2013).

Watson's view of classical conditioning continues as a foundational element of learning behavior. This refers to any learning that occurs when a neutral stimulus acquires the capacity to elicit a response that was originally elicited by another stimulus. It is also a widely accepted explanation for how individuals acquire emotional responses such as fear and anxiety (Ashford & LeCroy, 2013). Consider an adult who enjoys taking long leisurely walks at night. On one occasion, the adult is out walking when a bicyclist suddenly comes up behind her unexpectedly. The bicyclist is moving so fast that the adult has no choice but to jump off the path, fracturing an ankle. Once the injury recovers, the adult refuses to take walks at night, feeling panicked at the thought of even leaving the house at dark. The previously neutral stimulus of a walk at night is forever associated with the negative experience of the ensuring accident.

Case managers experience classical conditioning through any one of a number of experiences and that can easily impact job satisfaction and retention. Consider the new case manager who is not oriented to the role, or educated on how to provide a thorough and appropriate clinical review. She is expected to complete several of these reviews her initial week on the job and does so, feeling like the proverbial "baptism by fire." The case manager finds herself with a series of denials, being yelled at by patients, their families, and physicians alike. As a result, the case manager becomes fearful and hesitant to complete even the simplest clinical update. She feels like a failure in the role and is dismissed because of not passing her probationary appraisal.

B.F. Skinner and Operant Conditioning

Skinner advanced on Watson's learning theory through the concept of operant conditioning, or a form of learning that occurs when responses are purely controlled by their consequences (Ashford & LeCroy, 2013).

Behavior is often repeated when followed by positive consequences such as the child who is praised for toilet training. The child who can demonstrate positive skill with this often challenging task for parents, is greeted with claps and strong demonstrations of positive acknowledgment by those around them, if not tangible rewards such as toys. Behavior is equally not repeated when followed by neutral or negative consequences. So the child who is unsuccessful with toilet training and may have accidents is punished. They may receive verbal expressions of frustration and discipline by parents. Skinner noted how when the consequences of rewards and punishments are made contingent on behavior, they can equally have a powerful influence on that behavior (Ashford & LeCroy, 2013).

Skinner saw both reinforcement and punishment as critical elements of operant conditioning and factors that contribute to longer-term learning. He identified that behavior can be influenced over the entire life course, simply by the positive and negative experiences one has.

Jean Piaget and Cognitive Processing

Biologist and psychologist, Piaget was focused on the relationship between how human beings develop and learn. This weave was integral to his theory of cognitive development, shown in Table 10-1.

He incorporated the process of how individuals adapt, as integral components of learning. Assimilation involves how new

TABLE 10-1 Piaget's Theory of Cognitive Development

Mental Stage	Age	Characteristics
Sensorimotor Period	Birth–2 years of age	Infants understand the world through their own individual movements and sensations. They recognize how individual actions can cause responses to occur in others (i.e., a burp elicits laughter or crying elicits nurturing). Learning occurs through assimilation and accommodation.
Preoperations Period	2–7 years of age	Children begin to use words and pictures to represent objects. They see the world through their own point of view only, in concrete terms.
Concrete Operations Period	7–11 years of age	Children begin to think logically about concrete events. They begin to use reasoning to understand what is happening.
Formal Operations Period	12 years of age and older	Growing into adolescence and young adulthood, they can think abstractly and reason about hypothetical situations. They consider the moral, ethical, philosophical, political, social implications of issues in their world.

Adapted from Ashford, J. B., & LeCroy, C. W. (2013). Human behavior in the social environment (5th ed.). Australia: Brooks/Cole Cengage Learning.

information can be brought into our internal world, or schemata, and used to change what is actually perceived. Individuals can also accommodate thought patterns into their schemata, or actually change what is thought about a certain situation.

Case managers both assimilate and accommodate their thought processes toward learning on a regular basis. Consider the assortment of organizational policies and procedures (P and Ps) that accompany any new job. On many occasions these P and Ps serve to structure how a case manager completes his or her assorted roles and functions. The revision of these P and Ps can and will occur at any point, with a domino effect that requires the need to assimilate the changes and accommodate how the changes impact their daily work. Changes in reimbursement pose a similar challenge for case managers and they wrestle with understanding and assimilating the actual change, such as the Medicare two-night rule, and then accommodating their practice in a way that allows them to address the concept. It might be that the case manager must allow extra time to discuss this concept with patients and families and provide them with altered options.

Carl Rogers and the Experiential Learning Movement

Carl Rogers saw experiential learning as equivalent to personal change and growth. Through his work as a therapist and researcher, Rogers came to view all human beings as having a natural propensity to learn. This was akin to the client-centered or person-centered therapy approach that he created. In this nondirective counseling approach, the client determines the course of treatment, while the therapist clarifies the client's responses to promote self-understanding using a series of attitudes: genuineness, unconditional positive regard, and empathy. These attitudes serve to foster a high-quality relationship between the therapist and client, which is paramount (Rogers, 1951)

Learning and the motivation to learn follow the same process to Rogers. Learning to learn and having an openness to change accompany the overall progression of learning. For the student learner, these are integral points of understanding. In defining accountability for the overall learning process, Rogers and Freiberg (1994) saw it as the teacher's role to facilitate learning when:

1. The student participates completely in the learning process and has control over its nature and direction.
2. It is primarily based on direct confrontation with practice, social, personal, or research problems.
3. Self-evaluation is the principal method of assessing progress or success.

One is reminded of the popular adage, you can lead a horse to water but you can't make it drink. Case managers are often provided with large volumes of diverse resources and content to advance their practice. Whether the materials are provided by organizational leadership, valued mentor, and/or through mandatory continuing education program, the onus is on each individual case manager to accept accountability for his or her own extent of learning.

Malcolm Knowles and Andragogy: Six Characteristics of Adult Learners

Malcolm Knowles accepted and promoted the concept of **andragogy**, a term originally used by Alexander Kapp, a German educator in the 19th century. Knowles, who was also an educator, heavily engaged with this practical approach of self-directed and autonomous learners and teachers as facilitators of learning. When one becomes an adult, they arrive at a self-concept of being responsible for their own lives and thus self-directing. He viewed this as a more appropriate mode for adult learners than other traditional models (Knowles et al., 2012).

Knowles et al. (2012) put forth a core set of six adult learning principles underlying andragogy. Their explanation and application to case management are shown in Table 10-2.

- Need to know of the learner
- Self-concept of the learner
- Foundation of the learner
- Readiness to learn
- Orientation to learning
- Motivation to learn

Howard E. Gardner's Seven Intelligences

Gardner (2006) is a developmental psychologist inspired by the work of Piaget. In 1983, Gardner identified seven distinct intelligences that contribute to understanding how people perceive the world. For the purposes of his work, Gardner (2011) recognized the importance of combining biological and cultural research toward promoting that reason, intelligence, logic, and knowledge are not synonymous. He defined **intelligence** as the capacity to solve problems or to fashion products that are valued in one or more cultural settings.

Gardner recognized the broad swipe of learning intelligences and a need to expand from the traditional views, which had included only two styles of learning, verbal and computational. An example of these traditional styles brings many back to the standardized tests that were administered during primary education (e.g., elementary and middle school) which focused on language and mathematical abilities.

Gardner's **seven intelligences** include seven styles, which are shown and explained in Table 10-3. He was clear that the list is not exhaustive and over time other models have evolved which provide additional styles and/or interpretations. One related example is the VARK, a learning questionnaire that provides users with a profile of their learning preferences, or how they take-in and give-out information. The VARK (2014) includes the four learning perspectives of:

- Visual: seeing
- Aural: listening
- Read/Write: as noted
- Kinesthetic: energy of doing

David Kolb's Experiential Learning Cycle

Based on the work of John Dewey, discussed in chapter 8, Kolb's Experiential Cycle is a model of cognitive processing, or how individuals process learning in the brain. It is a fluid process where knowledge is created through the transformation of experience (Kolb, 1983). Kolb's work provides a solid and usable framework that translates to the present generation of students, in how it emphasizes the critical linkages among education, work, and personal development.

The workplace is seen as a learning environment that serves to both enhance and supplement formal education and foster meaningful work and career development opportunities. From Kolb's perspective, formal education plays a valuable role in LLL and the development of individual to their full potential as citizens, family members, and human beings (Kolb, 1983).

TABLE 10-2 Knowles's Six Assumptions Underlying Andragogy with Case Management Examples

Principle	Concept	Case Management Example
Need to know	Adults need to know the reason why they are learning.	Case managers are offered a new training focused on the HIPAA Omnibus rule because of a recent breach at their organization.
Self-concept of the learner	Adults become more self-directed and independent as they mature. They also become more actively involved in what they want to learn.	A case manager makes use of the expanded options for interactive learning. She/he especially enjoys breakout groups to strategize and apply concepts presented in the session.
Foundation of the learner	An adult's experience provides the basis for learning.	An experienced case management staff attend an interactive round-table discussion on "What contributes to a High-Power Case Management Department."
Readiness to learn	Adults are ready to learn dependent on what knowledge they identify they need to deal with current life circumstances.	Case managers attend a training on integrated behavioral health programs and ACO's upon passage of the PPACA.
Orientation to learning	Adult learning is problem-centered rather than content-oriented.	Case management staff attend a training focused on managing difficult team members.
Motivation to learn	Adults respond to internal vs. external motivation to learn.	Case managers are offered the ability to attend one of three concurrent tracks at a state conference: hospital case management, community-based case management, advancing from case manager to case management leader.

Adapted from Knowles, M., Holton, E. F., & Swanson, R. A. (2012). The adult learner (7th ed.). London, New York: Taylor and Francis.

TABLE 10-3 The Seven Intelligences

Intelligence	Learning Style
Body—kinesthetic	Use your body, hands, and sense of touch
Personal	
Interpersonal	Learn in groups or with people
Intrapersonal	Work alone and use self-study
Linguistic	Use words, both in speech and writing
Logical—mathematical	Use logic, reasoning, and systems
Musical—rhythmic	Use sound and music
Visual—spatial	Use pictures, images, and spatial understanding

Adapted from Gardner, H. E. (2011). Frames of mind: The theory of multiple intelligences (3rd ed.). New York, NY: Basic Books.

From Kolb's (1983) perspective, effective learning occurs when an individual advances through a cycle of four experiential stages as shown in Figure 10-1. The stages serve as action-oriented opportunities during which the learner must:

- Be willing to be actively involved in the experience
- Be able to reflect on the experience
- Must possess and use analytical skills to conceptualize the experience, and
- Must possess decision-making and problem-solving skills to use the new ideas gained from the experience.

Kolb then identified four learning styles that correspond to each of the four stages. The styles highlight conditions under which learners learn best. The styles are:

- Diverging
- Assimilating
- Accommodating, and
- Converging

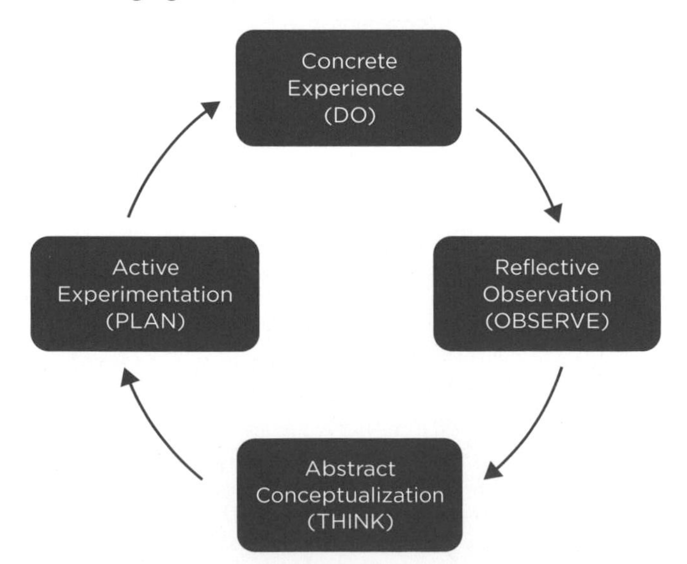

Figure 10-1. Kolb's Experiential Cycle. (Adapted from Kolb, D. (1983). *Experiential learning: Experience as the source of learning and development*. Englewood Cliffs, NJ: Prentice Hall.)

A combined representation of styles and associated modes are presented in Figure 10-2. Case managers are encouraged to consider for themselves which of the learning styles are most applicable to how they learn.

NURSING

Nursing's Competency Heritage

Nursing has embraced a solid competency-based learning framework to guide practice for decades. Examples of these approaches appear across Part 1, particularly in chapter 5

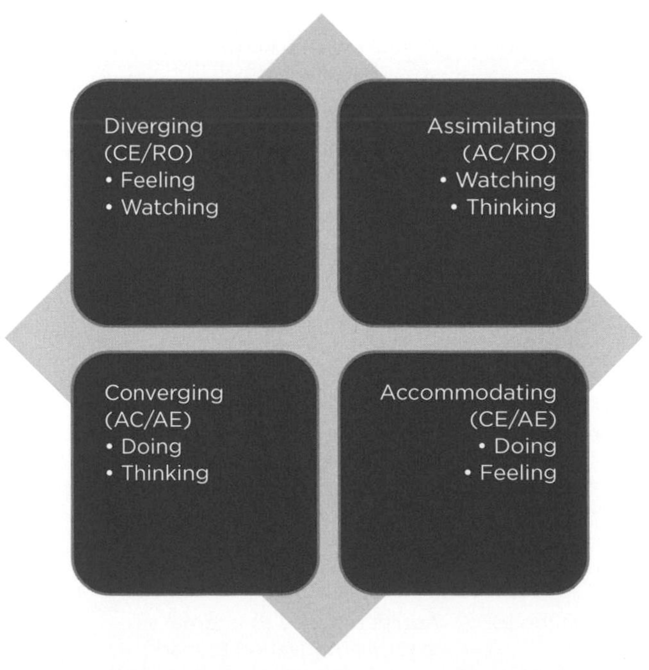

Figure 10-2. Kolb's Learning Styles. AC, astract conceptualization; AE, active experimentation; CE, concrete experience; RO, reflective observation. (Adapted from Kolb, D. (1983). *Experiential learning: Experience as the source of learning and development*. Englewood Cliffs, NJ: Prentice Hall.)

through the many models that serve as templates for the professional continuum. These extend from higher education up through most professional levels of licensure (American Association of Colleges of Nursing, 2014; QSEN, 2014).

Professional Standards

The nursing profession incorporates an abundance of professional and specialty organizations, which view it as a responsibility to both its members and the public to define the scope of practice and the standards of practice (American Nurses Association [ANA], 2014). These professional standards set the tone and context for how nursing is understood and practiced across the diverse specialties which transverse the industry. A representative listing of resources appear in Box 10-1. The standards for each entity offer a consistent understanding of the commonalities and distinctions in specialty practice roles across the nursing profession. They are also used to define position statements among the industry and its stakeholders (ANA, 2014).

BOX 10-1 Nursing Specialty Practice Standards

The American Academy of Nurse Practitioners Publishes Standards of Practice for Nurse Practitioners

- Anesthesia: The American Association of Nurse Anesthetists (AANA) publishes Scope and Standards for Nurse Anesthesia Practice as well as a number of position statements that serve to define scope of practice.
- Critical Care: The American Association of Critical Care Nurses (AACN) publishes a number of practice resources.
- Midwifery: The American College of Nurse-Midwives (ACNM) publishes Core Competencies for Basic Midwifery Practice and Standards for the Practice of Midwifery.
- Oncology: Oncology Nursing Society (ONS) publishes Oncology Nurse Practitioner Competencies. This document outlines specialty entry-level competencies for Oncology Nurse Practitioners (ONPs) who care for adult and late-adolescent patients throughout the continuum of cancer care.
- Pediatrics: National Association of Pediatric Nurse Practitioners (NAPNAP)
- Pediatric Nursing: Scope and Standards of Practice is a collaborative effort of the ANA, the Society for Pediatric Nurses (SPN), and NAPNAP.
- Psych/Mental Health: The American Psychiatric Nurses Association (APNA) Web site provides information about the role of the advanced practice psychiatric nurse organized by topic, workplace setting, and/or specialty.

Adapted from American Nurses Association. (2014). Scope and standards of practice. Retrieved September 7, 2014, from http://nursingworld.org/scopeandstandardsofpractice

Nursing and Credentialing Standards

Several nursing certifying bodies contribute to providing oversight for the nursing professions' numerous certifications. Although state licensure provides the legal basis for nursing practice, a growing number of states require additional certifications to grant practice privileges (e.g., the American Midwifery Certification Board). A list of those credentials provided through the American Nurses Credentialing Center (ANCC), appears in chapter 4. A global list of certifying bodies appears in Box 10-2.

BOX 10-2 Nursing Certifying Entities

American Academy of Nurse Practltioners Certification Program (AANPCP) Administers Programs for

- Adult Nurse Practitioner (NP)
- Gerontologic NP
- Family NP

American Nurses Credentialing Center (ANCC) Administers ProgramS for the Following Certifications

- Acute Care NP
- Adult NP
- Adult Psychiatric and Mental Health NP
- Diabetes Management—Advanced
- Family NP
- Family Psych and Mental Health NP
- Gerontolgoical NP
- Pediatric NP
- School NP

ANCC Administers Programs for the Following Clinical Nurse Specialist Certifications

- Adult Health CNS
- Adult Psychiatric and Mental Health CNS
- Child/Adolescent Psychiatric and Mental Health CNS
- Diabetes Management—Advanced
- Gerontological CNS
- Home Health CNS
- Pediatric CNS
- Acute Care Nurse Practitioner (ACNP)

American Midwifery Certification Board (AMCB) Administers Programs for

- Certified nurse-midwife (CNM)
- Certified midwife (CM)

National Board On Certification and Recertification of Nurse Anesthetists (NBCRNA)

- Certified Registered Nurse Anesthetists (CRNA)

(continued)

BOX 10-2 Nursing Certifying Entities (*Continued*)

National League for Nursing

Certification for Nurse Educators (CNE)

Oncology Nursing Certification Corportation (ONCC) Administers Certification for

Oncology Certified Nurse (OCN)

Certified Pediatric Hematology Oncology Nurse (CPHON)

Certified Breast Care Nurse (CBCN)

Advanced Oncology Certified Nurse Practitioner (AOCNP)

Advanced Oncology Certified Clinical Nurse Specialist (AOCCNS)

Blood and Marrow Transplant Certified Nurse (BMTCN)

Pediatric Nursing Certification Board (PNCB)

Pediatric Nurse Practitioner (PNP)

Certified Pediatric Emergency Nurse (CPEN)

Acute Care Certified Pediatric Nurse Practitioner (CPNP)

Adapted from American Nurses Association. (2014). Scope and standards of practice. *Retrieved September 7, 2014, from http://nursingworld.org/scopeandstandardsofpractice; National League of Nursing. (2014).* Certification for nurse educators. *Retrieved September 8, 2014, from http://www.nln.org/certification/index.htm*

A Need to Educate the Educators

Despite what presents as fluid change in the industry, it has been suggested that nursing education has not really fundamentally changed for the past 50 years (Tanner in Larson, 2010). One mandated task involves educating the educators. Although there may be an abundance of new knowledge available, those teaching the content may not be as up to speed as mandated (Larson, 2010).

Building faculty capacity in nursing education programs is a key factor in transforming nursing education (Halstead, 2012). Four priority areas are identified to achieve this end (Halstead, 2012), with examples are further elaborated in Table 10-4:

1. Building faculty capacity;
2. Designing new models of clinical education;
3. Developing innovative models of academic/practice collaboration; and
4. Advancing the science of nursing education through research.

(Halstead, 2012)

Nursing faculty specifically must be able to help students develop excellent clinical judgment, plus evidence-based practice skills. To accomplish this goal faculty must employ a combination of in-depth clinical knowledge and the ability to teach nursing. Incorporating technology, for example, is required (Larson, 2010). The education realm must more

TABLE 10-4 Building a Meaning Transformation of Nursing Education Models

Priority Area	Contributing Factors	Recommendations
Build faculty capacity that grows the professions	Aging faculty workforce. Compensation not competitive with practice settings. Insufficient pipeline of nurses qualified to teach in academic programs.	Emphasize academic preparation in nursing education and faculty development to help novice educators develop teaching skills in interactive environments. Retool current faculty who are being challenged to teach in a changing and increasingly complex health care environment where they do not have extensive practice experience.
Design new models of clinical education	The fragmented approach to clinical education is failing to adequately prepare graduates for transition into practice.	Design evidence-based learning experiences to prepare nurses to work in interprofessional health care teams and manage care transitions among settings.
Develop innovative models of academic/practice collaboration	The education and practice silos of the part are less prevalent in practice.	Great focus on building partnerships to leverage the expertise and resources of academic and practice settings.
Develop innovative models of academic/practice collaboration	Learning outcomes must be associated with new education to meet the emerging health care needs.	Base practice as educators on evidence. Use national research priorities defined by the National League for Nursing (2012). Use federal funding initiatives to support education research in nursing and other health professions that build a competent health care workforce and demonstrate the linkages between education and quality patient-care outcomes.

Adapted from Halstead, J. (2012, September 24). Transforming nursing education to meet emerging health care needs [Robert Wood Johnson Foundation Human Capital Blog]. Retrieved September 5, 2014, from http://www.rwjf.org/en/blogs/human-capital-blog/2012/09/transforming_nursing.html

accurately reflect the newest realities of interprofessional teams and practice, fluid and smoother transitions of care, as well as quality-driven evidenced-based efforts.

SOCIAL WORK

The Council on Social Work Education (CSWE) EPAS competencies (2008), presented in chapter 8, are one mechanism by which social workers are provided guidance with respect to expected learning goals and behaviors across higher education, and ultimately the professional realm. There are other valuable compilations that are used to define priorities for social work practice, plus acceptable standards for that practice.

Social Work Speaks

The National Association of Social Workers (NASW) Delegate Assembly is tasked every 3 years with meeting to discuss and define key areas of policy development and advocacy for the social work profession. Comprised of a defined number of elected state and territory delegates, these individuals are tasked with approving a varying number of identified policy statements specific to a range of populations and issues.

Published as Social Work Speaks (NASW, 2012), this list varies with each Delegate Assembly and in recent years has included a variety of changes, from revised titles from the prior edition for several topic areas to the more complex task of developing new content to address emerging populations of focus. The latter task is accomplished by assigning delegates to serve as designated subject matter experts.

There are 18 distinct population topic areas, shown in Box 10-3, with 64 policy statement titles spanning them. The individual policy statements include the spectrum of social work practice across the wide berth of intervention. This includes, but is not limited to, adolescent and young adult health, aging and wellness, capital punishment and the death penalty, professional self-care, immigrants and refugees, hospice care, rural social work, family violence, and voter participation, to name a few.

The importance of Social Work Speaks to the competency of LLL is especially vital. For the value it serves as an integral resource to define the professional social work's position on current critical issues. There is also significance derived from having access to the changing areas of professional focus. These impact workforce and employment trends plus can be used toward developing organization responses to policy issues and conducting policy analysis and study (NASW, 2012).

NASW Practice Standards

Box 10-4 shows the listing of current available professional standards of practice through NASW. These documents serve to set key definitions, guiding principles, goals, and unique standards to guide social work professionals who may choose to focus on specific populations and/or types of practice (e.g., case management). The body of each standard addresses LLL through providing a consistent understanding

BOX 10-3 Social Work Speaks Policy Statement Topic Areas

Adolescents
Aging
Behavioral health
Child welfare
Community
Discrimination and equity issues
Education
Employment
Ethnicity and race
Families and children
Family planning
Gender issues
Health
Macro issues
Political action
Social work professional statements
Substance use
Violence

Adapted from National Association of Social Workers. (2012). Social work speaks: NASW policy statements, 2012–2014 (9th ed.). Washington, DC: NASW Press.

BOX 10-4 National Association of Social Workers Practice Standards

NASW and ASWB Best Practice Standards in Social Work Supervision
NASW Guidelines for Social Worker Safety in the Workplace
NASW Standards for Social Work Case Management
NASW Standards for Social Work with Service Members, Veterans and Their Families
NASW Standards for School Social Work Services
NASW Standards for Social Work Practice with Family Caregivers of Older Adults
NASW Standards for Social Work Practice with Clients with Substance Use Disorders
NASW and ASWB Standards for Technology and Social Work Practice
NASW Standards for Social Work Practice in Health Care Settings
NASW Standards for Clinical Social Work in Social Work Practice
NASW Standards for Social Work Practice in Child Welfare
NASW Standards for Social Work Practice in Palliative and End-of-Life Care
NASW Standards for Social Work Services in Long-term Care Facilities

(continued)

BOX 10-4 National Association of Social Workers Practice Standards (*Continued*)

NASW Standards for Continuing Education and the Social Work Profession
NASW Standards for the Practice of Social Work with Adolescents
NASW Standards for Integrating Genetics in Social Work Practice
NASW Standards for Cultural Competence in Social Work Practice
NASW Standards for Indicators for Cultural Competence in Social Work Practice

Adapted from National Association of Social Workers. (2014). Professional standards. *Practice page. Retrieved September 3, 2014, from http://www.naswdc.org/practice/default.asp?topic=standards#swtopics*

of the historical relevance and knowledge expectations across the profession. Box 10-5 provides the outline content for the NASW Practice Standards for Social Work Case Management (2013) as a relevant template example.

BOX 10-5 National Association of Social Workers Practice Standard Content Inclusion, Standards for Social Work Case Management

Standards for Social Work Case Management
Introduction
Background
Goals of the Standards
Definitions
Guiding Principles
Standards with Interpretations
- Standard 1: Ethics and Values
- Standard 2: Qualifications
- Standard 3: Knowledge
- Standard 4: Cultural and Linguistic Competence
- Standard 5: Assessment
- Standard 6: Service Planning, Implementation, and Monitoring
- Standard 7: Advocacy and Leadership
- Standard 8: Interdisciplinary and Interorganizational Collaboration
- Standard 9: Practice Evaluation and Improvement
- Standard 10: Record Keeping
- Standard 11: Workload Sustainability
- Standard 12: Professional Development and Competence

References
Acknowledgments

Adapted from National Association of Social Workers. (2013). NASW standards for social work case management. *Washington, DC: National Association of Social Workers.*

GO FAR: An Action-Oriented Learning Framework

A fresh model for learning and career success appeared in Spring 2014 when Williams, director of Social Work at Idaho State University, put forth the GO FAR framework (2014). It acknowledges how overwhelmed students can become as they struggle to remember and apply the vast amount of information required to be effective and successful practitioners. This struggle continues, as graduates enter the workforce and become the next generation of practitioners. More experienced social workers equally wrestle with incorporating the most current knowledge into their professional lexicon over their careers. They must constantly work to stay up to speed on new populations, treatment interventions, and protocols, as well as new standards and competency expectations that emerge across the industry (Williams, 2014).

The GO FAR acronym is presented in Figure 10-3. The framework combines social work's didactic theories, concepts, and established resources with the more experiential learning components of professional identity and authenticity, to name a few. The text of books and theories is but a starting point, creating additional opportunities for more experiential learning (Daum, 2014).

This approach is applicable across the experience continuum from student to more seasoned professional, given the differing knowledge levels mandated for social workers to competently progress over the tenure of their career. Each letter of the acronym stands for a vital element of learning that contributes to a social worker's overall professional success. This framework is a practical approach to the knowledge base that supports a social worker's ability to be genuine, liberally express optimism, have fun personally and professionally, be accountable, and practice with rigor function together to help structure professional knowledge and gently move it into the realm of practice. GO FAR unites the acquisition of knowledge with the individual motivation to learn. It reflects the art of more intensive learning models that make the overall learning process as energizing and efficient as possible (Daum, 2014).

The GO FAR framework easily applies to case management, as the content in the acronym relates to most, if not all, health and human service professionals. Being authentic and genuine in practice, allows case managers to engage and establish rapport with their diverse range of clients. The attention to optimism and fun is solid reminder to the occupational hazards which comes with most health and human service professionals, of attending to others before and instead of themselves (Fink-Samnick, 2007). Being accountable to professional boundaries underlies most, if not all, professional standards, regulations, and codes. These assure that case managers do not engage in social relationships with patients or family members that could impact their objectivity and professionalism. This directly leads to the Rigor, and the attention to the established professional knowledge base and resource toolbox that enters the workplace with each case manager.

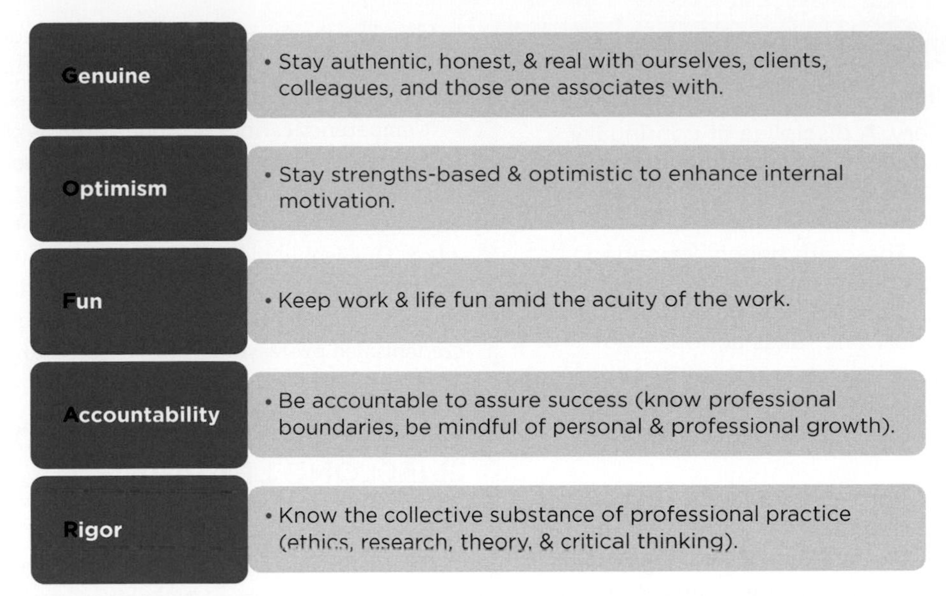

Figure 10-3. The GO FAR framework. (Adapted from Williams, D. J. (2014, Spring). *GO FAR! A useful framework for developing career success in social work*. The New Social Worker. Retrieved September 4, 2014, from http://www.socialworker.com/feature-articles/career-jobs/go-far-useful-framework-for-developing-career-success-social-work/)

GENERAL PERSPECTIVES

Senge and the Fifth Discipline: A Cornerstone of Learning Organizations

Peter Senge's (2006) work has served as a powerful influence in the areas of management and leadership, though has particular relevance to LLL. An American systems scientist, Senge morphed his background in aerospace engineering, philosophy, and social systems modeling to emerge as a major figure in organizational development.

He developed the concept of learning organizations, where:

- People continually expand their capacity to create the result they truly desire,
- New and expansive patterns of thinking are nurtured,
- Collective aspiration is set free, and
- People are continually learning to see the whole together.

In addition, Senge details two conditions which must be met in order for an entity to be known as learning organization. First, the organization must match the intended or desired outcomes defined. Second, an organization must have the ability to recognize when the initial direction of the organization is different from the desired outcome and follow the necessary steps to correct the disparity. Successful learning organizations engage in systems thinking, a framework for seeing interrelationships rather than things, for seeing patterns of change rather than static snapshots (Senge, 2006).

Amid his strong emphasis on management, Senge wove the strong role learning plays to the development of what he frames as a "learning organization." Three core learning capabilities of teams were represented by a three-legged stool to visually convey the importance of each concept (leg). Included are the capabilities of fostering aspiration, developing reflective conversation, and understanding complexity. Ultimately, the stool is unable stand on its own if any of the three capabilities are missing (Senge, 2006).

Senge's five disciplines represent the approaches (theories and models) that organizations should use toward developing the core learning capabilities. He aligned the two concepts to emphasize their interrelationship, with a depiction shown in Figure 10-4. Senge's five disciplines are further detailed in Box 10-6 along with the 11 Laws of the Fifth Discipline.

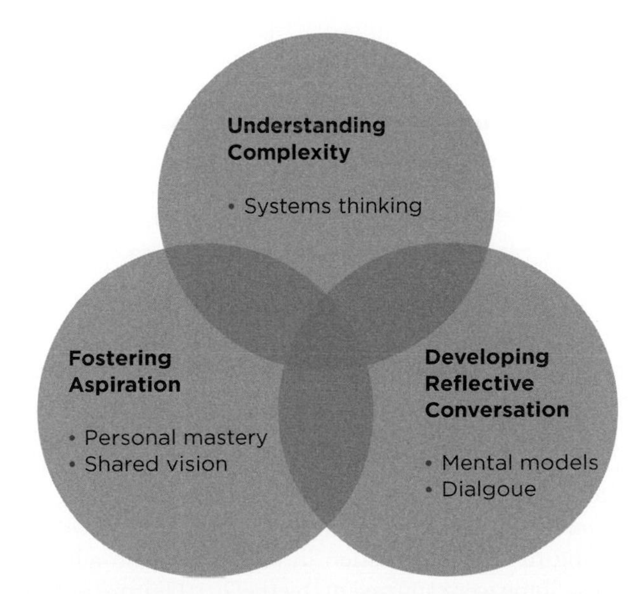

Figure 10-4. Core learning capabilities for teams with five disciplines. (Adapted from Senge, P. M. (2006). *The fifth discipline: The art and practice of the learning organization* (2nd ed.). New York, NY: Currency: Doubleday.)

BOX 10-6 Senge's Five Disciplines Model

The Five Disciplines

1. Personal mastery: A discipline of continually clarifying and deepening personal vision, of focusing energies, of developing patience, and of seeing reality objectively.
2. Mental models: These are deeply ingrained assumptions, generalizations, or even pictures of images that influence how one understands the world and how one takes action.
3. Building shared vision: A practice of unearthing shared pictures of the future that foster genuine commitment and enrollment rather than compliance.
4. Team learning: Starts with dialogue, the capacity of members of a team to suspend assumptions and enter into genuine thinking together.
5. Systems thinking: The fifth discipline that integrates the other four.

The 11 Laws of the Fifth Discipline

1. Today's problems come from yesterday's "solutions."
2. The harder you push, the harder the system pushes back.
3. Behavior grows better before it grows worse.
4. The easy way out usually leads back in.
5. The cure can be worse than the disease.
6. Faster is slower.
7. Cause and effect are not closely related in time and space.
8. Small changes can produce big results, but the areas of highest leverage are often the least obvious.
9. You can have your cake and eat it too, but not all at once.
10. Dividing an elephant in half does not produce two small elephants.
11. There is no blame.

Adapted from Senge, P. M. (2006). The fifth discipline: The art and practice of the learning organization (2nd ed.). New York, NY: Currency: Doubleday.

21st Century Skills

This term, 21st Century Skills, refers to the new generation of core competencies that education advocates view as essential for students to be successful in the workforce. Included are the competencies of collaboration, digital literacy, critical thinking, and problem solving (Education Week, 2010). Case managers are a growing number of professionals who are returning to higher education in order to obtain advanced degrees. Some were spurred on by the 2010 Future of Nursing Report completed by Robert Wood Johnson Foundation (RWJF) in partnership with the Institute of Medicine (IOM), which called for registered nurses to climb the educational ladder. The report was specific that a more highly educated nursing workforce can help ensure the nation's population has access to high-quality, patient-centered care (IOM, 2011).

Competency cannot be underrated. A case manager's ability to use a checklist does not always demonstrate proficiency in clinical assessment of pathophysiology or psychopathology. It does, however, denote the skill of placing a check in a box. One would like to think that consumers of health and behavioral health care deserve a more accurate evaluation of their presenting problem. Otherwise, why would competent credentialed professionals be so necessary?

CONTEXT FOR COLLLABORATE LIFELONG LEARNING

LLL is an unwritten component of each distinct COLLABORATE competency. It can serve to trigger a case manager's intellectual commitment or habit, a key definition related to CT (critical thinking), and a concept to be addressed in chapter 14, Organized. LLL impacts a case manager's efficiency and competence with outcomes measurement and defining return on investment, as focused on in chapter 9. It can temper one's knowledge of and effectiveness with resource awareness, as you will read about in chapter 15. Limited motivation to learn can detract from a case manager's leadership value to the patient as an advocate and or the transdisciplinary team that individual is often tasked to coordinate. A case manager not proficient in his or her requisite knowledge base will be ineffective as an out-of-the-box thinker he or she often needs to be in the fluid health care arena. Lack of accountability to learn can translate to limited proactivity and/or anticipatory action, which can also impact a case manager's skill in engaging in ethical–legal analysis and decision making. The bar has been set higher by social media and the need for case managers to demonstrate the highest levels of awareness to professional boundaries.

Reflect on the individual application in how any COLLABORATE competency is enhanced by a case managers skill to utilize new knowledge, skills, and the requisite training toward quality-driven professional practice.

KEY ELEMENTS OF THE LIFELONG LEARNING COMPETENCY

The key elements of the LLL competency value:

- Academia and advanced degrees;
- Professional development;
- Evolution of knowledge requirements for new and emerging trends (e.g., technology, innovation, reimbursement);
- Practicing at the top of licensure and/or certification; and
- Acknowledging no one case manager can and does know all.

Academia and Advanced Degrees

An increasing number of case managers are also in roles as students. Many are applying to degree programs to gain new knowledge plus those who are seeking promotional opportunities (e.g., those who obtain masters in business administration (MBAs). A recent trend includes those who are enrolling in programs due to changes in regulatory requirements. This includes recent state board mandates for those nurses with associates' degrees to now obtain a bachelor of science degree (Pace, 2014). This change in nursing requirement is based on the IOM recommendation (2011) for 80% of all nurses to have a 4-year degree by 2020, a move that is expected to enhance quality.

Health care professionals are applying in droves to certificate and degree programs in clinical informatics, one of the top areas of employment growth areas. Since 2007, postings for health informatics jobs have increased 10 times faster than health care jobs overall (Monegain, 2013). Many take certificate programs to obtain proficiency of the Patient Affordable Care Act, as it changes the rules for patients, managers, doctors, and other health professionals (Korkki, 2014).

As Lynn Munson, President and Executive Director of the Common Core states:

> Today's students are fortunate to have powerful learning tools at this disposal that allow them to locate, acquire and even create knowledge much more quickly than their predecessors. But being able to Google is no substitute for true understanding.
>
> *Munson, in Education Week, 2012*

Independent of the chronological age of the student, it is understood that technology proficiency will be part of their toolbox. Technology promotes 24/7 entries to information outside the brick and mortar of the traditional library or set of encyclopedias. Digital access provides information that is far more relevant and accurate. The opportunities afforded by technology should be used to reimagine 21st century education, focusing on preparing students to be learners for life (Cantor in Education Week, 2010).

Professional Development

Few would argue the amount there is to continuously learn in the health care industry. Knowledge is power so it is not surprising how many individuals take pride on being avid learners. This may be driven by adherence to any one of many professional standards and codes of professional conduct in the industry.

The Case Management Society of America (2010) Standards of Practice for Research and Research Utilization presents a case manager's responsibility to maintain familiarity with current research findings and be able to apply them, as appropriate, in his or her practice. Perhaps it might relate to the Commission for Case Manager Certification's (2009) Code of Professional Conduct, which speaks to certificants maintaining their competency at a level that ensures each of their clients will receive the benefit of services appropriate and consistent for their conditions and circumstances. The NASW Code of Ethics and the administrative regulations that underlie social work clinical licensure are clear in their direction to the workforce. Both mandate that each professional should advance their knowledge base, develop and enhance professional expertise, and continually strive to increase professional knowledge and skills to apply them in practice (NASW, 2008).

Evolution of Knowledge Requirements for New and Emerging Trends

Technology Proficiency and Innovation

LLL includes case managers being accountable for prioritizing and attaining knowledge proficiency of the abundance of new industry trends. Technology proficiency is a factor many have embraced, although others have resisted. Many case managers are among the 47% of health care professionals who are **digital omnivores**, using three screens daily to view patient information (Terry, 2013). This extends from entering and/or reviewing documentation in an electronic health record to contacting a colleague via a mobile device for consultation. Many professionals continue to feverishly grasp the full scope of Health Insurance Portability and Accountability Act of 1996 (HIPAA)–Health Information Technology for Economic and Clinical Health (HITECH) 1, 2, and now final rule with HITECH 3 released in January 2013. There are few who believe that this latest HIPAA is truly the final version, with most professionals anticipating further legislation miles to be paved as the industry moves down the HIPAA highway.

Recent studies validate that innovation is here to stay and only amplify in importance to the health care industry and its consumers. The value of the global telemedicine market grew from $11.6 billion in 2011 and is expected to hit $27.3 billion by 2016, an estimated compound annual growth of 18.6% over the next 5 years. About 2.8 million patients are being remotely monitored (Lewis, 2012), with the number continuing to rise exponentially for the future.

These new technologies bring a list of endless opportunities for case managers are finding case managers at opposite ends of a spectrum. On one end are those who are actively obtaining additional education and training in specialty areas such as informatics. This is one of the fastest growing arenas for practice, especially for nurses and other health care professionals who seek to bridge that gap between clinical care and technology. This is particularly valuable given the new wave of implementation and optimization of information systems and applications that include clinical documentation, computerized practitioner order entry (CPOE), and electronic medical records. Recent numbers from the Health Information Management and System Society's (HIMSS) 2014 Nursing Workforce Survey show dramatic growth in this field with 70% of the 1,000 surveyed having titles that specified an informatics position, with increases in salaries and continued interest in pursuing further training in this field (HIMSS, 2014).

On the other end of the spectrum are those case managers who project blame on the technology evolution as a precipitator for their early retirement (Treiger & Fink-Samnick, 2013).

This arena can be a staunch learning curve for case managers as they strive to master the new scope of health information technology and mobile device management—from password protection, to remote access and encryption, to understanding how new versions of products and regulations differ from each other (Fink-Samnick, 2013).

Changing Population Demographics and Health Literacy

Much has been written the last decade about the changing demographics of the population, and the relationship of these changes to health literacy. The PPACA defines health literacy as the degree to which an individual has the capacity to obtain, communicate, process, and understand basic health information and services to make appropriate health decisions (Centers for Disease Control and Prevention, 2014).

A variety of reports cite that health information is not presented in a way that is usable by most Americans, with nine out of 10 adults experiencing difficulty with basic information provided from test results, to consultation and treatment recommendations, and even medication management. This leads to increased emergency room usage, challenges in managing chronic diseases, and less-than-optimal outcomes and higher costs (U.S. Department of Health and Human Services, 2010).

The National Plan to Improve Health Literacy cites seven goals to improve health literacy and strategies to achieve them, as shown in Box 10-7. These can be especially robust challenges for case managers who are on the frontlines of intervening effectively in the patient-centered care culture. Particularly in light of the fact that one in two American adults are unable to read above a fifth grade level, solutions must be found. Case manager's part is a valuable part of the solution. Raising awareness of the scope of low literacy among patients is critical for any practice. Implementing basic practices to ensure effective communication will increase the likelihood of patient compliance and successful outcomes (Villaire & Mayer, 2007).

BOX 10-7 National Action Plan to Improve Health Literacy

Vision

- Provides everyone with access to accurate and actionable health information.
- Delivers person-centered health information and services.
- Supports lifelong learning and skills to promote good health.

Seven Goals

1. Develop and disseminate health and safety information that is accurate, accessible, and actionable.
2. Promote changes in the health care system that improve health information, communication, informed decision making, and access to health services.
3. Incorporate accurate, standards-based, and developmentally appropriate health and science information and curricula in child care and education through the university level.
4. Support and expand local efforts to provide adult education, English language instruction, and culturally and linguistically appropriate health information services in the community.
5. Build partnerships, develop guidance, and change policies.
6. Increase basic research and the development, implementation, and evaluation of practices and interventions to improve health literacy.
7. Increase the dissemination and use of evidence-based health literacy practices and interventions.

From U.S. Department of Health and Human Services. (2010). National action plan to improve health literacy, office of disease prevention and health promotion. *Retrieved September 5, 2014 from http://www.health.gov/communication/HLActionPlan/*

THE IMPACT OF THE PATIENT PROTECTION AND AFFORDABLE CARE ACT

This content has been broached in assorted chapters of this book, including this one. From health care reimbursement to mental health parity there is a vast learning curve required for anyone within the industry to achieve a minimum standard of understanding of PPACA's impact; practitioners, providers, product developers, and consumers alike. There are shared challenges and frustrations as newly insured individuals ask providers how to access care. Fourteen states continue to work through developing their own health insurance exchanges courtesy of the technical glitches that led to nonfunctional systems (Ellison, 2014). Twenty-three states continue to reject Medicaid expansion and can expect to contribute $152 billion over the next 10 years to states that will take federal money. Pennsylvania, Arkansas, and Iowa are setting up unique variations on Medicaid expansion that extends subsidies for private insurance to cover their state's poorest adults (Helms & Pugh, 2014).

The Mental Health Parity and Addiction Equality Act (MHPAEA) of 2008 (United States Department of Labor, 2014) allegedly required health plans offer mental health and substance use disorder benefits to cover on par with their medical/surgical benefits coverage. However, implementation of this act did not consistently occur as intended. Under PPACA, mental health is now a mandated benefit on plans purchased in the individual and small group marketplaces. Those with a history of mental illness can also no longer be denied covered for having a preexisting condition (Gold, 2014). The verdict is out across the industry on whether or not full adherence with both laws will occur as intended.

PPACA was intended to help standardize important parts of the (health care) system, by imposing common rules across the entire country and by providing federal financing to help residents in all states afford insurance coverage. Instead there is a hodgepodge of coverage and a wide variance (Shuman, 2014). Experts are clear that the country's health will never be whole until we insist that mental health be seen along with physical health as fundamental to our overall well-being, and funded as such (Ronan in Cullen, 2014). As a result, case managers will equally struggle with fight to reconcile appropriate benefit provision and access to identified health and mental health care for patients, clients, members, and consumers alike.

Practicing at the Top of Licensure and Certification

These are among the most competitive times for professional case management practice. This competition has contributed to expanded achievement of a proverbial professional "alphabet soup" to accompany a case manager's name. Although the importance of licensure and certification, and the expansion of credentialing have been discussed in chapter 4, it bears repeating as an issue of vital importance for the LLL competency.

There is one constant amid the wide variation in case management credentials, degrees, job titles, and names which are now adorn the industry. Certified case managers can present as more experienced than their uncertified peers, with the quality of these individuals and the depth of their professional development making them more compelling hires (Carter, 2009). The caution remains that the passing of an evidenced-based examination should not be the sole indicator of a case manager's ability to demonstrate competence and mastery of professional practice. However, it can be used as one of several factors to appraise and evaluate that practice.

Case managers are beholden to practice at the top of their requisite licensure and certification. This language appears in a majority of the established resources that guide professional case management practice across industry's many standards, codes, and regulations (ACMA, 2013; CMSA, 2010). Principle 5 of the Commission for Case Manager Certification's Code of Professional Conduct (CCMC, 2009) is specific that certificants will keep their competency at a level that ensures each of their clients will receive the benefit of services that are appropriate and consistent for the client's conditions and circumstances. Health care consumers deserve the highest level of professional knowledge, training, and skills that can be delivered to them by the case management workforce.

Acknowledging No One Case Manager Can and Does Know All

It is impossible that any single case manager can be the possessor of ALL that is case management. Whether an individual has longevity in the industry or is a "newbie," LLL is a must.

The COLLABORATE approach recognizes the fluid quantity of knowledge for case managers to acquire toward the purpose of assuring their workplace knowledge proficiency. This extends across the new practice trends and innovative models of health care delivery, to fluid patient demographics, advancing clinical pathophysiology and psychopathology, medication reconciliation models, and treatment protocols. Add in varying reimbursement models, overarching regulations, and changing psychosocial stressors for patients and families plus the accompanying dynamics.

The diversity of patient needs mandates a diverse professional case management workforce. Why would any single case manager claim the role of chief cook and bottle washer when the professional expertise of colleagues is at their disposal? The COLLABORATE LLL competency emphasizes the goal of addressing a patient's global issues through recognizing the value which can come when professionals of varied disciplines intentionally working together (IPEC, 2011). One wonders about the ultimate disservice of the mindset where one case manager need be responsible for any and all knowledge used. This serves as a setup of insurmountable expectations for any case manager, plus contributes to less-than-optimal outcomes for health care's stakeholders and consumers.

IMPLICATIONS FOR PRACTICE

LLL has a diverse scope of implications for case management practice.

Alignment Across the Case Management Process

First, it plays an integral role across each phase of the case management process. Consider the potential consequences for patients when case managers do not take either accountability for or initiative to maintain the most accurate and current knowledge base. There are ramifications in not being able to accurately define the most appropriate targeted populations to benefit from intervention, or available grant funding opportunities to finance new programming designated for those populations. A poorly organized assessment will cause a ripple effect in defining treatment plans, advocating with team members and other treatment providers for recommended patient needs that promote individualized, safe and quality-driven care. When a case manager lacks awareness of new diagnoses and treatment parameters across health and/or behavioral health for patients, how can they possibly advocate effectively with insurance companies, and resource providers for requisite needs across the transitions of care to optimize the patient's ability to reach the highest level of functioning.

Juggling Diverse CEU Requirements

Next, the CEU requirements for those professionals who comprise case management are diverse for they are managed across a fragmented licensure system and sundry assortment of certification entities. How can case managers develop a solid and comprehensive understanding of their learning needs amid a disjointed professional, and at times, contentious environment, one where team members squabble about whose competencies and which skill set and/or discipline make for the "best case manager?" This leads directly to the third point.

Reconciling Formal Framework for Research and Research Utilization

Professional case management as an industry must do a better job documenting a formal framework for research and research utilization. Although this topic is discussed in chapter 9, it is a point that bears repeating through alignment with LLL. For case management to be viewed as a profession it must encompass the many disciplines to comprise professional case management's workforce. This has now expanded beyond the traditional composition of nursing, social workers, professional counselors, and rehabilitation professions. Pharmacists have integrated themselves into collaborative teams and are expected to expand their role throughout the continuum of care (Cherian, Patel, & Reed, 2014). How can case management have a fighting chance for growth and sustainability without consensus in accepting who is welcome to sit at its ever-expanding table?

With no formal agreement across the case management industry as to best practice for measuring case management outcomes, the utilization of research findings is equally ill-defined. As a result, LLL becomes lost amid the mass of mandatory CEUs required across the diverse range of professional boards, certification entities, and higher education providers. Although there is great value in the abundance of professional standards of practice and ethical codes of professional conduct that exist, none of them serve as performance mandates for employers and/or case managers to follow. Mandates of this nature can only be reinforced by legal sanction.

Although the literature is full of quotes citing the critical importance of professional development and continuing education, there is little consensus on what that foundational based on research should consist of. Some indicate this should be evidence-based and/or outcomes-driven. Extensive knowledge is as vital a factor, as experience and interdisciplinary communication toward the goal of case managers working together to transition patients through the continuum of care (Nailey, 2012). Yet with multiple disciplines involved in the decision-making process, there continues to be little consistency and/or consensus about what exactly should comprise this holy grail of case management wisdom.

There is value in a cue to that work by the work of the World Health Organization (WHO) (2010) that helped to foster IPE plus trigger change in how health care professionals are educated. IPE serves as an opportunity to not only change the way the industry thinks about educating future health workers, but also to step back and reconsider the traditional means of health care delivery. "There needs to be a change in educational practice, plus the culture of medicine and health care" (WHO, 2010). There are grand lessons for case management amid how the WHO, CIHC, IPEC, and IOM ultimately crafted and facilitated new models of competency-based IPE. Each entity has been able to break through those solid walls among health care's disciplines to foster a collective approach to learning and providing care. In this way students from diverse health care professions learn as early as possible about, from, and with each other to enable effective collaboration and improve health outcomes (WHO, 2010).

Imagine a research agenda for professional case management that stems from a greater effort by its involved professional disciplines, one where those involved intentionally work together toward that purpose of safe, competent, and quality patient-centered care. What a powerful foundation would exist for this research agenda and its manifesting framework.

MENTORING'S INFLUENCE

Mentoring is a potent means to enhance and assure the highest quality of professional intervention. Defined as an experienced and trusted advisor (Oxford Dictionaries, 2014), the role of mentor is one of tremendous influence.

Commons and Snowden (2010) pose how mentoring has emerged as one of the most valuable roles one can perform in the workplace. Through case managers serving as role models, they are in a position to provide feedback, nurture talent, inspire individual development, and facilitate excellence.

The literature notes how the newest generation of case managers prefer the trendier buzzwords of "professional coaching," "advising," or "precepting" (Powell, 2013). Getting lost amid the weeds of names can and will devalue the ultimate purpose of the mentoring goal. It is the wisdom of experience that gives case managers a valuable professional mirror by which to reflect on their actions and expand on their skills and expertise. The sharing of both experiential and didactic learning is profoundly important not only to facilitate the growth of individual case managers, but also to evolve and advance case management practice itself beyond what it is today.

SUMMARY

Peter Drucker's (2003) words resonate: "Every enterprise is a learning and teaching institution. Training and development must be built into it on all levels—training and development that never stop." LLL is multifaceted with case managers having accountability for competent and quality-motivated practice.

Moving forward it is imperative that case management, as the profession it yearns to be, accepts overarching responsibility to develop strategic research agendas that weave across the macro worlds of regulatory boards, legislative and educational institutions, plus health care organizations. On the micro level, case managers must be motivated to excel in their respective pursuit of knowledge, both didactic and experiential, to assure a maximum standard of LLL, one that encourages responsibility for their new and continued learning. In turn, a case manager's individual LLL competence should contribute to greater consumer confidence among the total stakeholders of the industry. Accepting and promoting this shared commitment to LLL excellence will strengthen the resolve of the professional case management workforce toward an ultimate paradigm shift to COLLABORATE.

References

American Association of Colleges of Nursing. (2014). *AACN synergy model of patient care*. Retrieved April 20, 2014, from http://www.aacn.org/wd/certifications/content/synmodel.pcms?menu=certification#Basic

American Case Management Association. (2013). *Standards of practice and scope of services for health care delivery system case management and transition of care (TOC) professionals*. Retrieved September 7, 2014, from http://www.acmaweb.org/forms/2013SoPBrochure_FINAL_Online.pdf

American Nurses Association. (2014). *Scope and standards of practice*. Retrieved September 7, 2014, from http://nursingworld.org/scopeandstandardsofpractice

Ashford, J. B., & LeCroy, C. W. (2013). *Human behavior in the social environment* (5th ed.). Australia: Brooks/Cole Cengage Learning.

Carter, J. (2009). Case management credentials: Sorting out certificates and certification. *Professional Case Management*, *14*(5), 267–270.

Case Management Society of America. (2010). *CMSA standards of practice for case management* (Rev.). Retrieved April 25, 2013, from http://www.cmsa.org/portals/0/pdf/memberonly/StandardsOfPractice.pdf

Center for Disease Control and Prevention. (2014). *Health literacy*. Retrieved September 5, 2014, from http://www.cdc.gov/healthliteracy/Learn/index.html

Cherian J., Patel, K. R., & Reed, M. (2014). Evolving role of pharmacists in care coordination—A national survey. *Therapeutic Innovation and Regulatory Science*, *48*(2), 266–271.

Commission for Case Manager Certification. (2009). *Code of professional conduct for case managers*. Retrieved April 26, 2013, from http://ccmcertification.org/content/ccm-exam-portal/code-professional-conductcase-managers

Commons, D., & Snowden, F. (2010). Who needs mentoring in case management, inside case management. *Professional Case Management*, *15*(1), 49–51.

Council on Social Work Education. (2008). *Education policy and accreditation standards (EPAS) implementation*. Retrieved July 14, 2014, from http://www.cswe.org/Accreditation/EPASImplementation.aspx

Cullen, K. (2014). *Parity in mental health care a must*. Retrieved August 17, 2014, from http://www.bostonglobe.com/metro/2014/08/16/mental-health-care-critical-for-rich-and-poor/ERQqZFoxNjSX4MviKYQjSK/story.html

Daum, K. (2014). *5 Things really successful learners do*. Retrieved August 28, 2014, from http://www.inc.com/kevin-daum/5-things-really-successful-learners-do.html

Dictionary.com. (2014a). Professional development (definition). Retrieved September 4, 2014, from http://dictionary.reference.com/browse/professional+development

Dictionary.com. (2014b). Contact hours (definition). Retrieved September 4, 2014, from http://medical-dictionary.thefreedictionary.com/Continuing+education+unit

Dictionary.com. (2014c). Continuing education units (definition). Retrieved September 4, 2014, from http://medical-dictionary.thefreedictionary.com/Continuing+education+unit

Drucker, P. F. (2003). *The essential Drucker: The best of sixty years of Peter Drucker's essential writings on management*. New York, NY: Collins Business.

Education Week. (2010). *How do you define 21st century learning*. Teacher Pd Sourcebook, Retrieved August 29, 2014, from http://www.edweek.org/tsb/articles/2010/10/12/01panel.h04.html

Ellison, A. (2014). *4 Challenges that could hinder PPACA success*. Becker's Hospital Review. Retrieved September 3, 2014, from http://www.beckershospitalreview.com/finance/4-challenges-that-could-hinder-ppaca-success.html

Fink-Samnick, E. (2007). *Fostering a sense of professional resilience: Six simple strategies*. Harrisburg, PA: The New Social Worker, White Hat Communications.

Fink-Samnick, E. (2013, November). Case management's ethical eight: Preparing for the next wave. *Dorland Case In Point*, *11*(11), 1–4.

Gardner, H. E. (2006). *5 Minds for the Future* (1st ed.). Cambridge, MA: Harvard Business School Press/Center for Public Leadership.

Gardner, H. E. (2011). *Frames of mind: The theory of multiple intelligences* (3rd ed.). New York, NY: Basic Books.

Gold, J. (2014). Report: Adults with serious mental illnesses face 80% unemployment. *Kaiser Health News*. Retrieved September 3, 2014, from http://capsules.kaiserhealthnews.org/index.php/2014/07/report-adults-with-serious-mental-illnesses-face-80-unemployment/?referrer=search

Halstead, J. (2012, September 24). Transforming nursing education to meet emerging health care needs [Robert Wood Johnson Foundation Human Capital Blog]. Retrieved September 5, 2014, from http://www.rwjf.org/en/blogs/human-capital-blog/2012/09/transforming_nursing.html

Healthcare Information and Management Systems Society. (2014). *2014 HIMSS nursing workforce survey results show growth in informatics specialty*. Retrieved September 3, 2014, from http://www.himss.org/News/NewsDetail.aspx?ItemNumber=28588

Helms, A. D., & Pugh, T. (2014). North Carolina's $10B medicaid challenge: Pay for other states or take federal money? *The Charlotte Observer/Kaiser Health News*. Retrieved September 3, 2014, from http://www.kaiserhealthnews.org/Stories/2014/September/03/North-Carolinas-10B-Medicaid-Challenge-Pay-For-Other-States-Or-Take-Federal-Money.aspx

Institute of Medicine. (2011). *The future of nursing: Leading change*. Washington, DC: Advancing Health/National Academies Press.

Knowles, M., Holton, E. F., & Swanson, R. A. (2012). *The adult learner* (7th ed.). London, New York: Taylor and Francis.

Kolb, D. (1983). *Experiential learning: Experience as the source of learning and development*. Englewood Cliffs, NJ: Prentice Hall.

Korkki, P. (2014). New health law is sending many back to school. *New York Times*. Retrieved August 29, 2014, from http://www.nytimes.com/2014/03/18/education/new-health-law-is-sending-many-back-to-school.html?_r=0

Larson, J. (2010). Pursuing new models in nursing education. *NurseZone.com*. Retrieved August 29, 2014 from http://www.nursezone.com/Nursing-News-Events/more-features/Pursuing-New-Models-in-Nursing-Education_35068.aspx

Lewis, N. (2012). *Global telemedicine market headed for 27 billion*. Retrieved April 28, 2013, from http://www.informationweek.com/healthcare/mobile-wireless/global-telemedicine-market-headed-for-27/232602930

Merriam-Webster. (2014a). Learning (definition). Retrieved August 27, 2014, from http://www.merriam-webster.com/dictionary/learning

Merriam-Webster. (2014b). Didactic (definition). Retrieved August 27, 2014, from http://www.merriam-webster.com/dictionary/didactic

Merriam-Webster. (2014c). Logic (definition). Retrieved September 4, 2014, from http://www.merriam-webster.com/dictionary/logic

Merriam-Webster. (2014d). Reason (definition). Retrieved September 4, 2014, from http://www.merriam-webster.com/dictionary/reason

Monegain, B. (2013). Health informatics jobs growing. *Healthcare IT News*. Retrieved August 29, 2014, from http://www.healthcareitnews.com/news/health-informatics-jobs-growing

Moon, J. (2004). *A handbook of reflective and experiential learning: Theory and practice*. (p. 126). London: Routledge Falmer.

Nailey, C. (2012). *Evidence-based case management*. Advance Healthcare Network. Retrieved August 27, 2014, from http://nursing.advanceweb.com/Features/Articles/Evidence-Based-Case-Management.aspx

National Association of Social Workers. (2008). *Code of ethics of the national association of social workers*. Retrieved April 28, 2013, from http://www.naswdc.org/pubs/code/code.asp

National Association of Social Workers. (2012). *Social work speaks: NASW policy statements, 2012-2014* (9th ed.). Washington, DC: NASW Press.

National Association of Social Workers. (2013). *NASW standards for social work case management*. Washington, DC: National Association of Social Workers.

Oxford Dictionaries. (2014). Mentor. definition. Retrieved September 7, 2014, from http://www.oxforddictionaries.com/us/definition/american_english/mentor

Pace, E. (2014). New rules send upstate nurses back to school. *WKRN-TV News Nashville*. Retrieved September 2, 2014, from http://www.wkrn.com/story/25919803/new-rules-send-upstate-nurses-back-to-school

Quality and Safety Education for Nurses Competencies. (2014). *Quality and safety education for nurses institute*. Retrieved April 30, 2014, from http://qsen.org/competencies/

Powell, S. (2013). Case managers' retirement: What has reverse mentoring got to do with it? *Editorial Column*, *18*(6), 271–272.

Rogers, C. R (1951). *Client-centered therapy*. Boston, MA: Houghton Mifflin Harcourt Press.

Rogers, C. R., & Freiberg, H. J. (1994). *Freedom to learn* (3rd ed.). Upper Saddle River, NJ: Pearson.

Senge, P. M. (2006). *The fifth discipline: The art and practice of the learning organization* (2nd ed.). New York, NY: Currency: Doubleday.

Shuman, L. (2014). Two Americas on health care, and danger of further division. The Upshot, *New York Times*. Retrieved September 7, 2014, from http://www.nytimes.com/2014/07/24/upshot/two-americas-on-health-care-and-danger-of-further-division.html?_r=0andabt=0002andabg=0

Terry, K. (2013). 47% of doctors use smartphone, tablet and PC. *InformationWeek*. Retrieved September 3, 2014, from http://www.informationweek.com/mobile/47--of-doctors-use-smartphone-tablet-and-pc/d/d-id/1111170?

Treiger, T., & Fink-Samnick, E. (2013). COLLABORATE: A universal competency based paradigm for professional case management, part 2: Competency clarification. *Professional Case Management*, *18*(5), 219–243.

The United States Department of Labor. (2014). Employee benefits security administration, *Mental health parity*. Retrieved September 3, 2014, http://www.dol.gov/ebsa/mentalhealthparity/

U.S. Department of Health and Human Services. (2010). *National action plan to improve health literacy, office of disease prevention and health promotion*. Retrieved September 5, 2014 from http://www.health.gov/communication/HLActionPlan/

VARK. A Guide to Learning Styles (2014a). *FAQs page*. Retrieved August 27, 2014, from http://www.vark-learn.com/english/page.asp?p=faq

Villaire, M., & Mayer, G. (2007). Low health literacy: The impact on chronic illness management. *Professional Case Management*, *12*(4), 213–216.

Williams, D. J. (2014, Spring). *GO FAR! A useful framework for developing career success in social work*. The New Social Worker. Retrieved September 4, 2014, from http://www.socialworker.com/feature-articles/career-jobs/go-far-useful-framework-for-developing-career-success-social-work/

World Health Organization. (2010). *Framework for action on interprofessional education and collaborative practice*. Health Professional Networks. Geneva, Switzerland: Nursing and Midwifery, Human Resources for Health, World Health Organization.

11 LEADERSHIP

OBJECTIVES

After studying this chapter, you will be able to:

1. Define leadership.
2. Distinguish leadership from management.
3. Describe various leadership theories.
4. Provide historical context to the development of leadership theories.
5. Describe the key elements of case management leadership.
6. Identify leadership opportunities available to nurses and social workers.

KEY TERMS

ANA Leadership Institute
ANCC Magnet
AONE competencies
Behavioral theory
Case Management Leadership Coalition
Center for Creative Leadership (CCL) Competency Library
Contingency theory
Council on Leadership Development
Human services management competencies
Leadership
Leadership for Academic Nursing Program
NLN Leadership Institute
Professional communication
Professional identity
Quantum theory
Self-awareness
Servant theory
Social Work Leadership in Health Care
The Future of Nursing: Leading Change, Advancing Health
Transactional theory
Transformational theory

The COLLABORATE model considers leadership a necessary foothold for establishing and advancing professional case management practice. It has little to do with organizational hierarchy or a self-aggrandizing personal agenda, but rather pertains to leveraging personal strengths as well as recognizing and converting weaknesses on the journey to best practice, optimal outcomes, and professional growth.

When contemplating the leadership competency, it is essential to remember that case management leadership occurs in every aspect of practice and professional identity, from academia to professional associations to work setting. While formal education and hands-on training provide theoretical and practical foundations, management coalesces with policy and procedure to reflect professional standards and establish evidence-based practice. Ultimately, leadership is at the frontline where the case manager blends skill, strengths, and abilities harmoniously with client and organizational goals to achieve success.

A leader, as described by Kotter (2011), recognizes the urgency of a situation and wants to make things happen. Being a leader requires vision and the ability to inspire people to reach beyond what they believed was possible. A leader empowers individuals around them to accomplish goals and surpass expectations. A leader has a sense of purpose primarily focused on advancement of the industry, rather than of personal gain. This chapter focuses on the points of impact where the leadership competency influences case management practice.

BOX 11-1 Leadership Perspectives

The only definition of a leader is someone who has followers. Peter Drucker	The first step to leadership is servanthood. John Maxwell
Leadership is invisible, a leader is best when people barely know he exists, when his work is done, his aim fulfilled, they will say: we did it ourselves. Lao Tzu	Leadership: the art of getting someone else to do something you want done because he (or she) wants to do it. Dwight D. Eisenhower
Leadership is the capacity to translate vision into reality. Warren Bennis	If your actions inspire others to dream more, learn more, do more and become more, you are a leader. John Quincy Adams
A leader is a dealer in hope. Napoleon Bonaparte	A good leader takes a little more than his share of the blame, a little less than his share of the credit. Arnold H. Glasow

DEFINITION

Usually the source of a definition influences the words selected to capture the specific application to the field, population, or specialty. Because case management is a multidisciplinary practice, the definitional source is an especially important consideration. The two major streams, which feed the case management river, are nursing and social work. One might expect to utilize definitions from those areas but that would be limiting. Many influences on case management practice are dependent on practice setting. So, how does one come to an acceptable definition of **leadership**? Many definitions exist; Box 11-1 provides a sampling from a variety of perspectives. Suffice to say, there are consistent elements in many of these definitions; however, a definition offered by Chemers (1997), "a process of social influence by which an individual enlists the aid and support of others in the accomplishment of a task or mission," has withstood the test of time and continues to be relied on across many sectors.

EFFORTS TO BUILD LEADERSHIP

Nursing

The Future of Nursing: Leading Change, Advancing Health report (Institutes of Medicine, 2011) issued specific key messages and recommendations as part of its nursing workforce study in order to define an action blueprint for change in policy at all levels of government, regulation, and organization. Key message #4 pertained to workforce planning and policy. Immediately following removal of scope-of-practice barriers, the committee recommended expanded opportunities for nurse leadership and diffusion of collaborative improvement efforts to include nurses. A call for action was issued to the Center for Medicare and Medicaid Innovation, private and public funding sources, health care organizations, nursing programs, and professional associations to step up the development of programs, tools, and opportunities to foster nurse leadership.

Leadership is defined or accounted for within the constructs of one's educational and experiential alignment. For nurses, the American Nurses Association (ANA), American Nurses Credentialing Center (ANCC), the National League for Nursing (NLN), the American Association of Colleges of Nursing (AACN), and the American Organization of Nurse Executives (AONE) are some of the strongest among many organizations devoting resources to building nursing leadership depth.

The ANA supports the Institute of Medicine (IOM) Future of Nursing report findings, which emphasizes the importance of developing nurse leadership in a variety of ways. The **ANA Leadership Institute** delivers educational programs for nurses and nurse leaders at all stages of a career development. In addition to online offerings, publications focus on various aspects of leadership through various guidebooks. The Institute's programs are designed using a collaborative, problem-based learning model that incorporates best practices and the knowledge and skill sets expected of nurse leaders. Each program offering is designed to improve outcomes based on competencies drawn from the **Center for Creative**

Leadership (CCL) Competency Library—an evidence-based process for tailoring competencies most relevant for leadership development at different stages of a career trajectory (ANA, 2014). Face-to-face immersion learning opportunities address advanced leadership needs.

The **ANCC Magnet** program model includes 14 Forces of Magnetism supporting practice excellence (see Figure 11-1). The emphasis on leadership is clear, as the first of these forces is Quality of Nursing Leadership. In this force, the nurse leader is a knowledgeable, strong, risk-taker. Nurse leaders follow a well-articulated, strategic, and visionary philosophy in the day-to-day operations of nursing services. Nursing leaders, at all organizational levels, convey a strong sense of advocacy and support for the staff and for the patient. The results of quality leadership are evident in nursing practice at the patient's side (ANCC, 2014).

The **NLN Leadership Institute** offers rigorous 3-year programs supporting leadership skills development in nurse faculty. The three programs focus on nurse educators, simulation educators, and senior deans and directors, respectively. The common denominator of these programs is a shared commitment to nursing education excellence with the long-term goal being a lasting transformative leadership-building experience.

Quality of Nursing Leadership
Organizational Structure
Personnel Policies & Programs
Professional Models of Care
Quality of Care
Quality Improvement
Consultation & Resources
Autonomy
Management Style
Community & Health Care Organization
Nurses as Teachers
Image of Nursing
Interdisciplinary Relationships
Professional Development

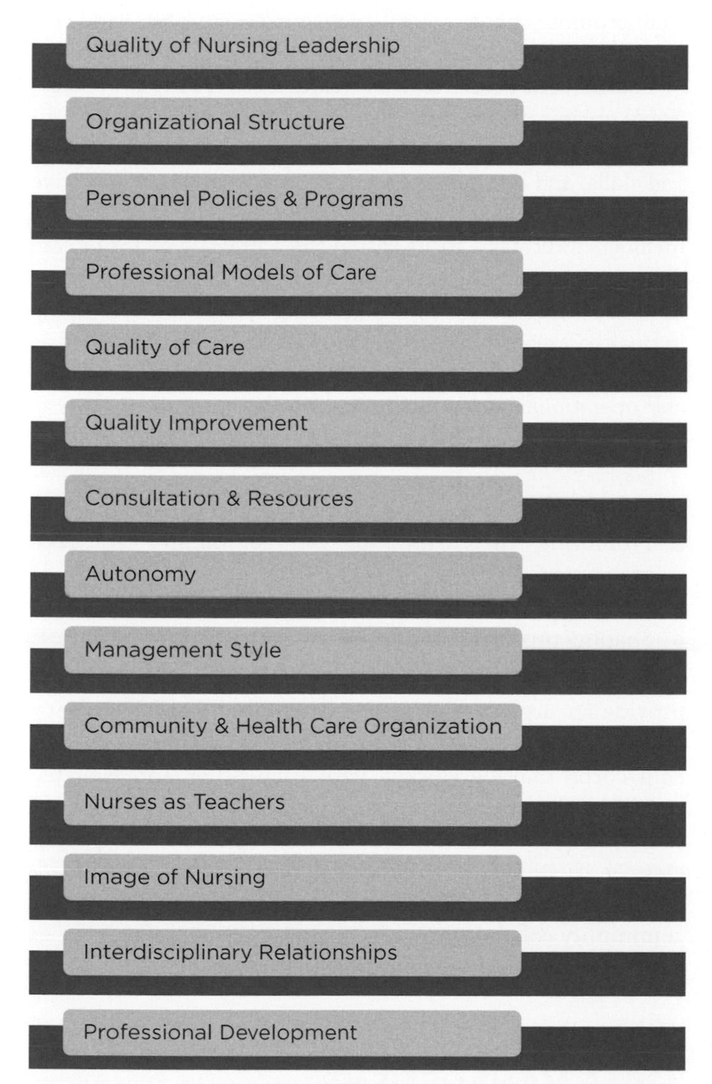

Figure 11-1. ANCC Magnet program forces of magnetism. (Adapted from American Nurses Credentialing Center. (2014). *Magnet recognition program model*. Retrieved June 30, 2014, from http://www.nursecredentialing.org/Magnet/ProgramOverview/New-Magnet-Model)

Support of leadership development has been a key element of the AACN mission since its inception over 40 years ago. AACN sponsors the **Leadership for Academic Nursing Program** (LANP), a fellowship for executive leadership targeting aspiring and new academic deans. The application process is competitive and admission is restricted to approximately 50 participants annually.

AONE recognizes that excellent leadership is essential to ensure excellent patient care. After publication of its role and function of nurse executives' study, **AONE competencies** for individuals in executive practice within the following skill domains (2005):

- Communication and relationship-building,
- A knowledge of the health care environment,
- Leadership,
- Professionalism, and
- Business skills.

AONE further delineates leadership as:

- Foundational thinking skills
- Personal journey disciplines
- The ability to use systems thinking
- Succession planning
- Change management

Devoting this level of support to nurse leadership skills development is not surprising in light of the fact that nurses make up the largest employee segment in health care, with more than 3.1 million registered nurses (RNs) nationwide. Of all licensed RNs, 2.6 million or 84.8% are employed in nursing (Health Resources and Services Administration, 2010). Nearly 58% of RNs worked in general medical and surgical hospitals (U.S. Bureau of Labor Statistics, 2010). Nurses practice independently yet collaboratively with other clinical professionals. The focus on leadership as a crucial need arises from the impact of significant changes that have occurred in the organization, delivery, and financing of health care during this turbulent period of time (Huber, 2010).

SOCIAL WORK

The history of social work in the United States is often portrayed as an altruistic venture taken on by individuals who delved into the plight of the most vulnerable populations and served as compassionate leaders committed to making a positive difference in their communities. These individuals led efforts to provide social services and give hope to the clients they served. Early pioneers, Jane Addams and Mary Richmond are noted in a previous chapter. There are contemporary organizations recognizing the importance of developing leadership in social work education and practice: the Council on Social Work Education (CSWE) (2014), the

Initiative 1

- Launched the CSWE Leadership Institute in Social Work Education, identified as a preconference educational event.

Initiative 2

- Launched the CSWE Leadership Scholars in Social Work Education Program. This program's purpose is to attract a small cohort of future leaders and provide them with targeted education, training, and mentoring. There is an application process and selected participants must make an 1-year commitment.

Initiative 3

- Launched the CSWE Leadership Networking Reception to support, encourage, and honor new leadership in the profession.

Figure 11-2. CSWE leadership initiatives. (Adapted from the Council on Social Work Education (2014). *Leadership institute*. Retrieved July 1, 2014, from http://www.cswe.org/CentersInitiatives/CSWELeadershipInst.aspx)

National Association of Social Workers (NASW), the Society for Social Work Leadership in Health Care, and the Network for Social Work Management (NSWM).

Under the umbrella of the CSWE, the **Council on Leadership Development** (CLD) established the Leadership Institute in 2008 with the support of the Commission on Professional Development. The CLD is responsible to set program and service policy relating to the development of social work education leaders. During 2008 to 2009, the Institute launched three initiatives, which promoted future leaders in social work education, higher education, and the social work profession (see Figure 11-2).

The NASW (2013) defines practice standards based on the area of specialization. The standards for social work case management practice combine advocacy and leadership in Standard 7, "The social work case manager shall advocate for the rights, decisions, strengths, and needs of clients and shall promote clients' access to resources, supports, and services." See Box 11-2 for the interpretation of Standard 7.

BOX 11-2 NASW Standard 7 Leadership Interpretation

Social work case managers exercise leadership by advocating for clients on the micro, mezzo, and macro levels. Microlevel advocacy may involve the following activities:

- Inclusion of clients in advocacy efforts and in program design, planning, and evaluation
- Promotion of clients' strengths, needs, and goals among colleagues and with other organizations
- Communication with other service providers and organizations to improve clients' access to resources, supports, and services

Adapted from National Association of Social Workers. (2013). NASW standards for social work case management. Retrieved April 25, 2013, from http://www.socialworkers.org/practice/naswstandards/CaseManagementStandards2013.pdf

Social Work Leadership in Health Care (2014) is a professional organization whose mission indicates its intent to support emerging leaders in all roles, provide leadership knowledge and skills, and be the force for advocacy through its collective leadership in all health care arenas. The concentration of board members indicates a focus within the acute care sector of care delivery. Social Work Leadership in Health Care offers publications and educational content, including Social Work Leadership in Health Care: Principles and Practice. This text is described as an exploration of how social work has and can provide invaluable operational leadership in tumultuous times, and includes:

- Characteristics of effective health care social work leaders,
- Effective management of complex health care systems,
- Promoting the health of the community and the institution,
- Education for leadership in health care social work, and
- Shaping professional destiny to secure your future.

The NSWM was launched in 1985, out of a desire to provide an organization devoted to social work managers. Among its foundational imperatives "to cultivate a leadership corps that networked with each other and elevated social work values into management decision-making" (2014). NSWM's **human services management competencies** are clustered into the four domains of executive leadership, strategic management, resource management, and community collaboration. See Figure 11-3 for competencies defined within executive leadership domain.

CASE MANAGEMENT

The prominent professional organizations in case and care management include the Case Management Society of America (CMSA), the American Case Management Association

Executive leadership

- Establishes, promotes, and anchors the vision, philosophy, goals, objectives, and values of the organization
- Possesses interpersonal skills that support the viability and positive functioning of the organization
- Possesses analytical and critical thinking skills that promote organizational growth
- Models appropriate professional behavior and encourages other staff members to act in a professional manner
- Develops and manages both internal and external stakeholder relationships
- Initiates and facilitates innovative change processes
- Advocates for public policy change and social justice at national, state, and local levels
- Demonstrates effective interpersonal and communication skills
- Encourages active involvement of all staff and stakeholders in decision-making processes
- Plans, promotes, and models lifelong learning practices

Resource management

- Effectively manages human resources
- Effectively manages and oversees the budget and other financial resources to support the organization's/program's mission and goals and to foster continuous program improvement and accountability
- Establishes and maintains a system of internal controls to ensure transparency, protection, and accountability for the use of organizational resources
- Manages all aspects of information technology

Strategic management

- Identifies and applies for new and recurring funding while ensuring accountability with existing funding systems
- Engages in proactive communication about the agency's products and services
- Designs and develops effective programs
- Manages risk and legal affairs
- Ensures strategic planning

Community collaboration

- Builds relationships with complementary agencies, institutions, and community groups to enhance the delivery of services

Figure 11-3. NSWM domains and competencies.

(ACMA), and the National Association of Professional Geriatric Care Managers (NAPGCM). None of the standards of practice documents for these organizations highlights leadership or the role of the case manager as a leader. ACMA advertises a Leadership Conference and Medical Director Forum in late 2014, the details of which are not yet publicly available. Some CMSA chapters offer leadership-focused conferences. For example, the New England chapter has offered an annual building strategies conference for the past 15 years.

The **Case Management Leadership Coalition** (CMLC) was formed in 2002 to bring together representatives of case management from across the health care industry. The intent seems to have been an opportunity to bring together case management leaders for discussion and consensus building with regard to current issues in case management. The group was also to address ways in which to replicate advances in the role and mission of case management. CMSA and the Academy of Certified Case Managers (ACCM) sponsored the CMLC. In 2005, there were reportedly 36 organizations participating in the CMLC. Documentation of the CMLC's work dates back to 2005; however, only a few references to this organization remain accessible via the Internet and the domain associated with this group (http://www.cmleaders.org) indicates it is currently for sale as of July 2014.

The Differences Between Management and Leadership

Drucker said that "Management is doing things right; leadership is doing the right things." A list distinguishing a leader from a manager was compiled by Warren Bennis (1989) in *On Becoming a Leader*, which is presented in Figure 11-4.

Past and Current Thinking

In order to establish edges to this sandbox, it is important to examine the evolution of leadership theory. Common elements capture and portray leadership as being a process inclusive influence, which requires a group context and the desire to attain a defined goal (Busse, 2014; Antonakis, Cianciolo, & Sternberg, 2004). However, leadership is quite complex and multifaceted. It is a phenomenon, which has been investigated ad infinitum; but despite numerous theories and volumes of research, little cumulative knowledge has been gained (Badshah, 2012).

Theoretical Underpinnings

So when narrowing down to a case management perspective, it is important to have an understanding of the theoretical

Leader	Manager
☐ Innovates	☐ Administers
☐ Is an original	☐ Is a copy
☐ Develops	☐ Maintains
☐ Focus on people	☐ Focus on systems & structure
☐ Inspires trust	☐ Relies on control
☐ Long-range perspective	☐ Short-range view
☐ Asks what & why	☐ Asks how & when
☐ Has eye on the horizon	☐ Bottom-line perspective
☐ Challenges status quo	☐ Accepts status quo
☐ Does the right thing	☐ Does things right

Figure 11-4. Bennis's leader versus manager comparison. (Adapted from Bennis, W. (1989). *On becoming a leader*. Reading, MA: Addison-Wesley.)

knowledge associated with general leadership in order to better transfer it from a 30,000-foot perch to a day-to-day perspective. A great many leadership theories can be grouped under major headings along a timeline. As a general review and for the purpose of this text, the following are included: behavioral, contingency, transactional, transformational, quantum, and servant theories.

Behavioral Theory

Behavioral theory offered the perspective that focused on behaviors of the individual rather than his or her characteristics (e.g., mental, physical, social characteristics). Behavioral theories of leadership are based on the belief that great leaders are made, not born. According to this theory, people can learn to become leaders through teaching and observation. Theories included in the behavioral category separated leaders by those concerned with tasks and those concerned with people. One's leadership style (e.g., dictatorial, democratic, laissez-faire) influenced group dynamics and outcomes. Studies conducted in Iowa, Ohio, and Michigan provided landmark findings that are still recognized today.

Contingency Theory

Contingency theory proposed that there is no one specific way in which to lead and that the manner of leadership varied based on circumstance. It focuses on environmental variables that influence a choice of leadership style, which may best suit a given situation. According to this theory, no one leadership style is applicable to all situations. Positive results depend on variables (e.g., leadership style, follower qualities, situational circumstance). The implication of this theory is that people perform optimally under certain conditions, but less so when not in an area of comfort.

Transactional Theory

Transactional theory highlights an exchange between leader and follower in which there is a positive and beneficial relationship for those involved. An effective transactional leader finds ways by which to meaningfully reward (or punish) the follower for performance. Also referred to as management theory, the focus is on the role of supervision, organization, and group performance. Transactional theory is frequently practiced in business settings.

Transformational Theory

The crux of **transformational theory** lies in the inspirational nature of the leader–follower relationship. There is a clear sense of belonging for the followers, who are able to identify with their leader. Also referred to as relationship or relational theory, transformational theory emphasizes the connection between leaders and followers. Transformational leaders motivate people through visualization of the importance and beneficial outcome of the work. These leaders are focused on the performance of both group and individuals.

Quantum Theory

In **quantum theory**, leadership addresses the organization holistically rather than as disparate, competing parts of a whole. Elements of quantum leadership include discovering, authenticity, passion, creating, relationship, inquiry, and fiscal astuteness. While traditional management theorists consider groups as hierarchical systems intent on goal accomplishment, quantum theory considers the organization–member dyad as interconnected and mutually influenced through collaboration and interaction. The relationship connections are neither linear nor hierarchical.

The quantum paradigm does not replace traditional frameworks, but it is very useful in situations that are dynamic and created from turbulence because quantum leaders are focused on the future and problem solving based on breaking conventional thinking to find solutions in fast-paced, continuously changing environments. Figure 11-5 displays Porter-O'Grady's principles of quantum mechanics as applied to nursing leadership.

Servant Theory

This leadership model focuses on the leader who focuses more on the needs of others ahead of his or her own needs. The concept of servant leadership extends back into century's old history. However, its contemporary application and the term itself was coined by Greenleaf (1977). The **servant theory** approach requires rethinking of the relationship between leader and follower. The leader is responsible for the promotion of employee performance and satisfaction.

This approach requires a leader to be introspective and self-aware in order to develop moral insight and core ethical beliefs. In this way, the leader must take the impact that their decisions and actions have on others into consideration as part of a decision-making process. Qualities and

All systems work from the inside out, not from the top-down or the bottom-up. Systems are cyclical and circular, not rectangular or pyramidal.

Relationship is as important as control to the effectiveness and sustainability of any system.

Vertical and horizontal integrations are necessary to the definition of a system. Vertical processes define control; horizontal processes define relatedness.

Systems are defined by a conception of the whole, not by an enumeration of the parts; they can be known only in understanding the whole, not by simply examining the parts.

All components of a system intersect and overlap, creating interdependencies that cannot be addressed separately or unilaterally, but only in the context of their relationship to each other.

When separate systems meet or intersect, they overlap and combine and become a new system. They do not remain what they once were when separate from each other.

All reality essentially is uncertain and cannot be predicted with any degree of assuredness. If we measure position (particle), direction becomes uncertain; if we measure direction (wave), position becomes uncertain.

The context of any situation, including our own expectations, influences what the quantum reality will become. Our expectations and participation alters our reality, yet this reality cannot be defined independent of them.

A system engages all of its components in undertaking a potential change; the potential is addressed from the perspective of every element, not simply from the direction provided by a select few.

The context of a system is forever in flux and working relentlessly at its borders, creating the conditions (potential) for the system's next shift in reality or form.

Healthy systems live in the tension between stability and chaos in a constant state of disequilibrium that creates the conditions and energy to ensure its response to the demand for evolution and change.

Engagement, investment, inclusion, and ownership are required throughout a system and are the conditions for any sustainable action within the system. Any rupture in any one part of a system means a break in the whole system.

Figure 11-5. Porter-O'Grady quantum principles and leadership impacts. (Adapted from Porter-O'Grady, T. (1997). Quantum mechanics and the future of healthcare leadership. *The Journal of Nursing Administration*, *27*(1), 15–20.)

characteristics of a servant leader include listening, empathy, healing, awareness, persuasion, conceptualization, foresight, stewardship, commitment to the growth of people, and building community (Spears, 2004).

CONTEXT FOR COLLABORATE LEADERSHIP

Leadership is less about a specific set of behaviors and more about creating an environment in which people are motivated to produce and move in the direction of the leader. In other words, leaders may need to concern themselves less with the actual behaviors they exhibit and attend more to the situation within which work is done (Horner, 1997).

Gardner's theory of leadership fits case management's purposes well. Gardner challenges the belief that leadership exists within a single designated person or situation. Instead, leadership exists in relationship to a goal or purpose and results from the efforts of multiple members of the group. Gardner sees the value of telling stories as part of the leadership process because he understands that most powerful lessons are often learned through the telling of stories. There are four factors which Gardner considers as indispensable for real leadership: a tie to a community or audience, a rhythm of life that includes isolation and immersion, a relationship between the stories leaders tell and the traits they embody, and arrival at power through the choice of the people rather than through brute force (Bennis, 1996). A case manager often uses stories as a means to communicate with clients in order to demonstrate an important point for educational or experiential purposes. The more effective stories are those that are authentic and have meaning to the individual.

From Gardner's (2011) perspective, a leader is someone who affects the thoughts, feelings, and/or behaviors of a significant number of individuals in a meaningful way.

Leadership may be direct (meaning face-to-face) or indirect. Indirect leadership is a situation in which an individual affects their audience via their work product. Regardless of approach, a leader's authenticity springs from the use of stories with which their audience identifies regardless of class, hierarchic, education, or other distinguishing level of sophistication. In case management, the means used to communicate with clients is expanding day-by-day and includes face-to-face, telephonic, instant messaging, texting, and video over Internet, as well as through tele-enabled or remote medical equipment (e.g., blood glucose monitor, weight scale). What we say, as well as what we do, matters a great deal to the outcome of a case management engagement.

Regardless of practice setting or administrative hierarchy, a case manager must regard himself or herself as a leader and demonstrate this attribute as an integral member of the health care team, as a professional colleague, and as a client advocate. COLLABORATE espouses that the professional case manager is a leader leveraging tools and resources to provide thoughtful case management interventions. Using this approach, case management adds value, rather than layers, to the delivery of health care services (Treiger, personal communication, 2008).

The professional case manager applies knowledge and experience along with sound clinical judgment to ensure optimal, cost-effective quality care to demonstrate leadership in facilitating care delivery. This is a key reason why nonclinical and/or underlicensed staff members should never serve as case managers; they have minimal to no specific educational or training basis on which to base their decision making.

As a leader, a case manager must provide valid authority and reasons that compel a client or caregiver to follow the path of supported care. Case management serves as a bridge, not a crutch (Treiger, 2012), supporting growth of independent, effective self-management. Rather than fostering dependent relationships, case manager-leaders foster self-confidence in others enabling them to do things they did not believe to be possible. The main ingredient for empowering others is a high belief in people. If you believe in others, they will believe in themselves (Maxwell, 2007). Rather than telling a client that she or he is going to or has already done something, the case manager works with client and care team on ways in which the task is completed, supporting the client to gradually take on more responsibility of completing tasks and ultimately contributing to the accomplishment of his or her own case management goals.

Within a corporate structure, providing fair and thoughtful leadership to a case management department is an essential quality for individuals pursuing traditional hierarchical management positions. Although staff members align within department management structure, that behavior relates more to positional power and is not to be confused with leadership. Although a degree of obedience results from this dynamic, the goal of a case manager-leader should be for staff to believe in the purpose of the department and actively engage in the delivery of high-quality service. This raises the topic of leaders as servants, which was discussed previously. It also presents an opportunity to address the differences between being a manager and being a leader.

LEADERSHIP CHARACTERISTICS

Clearly, many great minds have addressed the topic of leadership. However, the ongoing need for clarity and understanding indicates leadership is more of a riddle. Rapidly changing business environments certainly influence this moving target. Discussion of certain aspects of leadership is especially important for case management because of the absence of sustained attention to the topic. There is no single, universally accepted and applied theory of leadership; even the theory of situational leadership with its flexible approach of style driven by circumstance has detractors. As a result, it is advisable to look through many lenses when examining which approach to leadership may be most beneficial in a case management environment.

Maxwell (1993) defined five levels of leadership. Chemers (1997) discussed zones of integrative leadership. Bennis (1989) described ingredients needed to be a leader. Gardner (2011) looked at factors and principles of leadership. The following sections provide the basic concepts of these theoretical aspects of leadership.

Maxwell's Levels of Leadership

Influence is an important force associated with leadership. When influence increases, so too does the potential for leadership. Understanding levels of leadership provides insight into how one may best exert influence (Figure 11-6).

Level 1: Position

As pertains to case management, leadership level influences the case manager–client dyad as much as it does the hierarchical structure of management and career development. As Maxwell (1993) noted, "the only influence you have is that which comes with a title.". As discussed numerous times in this text, the case manager title is less impactful due to its widespread misuse. The position level is overweighted with individuals focused more on their territory and how much more they know than do their coworkers. Protocol and process have a place, but a leader at this level clings tightly to these constructs in an effort to exert control.

Consider the information hoarder. Every office seems to have one person who simply loves the fact that she or he seems to know more about everything than anyone does. Usually it is someone with so many years of working experience in the same job she or he has a "senior" designation in a job title. In an unusual transaction, this is the go-to person. You tentatively walk toward her or his cubicle. As she or he peers over thick-rimmed bifocals at you so condescendingly that you might even feel like Oliver Twist having to beg for help. Eventually you get the answer but not until everyone in the office knows how helpful she or he has been,

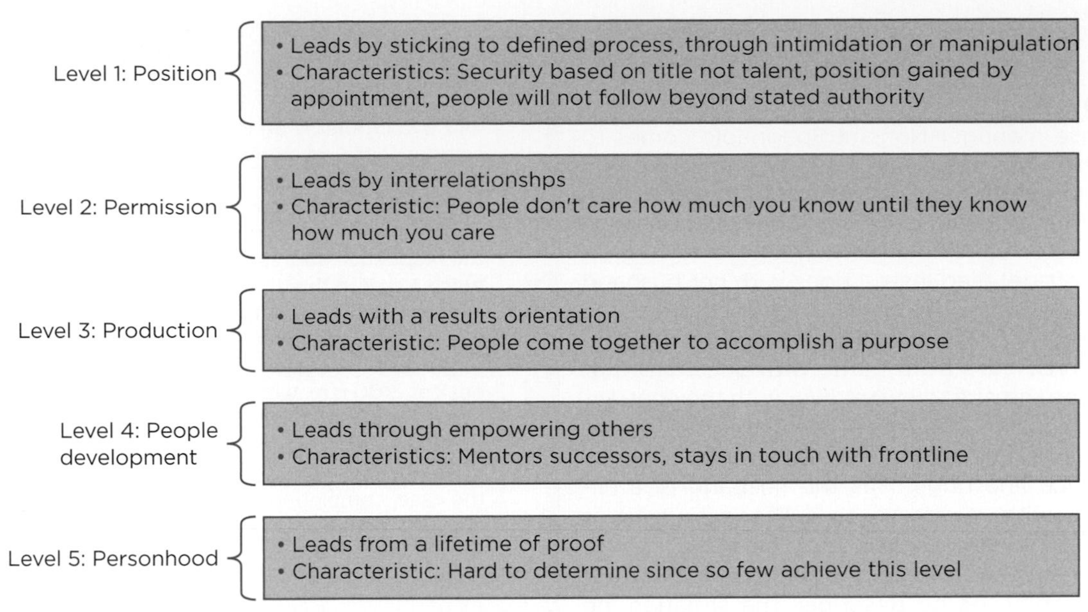

Figure 11-6. Maxwell's five levels of leadership. (Adapted from Maxwell, J. C. (1993). *Developing the leader within you*. Nashville, TN: Thomas Nelson.)

how indispensable she or he is to the team. This person's power is borne solely from the title granted due to her years of service. It is likely that senior management realized her or his leadership limitations, which is why there was no climb into management. This person is difficult to work with and will not have followers beyond the tight sphere of control in which she or he operates.

One of the great points of a case manager's value is in her or his generosity of sharing information and resources, be it with a client, caregiver, or colleague.

Level 2: Permission

Clients will not care about how much you know until they know how much you care (Maxwell, 1993). Permission is the next level of leadership, which begins within meaningful relationships. While overreliance on guidelines and procedures rule level 1 leadership, once in level 2, the individual focuses on building relationships and facilitating the development of those around him or her. Relationships require time, attention, and compassion during wwhich roots strengthen and spread.

Case managers working in environments where they are able to establish longer-termed relationships with clients have an opportunity to grow into level 2 leaders. However, it is essential that one go beyond the artifice of a title to the realization that authentic leadership has nothing to do with an organizational chart. It is about the knowledge and qualities possessed which makes it worthwhile for someone to follow. Initially, an individual may follow because of the client—case manager relationship but it is in the relationship dynamic where trust is established. At some point along the way, the interaction goes from being an obligation to one of an authentic desire to follow (Treiger, 2014).

Level 3: Production

Maxwell (1993) describes level 3 as the one in which morale is high, turnover is low, needs are met, and goals are realized. This is a high-efficiency atmosphere and all cylinders are firing. There is tremendous momentum established; people work together with a purposeful desired outcome. This is a results-oriented environment.

A case manager leading at level 3 has established his or her approach to work as joyful, rather than judgmental. When problems arise, they are seen as opportunities to learn something new. For case managers working in supervisory positions, the managerial tasks work may cause interruptions in the day but these are part of the job addressed promptly and professionally. Box 11-3 provides a scenario demonstrating the difference in approach of a case manager-leader functioning at level 1 versus level 3.

Level 4: People Development

At level 4 leadership, an individual obtains consistently superior performance from followers because of the ability to empower those around her or him. When individuals grow through the mentoring and assistance of a leader, loyalty is at its highest. It is important that individuals continually seek to foster growth in others by investing time and effort to help others, be they colleagues, staff, or clients.

Many case management departments exist within the traditional hierarchical bureaucracy. Although somewhat restrictive, this presents a perfect opportunity to establish an environment of mutual mentoring. Every individual in a management or supervisory position should mentor at least one person who is interested in career growth and advancement. Loyalty extends through an entire operation when

BOX 11-3 Distinction Between Leadership Levels 1 and 3

The Scenario

Senior case manager Nancita Spagnuolo comes to work rather distracted and frazzled. Work is being done at home but she is unable to personally oversee it. Instead, she had numerous conversations with the contractor to review her expectations. In addition, she left detailed instructions with her husband in case questions arise. At 8:00 a.m. she arrives to her office at XYZ Managed Care. Within 2 hours, she receives three calls from home with questions that she believes she already went over with the contractor; her stress level mounts as she begins to believe her husband is not able to oversee the work.

The office line rings. It is the husband of a client calling with regard to an authorization. He is frustrated with the process delay because his wife is experiencing more pain and her condition worsens by the day. As he describes the situation, he hears musical ringtone in the background. He is not pleased when Nancita abruptly cuts him off and places him on hold. It occurs to him that instead of addressing his situation, she is answering a personal call.

It takes 5 minutes for Nancita to get back to the business call. By the time she does, the client's husband has already hung up. She glances at the case notes. The request arrived 3 days earlier. The delay appears to be the result of missing information. Notes indicate an outgoing request for information was made according to office protocol.

The Difference in Action Taken

A Level 1 Leader Would . . .	A Level 3 Leader Would . . .
Review the written process and proceed to step two, a call to the doctor's office to make a second request. The level 1 leader leaves a voicemail message asking for the exact information needed and proving the company fax number to which it should be sent. She documents her actions and continues on to her other work. Someone from the doctor's office transcribes the voicemail message and forwards it to the office nurse. The next day, the office nurse reviews the record, finds the additional information, and sends a copy to XYZ Managed Care's main fax line. XYZ's fax router is offline so administrative staff must sort incoming documents into folders which are delivered to the respective addressee twice a day. In this situation, the necessary information arrives back to the level 1 leader's desk at 3:00 p.m. with five other faxes. It sits another day before the level 1 leader addresses the case, completing the approval and initiating an approval letter back to the originating office. All of this is in accordance with documented company procedure.	Understand the written process and call the doctor's office. Instead of voicemail, the level 3 leader already has a point of contact at this busy surgical practice. She asks to speak to the doctor's nurse who recognizes her name and takes the call. The office nurse explains the details that were missing from the original request which the level 3 leader transcribes into the case notes. She asks a few additional questions and adjudicates the decision, providing the authorization number to the office nurse while still on the call. She identifies the clerk who will schedule the appointment and write down her name and direct number. The level 3 leader then calls the husband to notify him of the approval and gives him the office number where a clerk is awaiting his call to make the appointment.

there is an authentic effort to help develop or personally reach out to individuals. Ways in which a leader in a large organization may accomplish this include:

- Learn people's names and greet them personally.
- Read and reply to emails personally.
- Attend department social events and work the crowd rather than staying cloistered with direct reports.
- Be systematic in mentoring individuals, introduce them to other leaders, and bring them to meetings and events.

Level 5: Personhood

This is a level reached by few. Only a lifetime of proven leadership will allow arrival (Maxwell, 1993). Although a number of individuals achieve recognition for contributions to a given field, these awards are not always objectively derived either in nomination or in selection process. One example is a situation in which an individual nominates a colleague for an achievement award. A few years later that colleague returns the favor and nominates that individual who nominated them for the same award. Another example is when recognition is achieved through a pay-for-self-nomination process. Although an expert panel may review the applications, the self-promotional aspect of the nomination cannot be ignored. Hence, touting oneself as a recipient of such an award does not necessarily reflect authentic widespread recognition for achievement.

Level 5 leadership goes beyond these scenarios to a circumstance in which leadership is recognized by a greater whole rather than within a cloistered subset. The characteristic embodiments of level 5 leadership are not fully discussed by Maxwell. Instead, this topic is left as a lifelong challenge yet an achievable goal.

Self-deployment

- Interface of leader & environment
- Causal process traces to leader personal orientations (e.g., values, needs, goals, habits, behavior) & demands of environment

Transactional relationship

- Dynamic interaction between leader/follower (L/F)
- L/F create understanding of relationship
- Interactions determine motivation, commitment, & satisfaction

Team deployment

- Systemic contingencies
- Objective situational demand

Figure 11-7. Chemers's zones of leadership. (Adapted from Chemers, M. M. (1997). *An integrative theory of leadership.* Mahwah, NJ: Lawrence Erlbaum Associates.)

Chemers's Zones of Leadership

In the integrative depiction of leadership, the model addresses interaction levels (e.g., individual, dyad, group, organization). Processes between these interaction levels are recognized in zones. The outcome associated with these interactions is driven by how well the parties are matched to each other as well as how well suited the resulting behavior is to the circumstance in which it occurs. Figure 11-7 highlights these zones.

The case management implications focus on the manner and quality in which interactions affect outcomes. The following considers the zones as applied to a case manager working in an acute care setting.

The zone of self-deployment considers the interplay between an individual's personal characteristics (e.g., values, needs, goals) and patterned habits of thought and/or behavior with the environment and demands of the situation (e.g., urgency of need for action, difficult client). When these forces are harmonious, it is considered to be "in-match." However, many circumstances affect interpersonal and inter-environmental harmony in a fast-paced setting. The case-manager-as-leader (CMAL) must remain mindful of these influences as his or her ability to control the environment is minimal. Figure 11-8 depicts two examples of CMAL match to environment.

The zone of transactional relationship addresses the interaction between leader and follower. The CMAL and the client-as-follower (CAF) create a dynamic, which may not be reflective of the situational reality observed by outsiders to the dyad. The CMAL's environmental match influences his or her interactions with CAFs. In the instance where the CMAL is not well suited to the challenges posed in a given situation, the lack of confidence and optimism influences his or her interaction with the CAF. Figure 11-9 depicts CMAL match impact on interaction and efficiency.

CMAL not-in-match	CMAL in-match
• Experienced in medical oncology • Covering orthopedic trauma unit	• Experienced in emergency dept. • Receives heavy throughput of multimorbid patients

Figure 11-8. CMAL environmental match.

The impact on transactional relationship influences both CMAL and CAF expectations. Situations in which the CMAL lacks confidence and becomes inefficient ultimately reflect in job satisfaction and fulfillment as well as influence behavior (e.g., anxiety, resentment toward management). Whereas the CAF expectations (e.g., quality–of-care level, staff competence) impact his or her behavior with respect to satisfaction survey, sharing personal opinion with family and friends, and more importantly, the ability to self-manage care. In instances with a highly involved caregiver, the CAF expectations apply to that individual as well.

The zone of team deployment influences various CAF factors, including, but not limited to, satisfaction, motivation, commitment, and goal achievement with each factor influenced by the CMAL. In the example provided, when a CMAL is not-in-match, the CAF suffers in many ways, including dissatisfaction with service, experiences knowledge gaps regarding health condition and follow-up needs, and lacks knowledge regarding his or her choices in transition plan options.

Bennis's Ingredients of Leadership

Bennis (1989) observed certain ingredients that appeared to be shared by leaders, including guiding vision, passion, integrity, trust, curiosity, and daring. Guiding vision implies clarity of personal and professional goals as well as persistence to continue moving toward those goals. Leaders love what they do and are able to impart that love through inspiring others. Knowing oneself, being truthful with oneself and others, and having the wisdom of experience combine to produce

CMAL not-in-match	CMAL in-match
• Training and experience in medical oncology • Temporarily covering orthopedic trauma unit • Unfamiliar with apparatus in use or forecast postacute needs • Uncomfortable addressing CAF questions relating to return home versus post acute admission • Unable to efficiently address transition needs of one CAF which affects ability to manage entire caseload	• Experienced in emergency dept. receiving heavy throughput of multimorbid patients • Understands interaction of multiple conditions, medications, and level of care requirements • Able to address CAF and caregiver questions regarding options for care • Effectively manages multiple CAF situations concurrently

Figure 11-9. CMAL match impact.

integrity, the foundation of trust. The leader continuously ponders the environmental issues, asks questions, and is not afraid to take risks, taking lessons from adversity and failure.

These ingredients evidence themselves in case management leadership when senior management supports case management effort and recognizes its value to the health care delivery chain. An individual who attains a management position without the skill of introspection likely lacks the personal and professional insight sufficient to generate an overall guiding vision for the department, nor have the stamina to power through challenging times. However, those who take the time to know themselves and understand the environment in which they exist possess the first ingredient for leadership success.

The second ingredient of leadership is passion. This applies to both life itself and one's work (Bennis, 1989). Leaders are able to communicate their own passion to their followers in order to enlist their active support of whatever issue or challenge presents. An example of passion personified is the case management director who is able to muster enthusiasm, rather than dread, for the changeover to a new information system. While many will be slow to adopt and/or adapt to the new system, the leader understands the various levels of acceptance and enlists staff support through positive, realistic messaging around benefits of the change.

The third ingredient of leadership is integrity, inclusive of self-knowledge, candor, and maturity (Bennis, 1989). Integrity evidences itself in difficult situations, such as a reduction in force. A leader faced with making a layoff announcement musters courage to be honest and forthright with staff. Candor in thought and action wins over those who initially balk. It will not soften the blow of job loss at an individual level, but the process will be handled with sensitivity and respect when a mature leader is at the helm.

Gardner's Factors of Leadership

The four factors Gardner identified as part of effective leadership are a tie to the community, a certain rhythm of life, an evident relation between stories and embodiments, and the centrality of choice. A review of each factor also reveals applicability to case management practice leadership.

Gardner and others note that a tie to the community is a critical factor in leadership. However, Gardner's (2011) point is that the relationship being ongoing, active, and dynamic. While it is easy for someone to sit and think to themselves "the people love me so I am a leader," if she or he is considering events which took place 20 years in the past, there is no actual leadership taking place. A true leader must demonstrate her or his concern for the community through thought and action on a continual basis. It is also imperative that the leader maintains a connection with current anecdotes. Recounting the same tired personal story or a participation in a project from glory of days gone by does not connect the leader to current issues facing the community. It is more reflective of a passive connection from the past in which the individual no longer truly connects with the frontline worker. For an active relationship to exist, active and ongoing nurturing requires a collaborative effort between the leader and the followers.

A certain rhythm of life means that the leader is a constant rather than an intermittent or inconsistent influence in the community. This requires balance between having time for maintaining oneself through self-knowledge, environmental awareness, and connection to mission, vision, and values (Gardner, 2011). The importance of striking a balance with connection versus time for inner self-maintenance varies according to the type of leadership. An indirect leader, such as one in a professional organization, connects to community through tools (e.g., newsletters, webinars) or smaller group activities. Finding time for inner self-maintenance is not as difficult as presents to a direct leader who must spend much of her or his time within the follower community. It is in striking the balance and finding the rhythm that fulfills the need for connectivity where success is forged.

Where stories and embodiments of leadership are concerned, the authentic leader must connect the two within his or her thoughts and actions. A person who tells stories that do not align with her or his actions loses credibility and influence over the followers. Examples of this are Reverend Jim Jones and

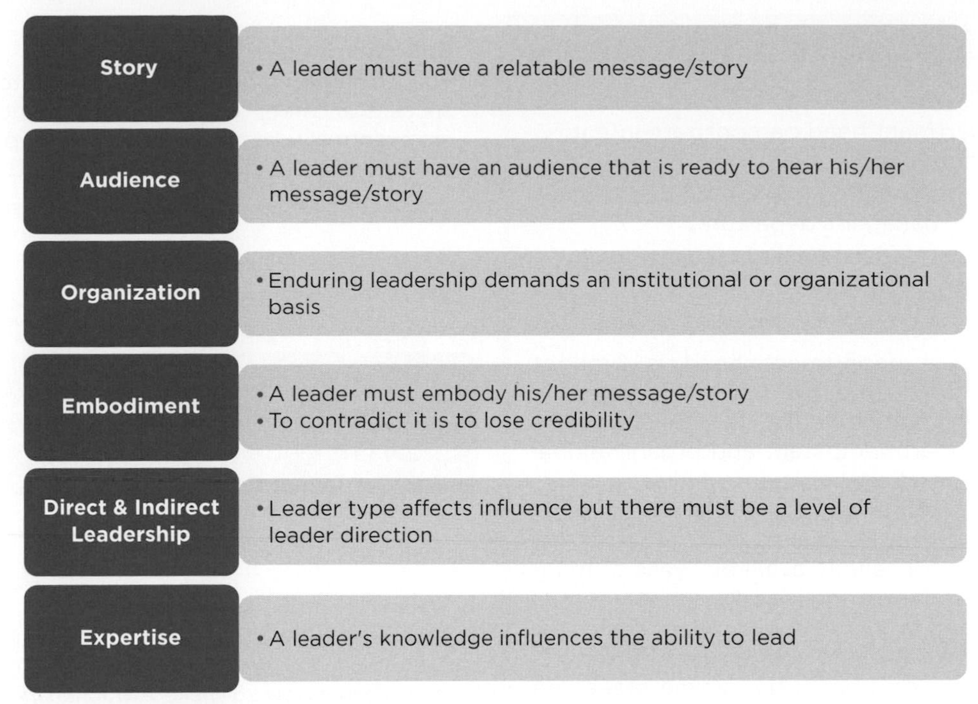

Figure 11-10. Gardner's six constants of leadership. (Adapted from Gardner, H. E. (2011). *Leading minds: An anatomy of leadership*. New York, NY: Basic Books.)

former President Richard Nixon. The incongruence between thought and deed engenders community hostility and ultimate rejection. The indirect leader who speaks to the point of professional unity yet actively attempts to discredit or disconnect individuals perceived as intellectual threats, demonstrates a disconnect between thought and action. Although this level of deception is uncommon, once revealed, the intended impact generally redirects to the originating source.

The final factor is that of centrality of choice. "Only in instances of leadership-through-choice does it make sense to think of stories being told, virtues being embodied or opinions being changed through example and persuasion" (Gardner, 2011). An example of this is an individual who achieves a leadership position through a manipulative approach. Although in a leadership position, their power lacks authenticity.

Gardner's Elements of Leadership

In studying 20th century leaders, Gardner noted the emergence of six constants of leadership. He looked at individuals considered leaders without discriminating on whether their outcome was positive or negative. He selected based on the impact the individuals had on thoughts, feelings, and behaviors of significant numbers (Gardner, 2011). Figure 11-10 describes the six principle findings of Gardner's work.

A leader must have a relatable story that is central to their cause for leadership. It should be a message that addresses follower current identity, as well as projects a promise for the future. The story need to be overly directive, but should put the follower on a path to think through to their own conclusion while at the same time be sufficiently inclusive that its theme is something the individual is able to associate to their personal frame of reference.

A leader must have a ready audience or organization, a group in want of a unifying force. The bigger challenge faces the individual who must unite a large group with a wider variance across the audience. Creating a new department within an existing organization presents such a challenge. However, the individual who comes into leadership of a large homogeneous, established group can exert governance with much less effort because an affinity already exists. An example of this type of leader is one elected to office in a professional association.

A leader must embody their story in an authentic manner. Although there need not be a reverential aspect to the story, the connection between leader and message must be true and clearly embedded in thought and action. As Gardner (2011) notes, the individual who does not embody her or his messages will eventually be discovered, even as the inarticulate individual who leads the exemplary life may eventually come to be appreciated. Box 11-4 recounts a tale of staff elimination in which the department head espoused organizational support and unity at the same time as he went about undercutting a capable manager for the desired result of forcing resignation.

PROCESS OF LEADERSHIP

The abundance of leadership theories indicates that there are as many variations on the process by which to work. However, there are leadership processes, which should be taken into consideration. Kouzes and Posner (2012) posited

BOX 11-4 A Tale of Staff Elimination

Consider the following story and ask:

1. Did the department head demonstrate integrity in thought or action?
2. How might this situation impact the department following the manager's departure?
3. Would this fact pattern result in a trusting environment in which to work?
4. What could the manager have done differently?

A newly hired department head is brought onboard by the vice president with great enthusiasm. During his initial weeks, he acquaints himself with the department, staff, and organizational structure and operational efficiency.

His manner is more aggressive than the department is accustomed. He makes daily requests for reports that are not readily available, yells at managers during staff meetings, assigns nonessential tasks (e.g., creating presentation slide decks for his use the next day), and rearranges the reporting structure moving previously topline managers to report to their fellow managers. He hires two new directors. Once they are in place, specific individuals are targeted for termination.

Over a period of a month, he creates a no-win situation for one manager. He conducts meetings with her staff to which she is not invited. Staff members are reassigned yet the positions are not backfilled; a request for overtime to address the growing backlog is rejected. Inventory mounts; turnaround times suffer. The manager, previously commended at "exceeds expectations" performance, receives verbal and written warnings for poor management. Her new director places her on a performance improvement plan.

Just prior to the holiday season, the department director informs everyone that instead of closing for Thanksgiving and Christmas, a small contingent of staff will be required; each director must designate staff to work. The manager under scrutiny is informed that she must work on Christmas Day. As she goes about her work on the holiday, the department head stops by her office and asks why she is at the office. The manager responds that she was told she had to work by the director, to which the department head replies, "No you never needed to be here."

Her work environment grows increasingly difficult. Another manager assigned to "mentor" her regarding backlog management provides suggestions, but all of them had been instituted. After another week of being deemed as showing no improvement, it is clear that the only remaining option is resignation. Over the weekend, she removes her personal belongings from her office. On Monday morning she arrives at work and hands her resignation letter to the human resources representative.

Epilogue

The manager who resigned went on to a fabulously successful career in case management. Senior leaders eventually discharged both the department head and director. Their current whereabouts are unknown.

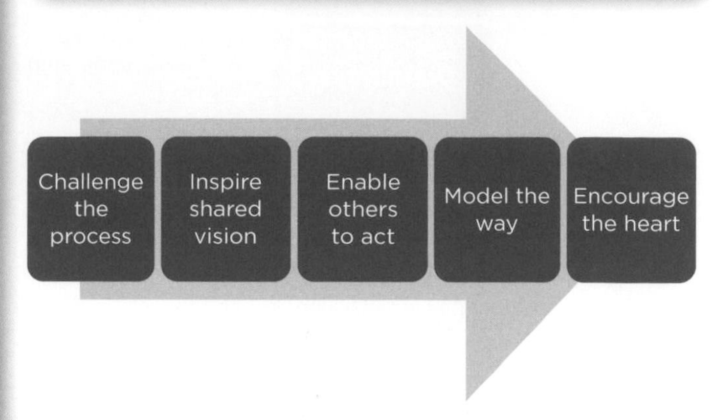

Figure 11-11. Kouzes and Posner leadership process model. (Adapted from Kouzes, J. M. & Posner, B. Z. (2012). *The leadership challenge: How to make extraordinary things happen in organizations* (5th ed.). San Francisco, CA: Wiley.)

a behavioral cycle associated with leadership excellence. The cycle included challenging the process, inspiring shared vision, enabling others to act, modeling the way, and encouraging the heart. This model is depicted in Figure 11-11.

Pierce and Dunham (1990) presented another leadership process model. The process depicts four factors, which are the leader, the follower, the context, and the outcome. Each of these factors is presented in Figure 11-12. This model highlights the interaction between leader, followers, and context to influence outcomes. The model also highlights the point that it be an active and continuing interaction. Being responsive to numerous variables allows the opportunity to produce better outcomes.

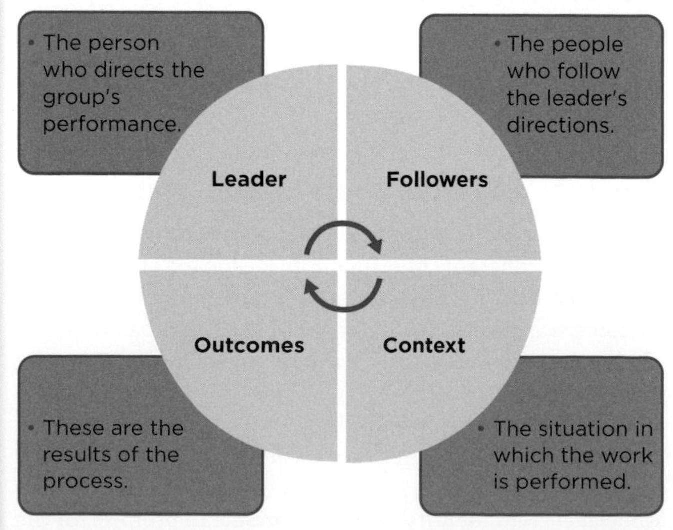

Figure 11-12. The process of leadership. (Adapted from Pierce, J. L. & Dunham, R. B. (1990). *Managing*. Glenview, IL: Scott Foresman & Co.)

LEADERSHIP'S KEY ELEMENTS

Professional Identity

Professional identity comes as a result of the developmental process facilitating one's understanding of self within one's field of work. This identity allows one to articulate her or his role to others both within and outside of the discipline (Brott & Myers, 1999; Smith & Robinson, 1995).

Regardless of practice setting or administrative hierarchy, a case manager regards herself or himself as a leader and demonstrates this attribute in serving as an integral member of the health care team and a client advocate. COLLABORATE places a spotlight on the practitioner who leverages the tools and resources at her or his disposal to provide thoughtful case management interventions adding value, rather than layers, to the delivery of health care services (Treiger, personal communication, 2008).

There are leadership opportunities presented each day. They need not be grandiose accomplishments either. It is through the little things, in being a better listener for a colleague experiencing a difficult challenge, being a more active coach to a client attempting to kick a bad habit, or making the effort to be more optimistic when caseload seems unbearable so as not to drag down a struggling team mate. The case manager-leader evidences herself or himself is subtle ways and in so doing weaves professional identity into every aspect of their work, utilizing knowledge and experience to ensure the delivery of high-quality health care. It is through consistent effort that each competency and key element combines into a strong fabric. Ultimately, the thread of professional identity creates cohesive synergy across disparate (and at times competing) agendas.

The leadership competency articulates points of consensus around the role of the case manager in order to articulate the value that professional case management holds to health care stakeholders. The leadership competency provides individual and organization with the underpinnings necessary to enable the advancement of professional practice.

Self-awareness

Self-awareness is considered the ability to engage in reflective awareness and is associated with executive processes essential to self-regulation. The self-aware individual is considered as controlled and intentional in his or her actions (Hull, 2007). The case manager-leader is mindful that every interaction leaves a lasting impression both of him or her as an individual and of case management.

One is reminded of both positive and negative call center experiences in which the manner of the customer service representative made a significant difference to satisfaction level, regardless of the final outcome. Always be aware of ones conduct because it leaves a lasting impression with the other party to the interaction.

Case management leadership is inclusive of the self-regulation concept. By definition, self-regulation means that society confers a group with the mandate to police itself. Because case management requires specialized knowledge for effective professional practice, it follows that case managers are in the best position to accomplish this oversight responsibility. This privilege is accompanied by immense accountability.

As leaders, we must address the wide variation in factors, such as scope of practice, licensure, methodical manner to ensure that every case manager is held to the standards of practice and ethical constructs of his or her respective license and to what governs case management practice. We continuously monitor ourselves (and our colleagues) to ensure practice within these limits.

As individuals, when we lack knowledge required for safe practice, we seek additional information to build and advance our competence level. The case manager is an important member of the care team; however, all other care team members need to understand case management's role within the team. Providing this overview reinforces one's self-awareness of role and function within a given situation. For example, the manner in which an initial introduction is conducted is essential to establishing the relationship ground rule basics. Box 11-5 provides a scenario for consideration.

BOX 11-5 The Self-Aware Case Management Introduction

The situation presented is the beginning of a conversation between a case manager-leader and a patient admitted to General Hospital. The self-aware case manager takes care to maintain the patient-centered focus in communicating with a recently admitted individual. He continually demonstrates respect for the patient asking permission to continue, providing opportunities for responses that go beyond simple yes and no.

Edward is a nurse case manager at General Hospital. He has reviewed his next patient's chart and does not see any diagnostic tests scheduled for the next hour. On entering a patient's semi-private hospital room, he notes the curtain is pulled around the patient's bed. Before pulling it open, he begins by introducing himself through the curtain, "Good morning, Mr. Cote. My name is Edward. I am a case manager here at General Hospital. May I come in to speak with you for a few minutes?"

Mr. Cote agrees. Edward pauses before stepping beyond the curtain and comes along the side of the bed, then adds, "I would like to share with you what I do here at General. Is now a good time for us to talk for about 10 minutes?"

Note: Edward asks Mr. Cote for permission twice before continuing. This demonstrates respect for the patient as an individual who with personal preferences (e.g., await caregiver arrival). Edward may or may not extend to shake the patient's hand depending on hospital policy. He does not carry a clip board or tablet, he makes eye contact when speaking.

(continued)

BOX 11-5 The Self-Aware Case Management Introduction (*Continued*)

Edward begins, "I am a case manager. What that means here at the General is I am here to coordinate services during your hospital stay and to make sure your needs are taken care of when it comes time for you to leave the General. For example, I arrange follow-up appointments; I make sure you have a supply of prescribed medications and help you with the things you need to know before you leave. Do any questions or concerns come to mind regarding what I have said so far?"

Note: Edward pauses again to allow Mr. Cote the opportunity to respond. "I do not know when you will be leaving the General. Do you have any immediate concerns or worries about leaving the hospital or in returning to your home?

Note: The conversation's focus is on the patient's perspective of need. This demonstrates a patient-centered approach to the transition process. Edward's communication style is open-ended, making the interaction more of a conversation than an interrogation or a lecture.

Edward continues, "I want you to think about a usual day in your life at home. What normally happens in terms of taking care of yourself, preparing meals, medications, etc.? How do you think your health condition may change the way you managed yourself and your day-to-day living?"

Note: The conversation continues to focus on the patient's perspective of daily living and helps to frame possible transition needs for his return home.

Before one asserts herself or himself as a leader, it is essential to know thyself. Self-knowledge takes a lifetime because from one moment to the next we are never exactly the same person. Perhaps most importantly, the only person who can teach you to be you is you. According to Bennis (1989), the four lessons of learning oneself are as follows:

- Be your own best teacher.
- Accept responsibility and do not place blame on others.
- Know that you can learn anything you want to learn.
- True understanding is born from reflecting on experience.

Learning is at the root of transforming oneself from what one is to what one wishes to be. It may come about as a result of a need to know something or as way in which to fill a gap between what one is versus what one can or should be. Learning is experienced as a personal transformation. A person does not gather learnings as possessions but rather becomes a new person with those learnings as a part of his or her new self. To learn is not to have; it is to be (Akin, 1987).

To be one's own best teacher, the case manager-leader must master the skill of learning. These concepts are also discussed in the chapter devoted to the lifelong learning competency. Akin (1987) also notes that the content of a learning experience may become less relevant. At a deeper level, however, the information that has been learned transforms the learner into a new person. The case manager-leader should not be afraid to change. This is at the heart of the personal transformative experience of knowing one's self. From the point of self-awareness, one is better able to contribute to the efforts of others, be they clients, an organization, or a whole industry.

Far too frequently, organizations tacitly foster a blaming culture. When something goes awry, the first impulse is to identify who did what wrong and issue a reprimand. In reality, there are few situations in which a single factor or person is to blame for an error. Staff are in fear of making a mistake and shrink up under their respective desks on realizing one has been made, secretly hoping it was their coworker in the next cubicle. This instills an individual competition atmosphere as opposed to a purpose-driven team approach.

W. Edwards Deming, the pioneer of using data to drive process, preached 14 points on which to found quality and process improvement initiatives. Driving out fear to enable a unity of effective purpose was sufficiently important that it was #4 on his list. Driving out the fear factor is both an organizational and an individual endeavor. The person afraid to make a mistake is frozen in place and may be unable to take action at all. Fostering a workplace environment of fear does not serve a useful purpose to an organization supposedly seeking growth. For the individual working in such an environment, there is a constant concern for making an error in judgment. The case manager-leader critically considers the options and impacts of words and actions. However, she or he is not fearful of taking action or making a statement.

The case manager exerts leadership by maintaining self-awareness in stressful situations, which can easily devolve into blame shifting. By avoiding the trap of affixing blame on others and remaining mindful of one's responsibility to the client, the case manager-leader regards poor results or bad news as an opportunity to improve and from which to learn. This is not intended to infer that below-par outcomes are acceptable. The case manager-leader leverages situations in order to gain insight into the factors contributing to the failure as well as how to improve the situation and avoid repetition.

Professional Communication

Professional communication refers to the manner in which the case manager interacts with others, verbally and nonverbally. As noted by Burgoon, Berger, and Waldron (2000), as an individual engages in social interaction, verbal and nonverbal communication channels afford her or him a wealth of potential information. The content, structure, and sequencing of verbal messages, as well as the paralinguistic cues, gestures, facial expressions, body movements, and cues provided by the physical environment that accompany verbal messages, all afford considerable grist for social actors' comprehension and interpretative mills. Certain work environments eliminate the dimension of face-to-face contact, placing the case manager at a disadvantage for

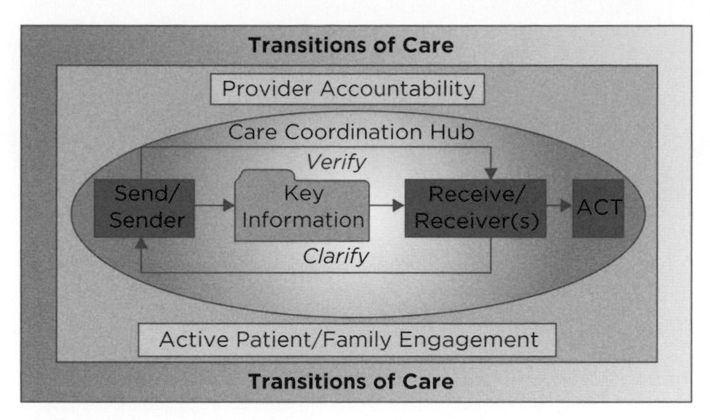

Figure 11-13. NTOCC's Model of Accountable Communication. Reprinted with permission from the National Transitions of Care Coalition.

having such a rich context from which to interpret another person's words and behaviors.

Important concepts within the context of professional communication include accountability and mindfulness. Taking responsibility for one's communication approach is a way in which a case manager demonstrates leadership and exhibits accountability of professional conduct.

Accountability means accepting responsibility for one's words, choices, actions, and outcomes. Assuming responsibility for another person's actions and consequences effectively eliminates that person's level of accountability. Although one cannot force accountability on another individual, it is possible to provide an atmosphere, which maximizes the potential for others to operate in an accountable manner. The case manager-leader does this by maintaining professional communication both verbal and nonverbal (e.g., written documents, body language, telephone contact).

The concept of accountable communication, as outlined in a 2008 National Transitions of Care Coalition white paper, provides a model on which a case manager-leader may fashion her or his own communication style (Figure 11-13). Consistently using this approach as a communication style model, the case manager ensures that information transfer is accurate, timely, and complete. Rather than a handoff of information in which the case manager acting as the sender, prepares a well-organized message (e.g., voicemail, email, information packet) prior to imparting it to the receiver. This accountable approach also requires a handover process in which the sender ensures receipt of information and interacts with the receiver to ensure all details and implications are understood. When the case manager is a receiver of information, she or he verifies message content, ensures clarity in meaning, and asks questions of the sender to avoid misunderstanding prior to taking action. Questions regarding message content are promptly addressed. These may be affected by timeliness standards (e.g., organization, regulatory, accreditation). Figures 11-14 and 11-15 provide two communication scenarios.

The first scenario depicts preparation of a thoughtful and organized message, followed by interaction between the sender and receiver. This interaction is intended to ensure not only that the message was received, but also that its content and intent was accurately understood. This period of interaction allows time for the receiver to ask questions of the sender and for the sender to ensure the receiver understands the message as intended. Ultimately, this model maximizes the potential for the interaction to produce the intended outcome. This model transcends all aspects of case manager-leader communication.

In the second scenario, there is no indication that the message was prepared; the sender transmits information in any given format. There is no interaction between sender and receiver; hence, no period during which receipt or comprehension of the message is validated. The receiver takes action based on her or his understanding of message meaning within her or his context. Ultimately, this communication process minimizes the potential for producing the intended outcome. Although the correct action and outcome may result, it is more likely to be a result of good fortune.

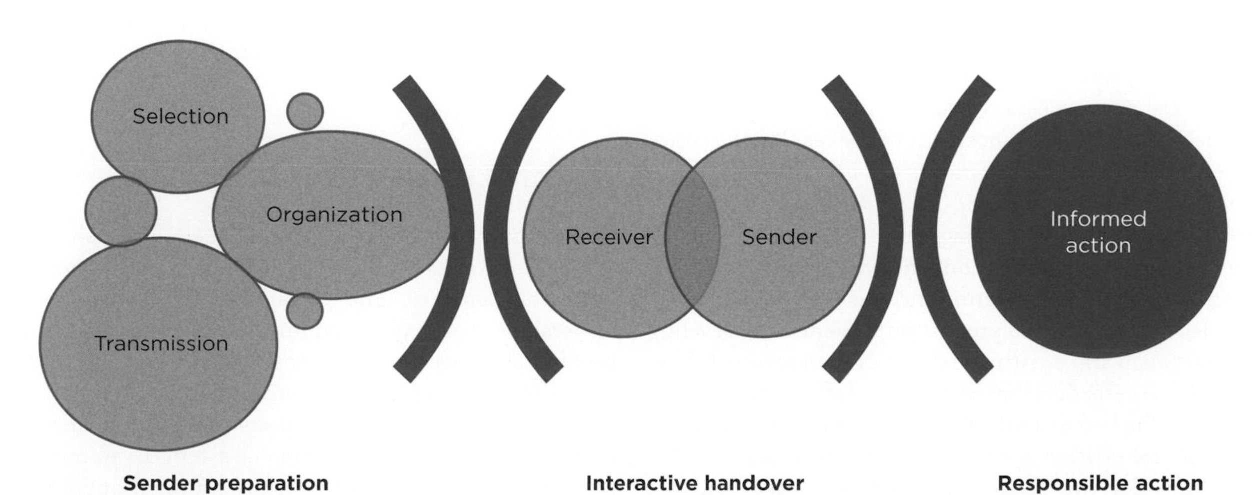

Figure 11-14. Accountable communication scenario A.

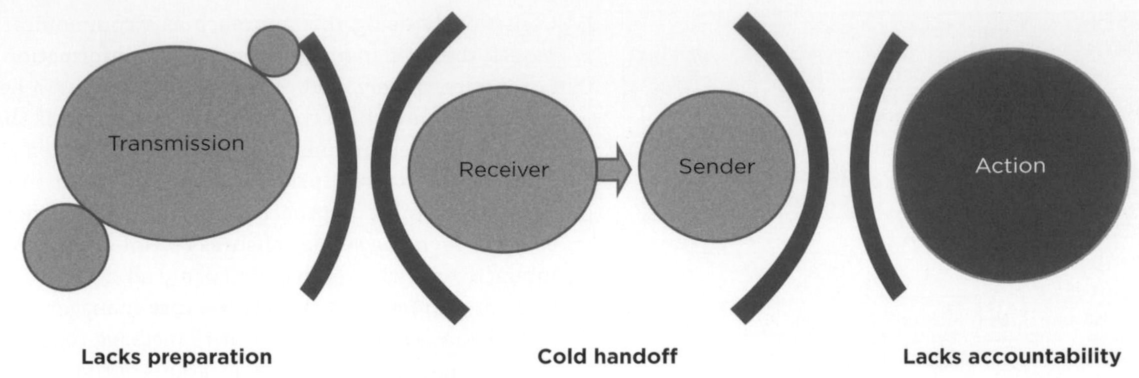

Figure 11-15. Accountable communication scenario B.

Team Coordinator: A Unifier Rather Than a Divider

The case manager-leader serves as a team unifier by minimizing unilateral actions based on limited information. Instead, she or he seeks consensus as a means of driving results-oriented, meaningful action. As a high-functioning member in any dyad or group (e.g., case manager–client, care team, functional team), the case manager-leader strives to work effectively and efficiently. In serving as a coordinator, a case manager facilitates the timely completion of activities through encouragement of others to take action rather than performing every action or intervention personally.

COLLABORATE implores a case manager to seek opportunities for discussion of important issues, setting priorities based on client need rather than care team convenience. This approach highlights the importance of advocacy competence, which is addressed in a separate chapter. Although this approach requires the investment of more time, it places the priority on patient-centered care delivery.

An example of this in an organizational setting is a situation in which a case management supervisor is tasked with cycle-time reduction of clinical information flow. Currently, the time from receipt of clinical information to decision point exceeds the regulatory mandate for timely authorization determinations. The supervisor who works as a unifier calls a team meeting to discuss the existing process and illicit suggestions for improvement, mapping out a revised process flow using sticky notes until achieving consensus. A few superusers test the new process revealing a 24-hour reduction in cycle-time. Following announcement of the results, the entire department successfully implements the new process.

Consider the above scenario in contrast to an authoritarian approach in which management determines process changes without consulting frontline workers. Information disseminates through email announcements. Staff promptly shoot holes in the intended process improvement by leveling derisive criticism and creating distrust of management. Irrespective of due consideration being placed into preparing the new process, the lack of unification in purpose runs contrary to the desire for efficiency and process improvement.

Now, consider the relationship between case manager and client who have worked out an action plan to address a care-plan obstacle. During the course of performing an intervention, the case manager also performs tasks previously deemed as client responsibilities. The rationale for completing the tasks was that she was working on a related activity so it was easier to do it herself. The client becomes upset when informed of the result, feeling betrayed because the case manager breached their previous agreement based on her own convenience. In addition, the achieved outcome was not exactly what he desired. The case manager realizes the misstep and reworks the care plan to allow the client an opportunity to achieve his desired goal of self-advocacy.

CASE MANAGEMENT PRACTICE IMPLICATIONS

Possession of competence in leadership transcends the entirety of case management practice. When contemplating the leadership competency, it is essential to remember that case management leadership occurs in every aspect of practice and professional identity, from academia to professional associations to work setting. While formal education and hands-on training provide theoretical and practical foundations, management coalesces with policy and procedure to reflect professional standards and establish evidence-based practice. Ultimately, leadership is at the frontline where the case manager blends skill, strengths, and abilities harmoniously with client and organizational goals to achieve success.

SUMMARY

This chapter explores the importance for leadership competence. Being a leader does not mean one is bossy of others, quite the contrary. The COLLABORATE model considers leadership as the glue required to establish and advance professional case management practice. One must discard conventional images of organizational hierarchy and apply concepts of leadership to all aspects of practice. Being a leader means that one cultivates personal strengths in oneself and others on the path to best practice, optimal outcomes, and professional growth.

References

Akin, G. (1987). Varieties of managerial learning. *Organizational Dynamics, 16*(2), 36–48. Retrieved July 3, 2014, from EBSCO 360 Link database

American Association of Colleges of Nursing. (2014). *Leadership for academic nursing*. Retrieved June 30, 2014, from http://www.aacn.nche.edu/lanp

American Case Management Association. (2013). *Standards of practice and scope of services for healthcare delivery system case management and transition of care professionals*. Retrieved April 25, 2013, from www.acmaweb.org/Standards

American Case Management Association. (2014). *Leadership conference and medical director forum*. Retrieved July 1, 2014, from http://www.acmaweb.org/map.aspx?mn=mn2

American Nurses Association. (2014). *Program offerings*. Retrieved June 30, 2014, from http://www.ana-leadershipinstitute.org/Main-Menu-Category/Offerings

American Nurses Credentialing Center. (2014). *Magnet recognition program model*. Retrieved June 30, 2014, from http://www.nursecredentialing.org/Magnet/ProgramOverview/New-Magnet-Model

American Organization of Nurse Executives. (2014). *Nurse executive competencies*. Retrieved June 30, 2014, from http://www.aone.org/resources/leadership%20tools/nursecomp.shtml

Antonakis J., Cianciolo A. T., & Sternberg R. J. (2004). *The nature of leadership*. Thousand Oaks: Sage.

Badshah, S. (2012). Historical study of leadership theories. *Journal of Strategic Human Resource Management, 1*(1), 49–59.

Bennis, W. (1989). *On becoming a leader*. Reading, MA: Addison-Wesley.

Bennis, W. (1996). The leader as a storyteller. *Harvard Business Review, January–February*, 154–160.

Brott, P. E., & Myers, J. E. (1999). Development of professional school counselor identity: A grounded theory. *Professional School Counseling, 2*(5), 339.

Burgoon, J. K., Berger, C. R., & Waldron, V. R. (2000). Mindfulness and interpersonal communication. *Journal of Social Issues, 56*(1), 105–127.

Busse, R. (2014). Comprehensive Leadership Review—Literature, Theories and Research. *Advances in Management, 7*(5), 52–66.

Case Management Leadership Coalition. (2014). *About CMLC*. Retrieved July 1, 2014, from http://www.cmsa.org/Consumer/NewsEvents/PressReleases/tabid/270/ctl/ViewPressRelease/mid/1004/PressReleaseID/18/Default.aspx

Case Management Society of America. (2010). *CMSA standards of practice for case management*. Revised 2010. Retrieved April 25, 2013, from http://www.cmsa.org/portals/0/pdf/memberonly/StandardsOfPractice.pdf

Chemers, M. M. (1997). *An integrative theory of leadership*. Mahwah, NJ: Lawrence Erlbaum Associates.

Council on Social Work Education. (2014). *Leadership institute*. Retrieved July 1, 2014, from http://www.cswe.org/CentersInitiatives/CSWELeadershipInst.aspx

Drucker, P. F. (2003). *The essential Drucker: The best of sixty years of Peter Drucker's essential writings on management*. New York, NY: Collins Business.

Gardner, H. E. (2011). *Leading minds: An anatomy of leadership*. New York, NY: Basic Books.

Greenleaf, R. K. (1977). *Servant leadership: A journey into the nature of legitimate power and greatness*. Mahwah, NJ: Paulist Press.

Health Resources and Services Administration. (2010, September). *The registered nurse population: Findings from the 2008 national sample survey of registered nurses*. Washington, DC: U.S. Department of Health and Human Services.

Horner, M. (1997). Leadership theory: Past, present and future. *Team Performance Management, 3*(4), 270–287.

Huber, D. L. (Ed.). (2010). *Leadership and nursing care management* (4th ed.). Maryland Heights, MO: Saunders Elsevier.

Hull, J. (2007). Self-awareness. In R. Baumeister & K. Vohs (Eds.), *Encyclopedia of social psychology* (pp. 791–793). Thousand Oaks, CA: Sage. doi:10.4135/9781412956253.n473

Institutes of Medicine. (2011). *The future of nursing: Leading change, advancing health*. Washington, DC: The National Academies Press.

Kotter, J. (2011). Change management vs. change leadership: What's the difference? *Forbes.com*. Retrieved April 15, 2013, from http://www.forbes.com/sites/johnkotter/2011/07/12/change-management-vs-changeleadership-whats-the-difference

Kouzes, J. M. & Posner, B. Z. (2012). *The leadership challenge: How to make extraordinary things happen in organizations* (5th ed.). San Francisco, CA: Wiley.

Maxwell, J. C. (1993). *Developing the leader within you*. Nashville, TN: Thomas Nelson.

Maxwell, J. C. (2007). *The 21 irrefutable laws of leadership: Follow them and people will follow you*. Nashville, TN: Thomas Nelson.

National Association of Social Workers. (2013). *NASW standards for social work case management*. Retrieved April 25, 2013, from http://www.socialworkers.org/practice/naswstandards/CaseManagementStandards2013.pdf

National League for Nursing. (2014). *NLN leadership institute*. Retrieved June 30, 2014, from http://www.nln.org/facultyprograms/leadershipinstitute.htm

National Transitions of Care Coalition. *Model for accountable communication*. Graphic reprinted with permission from the National Transitions of Care Coalition, 750 First St, NE Suite 700, Washington, DC 20002, www.ntocc.org

Network for Social Work Management. (2013). *Human services management competencies*. Retrieved July 3, 2014, from https://socialworkmanager.org/competencies

Pierce, J. L. & Dunham, R. B. (1990). *Managing*. Glenview, IL: Scott Foresman & Co.

Smith, H. B., & Robinson, G. P. (1995). Mental health counseling: Past, present, and future. *Journal of Counseling & Development, 74*(2), 158–162.

Society for Social Work Leadership in Health Care. (2014). *Publications*. Retrieved July 1, 2014, from http://www.sswlhc.org/html/publications.php

Spears, L. C. (2004). Practicing servant-leadership. *Leader to Leader, 34*, 7–11. Retrieved July 9, 2014, from Proquest database

Treiger, T. M. (2012). *Meet healthcare case management manager Teresa Treiger: Helping clients bridge gaps to self-advocacy, self-management* [interview]. Health Information Network. Retrieved July 1, 2014, from http://hin.com/blog/2012/09/14/meet-healthcare-case-management-manager-teresa-treiger-helping-clients-bridge-gaps-to-self-advocacy-self-management

Treiger, T. M. (2014). The importance of leadership followership. *Professional Case Management, 19*(2), 93–94.

U.S. Bureau of Labor Statistics. (2010, May). *Occupational employment and wages for 2009*. Retrieved from, http://www.bls.gov/oes

12 ADVOCACY

OBJECTIVES

After studying this chapter, you will be able to:

1. Define advocacy.
2. Discuss the scope of advocacy related to micro, mezzo, and macro practice.
3. Provide a historical context for advocacy.
4. Identify specific models of advocacy used to advance professional case management practice.
5. Discuss current challenges and implications related to advocacy as professional competency.
6. Understand the key elements of the advocacy competency.

KEY TERMS

Advocacy
Advocate
Client advocacy
Community advocacy
Critical theory
Empowering
Global advocacy
Lobbying
Macro
Mezzo
Micro
Navigator
Negotiation
Organizational advocacy
Out-of-contract
Out-of-network
Paternalistic
Patient-centered care
Shared responsibility
Social change

Amid health care's long and winding road of unpredictable detours and obstacles, advocacy has wound its way into the forefront of practice. A daily review of news stories across the industry yields an unparalleled need for advocacy at every crucial turn. Unprecedented changes impact care in all practice settings. These include financial pressures, uncertainty of the direction of health care reform, mandates from regulatory agencies to improve quality and patient safety, advancing technology, looming workforce shortages, and changes in the patient population (Tomajan, 2012).

Industry consensus for health care that is patient-centered serves as additional incentive for advocacy by the current generation of industry consumers. New and evolving technologies impact the many dimensions of care delivery (e.g., telehealth and remote health). As a result, the professionals rendering this care must lobby for regulatory changes to assure both proper reimbursement and the ability to provide the requisite interventions. In a perfect health care world, all populations have access to high-quality information when they need it, services are better coordinated, and medical errors are avoided through careful surveillance (Earp et al., 2008). Yet, industry stakeholders continue to be eons away from even a minimal standard of care delivery.

Advocacy's scope and importance within the health care industry has evolved over time. What began as an established professional value and moral obligation (Epstein, 2010; National Association of Social Workers [NASW], 2014; NursingLink, 2014) has expanded to diverse formal credentials, professional training, and, most recently, development of a federally designated title. Each of these contributions reinforce why advocacy's inclusion within the COLLABORATE paradigm is imperative.

DEFINITIONS

Advocacy is the act or process of supporting a cause or proposal (Merriam-Webster's Online Dictionary, 2014a). It can happen on any scale and/or location, from college students who attend a campus rally in opposition of tuition increases to the parents of a child diagnosed with intellectual disabilities who actively work with the school to obtain home-based education through an individualized education plan.

An **advocate** is defined as that person who argues for, defends, maintains, supports, and promotes the interests of another (Merriam-Webster's Online Dictionary, 2014b). Case management professionals often function as advocates, spending a large percentage of their day promoting the identified needs for clients at the service-delivery, benefits-administration, and policy-making levels (The Case Management Society of America (CMSA), 2010). In the health care arena, advocacy is predominantly client-focused rather than provider-driven; in fact, it is provider (case manager)-facilitated (Tahan, 2005). Six methods of how this standard can be demonstrated resonate across practice settings, as seen in Table 12-1.

Negotiate refers to discussing or conferring with another person so as to arrive at the settlement of a matter (Merriam-Webster's Online Dictionary, 2014c). This is a significant way case managers demonstrate advocacy in their work with clients.

TABLE 12-1 Application of CMSA Standard L: Advocacy

Demonstrated by	Example
1. Promotion of the client's self-determination, informed and shared decision making, autonomy, growth, and self-advocacy	The case manager for an acute ventilator weaning program reviews the advanced directives of a patient at the weekly team care coordination conference. Family members are also invited at the patient's request.
2. Education of other health care and service providers in recognizing and respecting the needs, strengths, and goals of the client	The case manager attends daily intensive care unit rounds to assure team members have current information on the full scope of a patient's wishes and family understanding.
3. Facilitating client access to necessary and appropriate services while educating the client and family or caregiver about resource availability within practice settings	The case manager coordinates a discharge meeting for a patient with a new diagnosis of renal failure and her caregivers. The patient is transitioning home following a lengthy hospitalization and will also be receiving outpatient dialysis.
4. Recognition, prevention, and elimination of disparities in accessing high-quality care and client health care outcomes as related to race, ethnicity, national origin, and migration background; sex, sexual orientation, and marital status; age, religion, and political belief; physical, mental, or cognitive disability; gender, gender identity, or gender expression; or other cultural factors	The case manager is working with a patient from another country who is admitted emergently from the airport while traveling. There are challenges with respect to health literacy and understanding of the patient's scope of care for both the patient and his daughter. The case manager is able to access a translation system to promote communication between patient, family, and team members, including care coordination with patient's embassy.
5. Advocacy for expansion or establishment of services and for client-centered changes in organizational and governmental policy	A case manager attends Public Policy Day for her professional association. She schedules individual meetings with both her home state senator and representative. Both support passage of a bill allowing for Medicare reimbursement of telehealth intervention by case managers.
1. Recognition that client advocacy can sometimes conflict with a need to balance cost constraints and limited resources. Documentation indicates that the case manager weighed decisions with the intent to uphold client advocacy, whenever possible.	A case manager reviews clinical documentation, and a cost-benefit analysis for a patient who suffered a C-1 level injury in a diving accident. With the patient currently a quadriplegic, the physician is requesting approval for his patient to trial an experimental exoskeleton.

Adapted from Case Management Society of America. (2010). CMSA standards of practice for case management. Revised 2010. Retrieved April 25, 2013, from http://www.cmsTBa.org/portals/0/pdf/memberonly/StandardsOfPractice.pdf

Negotiations often involve discussions around going out-of-network. In the context of health care, **out-of-network** refers to a patient seeking care outside the network of doctors, hospitals, or other health care providers that the insurance company has contracted with to provide care. It often applies to health maintenance organizations and preferred provider organizations. If a patient does seek out-of-network care, those services may only be partially covered or not covered at all, depending on the insurance plan (Medicare Newsgroup, 2014).

Out-of-contract is another term used in the negotiation arena that is familiar to case managers. It is distinct from a treatment or service provider being outside of network in that the item, service, and/or level of care being requested is simply not a covered benefit. The involved case manager will work to create a benefit or potentially transfer the dollars from another benefit not currently being used, such as in the case scenario in Box 12-1.

When advocacy is used within the public policy realm, it can involve **lobbying**. Political folklore has it that lobbying originated during the presidency of Ulysses S. Grant. By history, he would sit in the lobby of his favorite hotel and wait for the public to come offering and asking for favors (Public Broadcasting System, 2014). Over time lobbying became seen as a more formal process influencing public and government policy at all levels including federal, state, and local. It is so essential to the proper functioning of the U.S. government that it is protected by the First Amendment: Congress shall make no law ... abridging the right of the people peaceably ... to petition the Government for a redress of grievances" (The Legal Dictionary, 2014).

Case managers are engaged in a number of lobbying initiatives. Examples include the efforts employed across individual states toward passage of the nurse licensure multistate compact and/or at the federal level to promote case management's positioning and reimbursement within health care reform.

BOX 12-1 Out-of-Contract Case Scenario

Jyneal is a case manager employed by an inpatient rehabilitation program. She is working with Randy, a client who has experienced a traumatic brain injury. The treatment team agrees that Randy no longer needs intervention at the acute level of care, though would benefit from a structured daily program offering the full scope of rehabilitation, including community reintegration.

Randy's wife Monica, is able to provide all the necessary care and supervision for him from 6:00 p.m. to 8:00 a.m. The couple has two sons who are both away at college. Monica is employed during the day and unable to adjust her work schedule to be in the home. With no insurance benefit to cover the recommended brain injury day program, a discussion between Jyneal and her counterpart at the managed care organization, Pat, ensues.

Pat reviews the documentation Jyneal has provided and recognizes the benefit a brain injury day treatment program would yield for Randy. She reviews the full scope of the insurance policy and identifies an option. Randy has a covered benefit for alcohol outpatient treatment that nobody anticipates will be used. Pat discusses her plan with her medical director, Dr. Gray. They recognize both the clinical appropriateness and cost-savings of moving forward with the out-of-contract plan.

Jyneal obtains approval from Pat to proceed with the referral. Randy is discharged home and scheduled to attend the brain injury day treatment program not far from where Monica works. The program also provides outpatient therapy so that Randy can complete any further recommended treatment following his discharge from day treatment. This consistent team approach has Randy back employed part-time within 2 months of his discharge from the inpatient program.

PAST AND CURRENT THINKING

Health care advocacy is demonstrated throughout contemporary history. The pinnacle of advocacy practice for many professionals, especially case managers, comes from being able to provide assurance and appropriate care to patients and their families during the most acute phases of an illness course. Consider the sudden emotion, whether anxiety or fear, which patients and their caregivers experience as they transition between all levels of care, as well as care settings. These key times serve as opportunities for professionals to render empathic and authentic intervention, often framed as advocacy. They extend from a physician office to hospital emergency admission, transfer to or from an intensive care unit, as a patient is wheeled into the operating room for elective surgery, or discharge home.

The industry boasts a robust history of those health care professionals who contributed to enhancing patient care and professional identity through advocacy. This section provides critical retrospective, inspiration, and a starting point for advocacy's sizeable scope.

NURSING

Advocacy has a strong heritage in the nursing profession, whether directed toward a greater voice in health care policy, expanded employment opportunities, and/or an enhanced professional image for the workforce (Benner, Stephen, Leonard, & Day, 2010). This legacy extends back to Florence Nightingale, who employed advocacy for individual patients and for the nursing profession (Selanders & Crane, 2012).

As intermediaries between the world of patients and medical institutions, nurses were among the first in health care to define their professional role in terms of advocacy (Earp et al., 2008). This results in literature that is robust in terms of applicable content and references. Most nurses are able to accept the advocacy role as it applies to their patients. Although there are a large number of definitions for and examples of advocacy in the nursing realm, a primary focus is the nurse's role in protecting the patients' autonomy. However, it also presents that the greater challenges with advocacy manifest when that scope of the (advocacy) effort is required on behalf of colleagues, the profession, and/or oneself (Tomajan, 2012).

Defined Advocacy Skills

A series of the models in nursing, as well as other disciplines, define the fundamental skills required for professionals to engage in advocacy activities on behalf of their clients or for public policy purposes.

Baldwin (2003) identifies three essential attributes of patient advocacy:

1. Valuing patients' right to self-determination,
2. Apprising patients through a combination of education and advising so that they can take part in decision making, and
3. Interceding for patient with others, including family members and physicians to ensure that patients' wishes are honored.

Reflect on the scenario found in Box 12-2 in which a case manager leverages Baldwin's attributes through her day.

BOX 12-2 Baldwin's Attributes Case Scenario

Sandy is a case manager for the oncology program of a bustling acute care hospital. She engages in Baldwin's three attributes many times over on a daily basis for each patient and family system she interfaces with. Consider her work with a 40-year-old patient who is newly diagnosed with stage 4 ovarian cancer.

The patient, Carol, has been notified of the diagnosis by her family physician, Dr. Jones, earlier in the day. She refuses to have further treatment. "I saw what my mother went through with this and I'm not subjecting my family to that level of suffering," Carol emphatically tells Sandy. She also informs Sandy that she would like to complete advanced directives. Sandy alerts Dr. Jones of Carol's request. Although he is initially puzzled why Carol would not want to expend some preliminary energy to fight the disease, he ultimately facilitates her request.

Sandy coordinates a referral to a hospice program of Carol's choosing, then schedules and co-coordinates a family meeting with the hospice intake nurse. Carol asks Sandy to attend the intake meeting, which she agrees to do. Sandy and the intake nurse manage the strong family emotions while simultaneously providing the necessary psycho-education and support of everyone who attends. They especially focus on defining how the care process will be coordinated from this point onward. Sandy then meets with Carol to support her in her dialogues with several family members who are in denial about the severity of the diagnosis, and also not in favor of Carol's preferred hospice plan.

Adapted from Baldwin, M. (2003). Patient advocacy: A concept analysis. Nursing Standard, 17(21), 33–39.

Sandy case scenario also serves as a solid example of why patient advocacy has its roots in specialty health care areas, such as those which involve end-of-life care. Professionals involved with this population often find themselves concerned with protecting and extending patients' comfort and autonomy. Critical to this effort are the additional considerations cited by the Institute of Medicine (IOM) (1998):

- The need to facilitate communication between patients and providers about treatment options and care preferences,
- The recognition and importance of cultural and spiritual dimensions of care, and
- The need for adequate pain management.

Although end-of-life care has changed dramatically since this report's publication, advocacy continues to be paramount theme for those professionals who engage with any patient who warrants this level of care. One prevailing dilemma involves how the health care system is still aimed at curative rather than supportive and comfort care (Hackethal, 2014). Advocacy skills must be actively engaged in by those involved in care coordination to ensure that a patient's right of self-determination is realized.

Nursing and Public Policy Advocacy

Tomajan (2012) speaks to the importance of using specific and tactical skills to facilitate the complex process of advocacy. These are deemed as an essential component of the job, particularly as point-of-care nurses expend their energy to develop and intentionally utilize advocacy. Advocacy can also occur incrementally, happening through a series of efforts over time (Tomajan, 2012). The four skills should be directed toward addressing workplace concerns, promoting positive work environments, as well as being an advocate for the profession.

The four skills of problem solving, communication, influence, and collaboration are presented in Figure 12-1. Each of these skills contributes to the overall effectiveness of advocacy. Box 12-3 highlights a scenario pertaining to nursing licensure portability, an issue of particular importance to nurses practicing in case management across state lines.

Advocacy Addresses the Patient-Centered Culture

In the early 1960s only a handful of hospitals had organized patient education programs. Professionals and patients alike recognized the seek to change the status quo which is often associated with the industry, making health care more responsive to the presenting needs (Earp et al., 2008). As both health care and time advanced from the 20th to 21st century, the reports of the IOM (1999, 2001, 2003) emerged fast and furiously. Each one captivated the attention of industry stakeholders by focusing on themes which served as calls for health care providers and organizations to take necessary action. They all emphasized the mandate for increased attention to patient safety and provision of quality care, with many of these discussed throughout the chapters in Part 1.

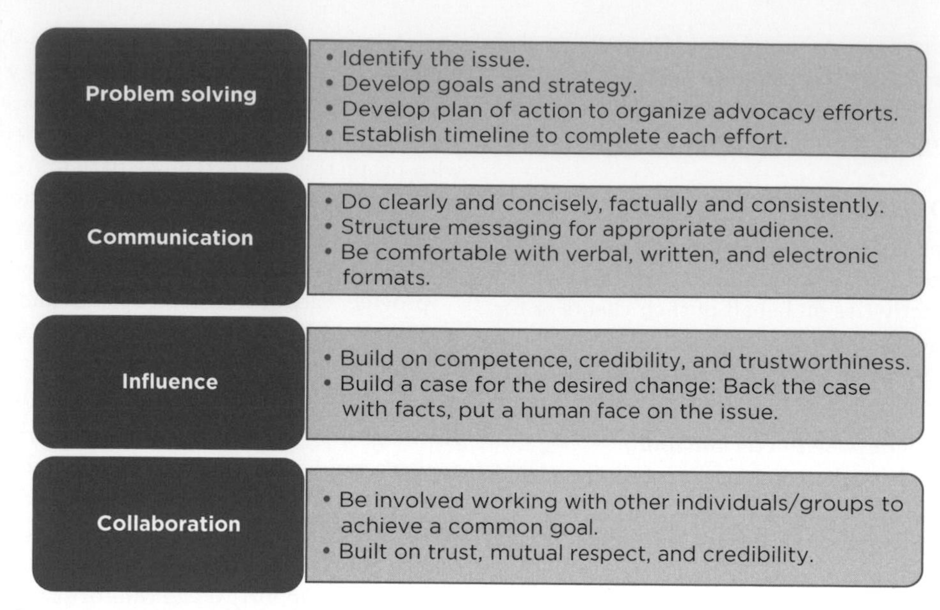

Figure 12-1. Four advocacy skills for nurses. (Adapted from Tomajan, K. (2012). Advocating for nurses and nursing. *OJIN: The Online Journal of Issues in Nursing. 17*(1), Manuscript 4.)

BOX 12-3 Nursing Public Policy Advocacy Case Scenario

Melinda is a senior case manager for a national workers' compensation management company. For the past 5 years she has been employed as a working manager who has assigned clients in one state. In addition, Melinda supervises 10 other case managers for the region.

Melinda receives an email from the regional director of case management informing her that the coverage area for all case managers will expand next month. It will now cross three states courtesy of several new payer contracts. Melinda will receive a raise for the increased responsibilities; however, there is one pitfall. She must obtain licensure in the two additional jurisdictions since the surrounding states have not passed the nurse licensure compact (NLC). Melinda is also informed that the cost of licensure application in these added states is one that she must incur. Furious at what she hears, Melinda focuses her energies. She will develop a plan to advocate for herself and her colleagues who are in this position:

1. Problem solving. Melinda contacts her manager colleagues, all who express their displeasure with paying personally for the additional licensure. Together they identify a list of those impacted, plus develop a strategic plan of action.
2. Communication. Melinda and two of her colleagues will develop a 60-second speech to advocate for employer reimbursement of additional state licensure, especially when it is mandated to do the job. Included will be a use of the NLC map posted on the National Conference of State Board of Nurses website.
3. Influence. Melinda will work with her colleagues, including senior case management leadership toward meeting with human resources at the corporate level, and organizational leaders.
4. Collaboration. As a member of a case management professional association, Melinda will be familiar with the status of the NLC in her neighboring states. She will contact the leaders of other initiatives that are in process to assure a consolidated and integrated versus fragmented approach. She will suggest the development of a coalition, comprised of interested stakeholders from the other initiatives to combine resources and energies toward ultimate resolution.

A new generation of health care delivery models emerged, one of which was **patient-centered care**, which is defined as "Providing care that is respectful of and responsive to individual patient preferences, needs, and values, and ensuring that patient values guide all clinical decisions" (IOM, 2001). The five attributes of patient-centered care identified in Table 12-2 highlight this model's support of health care advocacy.

Since the appearance of the phrase, patient-centered care, it has become the new mantra, if not battle cry, of many strategic planning efforts across health care organizations and programs. With respect to health advocacy, patient-centered care is but one of several overarching goals; this in addition to safer medical systems, and greater patient involvement in health care delivery and design (Earp et al., 2008).

The nursing profession places significant importance on advocacy, particularly through dedication to patient safety and nursing quality. The number and scope of

TABLE 12-2 Patient-Centered Care Attributes

Attribute	Explanation
"Whole-person" care	Providers of care need to take the time to get to know the patient and the involved family and/or support system.
Coordination and communication	1. Active responsibility by involved clinicians for coordinating care across settings and services in collaboration with the patient and family. 2. This is further enhanced by meaningful communication by all involved treatment providers including open dialogues about test results, treatment recommendations, and transitions of care.
Patient support and empowerment	1. A strong sense of partnership 2. Support for patient self-management, trust, and respect
Ready access	1. Obtain access to prompt care, with appropriate awareness of need for accommodations from physical disabilities, cognitive impairment, language barriers, and cultural differences. 2. Primary care teams are the trusted gateway to other professionals and needed services rather than simply gatekeepers.
Autonomy	Truly patient-centered health care must be designed around what patients say is important to them.

Adapted from Betchel, C., & Ness, D. L. (2010, May). If you build it, will they come? Designing truly patient-centered health care. Health Affairs, 29(5), 914–920.

ANA-sponsored advocacy initiatives continues to evolve. Recent activities focus on bullying in the workplace, safe staffing levels, and support for funding workforce development.

SOCIAL WORK

Advocacy, case management, and the social work profession share a common heritage that dates back to the late 19th century. Poverty was rampant in society along with diverse social problems associated with industrialization, urbanization, immigration, and population growth (NASW, 2013). During this time, social work pioneers Mary Richmond and Jane Addams engaged in their respective work, which so heavily influenced case management.

Jane Addams is often referred to as an advocate for the poor and activist for peace (Kelly, 2012). Through her work with Hull House and the surrounding community, Addams engaged in advocacy that was both client- and profession-focused. She was also instrumental in lobbying the state of Illinois to re-think laws governing child labor, and the factory inspection system to increase worker safety (Kelly, 2012).

Mary Richmond advocated for the establishment of social work professional schools and lobbied for legislation to address housing, health, education, and labor (The Social Welfare History Project, 2014). Richmond's work with the Charity Organization Societies provided her the opportunity to advocate for enhancing the human condition through direct client practice.

Although these distinct contributions are discussed extensively in chapter 1, they also demonstrate how the dual dimensions of advocacy manifest in the professional realm and across social work especially.

Advocacy Across Practice Concentrations

Advocacy and social work are aligned by virtue of the profession's definition:

> Social work is a practice-based profession and an academic discipline that promotes social change and development, social cohesion, and the empowerment and liberation of people. Principles of social justice, human rights, collective responsibility and respect for diversities are central to social work. Underpinned by theories of social work, social sciences, humanities and indigenous knowledge, social work engages people and structures to address life challenges and enhance well being.
>
> *IFSW, 2014*

The concept of advocacy particularly resonates through social work's two major practice specializations. **Macro** practice focuses on larger-scale societal and institutional influences of regulation and legislation, public policy, funding, and reimbursement that directly impact clients. This concentration is also known by other names such as **social change** and social policy change. **Micro** social work is the most common type of practice, focusing on the direct interventions that occur with individual clients and/or families and groups, often through therapy, counseling, and related clinical modalities (Social Work Licensure Map, 2014).

A third level of **mezzo** social work practice is sometimes identified, though is not a distinct academic area of academic specialization for masters' level preparation. Work in the mezzo level is usually divided between micro and macro realms. It involves interventions with small-to-medium-sized groups such as neighborhoods, schools, or local organization (e.g., community organizing, management of social work organizations, or working toward institutional or cultural change) (Social Work Licensure Map, 2014). For the purposes of this chapter, the focus will strictly be limited to micro and macro practice.

Most social work practitioners engage in advocacy for clients, independent of whether their role is primarily macro- or micro-focused. The larger-scale macro realm directly influences the more direct intervention of the micro practitioner. For example, social workers employed as behavioral case managers for a managed care organization (MCO) strive to understand how new legislation, as the Patient Protection and Affordable Care Act (PPACA) and the Mental Health Parity and Addiction Equality Act (MHPAEA), will affect their clients. New provider contracts will be developed and new benefits will be administered. How will clients be impacted by this change? Will the laws enhance or further restrict clients' access to their health and mental health care? MCO case managers may find themselves advocating on behalf of their clients directly with providers to assure appropriate approval for services, as well as payment and reimbursement.

For those social workers employed in the macro intensive role of a fundraising department at a not-for-profit health care system, PPACA and MHPAEA hold different implications. Increased care delivery models and program reimbursement will drive the need to develop new initiatives and/or expand existing programs. Attention will be prioritized on exploring grants or other income sources to cover the necessary organization growth. Although these social workers are not directly involved with patient interventions, their actions will influence how patients access care. How many new case managers will need to be hired? How will the strong focus on integrated behavioral health, impact the qualifications for those who are hired? Many questions beckon at the macro level of practice for it directly influences the micro level of patient care.

Critical Theory Bridges the Micro and Macro Advocacy Chasm

One of the defining characteristics of social work is how it addresses the existing gaps between the human condition and members of society. Case managers who advocate on behalf of clients in need of housing or out-of-contract benefits for addiction day treatment programs exemplify this concept. Bridging that chasm between macro-affiliated social programs or legislation and micro-aligned clinical intervention is how social workers understand their role within case management.

"With its strengths-based, person-in-environment perspective, the social work profession is well trained to develop and improve support systems (including service-delivery systems, resources, opportunities, and naturally occurring social supports) that advance the well-being of individuals, families, and communities" (NASW, 2013).

Yet, it has been implied that social work is amid a monumental practice dichotomy of its own, between those who provide services to the individual and those who seek a different level of change effort as they work to change the overall environment (Salas et al., 2010). This has become a common discussion across social work classrooms and professional meetings.

On one side of this argument are those who subscribe to the heritage of social work practice dedicated to advocating for the poor, disabled, and disenfranchised. They seek to influence social policies through lobbying and other methods. On the other side are social workers who follow the behavioral health path to private practice. Because of their education and training in clinical concepts (e.g., psychopathology, assessment, interventions, treatment planning), these professionals usually engage in roles that mandate licensure for independent practice, such as private practice, or professional case management. Their focus is on more fiscally driven models of payment and reimbursement, an act often viewed as counter to social work culture for it speaks to a for-profit mindset.

Critical theory has been touted as the perspective to bridge the dichotomous approach to macro and micro social work practice (Salas et al., 2010). The criteria for critical theory speak to a more comprehensive and timely integration of professional perspectives, and is shown in Figure 12-2. This theory offers a framework to engage the professional in purposefully considering multiple influencers on the client's situation. There is an opportunity to reflect on each of the contributing factors from both an organized and systematic approach as well as the individual context of the client(s) (Salas et al., 2010), thus no cookie cutter approach to care.

Professionals using critical theory are able to reflect on the needed interventions from two fronts: through assessing the client's individual clinical presentation plus how the larger-scale environmental issues have potential to impact this presentation. For example, a case manager involved with two distinct clients who have each experienced the sudden death of a parent, will express their grief differently. On the micro level, the case manager may have to assess the strong visceral reactions for one client as opposed to a stoic response for the other. There may need to be exploration of the unique relationship between each client and parent, along with other family dynamics. On the macro level, there could be attention to how the individual cultural communities of each client view death as a concept. This can provide a context for why the grief manifests so differently for each person. There may also be larger issues specific to how the spiritual and religious communities of each client bear on the situation. Even the concept of how assorted cultures communicate with health care professionals, can come into play for some.

In using this approach, professionals must also be comfortable with internal and ideological contradictions (Salas et al., 2010). Individuals must be as skilled to explore the dynamics and factors impacting each individual client who has experienced a traumatic event (e.g., sudden death, domestic violence) as they are in looking at the broader community, gender, and/or ethnic historical influences associated with the event, such as oppression, power, and control. A case

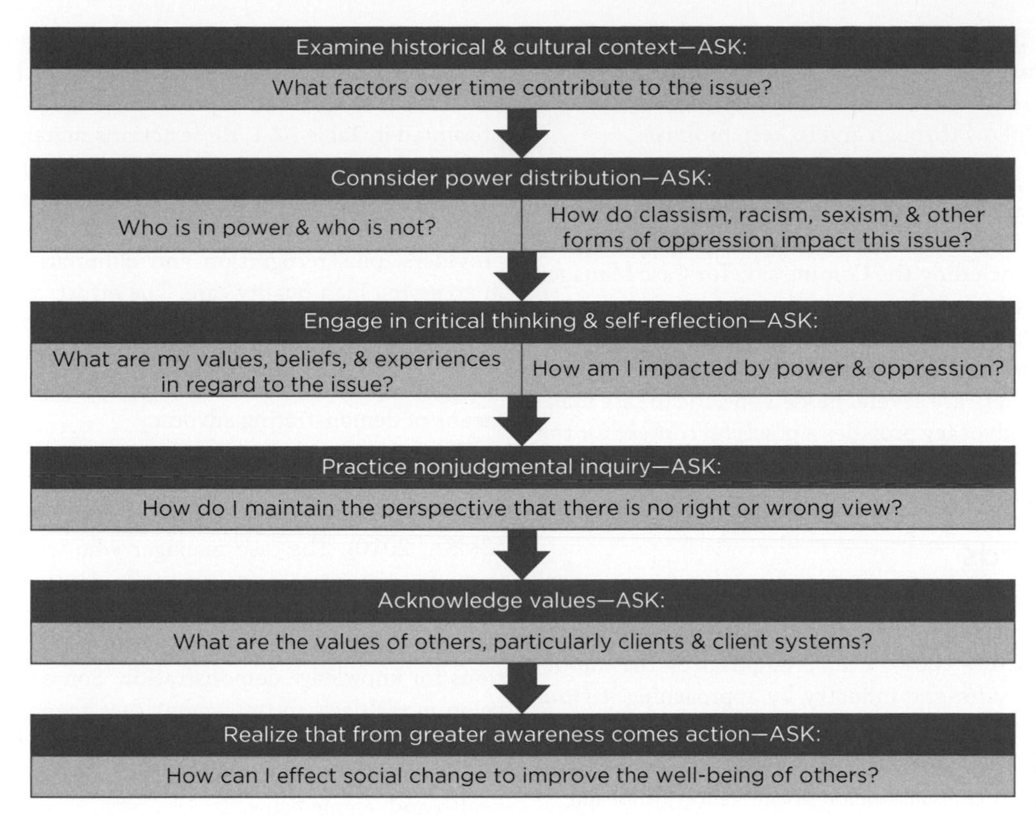

Figure 12-2. Critical theory criteria. (Adapted from Salas, L. M., Sen, S., & Segal, E. (2010). Critical theory: A pathway from dichotomous to integrated social work practice. *Families in Society*, *9*(1), 91–96.)

manager can feel as if he or she is being biased when assessing why families of different cultures and circumstances respond so very differently.

The use of critical theory integrates and emphasizes the deeper level of thinking associated with critical thinking (CT), another COLLABORATE competency. This is accomplished by assuring the involved professional has the insight to ask vital questions, plus gather and assess relevant information. Through processing the client circumstances at a deeper level and using CT, the ability of a professional is optimized, fostering his or her ability to recognize underlying bias, implications, and consequences of his or her thought process (Salas et al., 2010).

CASE MANAGEMENT

Interpretations vary on how advocacy is implemented by case managers. A range of case management standards now exists across professional associations and credentialing bodies. More alignment than distinction exists among these documents with the standards presented in Table 12-3.

With advocacy considered a moral obligation of professional practice (NursingLink, 2014), a natural weave exists between this COLLABORATE competency and both the values and ethics underlying case management practice.

- Beneficence: To do good.
- Nonmalfeasance: To do no harm.

TABLE 12-3 Advocacy across Professional Standards of Practice: Case Management

CMSA Standards of Practice for Case Management (2010)	ACMA Standards of Practice & Scope of Services for Health Care Delivery Systems Case Management and Transitions of Care (TOC) Professionals (2013)	NASW Standards for Social Work Case Management (2013)
Standard L: Advocacy	Standard V: Advocacy	Standard 7: Advocacy & Leadership
The case manager should advocate for the client at the service-delivery, benefits-administration, and policy-making levels.	Advocacy is the act of supporting or recommending on behalf of patients/family/caregivers and the hospital for service access or creation, and for the protection of the patient's health, safety, and rights.	The social work case manager shall advocate for the rights, decisions, strengths, and needs of clients and shall promote clients' access to resources, supports, and services.

- Autonomy: To respect individuals' rights to make their own decisions.
- Justice: To treat others fairly.
- Fidelity: To follow through and to keep promises.

(CMSA, 2010)

To this end, several professional entities include the advocacy standard within their Code of Professional Conduct and Code of Ethics, including the Commission for Case Manager Certification (CCMC) and the American Nurses Association (ANA), respectively. Advocacy from the lens of ethical and/or professional conduct is shown in Table 12-4.

In addition, there are several models specific to case management where advocacy provides a powerful context for the many tasks, roles, functions, and responsibilities of the case managers (Tahan, 2005).

The Standards

CCMC. As a process, advocacy promotes beneficence, justice, and autonomy for clients that aim to foster the client's independence (CCMC, 2009). CCMC emphasizes the importance of advocacy for the industry by approaching it from two fronts. First, they provide a definition in their Code of Professional Conduct (2009), which reads:

> Advocacy – a process that promotes beneficence, justice and autonomy for clients. Advocacy especially aims to foster the client's independence. It also involves educating clients about their rights, healthcare and human services, resources, and benefits, and facilitating appropriate and informed decision-making, and includes considerations for the client's values, belies and interests.
>
> *CCMC, 2009*

The meaning and direction for those certified by CCMC is clear that advocacy is a multifaceted process that occurs over the tenure of the case manager's relationship with his or her client.

Second, CCMC integrates advocacy as a case manager's ethical obligation toward the purposes of respecting client integrity and self-determination in the decision-making process. This is a strategic move that integrates the concept of advocacy in accordance with a certified case manager's professional conduct. Further elaboration on the ethical–legal fundamentals of case management practice will be explored in chapter 18.

CMSA. As an action-oriented case management function, the CMSA frames a detailed standard which demonstrates how case managers are expected to engage in advocacy. As presented in Table 12-1, these actions materialize across the diverse practice settings and roles which case managers are in. These include ensuring client self-determination, shared decision making, education of other involved health care providers, plus recognition and elimination of disparities in accessing high-quality care. The efforts engaged in by an MCO-based case manager who contacts her patients to assure they receive both appropriate and timely information on the proper mechanism for appealing a decision, is one means of demonstrating advocacy.

Other case managers participate at the macro level in working to expand or establish services and for client-centered changes in organizational and governmental policy (CMSA, 2010). The case manager who writes examination items for a new case management credentialing examination engages in advocacy by assuring the minimal professional practice standard is upheld through the industry expectations for knowledge demonstration. Some professionals develop model laws to implement case management practice and spearhead state and federal initiatives to support laws which speak to reimbursement of case managers under telehealth and telemedicine.

The American Case Management Association (ACMA). ACMA provides an equally detailed list of 10 specific ways in which advocacy is expected to be operationalized by the industry workforce. With a majority of ACMA members employed in hospital-based environments, the scope of the framing of each example is most applicable to that focus of practice. For example, the case manager:

- Identifies the legal decision maker (patient or surrogate)
- Promotes culturally competent care
- Provides patient/family/caregivers available tools/resources to make informed choices
- Utilizes the ethics committee or other resource to resolve conflict or challenges regarding patient care
- Promotes the understanding and use of advanced directives and ensures patient wishes are respected

(ACMA, 2013)

TABLE 12-4 Advocacy Across Ethical Codes

CCMC, Standards for Professional Conduct (2009)	ANA, Codes of Ethics for Nurses, with Interpretive Statements (2001)
Section 1: Advocacy, S1-The Advocate	Provision 3
Certified case managers will serve as advocates for their clients and ensure that: a. a comprehensive assessment will identify the client's needs b. options for necessary services will be provided to the client c. clients are provided with access to resources to meet individual needs	The nurse promotes, advocates for, and strives to protect the health, safety, and rights of the patient. 3.1-Privacy 3.2-Confidentiality 3.3-Protect of participants in research 3.4-Standards and review mechanisms 3.5-Acting on questionable practice 3.4-Addressing impaired practice

The NASW Standards for Social Work Case Management. When NASW released their revised standards for social work case management in 2013, they included a separate standard for advocacy. However, the standard combines the advocacy role with that of leadership. This is explained in the interpretation through affirming that "social work case managers exercise leadership by advocating for clients on the micro, mezzo, and macro levels" (NASW, 2013). Elaboration is provided to assure full understanding of the full scope of case management roles that social workers engage in. At the micro level, it is understood that social workers will communicate with the providers of treatment and services at other organizations where mutual clients are seen for the purpose of enhancing the clients' care. For example, the case manager for an oncology unit at a large hospital will dialogue with the care team at a hospice program where a mutual patient will be transferred for palliative or end-of-life care.

For macro-level advocacy, case managers explore ways to bridge the gaps in medical care for older and/or disabled adults in need of transportation for appointments.

Advocacy Defined for Case Management

Hellwig, Yam, and DiGuilio (2003) shed an important and contemporary light on advocacy as an important competency for case managers. Because of case management's history in managed care, the workforce has a profound appreciation for finding innovative strategies to benefit the best interests of patients while adhering to the increasingly stringent utilization review guidelines and cost constraints of managed care (Hellwig et al., 2003). This is a juggling act that many case managers sought to master during their tenure on those managed care frontlines and is explored in chapter 1.

By exploring advocacy's history and manifestation across the industry, the authors were able to break down advocacy into two perspectives: traditional **paternalistic** and **empowering**. The traditional paternalistic assumes the stance that the health professional, if not the case manager, has far greater knowledge about the complexities that underlie the overall health care system. This perspective also notes that the patient either does not want information or is incapable of understanding that information if it is provided. As a result, this professional is in a greater position to decide what is in the patient's best interests (Hellwig et al., 2003).

A case manager is meeting with a patient around the current options for transfer to acute as opposed to subacute rehabilitation programs. The case manager is aware that the patient can complete the minimum amount of therapy daily, perhaps no more than 2 hours. Although the patient has the best intent to do more, it is not possible at the present time. The rehabilitation team indicates that although the prognosis is uncertain, there is good potential for the patient to engage in a higher level of treatment at a future point. In this approach, the case manager facilitates the appropriate transfer. However, it should be noted that this does not mean that no communication should occur with either the patient (as appropriate) or the family (if involved) of the options, alternative settings, information about how the application process unfolds, and the arrangements for transfer. There might also be a dialogue of potential acute rehabilitation options for future consideration.

In the empowerment perspective, knowledge is viewed as that valuable commodity which enables a patient to act as an empowered and informed participant of the process. The scope of this information can involve when patients and families take that information to directly advocate in pursuit of specialty programs or treatment alternatives they may have been originally rejected. This could include the explanation of the appeal processes that patients capable of doing so or their family members engage in to access treatment, obtain out-of-network benefits or providers, or related situations (Hellwig et al., 2003).

Let us re-address the prior case scenario and apply the empowerment perspective. The case manager begins with that often tough dialogue between patient and family around the guidelines for acute rehabilitation program, which include the benefit of starting rehabilitation at a slower pace reflective of where the patient is at, so as not to sabotage his or her efforts. The patient and family are not in agreement and want to "push the envelope," so get on the phone with prospective rehabilitation programs and potentially the group administrator for the patient's group-managed insurance as applicable. The patient is viewed as the key architect of his or her own life, and lifestyle choices. Both roles stress the importance of the case manager's role as a client educator and supporter (Tahan, 2005).

The Four Classes of Advocacy

Tahan (2005) refers to advocacy as the essence or core of the client–case manager relationship. It can be very unclear just how much, how often, and to what degree case managers must be involved in each individual client's advocacy. The variation is immense across professional practice, with a series of variances at issue including, but not limited to, the:

- Context of practice (setting)
- Case manager's skills, knowledge, and competences
- Client's level of functioning, cognition, alertness, interests, and willingness, and
- Situation at hand

(Tahan, 2005)

Although Tahan affirmed the two perspectives of traditional paternalistic and empowering cited by Hellwig et al., he then identified a vital third one, that of **shared responsibility** (Taylor, 2005). In shared responsibility, the important values of moral commitment to client autonomy and client-determination are present. These three perspectives unite to form a commanding foundation for how case managers can comprehend advocacy across their diverse roles and functions.

Four distinct classes of advocacy are identified which prevail across case management practice (Tahan, 2005). These include:

- **Client advocacy (individual)**
- **Organizational advocacy (service)**
- **Community advocacy (population)**
- **Global advocacy (state/national)**

TABLE 12-5 Four Classes of Advocacy

Advocacy Skill	Explanation	Application
Client/Individual	Occurs at the level of a single client Simple complexity in scope Client behaviors impact one person at a time, and integral to the case manager–client relationship. They also vary based on the needs of the individual client.	A case manager (CM) at an acute rehabilitation hospital meets a new admission to conduct the intake assessment. The patient verbalizes concern about his prognosis and requests to meet with the treatment team sooner than later. The CM contacts the team and physician to confirm when the initial evaluations will be completed. The team conference is in turn scheduled for the next afternoon.
Organizational/ Service	Occurs at the level of a health care organization or program within that organization Moderate complexity in scope Involves actions that improve the efficacy and efficiency of services and systems of care delivery	The patient and his brother attend the team conference, anxious to hear from the team. The CM notified the physical therapist (PT) and occupational therapist (OT) are unable to attend but sent progress notes. The CM is aware of this pattern and furious. She meets with her director plus the medical director of rehabilitation. The family complains to the physician and CM, plus file a complaint with the regulatory entities including Joint Commission and CARF International (The Commission on Accreditation of Rehabilitation Facilities). A meeting is scheduled for involved department directors to develop a strategic plan to resolve the problem.
Community/ Population	Occurs at the level of the community at large served by the individual health care organization Moderate-to-high complexity in scope Involves proactive actions to improve the health of the community	Changes in the community surrounding the hospital and rehabilitation program evoke concern by the parent company. Administration discloses efforts are underway to either potentially sell the facility or close it. Hospital staff and governing board meet with community leaders to develop an action plan to halt any closure efforts.
Global or State/ National	Occurs at the broader scope that influences the health of the public at large High complexity in scope Involves proactive and reactive actions that improve the health of the public, independent of geographical boundaries	A series of public hearings are held to address the potential closure of the hospital. The CM contacts prior patients to provide public testimony to support the community's need for both the hospital and rehabilitation programs. Hundreds of former patients, staff, and stakeholders turn out at the state capital to testify and protest closure. The actions contribute to keeping the facility open.

Adapted from Tahan, H. (2005). Essentials of advocacy in case management. Professional Case Management, 10*(3), 136–145.*

The four classes of advocacy are presented in Table 12-5 with a case scenario to demonstrate their individual application. They are reminiscent of the macro, mezzo, and micro concepts utilized in social work, though provide a further distinction at the mezzo level. In this way, there is a further separation of the advocacy occurring at the organizational or program level from that of the involved community or target population addressed.

Application of the four classes model has profound significance to case management, particularly with the expanding industry focus on population health management initiatives and next generation of care coordination programming. Utilization of the four classes identified through the model provides case managers the opportunity to critically consider the dimensions of their advocacy. They are also able to advance the potential scope of their case management practice through the continuum of professional practice.

PROFESSIONAL PATIENT ADVOCATES

Patient advocate is a broad title that encompasses many types of services for patients, typically working independently of a health care system or hospital, on behalf of the patient (Torrey in Murphy, 2013). These individuals are viewed as professionals who come from a broad spectrum of health-related degrees across the care team and possess skills to assist patients and their families maneuver the complex health care system. The exhaustive list of involved professional disciplines includes, but is not limited to, case managers, nurses, disability management specialists, physicians, pharmacists, nurse practitioners, physician assistants, psychologists, nurse **navigators**, geriatric care managers, life-care planners, rehabilitation nurses, financial/insurance/billing advocates, behavioral health specialists, and social workers (PPAI, 2014).

There is no universal certification for patient advocacy, though many individuals have sought certification from the expanding list of credentialing entities. Most of these provide a certificate following completion of defined coursework which is offered through a variety of modes (e.g., strictly online, in-person or hybrid models which provide both types of learning opportunities).

A new generation of degree programs is appearing in higher education such as those through Southern Vermont College and the University of Arizona College of Nursing-RN Patient Advocates, to name a few (APHI, 2014b). Table 12-6

TABLE 12-6 Professional Patient Advocate Certifications

Certification Entity	Certification	Eligibility Requirements
Professional Patient Advocate Institute (PPAI, 2014)	Hospital Patient Advocacy 9 courses E-learning	Open to all who want an introduction to the field or organizations, who want to use the program to provide common ground for which all members of the health care team can work together to improve the patient experience
	Patient Advocacy 11 courses In-person and/or E-learning	Licensed health care professionals National health care education in a health and human service discipline whose scope of practice allows for independent assessment Those with a baccalaureate, graduate degree of PhD in social work (or another health and human service field that promotes the physical, psychological, vocational well-being of those served) Financial professionals and/or professional coders
UCLA Extension: Patient Advocacy Certificate Program (APHI, 2014)	Patient Advocacy 8 courses + Seminar: In-person and E-learning	Minimum of bachelor's degree in any field, or associate's degree in nursing, respiratory, occupational, or physical therapies, emergency medical technician (EMT)
Southern Vermont College (APHI, 2014)	Bachelor of Science Degree in Healthcare Management and Advocacy 48 core credits 36 course credits 12 concentration credits 32 elective credits Capstone course project	General core requirements: Interviewing/counseling Psychology Algebra Pre-Practicum Practicum Major requirements: Organizational Finance Macro-Economics Intro to Health Care I Intro to Health Care II Health Care Law Health Care Insurance Topics in Health Care Mgmt./Advocacy Organizational/Mgmt. Theory Marketing Psychology Case Management Ethics in the Helping Professions Social Research Conflict Resolution

compares several certificate and degree options, with a more comprehensive master listing of programs available in the website resources appendix.

PATIENT NAVIGATION

Patient navigation emerged on the health care horizon in the early 1990s. There has been considerable industry confusion between the role of patient navigator and that of patient advocate, despite clear definitions to distinguish between the two roles. This becomes evident through the most basic of language used on websites and other promotional materials for the advocacy and navigation roles. The Alliance of Professional Health Advocates (2014a), a membership association to support the business needs of professional advocates, uses the following language on their home page:

> The organization provides independent patient advocates and navigators, and those interested in exploring this profession with the support they need to start and grow a successful advocacy practice.

Can a professional health advocate also be a patient navigator? If there is a defined answer, one has to wonder if the industry is aware of what that (answer) may be. The answer may be a moot point, for some suggest that everyone involved in a patient's care has a role within the navigation process (Academy of Oncology Nurse and Patient Navigators [AONN], 2014).

A diverse group of programs and certifications have emerged encompassing the roles engaged in by the two types of navigators. There are those who maintain a clinical focus and are involved in patient assessment and coordination of care. These navigators are unrelated to health insurance exchange navigators, though their presence has been boosted by a mandate tied to federal grant money, expected future accreditation requirements, and research that backs the concept (Kreimer, 2014). A number of hospitals and health care organizations and programs have instituted formal clinical patient navigator roles, such as for oncology and other specialty programs. The AONN (2014) provides the following definition:

> A navigator is a medical professional whose clinical expertise and training guides patients and their caregivers to make informed decisions, collaborating with a multidisciplinary team to allow for timely cancer screening, diagnosis, treatment, and increased supportive care across the cancer continuum.

Although AONN also extends the definition to cover those in lay navigator roles, they make a clear designation between those actions engaged in by a medical professional, implying the mandate for a license. There are also navigators who are lay persons and focus on nonclinical tasks such as facilitating transportation to appoints, providing patients resources, and assuring availability of patient's medical records treatment providers (Murphy, 2013).

Despite the variation in scope of the two types of navigation roles, a common link exists between them. This encompasses the personalized assistance and support offered to patients, families, and caregivers to help overcome health care system barriers (e.g., fragmented care) and/or personal barriers (e.g., cultural, financial, educational, spiritual, psychosocial), and facilitate timely access to quality health and psychosocial care (AONN, 2014).

Harold P. Freeman Patient Navigation Institute

Harold Freeman is often referred to as the father of patient navigation. Dr. Freeman is a physician who in 1989 was serving as the president of the American Cancer Society. The organization held a series of hearings to explore the prevention and treatment needs of underserved cancer patients, identify potential barriers to care, and define programs and strategies to manage those barriers.

Testimony from patients living with cancer revealed a disparity in treatment, compared to other populations. The key findings included that economically disadvantaged patients:

- Endure greater pain and suffering
- Make extraordinary personal sacrifices to obtain and pay for care
- Face substantial obstacles in obtaining and using health insurance
- Do not seek care if they cannot pay for it
- Encounter education programs that are culturally insensitive and irrelevant to their situation
- Have fatalistic feelings about diagnosis and treatment

(American Cancer Society, 1989)

Dr. Freeman spearheaded the efforts to reduce these disparities for the residents of Harlem, NY, and began a program at Harlem Hospital Center. Funded through a grant from the Amgen Foundation and the Ralph Lauren Center for Cancer Care and Prevention, Harold P. Freeman Patient Navigation Institute (HPFPNI) was established to support the training of individuals who are associated with organizations (HPFPNI, 2014a) to work with patients who otherwise would not tend to obtain the medical care they needed.

The program has evolved to include the movement of an individual across the entire health care continuum. This includes prevention, detection, diagnosis, treatment, support, and end-of-life care (HPFPNI, 2014b), all critical components of effective population management. Potential barriers which patient navigation addresses include:

- Financial (including uninsured and under insured)
- Communication (e.g., lack of understanding, language/cultural)
- Medical system (e.g., fragmented medical system, missed appointments, lost results)
- Psychological (e.g., fear and distrust)
- Other (e.g., transportation and need for child care)

In 2005, the Patient Navigator Outreach and Chronic Disease Prevention Act was passed to fund and further expand the program to low-income areas across the United States. Navigators continue to help uninsured patients evaluate treatment options, enroll in clinical trials, obtain referrals, and apply for financial assistance (Howard University, 2005).

The PPACA and the Health Insurance Exchange Navigator

The passage of PPACA brought heightened attention to the navigator role. From the perspective of health care reform, navigator refers specifically to an individual or organization trained to help consumers, small businesses, and their employers as they look for health coverage options through the marketplace. This role is a free service provided to consumers and includes completing of eligibility and enrollment forms (Healthcare.gov, 2014).

The requirements for this role include:

- Completing up to 30 hours of training,
- Passing an Health and Human Services (HHS)-approved certification test, and
- Having the ability to provide culturally and linguistically appropriate services to individual and small business exchanges.

(Centers for Medicare and Medicaid Services, 2013)

Much of the controversy surrounding the navigator program has originated with the insurance industry. Insurance agents and brokers view the navigator role as impinging on their turf. The agents are concerned that they will lose the commissions they are entitled to when navigators help consumers enroll in insurance plans. There is an additional concern that if unqualified navigators or other assisters are allowed to recommend insurance products to consumers, consumers may purchase products that do not meet their needs (Jost, 2013).

There has been considerable lobbying of state legislatures to assure a minimum standard of navigator practice through licensure, and other eligibility requirements beyond the preliminary mandatory training (Jost, 2013). Proposed regulations include the development of clear standards for the navigator program in the federal exchange, and clarification of the extent to which states can license navigators in federal and state exchanges.

CONTEXT FOR COLLABORATE ADVOCACY COMPETENCY

From the COLLABORATE approach, advocacy is that strong and steady pulse which gives life to a case manager's multifaceted professional soul. The force of this competency provides the impetus for the wide array of endeavors that serve as vital elements of the case management profession. These span the distinct domains where case managers engage across those of the client, organization, community, and global (Tahan, 2005).

KEY ELEMENTS OF ADVOCACY COMPETENCY

The key elements of the advocacy competency include:

- Patient,
- Family/support system, and
- Professional—the individual and the profession.

Patient and Family/Support System

A majority of professional case managers know how to advocate for those who they intervene on behalf of and aspire to do so. This level of direct patient interaction is the one which is the most comfortable for many health care professionals (Morse, 2008; Tomajan, 2012). With respect to case managers, it is the development and implementation of a unique plan that serves to energize and inspire them unlike any other activity. In dialoguing with professionals across the industry, discussions about strategically executed case management processes often yield the most motivational reflections for many.

However, another reality for most case managers involves the lengthy list of impeding priorities that can hijack their day. These activities can all too often negate any positive feelings that they may have otherwise experienced in working with their target population. These priorities impact a professional's ability to effectively fulfill the goals defined in treatment plans for clients. During a day consumed by the paramount responsibilities of clinical reviews, data entry, and outcomes completion, any additional time and energy needed to advocate for others falls to the bottom of the "to do" list.

From the COLLABORATE approach the professional case manager focuses on the advocacy efforts needed to address issues for the patient, family, and/or support system. There is an ability to also anticipate the realities, which can and do present with potential to impede the process. This will be further addressed in the Anticipatory Competency, chapter 16.

There is a proactive effort by the case manager to recognize that despite the best efforts of efficiency and effectiveness, the unexpected occur to impede their well-planned advocacy. A reaction, with the accompanying emotions, frustrations, and often tantrums, has no benefit other than to compromise and delay needed intervention. Consider the case scenario in Box 12-4 to demonstrate how this element plays out.

Professional

This element cuts to the core of a case manager's professional identity. It involves how to put that professional foot forward consistently to address the needs of the patient as well as the case management profession itself. A case manager's adherence to advocacy as a competency can be enhanced through his or her commitment to achieve balance between occupational stressors and life challenges while fostering professional values and career sustainability (Fink-Samnick, 2009). This is yet another opportunity to commit to a specific habit, in this instance to acknowledge there will always be stresses and strains to challenge work performance. Yet case managers have a choice, no matter what challenges manifest. They can present as polished, posed professionals or the antithesis of emoting and reactionary amateurs.

The Individual. Individual leadership (self-leadership) starts with each case manager recognizing the importance of how to present as a health care professional. This involves

BOX 12-4 COLLABORATE Approach, Case Scenario Patient and Family Support System Element

Melisa is a case manager for an acute rehabilitation hospital. She is working with Mark, an adult who has suffered a traumatic brain injury. Mark's family is supportive, though having a difficult time adjusting to the patient's unknown prognosis. Their frustration is directed at the team, the case manager, the system, and anyone else they can think of.

The treatment team has defined that Mark would benefit from an additional week before transitioning home. The family reluctantly agrees and receives training to enhance their confidence with the patient's scope of care. The worker's compensation case manager, Beth, leaves you a voicemail saying "Mark can accomplish the remaining goals defined at a lower level of care, which is more cost effective. It is the strong recommendation of our medical director that Mark be transferred tomorrow to a local subacute nursing home for the next 2 weeks. They can address the remaining goals needed to discharge him directly home.

It might present this is the answer to Melisa's prayers, especially amid three new admissions and four other discharges that day. Although this plan is wrapped-up with a bow, Melisa knows it is far from Mark's best interests that he be forced to orient to a new treatment environment and new team members. Mark's family is horrified and concerned about the transfer. Melisa defines an advocacy plan with the transdisciplinary team to:

1. Review the fiscal disincentives of the transfer including potential treatment time lost for Mark in the context of his diagnosis. She adds in the daily cost to the payer to denote a potential return on investment.
2. Define goals and objectives for each discipline involved, with team coordination to address specific issues such as compensatory strategies to maximize external distractions impacting functional ambulation to manage steps, curbs, home safety, and other issues, which would promote further self-sufficiency for the patient.
3. Discuss out-of-contract benefits to cover the continued stay, or agree to negotiate the current per diem rate as required.
4. Facilitate communication between Mark's attending physician and the medical director of the insurance plan.
5. Involve Mark's family in the process so they feel empowered. In this way they can advocate for Mark while Melisa advocates for all of them.
6. Melisa explains the strategy: if the plan to extend Mark's stay is not approved, his family will spring into action and contact his employer. As a group administered policy, covering over 450,000 lives in the region, the employer group administrator has offered to contact the insurance company to mandate they extend the benefit to cover the continued days.

implementation of solid and eloquent communication with anyone whom he or she interacts. It also takes into account whether that communication occurs through written, verbal, or nonverbal messaging. That old adage "it's not what you say but how you say it" rings true.

This element also extends to those skills and strategies used to effectively manage and lead a transdisciplinary team. Case managers are viewed as team leaders and expected to facilitate the care coordination process. This involves any and all dialogues the case manager has with team members or other stakeholders of the process. It can include the skillful art of negotiation to obtain authorization for extended days, treatments, or other identified resources for patients. How a case manager connotes unique expertise is critical to the success of his or her individual professional effort.

The Profession. There are many ways in which case managers advocate for the profession. This book is one means to accomplish advocacy given the theme involves motivating and establishing a competency-based framework to move from advanced practice to profession. Some case managers join professional association public policy committees. This affords the opportunities to contribute to initiatives dedicated to title protection, licensure portability, defined competencies, and other means to promote the concept of professional case management.

IMPLICATIONS FOR PRACTICE

Advocacy provides a powerful context for the many tasks, roles, functions, and responsibilities of case managers (Tahan, 2005). To this end, there is agreement across industry stakeholders. However, a series of influencers yield powerful implications for how case managers understand and actively engage in advocacy. Although the story for each continues to unfold, they bear preliminary identification for case management's consideration moving forward.

PROFESSIONAL TITLE/DESIGNATION OPPOSED TO ROLES/FUNCTIONS

What's in a name? With consumer protection, a current goal across the industry, it is presumed that advocacy will be a function of most, if not all, health care roles. A nurse who seeks to clarify a physician's order for a change of a medication dosage advocates for her patient as readily as the case manager who seeks approval for that patient's home-based intravenous medication management. Why must competition for the competent delivery of advocacy invade the effort? It was identified earlier in chapter 4 how too many certifications can fragment as opposed to integrate a profession. What is the true benefit of adding a patient advocacy certification and a rash of new titles to the already massive credentialing conundrum in the health care world?

Why does a professional's adherence alone to the range of advocacy standards and ethical principles present as insufficient? One has to wonder what the real value of the industry's established standards and principles are, especially when they are so casually usurped by newer certifications, designations, and even more letters to appear after a professional's name.

PROTECTING THE PUBLIC: A PROFESSIONAL PRIORITY AND MANDATE

There has been heightened attention to the concept of protecting the public across the industry through the full scope of health care stakeholders, including credentialing bodies. To this end, distinct certifications and licensure boards view protecting the public as a professional mandate. Why this presents as an obsolete or forgotten tenet is concerning. Perhaps, it provides validation for why there has been a need to develop additional specialty certifications and degrees which speak directly to the concept of advocacy. How does this assure the public that consumers can untangle the quagmire of their health care experience any easier? The verdict is out on this decision.

Professional associations are focused on improving the way all people interact with and experience the health care system by supporting public education to foster effective self-advocacy (National Association of Healthcare Advocacy Consultants, 2013). The National Association of Healthcare Advocacy Consultants and the Professional Patient Advocate Institute (2014) support the inclusion of all interested professionals across the myriad of involved disciplines of origin.

The importance of consumer advocacy in the health care realm is a focus endemic to licensed professionals, and embedded in a case management's professional core. To have consumer advocacy further emphasized by added credentialing and programming presents as an unnecessary duplication of time and effort, that which the industry cannot afford.

SUMMARY

Throughout the varied and robust content of this chapter, one critical theme rings true. As the health care system becomes more complex, the concept of advocacy has probably never been more important (Morse, 2008). Advocacy will most likely continue to evolve as it strives to meet the emerging demands of those who rely on its underlying purpose, whether referred to as patients, clients, members, or consumers. Advocacy is an integral competency which holds unique significance for professional case management as a COLLABORATE competency.

References

Academy of Oncology Nurse and Patient Navigators. (2014). *Definition*. Retrieved September 29, 2014, from https://www.aonnonline.org

Alliance of Professional Health Advocates. (2014a). *Home page*. Retrieved September 17, 2014, from http://aphadvocates.org

Alliance of Professional Health Advocates. (2014b). *Master list of patient advocacy educational courses, programs and organizations*. Retrieved September 18, 2014, from http://healthadvocateprograms.com/masterlist.htm

American Cancer Society. (1989). A summary of the American cancer society report to the nation: Cancer in the poor. *CA: A Cancer Journal for Clinicians, 39*(5), 263–265.

Baldwin, M. (2003). Patient advocacy: A concept analysis. *Nursing Standard, 17*(21), 33–39.

Benner, P., Stephen, M., Leonard, V., & Day, L. (2010). *Educating nurses: A call for radical transformation*. San Francisco, CA: Jossey Bass.

Case Management Society of America. (2010). *CMSA standards of practice for case management* (Rev. ed.). Retrieved April 25, 2013, from http://www.cmsa.org/portals/0/pdf/memberonly/StandardsOfPractice.pdf

Centers for Medicare and Medicaid Services. (2013). *PPHF—2013—Cooperative agreement to support navigators in federally—Facilitated and state partnership exchanges* [Navigators and other marketplace assistance programs]. Retrieved September 17, 2014, from http://www.cms.gov/CCIIO/Resources/Funding-Opportunities/Downloads/2013-navigator-foa-4-9-2013.pdf

Commission for Case Manager Certification. (2009). *Code of professional conduct for case managers*. Retrieved September 10, 2014, from http://ccmcertification.org/content/ccm-exam-portal/code-professional-conduct-case-managers

Earp, J. A., French, E. A., & Gilkey, M. B. (2008). *Patient advocacy for health care quality: Strategies for achieving patient centered care*. Sudbury, MA: Jones and Bartlett.

Epstein, E. G. (2010, September). Moral obligations of nurses and physicians in neonatal end-of-Life care. *Nursing Ethics, 17*(5), 577–589. Retrieved September 13, 2014, from NIH Public Access, http://www.ncbi.nlm.nih.gov/pmc/articles/PMC3615421/

Fink-Samnick, E. (2009). The Professional Resilience Paradigm: The next dimension of professional self-care, *Professional Case Management, 14*(6), 330-332.

Hackethal, V. (2014). *'Dying in America' IOM Report calls for major reform, medscape*. Retrieved September 19, 2014, from http://www.medscape.com/viewarticle/831935

Harold P. Freeman Institute for Patient Navigation. (2014a). *About us*. Retrieved September 17, 2014, from http://www.hpfreemanpni.org/about-us/

Harold P. Freeman Institute for Patient Navigation. (2014b). *Our model*. Retrieved September 17, 2014, from http://www.hpfreemanpni.org/our-model/

Healthcare.gov. (2014). Navigator. Retrieved September 17, 2014, from https://www.healthcare.gov/glossary/navigator/

Howard University. (2005, June 30). *Press release*. Washington, DC: Howard University Newsroom.

International Federation of Social Workers. (2014). *Global definition of social work*. Retrieved September 29, 2014, from http://ifsw.org/get-involved/global-definition-of-social-work/

Institute of Medicine. (1998). *Approaching death: Improving care at the end of life*. Washington, DC: Institute of Medicine, National Academy of Sciences.

Institute of Medicine. (1999). *To err is human: Building a safer healthcare system*. Washington, DC: National Academies Press.

Institute of Medicine. (2001). *Crossing the quality chasm: A new health system for the 21st century*. Washington, DC: National Academies Press.

Institute of Medicine. (2003). *Health professions' education: A bridge to quality (The Quality Chasm Series)*. Washington, DC: The National Academies Press.

Jost, T. (2013, April 4). Implementing health reform: Proposed Regulations For Exchange "Navigators". [Health Affairs Blog]. Retrieved September 18, 2014, from http://healthaffairs.org/blog/2013/04/04/implementing-health-reform-proposed-regulations-for-exchange-navigators/

Kelly, K. (2012). Influential women. *AmericaComesAlive.com*. Retrieved October 8, 2014, from http://americacomesalive.com/2012/03/14/jane-addams-1860-1935-advocate-for-the-poor-and-activist-for-peace/#.VDWUsb7F-JU

Kreimer, S. (2014, July). Patient navigator role growing in popularity. *Hospitals and Health Networks Magazine*, Retrieved September 18, 2014, from http://www.hhnmag.com/display/HHN-news-article.dhtml?dcrPath=/templatedata/HF_Common/NewsArticle/data/HHN/Magazine/2014/Jul/patient-navigators

Legal Dictionary. (2014). Lobbying. Retrieved September 25, 2014, from http://legal-dictionary.thefreedictionary.com/Lobbying

Medicare Newsgroup. (2014). *Out of network*. Retrieved September 25, 2014, from http://www.medicarenewsgroup.com/news/medicare-faqs/individual-faq?faqId=edf1b895-b883-4078-a3e6-fcd7216ad1aa

Merriam-Webster's online dictionary. (2014a). Advocacy. Retrieved September 9, 2014, from http://www.merriam-webster.com/dictionary/advocacy

Merriam-Webster's online dictionary. (2014b). Advocate. Retrieved September 13, 2014, from http://www.merriam-webster.com/dictionary/advocate

Merriam-Webster's online dictionary. (2014c). Negotiate. Retrieved, September 25, 2014, from http://www.merriam-webster.com/dictionary/negotiate

Morse, K. (2008). Patient advocacy: New skill or core competency? *Editorial, Critical Care*, *3*(3), 4.

Murphy, D. (2013). *What is a patient navigator, surround health*. Retrieved September 17, 2014, from http://surroundhealth.net/Topics/SurroundHealth-Members-Lounge/The-Lounge/Articles/What-is-a-Patient-Navigator.aspx

National Association of Healthcare Advocacy Consultants. (2013). *Organizational website*. Retrieved April 26, 2013, from http://nahac.memberlodge.com

National Association of Social Workers. (2013). *Standards for social work case management*. Retrieved October 6, 2014, from http://socialworkers.org/practice/naswstandards/CaseManagementStandards2013.pdf

National Association of Social Workers. (2014). *Advocacy and organizing*. Retrieved April 26, 2013, from http://socialworkers.org/pressroom/features/issue/advocacy.asp

NursingLink. (2014). *Patient advocacy: Barriers and facilitators, nursing management*. Retrieved September 11, 2014, from http://nursinglink.monster.com/training/articles/929-patient-advocacy-barriers-and-facilitators

Professional Patient Advocate Institute. (2014). *About us*. Retrieved September 18, 2014, from http://www.patientadvocatetraining.com/?page=about_us

Public Broadcasting System. (2014). *Moyers on America: The land of Lobby*. Retrieved October 7, 2014, from http://www.pbs.org/moyers/moyersonamerica/capitol/lobby.html

Salas, L. M., Sen, S., & Segal, E. (2010). Critical theory: A pathway from dichotomous to integrated social work practice. *Families in Society*, *9*(1), 91–96.

Selanders, L., & Crane, P. (2012). The voice of Florence nightingale on advocacy. *OJIN: The Online Journal of Issues in Nursing*, *17*(1), Manuscript 1.

The Social Welfare History Project. (2014). *Mary Richmond*. Retrieved October 8, 2014, from http://www.socialwelfarehistory.com/people/richmond-mary/

Social Work License Map. (2014). *Macro, mezzo and micro social work*. Retrieved September 29, 2014, from http://socialworklicensemap.com/macro-mezzo-and-micro-social-work/

Tahan, H. (2005). Essentials of advocacy in case management. *Professional Case Management*, *10*(3), 136–145.

Taylor, C. (2005). Ethical issues in case management. In E. Cohen & T. Cesta (Eds.), *Nursing case management: From essentials to advanced practice applications* (chap. 33, pp. 361–379). St. Louis, MO: Elsevier Mosby.

Tomajan, K. (2012). Advocating for nurses and nursing. *OJIN: The Online Journal of Issues in Nursing*. *17*(1), Manuscript 4.

13 BIG-PICTURE ORIENTATION

OBJECTIVES

After studying this chapter, you will be able to:

1. Define assessment.
2. Distinguish between psychopathology and pathophysiology.
3. Discuss the biopsychosocial perspective of assessment.
4. Demonstrate application of the Global Assessment Lens.
5. Understand the key elements of the Big-Picture Orientation competency.

KEY TERMS

Assessment
Biopsychosocial framework
Behavioral health
Clinical reasoning
DSM-5
Global Assessment Lens
Human behavior in the social environment
Mental health
Mental illness
Pathophysiology
Psychopathology
Psychosocial stressors
Strengths-based helping
The nursing process

The overall effectiveness of each case manager's interventions is directly related to the size, scope, and accuracy of the picture that he or she can obtain about the patient. There is a great variation in exactly what information should be included in that picture and the mechanisms by which that information should be obtained, whether use of technology or traditional interviewing. However, industry consensus prevails about the critical value of the assessment process overall (Ashford & LeCroy, 2013; Bond, 2010; Campbell, Webster, & Glass, 2009; Watson, 2006).

Many factors impact how each case manager approaches an assessment. Practice setting and the scope of practice for a case manager's professional discipline will impact what content is included. Add the emerging population-based foci of behavioral health, immigration, and increased attention to health literacy to the growing list of valuable content. Case managers also must consider global constructs of ever-changing fiscal reimbursement, availability, and emergence of new technologies to render and document care, as well as access to care by distinct patient populations.

What emerges is the mandate for case managers to view patients from a perspective that promotes attention to a large volume of evolving concerns across biological, psychological, sociological, and spiritual domains of professional practice.

DEFINITIONS

Assessment is the act of making a judgment about something (Merriam-Webster, 2014a). This is a general and simple definition for a word used so frequently in the health care industry. Anything and everything easily become the focus of a case manager's assessment.

Specific to the health care arena, assessment is a systematic and dynamic way to collect and analyze data about a client (American Nurses Association, 2014). Case managers spend a majority of their day assessing a broad range of data about a patient. First, there will be exploration of the clinical status of a patient, perhaps to verify the patient's appropriateness for intervention and/or continued stay in a facility. The word *clinical* pertains to the actual observation and treatment of patients as distinguished from *theoretical* or *basic sciences* (Dorland Medical Dictionary, 2007). However, there are especially varied applications of how a clinical assessment is understood in health care. This due, in part, to different interpretations of the word, dependent on the case manager's professional discipline of origin, if not also scope of practice.

Those with a nursing or medical degree might explore the clinical status of a patient specific to their **pathophysiology**, the functional changes that accompany a particular syndrome or disease (Merriam-Webster, 2014b). Understanding routine laboratory values, vital signs, and symptoms of disease are commonly used examples. A case manager with professional education in a mental health field, such as a social worker or counselor, might engage in a patient's clinical assessment by exploring the **psychopathology**, which includes the study of psychological and behavioral dysfunction occurring in mental disorders or in social disorganization (Merriam-Webster, 2014c). Examples include the patient's orientation, potentially the presence of psychotic or potentially suicidal thoughts, and history of substance use.

Exploration of a patient's **psychosocial stressors** might be warranted. These are major life-influencing events that lead to intense stress so profound that they can contribute to the development or aggravation of an existing psychological disorder (Psychology Dictionary, 2014). Included in this list could be the death of a loved one, divorce, domestic violence or sexual assault, loss of one's home, or even sudden, unexpected unemployment.

Prevailing psychosocial stressors could yield the need for assessment of a patient's **mental health** and/or **mental illness**. These two terms are often used interchangeably, yet there are defined distinctions identified between them. Mental health refers to a broad array of activities directly or indirectly related to the mental well-being component included in the World Health Organization's (WHO) definition of health: "A state of complete physical, mental and social well-being, and not merely the absence of disease." It is related to the promotion of well-being, the prevention of mental disorders, and the treatment and rehabilitation of people affected by mental disorders (WHO, 2014).

In contrast, mental illness refers to the disorders generally characterized by dysregulation of mood, thought, and/or behavior, as recognized by the *Diagnostic and Statistical Manual*, 5th edition (*DSM-5*) of the American Psychiatric Association (Centers for Disease Control and Prevention, 2014). The ***DSM-5*** is the standard classification of mental disorders used by mental health professionals in the United States. It includes a listing of diagnostic criteria for every psychiatric disorder recognized by the U.S. health care system (American Psychiatric Association, 2013).

Behavioral health is a term frequently used across the industry to denote mental health concerns. There is no industry consensus on the meaning, or usage. Many view the term of behavioral health to be interchangeable with mental health while others suggest distinctions. Behavioral health can convey less stigma, since a behavior is an aspect of an individual's personality which can be changed. As a result, the term behavioral health presents a more optimistic view for those who experience mental illness or addiction and who may have felt that these diseases were permanent parts of their lives (Sandler, 2009). It has also been presented that behavioral health is a more inclusive term since it not only includes ways of promoting well-being by preventing or intervening in mental illness, but also has an aim of preventing or intervening in substance use or other addiction (Sandler, 2009).

PAST AND CURRENT THINKING

An exhaustive number of patient assessment models appear across the health care industry. The identification and gathering of pertinent information to be included in an assessment is a paramount first step in defining a patient's status and the extent of his or her needs. The importance of a thorough and accurate assessment to the overall care process is a common thread across all transitions of care, independent of a case manager's professional discipline or origin or the setting in which he or she practices.

The case manager's initial assessment opens a window into the unique world of the patient and family system. The size and scope of that assessment are subject to a variety of factors including, but not limited to, a case manager's practice setting, role and functions, professional discipline, as well as the legal scope of practice associated with an individual's licensure and/or certification.

The amount of information included in an assessment about each patient and family system is equally diverse and can feel never-ending. There is an exhaustive list of items for consideration by case managers, including, but not limited to, patient pathophysiology, clinical psychopathology and behavioral health history, family relationships and dynamics, treatment adherence history, cultural diversity, plus suicidality and risk, to name a few. The mode by which the information for each assessment is captured is also a vital factor for consideration, particularly in the present context of technology's permeation of the industry.

NURSING

A Paramount Responsibility: Assessment and Patient Safety

Assessment is viewed as the key to safety, accuracy, and efficiency (Alfaro-LeFevre, 2014). Historically, the role of the nurse has been to record but not interpret observations including blood pressure, pulse, temperature, respiratory rate, and consciousness level. By accurately recording this information, the nurse is able to prioritize patient care (Watson, 2006). This is conducive to the traditional role of nurse as caregiver, where a basic premise of nursing care is the prevention of noxious influences and the provision of life-sustaining resources (Newell, 1996).

The importance of a nurse's accountability for the completion of an accurate patient assessment is delineated by the concept's presentation as the first professional standard of practice,

> Standard 1: Assessment,
> The registered nurse collects comprehensive data pertinent to the healthcare consumer's health and/or situation.
>
> *American Nurses Association, 2010*

Critical consideration of the infinite amount of information to be gathered is identified through the requisite competencies associated with the assessment standard, which are shown in Box 13-1. Emphasis on the differing practice scope expectations is also accounted for by the presence of additional dedicated competencies for graduate-level-prepared specialty nurses and the advanced practice registered nurse (APRN).

With a patient's status ever-evolving and changing, assessment becomes the nurse's (if not any case management professional's) first line of defense to ensure that information is correct, and planned care is safe and appropriate (Alfaro-LeFevre, 2014). The Institutes of Medicine (IOM) identified the importance of solid assessments as a factor to influence quality-driven patient-centered care (IOM, 1999, 2000, 2001, 2003, 2011). Patient safety remains one of the most critical issues facing health care and the nurses are the health care professionals most likely to intercept errors and prevent harm to patients (Hughes, 2008).

The IOM's Six Aims (2001) which are discussed earlier in this text, propose that health care be safe, effective, patient-centered, timely, efficient, and equitable. The successful attainment of the aims lies in the ability of all professionals to document and assure knowledge of information exclusive to a patient, such as allergies, medications, diagnostic and treatment plans, and any other specific needs as available. In a safe system, information is not lost, inaccessible, or forgotten in transitions (IOM, 2001).

The Pennsylvania Patient Safety Advisory brief on Medication Errors Associated with Documented Allergies (2008) reviewed over 3,800 reports of cases in which patients received medications to which they had documented allergies. Large numbers of errors were associated with breakdowns in patient information, including allergies, diagnosis, comorbid conditions, current medication lists, and laboratories. These breakdowns manifested at each level of the medication-use process including when practitioners:

- Obtain information from patients, caregivers, or other health care facilities during the reconciliation process;
- Document the information into paper-based and electronic records;
- Write orders for medications or enter orders into computerized prescriber order entry systems;
- Enter orders into the pharmacy order entry systems and dispense medications; and
- Obtain and administer medications.

BOX 13-1 Competencies for Standard 1: Assessment, Nursing Standards of Practice

Competencies

The registered nurse:

- Collects comprehensive data including, but not limited to, physical, functional, psychosocial, emotional, cognitive, sexual, cultural, age-related, environmental, spiritual/transpersonal, and economic assessments in a systematic and ongoing process while honoring the uniqueness of the person
- Elicits the health care consumer's values, preferences, expressed needs, and knowledge of the health care situation
- Involves the health care consumer, family, and other health care providers as appropriate, in holistic data collection
- Identifies barriers (e.g., psychosocial, literacy, financial, cultural) to effective communication and makes appropriate adaptions
- Recognizes the impact of personal attitudes, values, and beliefs
- Assesses family dynamics and impact on health care consumer health and wellness
- Prioritizes data collection based on the health care consumer's immediate condition, or the anticipated needs of the health care consumer or situation
- Uses appropriate evidence-based assessment techniques, instruments, and tools
- Synthesizes available data, information, and knowledge relevant to the situation to identify patterns and variances
- Applies ethical, legal, privacy guidelines, and policies to the collection, maintenance, use, and dissemination of data and information
- Recognizes the health care consumer as the authority on her or his own health by honoring their care preferences
- Documents relevant data in a retrievable format

Additional competencies for the graduate-level-prepared specialty nurse and the advanced practice registered nurse:

- Initiates and interprets diagnostic tests and procedures relevant to the health care consumer's current status
- Assesses the effect of interactions among individuals, family, community, and social systems on health and illness

Adapted from American Nursing Association. (2010). Nursing, scopes and standards of practice (2nd ed.). Author. Retrieved from Nursebooks.org

A review of the admission notes from over a 3-month period, evaluated the completeness and accuracy of drug allergy documentation by primary care nurses, along with medical residents. The results of this review showed that approximately 20% of the health care professionals failed to document drug allergies in their admission notes alone (Pennsylvania Patient Safety Authority, 2008). Allowance of any information that fails to reflect the most accurate portrait of the patient, will surely result in care that is less-than optimal and far from safe.

The quality of the individual patient assessment bears directly on an organization's ability to meet these six aims, both individually and collectively. Case management serves a pivotal role in these efforts by assuring the gathering and transmission of information exclusive to the patient is not only accurate, but is in turn appropriately conveyed to all who render care.

The Nursing Process

The nursing process is a problem-oriented model that breaks down symptoms into nursing problems utilizing nursing diagnosis (Yildirim & Özhahraman, 2011). This structured and methodical approach to assessment is one which resonates with case management. Viewed as the common thread uniting different types of nurses who work in varied areas, the nursing process is seen as the essential core of practice for the registered nurse to deliver holistic, patient-focused care (ANA, 2014). It also has the distinction of being seen as an integral decision-making approach that promotes critical thinking, the initial COLLABORATE competency (Yildirim & Özhahraman, 2011).

Assessment is the foundation of the nursing process, for it is recognized as the first critical step to determining health status and identifying actual and potential problems (Alfaro-LeFevre, 2014). Consider how the effectiveness of many a patient care process becomes easily compromised as a result of missing vital information from the assessment. The Pennsylvania Patient Safety Authority Advisory (2008) showed that as many as 18% of serious, preventable adverse drug events stem from practitioners having insufficient information about the patient before prescribing, dispensing, and administering medications. Perhaps copies of the advanced directives were not obtained or documented with a patient unnecessarily intubated during a sudden event, as a result. The safety, accuracy, and efficiency of all other phases of the nursing process depend on the ability of a nurse to gather accurate, relevant, and complete assessment data (Alfaro-LeFevre, 2014). Special emphasis is placed on the utilization of assessment through the six critical elements that comprise the nursing process, as shown in Figure 13-1.

Alfaro-Lefevre (2014) denotes the importance of an assessment being viewed as a distinct process, with six individual phases that are interrelated and dynamic:

1. Collecting data
2. Identifying cues and making inferences
3. Validating (verifying) data
4. Clustering related data
5. Identifying patterns/testing first impressions
6. Reporting and recording data

Clinical reasoning serves as the bridge to connect assessment and the second stage of the nursing process, diagnosis. It is comprised of the actions of analyzing, synthesizing, reflecting, and drawing conclusions from the information gathered during the assessment. When case managers can engage in the keen act of clinical reasoning, the stage is set for their ability to pull together the critical puzzle pieces of a patient's situation, and then discourse with the care team in

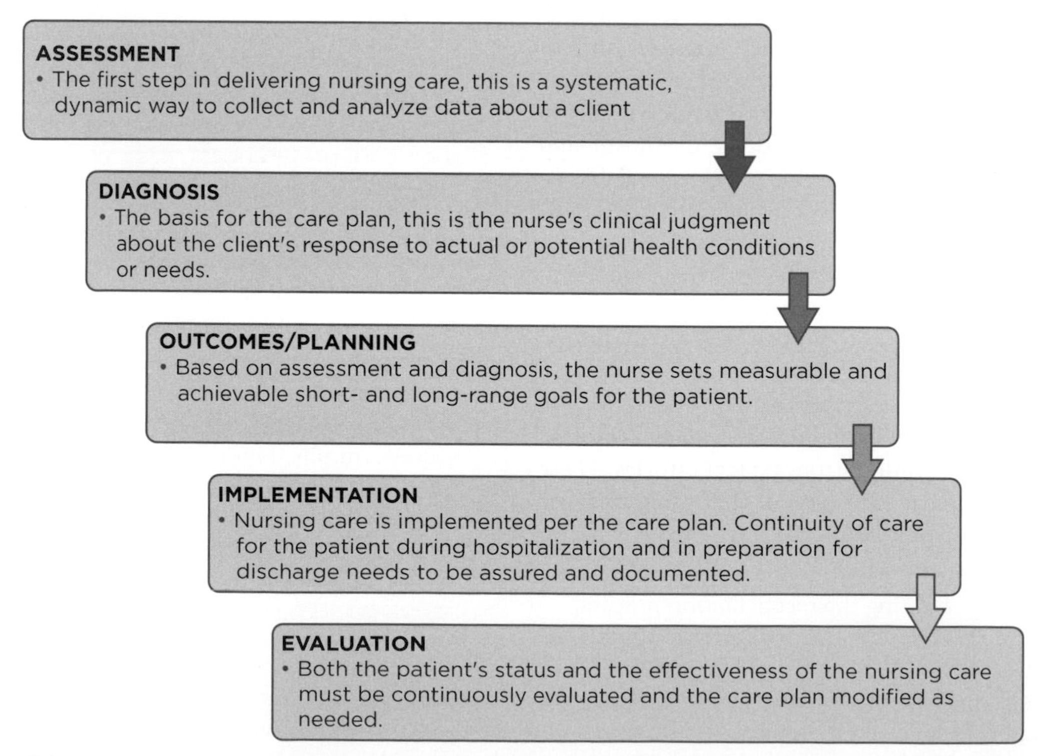

Figure 13-1. The nursing process. (Adapted from American Nurses Association. (2014). *The nursing process, nursing world.* Retrieved October 9, 2014, from http://www.nursingworld.org/EspeciallyForYou/What-is-Nursing/Tools-You-Need/Thenursingprocess.html)

order to properly diagnose the patient, and define the next steps of treatment planning.

SOCIAL WORK

Council on Social Work Education EPAS Competency: Assessment

The Council on Social Work Education (CSWE) views assessment as one of the mandated competencies of professional practice. As shown in Box 13-2, Educational Policy 2.1.10 includes the key principles that span a social worker's relationship with individuals, families, groups, organizations, and communities. The scope of practice behaviors aligned with the assessment competency, afford case managers a comprehensive means to gather the necessary information to formulate a patient's goals, objectives, and subsequent treatment plan.

Biopsychosocial Assessment: Human Behavior in the Social Environment

Biopsychosocial assessment is the foundation of the social work case management (NASW, 2013). Generations of professionals have grounded their professional practice by examining patients through use of this perspective, also known as **human behavior in the social environment** (HBSE). This **biopsychosocial framework** is based on principles from systems thinking which assume that each person is composed of molecules, cells, and organs; each person is also a member of a family, community, culture, nation, and world. As a result, professionals analyze patients within their exclusive environment through a framework including the biological (or biophysical), psychological, and social (including cultural and spiritual) dimensions (Ashford & LeCroy, 2013). Figure 13-2 presents each dimension with its included components.

The HBSE perspective takes the stance that:

1. The three dimensions are conceptualized as a system of biopsychosocial functioning.
2. This system involves multiple systems that are organized in a hierarchy of levels from the smallest (cellular) to the largest (social).
3. This ascending hierarchy of systems is in a constant state of interaction with other living systems and with other nonliving components of the systems' physical environment.

(Ashford & LeCroy, 2013)

Attention to how human behavior manifests across the developmental life stages, is an additional component of HBSE. This concept reflects Erik Erikson's stages of psychosocial development, where each stage contains specific life tasks that need to be achieved for optimal development (Ashford & LeCroy, 2013). These life stages extend from infancy through to early childhood, middle childhood, adolescence, young adulthood, middle adulthood, and then older adulthood. Each individual stage of development should be viewed as a psychosocial crisis of conflicting forcers such as the first stage of trust versus mistrust.

In each stage a person confronts and hopefully masters new challenges. Each stage builds upon the successful completion of earlier stages, though mastery of the tasks for each stage is not necessary to advance to subsequent stages. In fact, problems are most likely to appear in future stages because of the failure to address them fully in a prior stage. Erikson's model is displayed in Table 13-1.

Professionals learn to integrate evidence-based findings from number of distinct realms including behavioral, functional, cognitive, as well as genetic, health, and social sciences toward assessing social functioning and other concerns. There is promise for utilization of this approach by case management, for it sets a more global perspective of how each patient could be assessed. Practitioners must be clear about how they will systematically assess, measure, or describe the characteristics of their clients and their various life troubles in the changing social and physical contexts (Ashford & LeCroy, 2013). When viewed collectively, the distinct realms of the biophysical, psychological, and social dimensions provide a fundamental template to ensure a thorough and comprehensive evaluation of a vital patient clinical pathophysiology and psychopathology.

Saleeby and the Strengths' Perspective

Case managers strive to look on the side of patient strengths as opposed to weaknesses, or at least believe they do. However, there is a tendency to fall short for a variety of reasons (Saleeby, 2012). Primarily, Saleeby (2012) noted how practitioners easily focus on presenting problems and as a result fail to accurately assess the critical areas of strength that can

BOX 13-2 Council on Social Work Education Educational Policy: Assessment

EP 2.1.10 Engage, Assess, Intervene, and Evaluate with Individuals, Families, Groups, Organizations, and Communities

Professional practice involves the dynamic and interactive processes of engagement, assessment, intervention, and evaluation at multiple levels. Social workers have the knowledge and skills to practice with individuals, families, groups, organizations, and communities. Practice knowledge includes identifying, analyzing, and implementing evidence-based interventions designed to achieve client goals; using research and technological advances; evaluating program outcomes and practice effectiveness; developing, analyzing, advocating, and providing leadership for policies and services; and promoting social and economic justice.

Educational Policy 2.1.10 (B) Assessment Practice Behaviors

32. Collect, organize, and interpret client data;
33. Assess client strengths and limitations;
34. Develop mutually agreed-on intervention goals and objectives;
35. Select appropriate intervention strategies.

CSWE, 2008

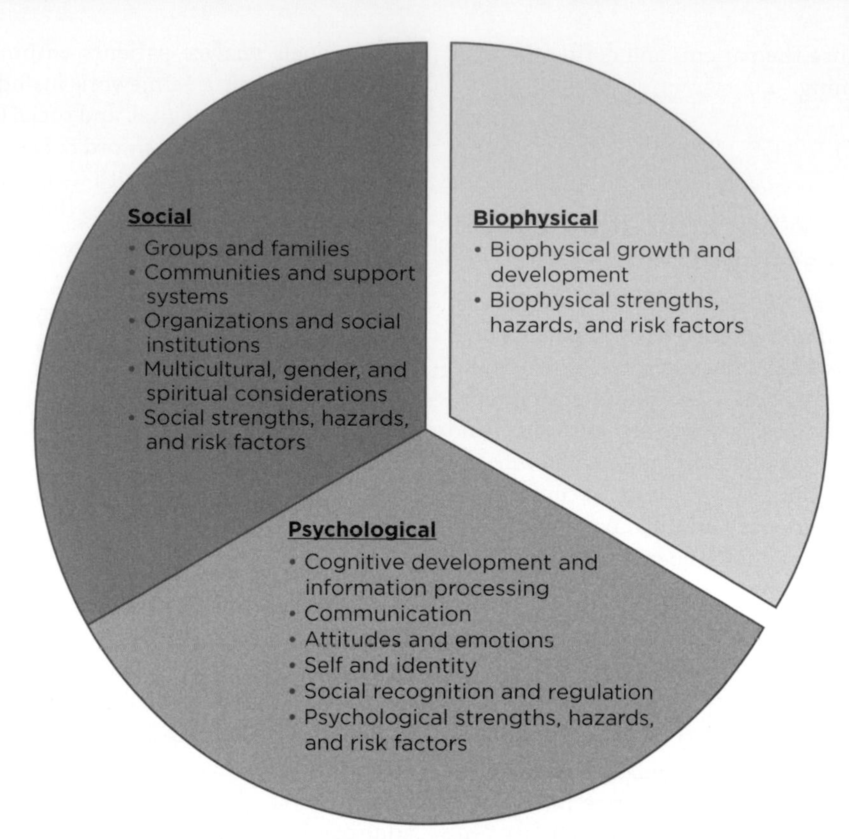

Figure 13-2. Multidimensional assessment approach. (Adapted from Ashford, J. B., & Lecroy, C. W. (2013). *Human behavior in the social environment: A multi-dimensional perspective* (5th ed.). Belmont, CA: Brooks/Cole, Cengage Learning.)

TABLE 13-1 Erikson's Stages of Psychosocial Development

Stage	Age	Existential Question
Trust vs. mistrust	Infancy	Who am I able to trust?
Autonomy vs. shame/doubt	Early childhood	How much control do I have?
Initiative vs. guilt	Play age	How much can I do, move, and act on my own?
Industry vs. inferiority	School age	How successful will I be in the world of people and things?
Identity vs. role confusion	Adolescence	Who am I? Who can I be?
Intimacy vs. isolation	Young adulthood	Am I capable of love and commitment?
Generativity vs. stagnation	Maturity	What type of legacy did I leave?
Integrity vs. despair	Old age	Did I live a fulfilling life or one of regret?

Adapted from Ashford, J. B., & Lecroy, C. W. (2013). Human behavior in the social environment: A multi-dimensional perspective (5th ed.). Belmont, CA: Brooks/Cole, Cengage Learning.

facilitate real change in a patient and their situation. This focus (or lack thereof) contributed to a somewhat biased view on the part of the professional toward the client—bias about the patient as a person and potentially that person's decision-making judgment.

Saleeby designed six principles of **strengths-based helping**, which appear in Figure 13-3. Assessing patients from this context fosters an approach that relies heavily on the ingenuity and creativity of both patients and the professionals who are involved. The strengths' perspective embraces the value of self-determination, for it honors the innate wisdom of the human spirit, the inherent capacity for transformation of even the most humbled and abused (Saleeby, 2012).

Saleeby was clear about the power of change that is derived when professionals are able to respect patient self-determination, often viewed as one of the toughest challenges that professionals face. Self-determination involves

1. Every individual, group, family, and community has strength
2. trauma and abuse, illness and struggle may be injurious, but they may also be sources of challenge and opporutnity
3. Assume that you do not know the upper limits of the capcity to grow and change, and take individual, group, and community aspirations seriously
4. We best serve clients by collaborating with them
5. Every environment is full of resources
6. Caring, caretaking and context

Figure 13-3. The six principles of strengths-based helping. (Adapted from Saleeby, D. (2012). *Strengths perspective in social work practice, advancing core competencies* (6th ed.). Pearson.)

maintaining healthy respect for patient decision-making processes, allowing that patient to engage on a treatment plan of his or her own definition. This plan may be in direct opposition to the one expertly designed and recommended by the case manager, physician, and treatment team. Self-determination is a foundational concept of professional practice and an integral value that exists across health care's many disciplines. Simply stated, it is about allowing the patient to be comfortable with where he or she is at as opposed to where the case manager or other health care professional wants that patient to be.

Consider you are case managing a male patient who has a history of chronic emergency department admissions for severe hypertension and obesity. That same patient refuses to make recommended changes to his diet, although he has begun a daily walk. While the walk is a start, you know that on its own it will be insufficient to yield optimal outcomes. You dialogue with the patient repeatedly, becoming frustrated about his adamant stance. Ultimately the patient refuses to dialogue with you at all.

Thus from Saleeby's perspective, change the situation by starting where the patient is, and support the small change in his behavior—the walk. You agree to disagree, which promotes respect for the patient's perspective. You are able to engage with the patient and engage with him on his level. Ultimately the patient agrees to make some subtle changes in his diet. Case managers deal with situations of this nature on a fairly regular basis.

Saleeby (2012) cued the industry that engaging in a focus on strengths does not mean one ignores the realities of those decisions individual patients will have to make regarding behaviors that may not be conducive to their wellness and the wellness and safety of others. In the era of managed care, the ultimate challenge is to balance attention to symptoms, problems, deficits, and medical necessity. In this way professional case managers can foster the development of individualized plans of care that demonstrate evidence that the intervention is making a difference (Saleeby, 2012).

CASE MANAGEMENT

Standards, Definitions, and Codes

The importance of assessment as a concept is delineated by its appearance at the front end of case management's definition: a collaborative process of assessment, planning, facilitation, care coordination, evaluation, and advocacy for options and services to meet an individual's and family's comprehensive health needs (CMSA, 2010).

Assessment serves a critical role to case managers. It provides a comprehensive means to gather the scope of information related to patient care (e.g., biopsychosocial intakes and history and physicals) as well as to assess other areas related to the patient care process. Consider the range of models and tools discussed in the other COLLABORATE competencies that involve assessment processes, such as those specific to critical thinking (chapter 8), outcomes-driven (chapter 9), and ethical decision making (chapter 18).

The industry's case management professional associations and certification bodies address assessment in many ways. One includes the concept with a unique definition (CCMC, 2009), while others have created a specific standard to address it (ACMA, 2013; CMSA, 2010; NASW, 2013). Several entities and experts view assessment as a continuous process that occurs across the full scope of case management practice (ACMA, 2013; CMSA, 2010; NASW, 2013; Powell & Tahan, 2008), while others see it as the process of collecting in-depth information about a person's situation and functioning to identify individual needs in order to develop a comprehensive case management plan that will address those needs (CCMC, 2009).

Recognizing that different types of licensed professionals are involved in the case management workforce, there is attention to assessing within the scope of one's professional licensure and a specific practice paradigm (NASW, 2013). The concept of a licensed professional being able to complete an independent assessment is addressed under the certification eligibility criteria for one organization and a standard

TABLE 13-2 Case Management Standards, Definitions, and Principles for Assessment

American Case Management Association: Standards of Practice and Scope of Services for Health Care Delivery System Case Management and Transitions of Care Professionals (ACMA, 2013)	**Commission for Case Management Certification: Code of Professional Conduct (CCMC, 2009, *2014)**	**Case Management Society of America: Standards of Practice (CMSA, 2010)**	**National Association of Social Workers: Social Work Standards of Practice for Case Management (NASW, 2013)**
Component: Case managers must have a defined case management assessment tool that expands the case managers' knowledge of the risks identified in the screening process and is complementary to the assessment of other clinical disciplines.	**Definition**: The process of collecting in-depth information about a person's situation and functioning to identify individual needs in order to develop a comprehensive case management plan that will address those needs. ***Eligibility:** Board-certified case managers must hold a current, active, and unrestricted licensure or certification in a health or human services discipline that within its scope of practice allows the professional to conduct an assessment independently.	**Standard B**—Client Assessment: The case manager should complete a health and psychosocial assessment, taking into account the cultural and linguistic needs of each client **Demonstrated by:** Documentation of client assessments using standardized tools, when appropriate. Documentation of resource utilization and cost management, current diagnosis(es); past and present course and services; prognosis; goals (short- and long-term); provider options; and available health care benefits. Evidence of use of relevant, comprehensive information and data required for client assessment from many sources **Standard I**—Qualifications: Case managers should maintain competence in their area(s) of practice by having one of the following: Current, active, and unrestricted licensure or certification in a health or human services discipline that allows the professional to conduct an assessment independently as permitted within the scope of practice of the discipline.	**Standard 5**—Assessment: The social work case manager shall engage clients— and, when appropriate, other members of client systems—in an ongoing information-gathering and decision-making process to help clients identify their goals, strengths, and challenges. **Interpretation:** Biopsychosocial assessment is the foundation of social work case management and is conducted in collaboration with the client. Assessment is an ongoing activity, not a one-time event. Reassessment serves both monitoring and evaluative functions, enabling the social worker and the client to determine whether services have been effective in helping achieve the client's goals.

for another (CCMC, 2014; CMSA, 2010). Table 13-2 provides a rendering of how assessment is viewed across the industry.

The Case Management Process

The case management process is much broader than the nursing process (Tahan, 2008). With case managers often identified as the leader of the care coordination effort, there is no doubt of the enormity of issues which can be identified throughout the care process.

The stage of assessment (and problem/opportunity identification) begins after the completion of the case selection and intake into case management, and occurs intermittently, as needed, throughout the case (Powell & Tahan, 2008). In this way, a case manager's assessment is understood to be a fluid representation of the patient within their illness course, disease process, and life circumstance. This also promotes a greater understanding and far more realistic representation of the patient. The assessment and problem identification step of the case management process is depicted in Box 13-3.

BOX 13-3 Assessment and Problem Identification—the Case Management Process

1. A thorough assessment must be done to determinate the needs of the patients, particularly as they relate to the treatment and transitional or discharge plans.
2. An inaccurate or poor assessment can lead to an unsafe discharge plan.
3. Sources of assessment data are:
   a. Patient and family/caregiver
   b. Family physician or primary care providers
   c. Office and hospital medical records, including old and current emergency department records
   d. Ancillary staff
   e. Employers
   f. Other external agencies such as extended/skilled care facilities and home care services
4. The assessment must be comprehensive and address the following:
   a. Patient's health and demographics
   b. Appropriateness for admission to the level of care or setting the patient is in
   c. Current medical status, including the chief complaint that prompted the patient to seek medical care
   d. Nutritional status
   e. Adjustment to illness
   f. Health education needs
   g. Medications assessment
   h. Financial assessment including health insurance, certification/authorization status
   i. Functional assessment and environmental factors
      I. Home environment assessment
      II. Activities of daily living and assessment (ADLs and IADLs)
   j. Psychosocial assessment, including family and support systems
   k. Cultural, spiritual, and religious characteristics
5. Based on the assessment data and findings, case managers are able to:
   a. Identify the actual and potential problems to be addressed
   b. Set the goals of treatment
   c. Identify the necessary interventions and strategies that will need to be incorporated in the case management plan of care in order to achieve the goals, and
   d. Determine the resources needed for addressing these problems.

From Tahan, H. A. (2008). The case management process. In S. K. Powell & H. A. Tahan. (Eds.), CMSA core curriculum for case management (2nd ed., pp. 177-189). Philadelphia, PA: Lippincott Williams & Wilkins.

INDUSTRY TOOLS AND TEMPLATES

As the continuum of health and behavioral health care has grown, a greater reliance and use of the care levels and programs have manifested. The transition of patients between so many levels of care has contributed the need for the industry to develop, implement, and use a variety of tools and templates to compile, track, and share patient information.

National Transitions of Care Coalition (NTOCC)

In 2006, CMSA and Sanofi-Aventis convened a group of concerned organizations and individuals to address the emerging problems associated with the movement of patients from one practice setting to another, transitions of care. During these transitions of care, poor communication and coordination between professionals, patients, and caregivers were leading to serious and even life-threatening situations. In addition, these inefficiencies wasted resources and frustrated health care consumers (NTOCC, 2014a).

Patient care during transitions can be rushed, with the responsibility for managing the sharing of information among multiple providers fragmented at best (NTOCC, 2014c). NTOCC has developed a number of tools and resources to enhance the communication process among the stakeholders involved with patients. Table 13-3 provides a listing of the tools available on the NTOCC website. Among those who benefit from these resources are patients themselves, their caregivers, health care professionals, and policy makers (NTOCC, 2014c).

NTOCC's is now viewed as an industry leader in developing tools, products, reports, and white papers on addressing the gaps that impact safety and quality of care for transitioning patients. Their board of directors works with over 30 professional associations, medical specialty societies, standards bodies, regulators, and government organizations. In addition,

TABLE 13-3 National Transitions of Care Coalitions Tools and Resources

Tool	Description
My Medicine List	Helps patients gather important information about their medications. Provides the ability to compile a list of medications to share with involved treating physicians, and health care providers. Awareness of the current medications on the list, and changes to the list, enhance patient understanding of the medications he or she should be taking.
Patient Bill of Rights During Transitions of Care	Patients and their families have the right to care transitions that are safe and well coordinated. This guide helps get the information and services needed by the patient, at every step along the way.
Taking Care of My Health	Developed as a guide for patients and their caregivers, this tool helps them be better prepared when they see a health care professional on what kind of information and questions they need to ask.
How to Implement and Evaluate a Plan	Is a guidebook that provides an implementation plan, with individual modules, plus an outline of the concepts, process, and "how to" on implementing and evaluating Transitions of Care plan. "Hospital to Home" and "Emergency Department to Home" are highlighted. Each transition point for the patient is treated as an "exchange" where communication and evaluation of the process may both occur.
Transitions of Care Checklist	This list provides a detailed description of an effective patient transfer between practice settings. Implementing this process can help to ensure patients and their critical medical information are transferred safely, timely, and efficiently.
Medication Reconciliation Essential Data Specifications	These consensus elements will help health care professionals collect, transmit, and receive critical medication information needed when patients move from one practice setting or level of care to another. The use of these elements in the reconciliation process required by the Joint Commission could help reduce medication errors.
Cultural Competence: Essential Ingredient for Successful Transitions of Care	This white paper provides information about culture and cultural competence, as well as strategies and resources to enhance professionals' capacity to deliver culturally competent services during transitions of care.

From National Transitions of Care Coalition. (2014b). Available tools and resources. Retrieved November 3, 2014, from http://www.ntocc.org/WhoWeServe/HealthCareProfessionals.aspx

they have over 450 organizations participating as associate members who review, test, and implement NTOCC's tools and resources across the industry. Another 3,200 individual professionals are enrolled as subscribers who receive news and materials on transitions of care improvement (NTOCC, 2014a).

The Society of Hospital Medicine: The 8Ps

The Society of Hospital Medicine (SHM) is a professional medical society which represents approximately one third of the 44,000 practicing hospitals in the United States (SHM, 2014a). Their focus is specific to the increasing generations of hospitalists, physicians who specialize in the practice of hospital medicine (SHM, 2014b).

With a strong focus on quality of care across care transitions, SHM developed Project BOOST: Better Outcomes by Optimizing Safe Transitions. The focus promotes the use of a robust series of tools and products, geared to provide the backbone of interventions that will improve the care transitions of hospitalized patients. Implementation is individualized based on a health organization's identified priorities and state regulations (SHM, 2014c). Led by national leaders across care transitions, hospital medicine, payers, and regulatory agencies, and sponsored in part by an unrestricted educational grant from the John A. Hartford Foundation, Project BOOST is geared to:

- Identify patients at high risk of rehospitalization and target specific interventions to mitigate potential adverse events
- Reduce 30-day readmission rates
- Improve patient satisfaction scores and H-CAHPS scores related to discharge
- Improve communication between providers and patients
- Optimize discharge processes

(SHM, 2014c)

One of the valuable tools is the Risk Assessment-8Ps, which provides a checklist of risks that should be identified and addressed to understand a patient's risk for adverse events after discharge. SHM contends that assessing patients through this lens, affords the interprofessional hospital team a proactive means to begin to mitigate those risks while the patient is hospitalized. A three-step process is used:

1. Identify: Screen the patient for specific risk factors known to be associated with adverse post-discharge events
2. Mitigate: Put in place risk-specific interventions that an organization believes will lessen the impact of the risk factor, and assure clarity about who on the care team is responsible for carrying out the intervention
3. Communicate: Recognizes that most interventions cannot eliminate the risk completely, and certainly not in the amount of time most hospitalizations offer. It is important to communicate the risk and intervention to the next providers of care, so efforts may continue to reduce the impact of risk on the patient's health.

(SHM, 2014d)

The eight risk factors which should be identified and addressed are shown in Figure 13-4.

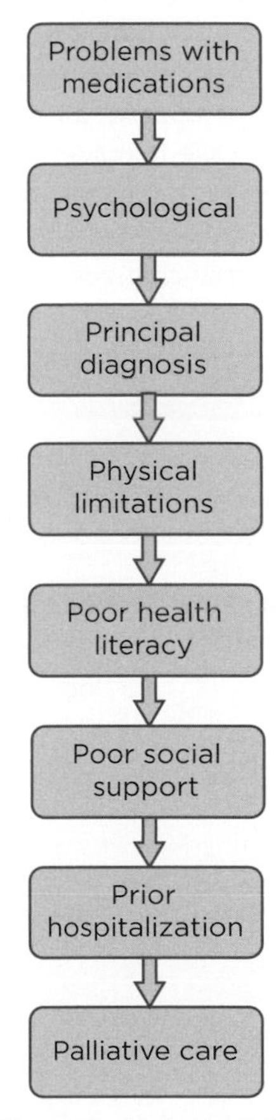

Figure 13-4. The 8P's tool. (Adapted from Society of Hospital Medicine. (2014d). *Project BOOST® Implementation Toolkit, Touch Points: Admission, During Hospitalization and Discharge*. Retrieved November 8, 2014, from http://www.hospitalmedicine.org/Web/Quality_Innovation/Implementation_Toolkits/Project_BOOST/Web/Quality_Innovation/Implementation_Toolkit/Boost/BOOST_Intervention/Tools/Risk_Assessment.aspx)

CONTEXT FOR COLLABORATE BIG-PICTURE ORIENTATION

The COLLABORATE approach starts from the premise that a case manager's intervention is only as solid as his or her preliminary assessment, whether that assessment involves a patient or an administrative or a programming decision. Case managers must be confident that they possess accurate, thorough, and comprehensive knowledge about each patient and issue(s) of concern along with the unique circumstances surrounding his or her health status. Each bit of information serves to further clarify the view that treatment providers have of the patient.

The big-picture orientation (BPO) competency does not portray assessment as a siloed or piecemeal view of the health care consumer. Instead, it acknowledges that big picture of a patient's real world, the one which the case managers must take into account when working to prioritize, coordinate, and ultimately collaborate with other professionals to define treatment plans that are individualized.

In an industry increasingly focused on assessments increasingly completed by checklists alone that can present as cookie cutter in nature, the BPO competency strategically engages in deliberate information gathering that aligns with critical thinking. Through this process, the finite and more obscure areas of focus can be merged just as individual pixels unite to form a rare, composite image. While the image will need to refocus as new pixels are added, ultimately a far clearer and complete representation of the patient's life is portrayed to those professionals able to view it.

From the COLLABORATE approach, knowing a patient's code status becomes as vital to the treatment team as the deciphering of applicable health care regulations and reimbursement. Prevailing family dynamics which may stress or support the care process is as critical to interpret as the patient's latest laboratory values. The religious and spiritual foundation becomes as important as the primary diagnosis prompting attention, as both will influence treatment. Health literacy issues must be explored and understood with the same diligence as a patient's history of suicidal ideation and manifesting psychopathology.

KEY ELEMENTS OF BIG-PICTURE ORIENTATION COMPETENCY

The key elements are the following:

- Bio-psycho-social-spiritual assessment
- Macro impact on micro interventions

Bio-Psycho-Social-Spiritual Assessment

Case managers possess expanded power when they are able to assess patients through the largest lens possible. From the COLLABORATE approach, it is understood that a case manager's licensure scope of practice may not allow for that professional to complete an actual assessment of a specialty area. For example, a nurse and a social worker may not have achieved proficiency with understanding a patient's laboratory work to fully grasp the dangerous implications of allowing that patient to be discharged with a grossly elevated white blood count. A nurse may be cautious about a patient who presents with suicidal ideation, though not skilled to complete a solid risk assessment of suicidality.

From the perspective of COLLABORATE, it is an asset for case managers to embrace a process that begins with a **Global Assessment Lens**. This broad perspective of assessment affords case managers the ability to be thorough and organized with respect to designing an appropriate treatment plan, one which reflects the clearest picture of each patient and their unique situation. When the distinct domains of the biophysical, psychological, sociological, and spiritual dimensions are viewed collectively, they provide a model to assure a thorough and comprehensive evaluation of vital patient clinical pathophysiology and psychopathology.

The Global Assessment Lens multidimensional assessment provides an all-inclusive template, which is shown in Table 13-4. This template is applicable and may be adjusted to any patient, in any practice setting across all transitions of care. The importance of a professional's scope of practice is accounted for, in that it is not expected case managers will complete a multidimensional assessment totally on their own. A key element from the lifelong learning competency has additional relevance in the BPO competency, acknowledgment that no single manager can and does know all.

Using the Global Assessment Lens will assure a case manager the ability to identify a greater scope of issues, but it is not expected the case manager will possess the clinical competency to assess each individual dimension on their own. Instead, the case manager should advocate for appropriate consultation by other professional disciplines as these specialty areas are identified for exploration. This also prompts a greater opportunity for the case manager to engage in interprofessional treatment team dialogues, a concept that will be further addressed in chapter 17, The Transdisciplinary Competency. The case scenario in Box 13-4 demonstrates how the Global Assessment Lens may be implemented.

In practice settings which involve a professionally diverse care coordination team, use of the Global Assessment Lens© offers a systematic and inclusive method to gather necessary and relevant patient data plus support system's pertinent information. Defined templates also support a case manager's ability to track outcomes, as addressed in chapter 9.

Macro Impact on Micro Interventions

Macro impact signifies those larger-scale policy implications and societal initiatives, all poised to greatly influence a case manager's micro or direct interventions. This involves any aspect of a case manager's role and associated functions, from quality of and access to appropriate patient care to assessing and intervening with patients across state lines to the lack of ability to obtain authorization for behavioral health care despite the presence of a benefit for it. How effective can any case manager be in planning and defining appropriate care options for patients without knowledge of relevant reimbursement for those options? What of the patient who is unable to be approved for inpatient psychiatric admission because the case manager lacks awareness of the current *DSM-5* treatment codes that went into effect?

It behooves case managers to stay aware of the current policy initiatives, industry changes, and relevant legislation

TABLE 13-4 Global Assessment Lens

Biophysical	Psychological	Sociological	Spiritual
Clinical acuity	Psychopathology	Family and support system —Dynamics among involved parties and systems —Cultural influences, values, beliefs, and mores	Religion
Pathophysiology	Cognition and mentation —Competence	Geographic and/or regional influences	Values, beliefs, and mores
Treatment protocols	Communication patterns —Listening skills and/or translation needs —Health literacy	Generational factors	Individual philosophical grounding
Treatment plan variances	Disability accommodation	Socioeconomic factors	
Disability accommodation	Developmental stages	Occupational system —Insurance —Entitlement eligibility	
Key treatment history and concerns	Psychosocial stressors	Government system —Legislation —Policies and procedures	
	Risk of suicidal/homicidal ideation and/or intent		

Adapted from Treiger, T and Fink-Samnick, E. (2013) COLLABORATE©: A Universal Competency-Based Paradigm for Professional Case Management, Part II: Competency Clarification, Professional Case Management, 18(5).

BOX 13-4 Global Assessment Lens Case Scenario

Marco is a 60-year-old man recently diagnosed with emphysema. He resides with his spouse, Luz and five of their six children, ages 15 to 28, in a private home. The couple's oldest son, Miguel, and his family live next door. Marco and Luz immigrated to the United States 30 years ago and were both granted citizenship last year. Their family mantra is, "work hard and success will be your reward." They own a successful restaurant in the community where all family members work. In addition, Marco works closely with his church to provide jobs to new immigrants from his home country of Chile.

Luz worries about her husband's strong work ethic, and his often 18-hour work days. However, she is proud of her husband, their community standing, and accomplishments. To family and community members, Marco is known as "the mayor."

One afternoon Miguel arrives at the restaurant and finds his father slumped in a chair. Unable to convince his father to contact his doctor, Miguel calls the paramedics who bring Marco to the hospital. Marco's oxygen saturation is 75% and his breathing shallow. A deeply religious man, Marco turns to Miguel and says, "Whether I live or die is decided by our Holy Father and not the doctors."

Dr. Fein is the emergency department (ED) hospitalist on call. Marco is resistant and adamantly refuses to let Dr. Fein examine him. "Who does this Lady Doctor think she is, telling me what to do? Not even my Luz would dare to do this." Marco says to his son.

Kara, the ED case manager, is finishing with another patient when Dr. Fein approaches her. "Kara, I need your big-picture orientation. My patient must be admitted for observation. Help me get through to him."

Kara meets with Miguel first, who introduces her to Marco. After 10 minutes Kara identifies the key issues using the Global Assessment Lens:

- **Biophysical**: Kara learns Marco sees Dr. Rodriquez in the community, a male physician who Marco trusts. She obtains permission from Marco for Dr. Fein to contact Dr. Rodriguez directly. Though not on staff at the hospital, Dr. Rodriguez agrees to speak with Marco on the phone about his current medical status, consequences of him leaving the hospital and his need for treatment.
- **Psychological**: Kara assesses that health literacy is a major factor for Marco. With emphysema a new diagnosis for Marco, Kara provides him information in his native language. In addition through the translation line at the hospital, Kara engages someone to answer Marco's questions about prognosis, and the importance of medication and treatment adherence.

Kara also finds out Marco is too proud to let Luz know his diagnosis, fearing it will make him look weak. Dr. Rodriguez is helpful in speaking with Marco on how to engage Luz in the treatment process.

- **Sociological:** Kara's discussion with Marco and Miguel validates the need for Dr. Fein to be respectful of Marco's concerns around trusting a new physician, who is also a female. Dr. Rodriguez assures Marco of Dr. Fein's competence.
- **Spiritual:** Since Dr. Rodriguez attends the same church as Marco, he is able to contact their priest, Father Juan, to visit Marco in the ED. Kara has worked with Father Juan on other patients and is confident he will address, support, and comfort Marco.

Marco agrees to be admitted for observation. Within 10 hours he is stable to return home. Kara facilitates his outpatient follow-up directly with Dr. Rodriguez. A grateful Luz meets Marco at the hospital to bring him home.

at the macro level. All of these actions have the potential to impact a case manager's individual practice, and most certainly his or her patient population. The case scenario in Box 13-5, demonstrates how a case management department engage in the COLLABORATE approach. Using organized and concerted efforts the case managers are able to assure their awareness of, education about, and attention to the macro impact on their distinct micro interventions.

BOX 13-5 Macro Impact Influences Micro Interventions: Case Scenario

The case managers for a Medicare advantage program engage in a series of actions to ensure education about new regulations (macro interventions) to directly impact their (micro) interventions with subscribers.

- All case managers set the calendar on their electronic tablets to alert them to complete a quarterly review of the home pages of their professional licensure boards. This keeps the workforce informed of new and relevant regulations.
- Upon email receipt of the digital edition of their professional organization magazine, each case manager reviews and bookmarks articles of potential interest to share with colleagues. Specific topics of interest are identified and updated quarterly (e.g., relevant legislation, new regulations for the Center for Medicare and Medicaid Services, and innovative care coordination models). The group distributes a list of the articles among themselves.
- Case managers each join one professional social media group focusing on issues impacting case management and the patient population (e.g., managing new disease-specific

(continued)

BOX 13-5 Macro Impact Influences Micro Interventions: Case Scenario (*Continued*)

populations, care coordination reimbursement, end-of-life and palliative care, and applicable resources).

- A peer-mentoring group is formed for case managers to engage in monthly. One staff member is chosen to lead each group, with a structured agenda defined in advance by all involved. Topics focus on new organizational policies in the workplace to impact their individual practice, and industry changes (i.e., new states to pass the Nurse Licensure Compact and start of a title protection initiative for case managers). This forum also provides the case managers an opportunity to discuss journal articles of mutual interest and advance their practice knowledge.

IMPLICATIONS FOR PRACTICE

Technology and Template Overreliance

Much has been written about the danger of a growing overreliance on assessment tools, particularly those appearing due to technology. Yet, while electronic health records health information technology plays an important role to cue the memory of the involved clinical professional of what to assess, accountability is still on that professional to learn the principles needed to collect, prioritize, and think about the data which is gathered (Alfaro-LeFevre, 2014).

There is industry concern of how vague, imprecise, tough to use, and impractical these electronic assessment tools can be (Bowman, 2013; KevinMD.com, 2014). The new generation of digitalized assessment tools has come with a price. There has been a steady stream of reports on EHR system design and improper use, which cause EHR-related errors that jeopardize the integrity of the information in the EHR. These factors contribute to errors that endanger patient safety or decrease the quality of care. These unintended consequences also may increase fraud and abuse and can have serious legal implications (Bowman, 2013).

"Medical errors happen every day. Few make the headlines, but when they do, almost everyone who chimes in to comment offers the same type of solution for avoiding them. Three of the most common are guidelines, decision support and checklists." (KevinMD.com, 2014)

Bowman (2013) further discusses how risks to documentation integrity result from the incorrect use of copy and paste functionality, including:

- Inaccurate or outdated information
- Redundant information, which causes the inability to identify the current information
- Inability to identify the author or intent of documentation
- Inability to identify when the documentation was first created
- Propagation of false information
- Internally inconsistent progress notes, and
- Unnecessarily lengthy progress notes

The ease with how easily patient documentation can be copied and pasted, leads to the concern about who is responsible for the completion of the patient assessment included within that documentation. As the use of checklists providing specific intervention activities expands, so does the risk of overlooking vital information that may not be collected by these efficiency-focused tools. These actions contribute to the defining, advanced intellectual and analytical skills that are the hallmark of an independent practitioner (Treiger & Fink-Samnick, 2014). The argument for the need of clinical professionals to balance keen assessment proficiency with new technologies, is noted by Bond (2010),

> In this age of 'big bad medicine,' which includes the latest and greatest in diagnostic machines, tests, and evaluations by multiple specialists, professionals are losing the ability to "see the forest for the trees" so to speak. (All) need to remember the basics of good medicine begin with proper, thorough and good assessment skills...Remember, if you don't assess properly, you can't treat properly.

Assessments are as much about identifying barriers and impediments to care for the patient, as they are about providing valuable information about the patient's illness history and course. Without the use of critical thinking, the ability to adeptly view such barriers in the context of patient safety and quality is further compromised (Treiger & Fink-Samnick, 2014). Case management becomes easily devalued from an advanced practice completed by expertly educated, trained, and licensed and certified health care professionals to one completed by nonclinical and underlicensed workers, those who lack the education and training that ground the critical thinking competency.

Although there is a definite role for nonclinical administrative support staff in the delivery of high-quality patient care, these valued members of the care team can never take the place of a professional case manager. The use of nonclinical staff, as well as licensed individuals without appropriate education or training, to perform case management assessments is already taking place. The impact that this approach to staffing has on quality of care or value for service delivered has yet to be clearly and consistently demonstrated (Treiger, 2011). It is nonetheless a huge concern in the scope of the assessment quandary as to who is most competently prepared to complete the requisite assessments on populations.

TRANSITION FROM TRADITIONAL HEALTH CARE ROLES TO CASE MANAGER

Many professionals enter case management after other traditional roles in the health care workforce, such as bedside or utilization nurses, therapists or direct practice social workers for hospitals or other community agencies. It is a common misperception that they adjust easily to the new job and functions because of their prior experience, particularly with patient assessment. Unfortunately, case management is a different animal of and unto itself. As nurses transition into case management, they face challenges their previous positions may not have prepared them for, such as agency politics, ethical dilemmas, and a broader sensitivity to health care issues (Henning & Cohen, 2008).

Schmitt (2006) identified how nurses' expectations about the role of case manager were closely tied to the promise it held for providing relief from the undesirable conditions of the roles they were exiting. These expectations included:

1. More flexible work schedule,
2. Less physically taxing job responsibilities,
3. Manageable workloads,
4. Opportunities to utilize nursing knowledge,
5. Better compensation, and
6. Job security.

In fact, nurses experienced feelings of inadequacy, if not competence, from adjusting to the role transition. This role strain centered around time-task orientation, interactions and relationships, business culture and objectives, and professional identity and self-image (Schmitt, 2006). Further explanation of these four areas is shown in Table 13-5.

Despite these expectations, nurses experienced substantial role ambiguity and role conflict in transitioning to the case manager role. This was primarily because of inadequate role definition, unexpected ethical challenges, and lack of prior insight into the case manager role (Smith, 2011).

EVOLVING SHIFTS IN DEMOGRAPHICS: HOW BIG WILL THE BPO BECOME?

Case managers are practicing in a world of continuous shifts in patient demographics, population-based health priorities along with fluid societal trends. As a result, there will always be new areas of attention to consider, credence to the mantra that the only constant is change. To this end, a challenge to the industry presents in considering how big will the BPO become?

It is evident that today's priority will be replaced by other more pressing needs. Infectious disease is an area of paramount concern. As this book is being published, Ebola is ravaging international populations. Immediate attention to treatment and prevention efforts is captivating health professionals and those who they treat, with new information developing daily.

The past several decades have witnessed a dramatic transformation in the response to intimate partner violence (Campbell et al., 2009). There are more than three to four million women in the United States abused annually, with 1,500 to 1,600) killed by their abusers. The challenge for those who encounter abused individuals is to identify those with the highest danger (Danger Assessment, 2014). Case managers can easily find themselves on the front line of these complex and often emotionally charged situations. As licensed health care professionals, case managers have an affirmative duty to report suspected acts of domestic violence,

TABLE 13-5 Transition From Bedside Nurse to Case Manager—Sources of Role Strain

Role Strain	Marked by
Time-task orientation	• Challenges from managing case over an extended period of time as opposed to completing care required by assigned patients on an 8-12 hour shift • Changes in the scope of how task accomplishment is defined between the two roles • Adjustment to the autonomy of the CM role and designing of own system to manage entire workload (e.g., calls to and appointments with clients, providers of care, completing time-sensitive file documentation). This is in contrast to role of the bedside nurse, which focused on immediate health needs of patients.
Interventions and relationships	• New dimensions of relationships with above populations led to unanticipated dynamics in those interactions (e.g., dealing with clients who lie to access benefits as opposed to address patient medical need, increased caution and resistance to engage by clients when in CM role. • New types of relationships with MCO-CM's adjustors mandate different communication skills from prior role. • Need to develop new strategies to engage and establish rapport with patients, physicians, nonmedical colleagues (team members), payer claims adjustors, and potentially managed care case managers (MCO-CMs)
Business culture and objectives	• Acclimating to the new work objectives, support structures, and tools of the CM role. • Challenge in the cost containment focus • Tension between prior role as patient advocate and CM role of impacting financial bottom line.
Professional identity and self-image	• Interpretation of CM role as less important and/or significant than nursing role • Requires a different skill set than prior role of bedside nurse • Role of CM in conflict with unbiased and apolitical image held in role as bedside nurse

CM, case manager; MCO, managed care organization

Adapted from Schmitt, N. (2006). Role Transition From Caregiver to Case Manager-Part II, Lippincott's Case Management, 11(1), 37-46.

also referred to as intimate partner violence, elder abuse, and child abuse (Muller, 2014).

The publication of *DSM-5* last year brought dramatic changes to the mental health community in terms of what disorders are included, how they are classified, as well as billing and coding issues, to name a few challenges. For example, Asperger syndrome is no longer included but a new autism spectrum is now included. Yet, not everyone previously diagnosed with Asperger syndrome would necessarily be diagnosed on the autism spectrum. If this presents as confusing to you, you are not alone.

As readily as the *DSM-5* is recognized as the universal authority for psychiatric diagnosis (American Psychiatric Association, 2013), a number of prestigious national and international entities have not accepted it for implementation, including the National Institutes of Mental Health, the world's largest funding agency for research into mental health (Lane, 2013). There continues to be dissension across the mental health industry about acceptance and implementation of the *DSM-5*.

Other important treatment concerns are reflected through a current review of health care news across the news and include opioid and pain management, the health care industry's continued attention to health literacy, cultural competence for professionals with new and emerging populations, and mental health parity with respect to the equitable reimbursement of behavioral health treatment.

There has been discussion throughout this book of new regulations and legislation, ever-shifting models of reimbursement, and a list of innovative care delivery models to account for. The verdict is out on how the Patient Protection and Affordable Care Act will actually play out. Will health care reform continue to reform? How will it ultimately reimburse providers for care? What new programming will be mandated and revised from prior versions of legislation?

A whole host of critical issues of concern will continue to manifest for case managers as they struggle to incorporate new information about these populations and potentially new means of assessment to their proverbial tool box. At what point does the scope of patient assessment become too large to account for? The correct answer may very likely be, never. Amid shifting world demographics there will always be new factors which need to be accounted for in the context of the health, safety, and well-being of populations. At the core of both patient centeredness and cultural competence is the importance of seeing the patient as a unique person (Campinha-Bacote, 2011).

SUMMARY

Case managers must be on a more uniform page of what to include and focus on during their assessment. They must be better able to dialogue, discuss, consider, and interact with colleagues to appropriately assess and identify key areas of needs for patients. Accepting and acknowledging the BPO competency is a substantial first step in accomplishing this goal.

By virtue of the rich interprofessional workforce that comprises case management, there is an opportunity to develop a thorough assessment lens by which to view the patient from. The BPO competency accomplished this by promoting a greater level of proficiency for case managers, with whatever societal factors and industry trends manifest. By doing so, case managers will possess an enhanced ability to see the biggest picture of professional practice from the most expansive and clearest lens.

References

Alfaro-Lefevre. (2014). *Applying Nursing Process: The Foundation for Clinical Reasoning* (8th ed.). Philadelphia, PA: Lippincott Williams & Wilkins.

American Case Management Association. (2013). *Standards of practice and scope of services for health care delivery system case management and transitions of care professionals.* Little Rock, AK: Author.

American Nurses Association. (2010). *Nursing, scopes and standards of practice* (2nd ed.). Retrieved from Nursebooks.org

American Nurses Association. (2014). *The nursing process, nursing world.* Retrieved October 9, 2014, from http://www.nursingworld.org/EspeciallyForYou/What-is-Nursing/Tools-You-Need/Thenursingprocess.html

American Psychiatric Association. (2013). *Diagnostic and statistical manual of mental disorders* (5th ed.). Washington, DC: Author.

American Psychiatric Association. (2014). *DSM 5 homepage.* Retrieved November 9, 2014, from http://www.dsm5.org/Pages/Default.aspx

Ashford, J. B., & Lecroy, C. W. (2013). *Human behavior in the social environment: A multi-dimensional perspective* (5th ed.). Belmont, CA: Brooks/Cole, Cengage Learning.

Bond, P. (2010). On the importance of good assessment skills. *Emergency Nursing Today.* Retrieved November 6, 2014, from http://emergencynursingtoday.com/?p=1784

Bowman, S. (2013). *Impact of Electronic Health Record Systems on Information Integrity.* Retrieved October 10, 2013, from http://perspectives.ahima.org/impact-of-electronic-health-record-systems-on-information-integrity-quality-and-safety-implications/#.UlUjnBYeZUS.

Campbell, J. C., Webster, D. W., & Glass, N. (2009). The danger assessment-validation of a lethality risk assessment instrument for intimate partner femicide. *Journal of Interpersonal Violence, 24*(4), 653–674.

Campinha-Bacote, J. (2011). Delivering patient-centered care in the midst of a cultural conflict: The role of cultural competence. *OJIN: The Online Journal of Issues in Nursing, 16*(2), Manuscript 5.

Case Management Society of America. (2010). *CMSA standards of practice for case management* (Rev.). Retrieved April 25, 2013, from http://www.cmsa.org/portals/0/pdf/memberonly/StandardsOfPractice.pdf

Center for Disease Control and Prevention. (2014). *Mental illness.* Retrieved November 9, 2014, from http://www.cdc.gov/mentalhealth/basics/mental-illness.htm

Commission for Case Manager Certification. (2009). *Code of professional conduct for case managers.* Retrieved October 31, 2014, from http://ccmcertification.org/ content/ccm-exam-portal/code-professional-conductcase-managers

Commission for Case Manager Certification. (2014). *Case managers.* Retrieved November 8, 2014, from http://ccmcertification.org/case-managers

Council on Social Work Education. (2008). *Education policy and accreditation standards.* October 31, 2014, from http://www.cswe.org/Accreditation/EPASImplementation.aspx

Danger Assessment. (2014). *What is the danger assessment?* Retrieved November 9, 2014, from http://www.dangerassessment.org/about.aspx

Dorland Medical Dictionary. (2007). Clinical, Dorland's medical dictionary for health consumers. Philidelphia, PA: Saunders, Elsevier.

Henning, S., & Cohen, E. (2008). The competency continuum: Expanding the case manager's skill set and competencies. *Professional Case Management, 13*(3), 127–148.

Hughes, R. G. (Ed.). (2008). *Patient safety and quality: An evidence-based handbook for nurses*. Rockville, MD: Agency for Healthcare Research and Quality.

Institutes of Medicine. (1999). *To err is human: Building a safer healthcare system*. Washington, DC: The National Academies Press.

Institutes of Medicine. (2001). *Crossing the quality chasm: A new health system for the 21st century*. Washington, DC: The National Academies Press.

Institutes of Medicine. (2003). *Health professions education: A bridge to quality (quality chasm series)*. Washington, DC: The National Academies Press.

Institutes of Medicine. (2011). *Clinical practice guidelines we can trust: Practice brief*. Washington, DC: The National Academies Press.

KevinMD.com. (2014). When checklists become chokelists. Retrieved November 3, 2014, from http://www.kevinmd.com/blog/2014/11/checklists-become-chokelists.html

Lane, C. (2013). NIMH withdraws support for DSM 5. *Psychology Today*. Retrieved November 8, 2014, from http://www.psychologytoday.com/blog/side effectside effects/201305/the-nimh-withdraws-support-dsm-5

Merriam-Webster'S online dictoinary. (2014a). Assessment.. Retrieved November 8, 2014, from http://www.merriam-webster.com/dictionary/assessment

Merriam-Webster'S online dictoinary. (2014b). Pathophysiology. Retrieved November 8, 2014, from http://www.merriam-webster.com/dictionary/pathophysiology

Merriam-Webster'S online dictoinary. (2014c). Psychopathology. *Psychopathology*. Retrieved November 8, 2014, from http://www.merriam-webster.com/dictionary/psychopathology

Muller, L. (2014). A case management briefing on domestic violence, legal and regulatory department. *Professional Case Management, 19*(5), 237–240.

National Association of Social Workers. (2013). *NASW Standards for Social Work case management*, Washington, DC: Author.

National Transitions of Care Coalition. (2014a). *About us*. Retrieved November 3, 2014, from http://www.ntocc.org/AboutUs.aspx

National Transitions of Care Coalition. (2014b). *Available tools and resources*. Retrieved November 3, 2014, from http://www.ntocc.org/WhoWeServe/HealthCareProfessionals.aspx

National Transitions of Care Coalition. (2014c). *Who we serve*. Retrieved November 3, 2014, from http://www.ntocc.org/WhoWeServe.aspx

Newell, M. (1996). *Using nursing case management to improve health outcomes*. Gaithersburg, MD: Aspen Publishing.

Pennsylvania Patient Safety Advisory. (2008). Medication errors associated with documented allergies. *Pennsylvania Patient Safety Advisory, 5*(3), 75–80.

Powell, S. K., & Tahan, H. A. (2008). *Case management society of America (CMSA) core curriculum for case management* (2nd ed.). Philadelphia, PA: Lippincott Williams & Wilkins.

Psychology Dictionary. (2014). Psychosocial stressors. Retrieved November 9, 2014, from http://psychologydictionary.org/psychosocial-stressor/

Saleeby, D. (2012). *Strengths perspective in social work practice, advancing core competencies* (6th ed.). Upper Saddle River, NJ: Pearson.

Sandler, E. (2009). Behavioral health versus mental health, does what we call it influence how people think about it? *Psychology Today*. Retrieved November, 9 2014, from http://www.psychologytoday.com/blog/promoting-hope-preventing-suicide/200910/behavioral-health-versus-mental-health

Schmitt, N. (2006). Role Transition From Caregiver to Case Manager-Part II, *Lippincott's Case Management, 11*(1), 37-46.

Smith, A. C. (2011). Role Ambiguity and Role Conflict in Nurse Case Managers: An Integrative Review, *Professional Case Management, 16*(4), 182-196.

Society of Hospital Medicine. (2014a). *About, society of hospital medicine website*. Retrieved November 8 2014, from http://www.hospitalmedicine.org/Web/About_SHM/About_SHM/About_SHM_Landing_Page.aspx?hkey=fea27f96-d2dc-419b-b0ea-48d9e7ddb09c

Society of Hospital Medicine. (2014b). *Definition of a hospitalist, society of hospital medicine website*. Retrieved November 8, 2014, from http://www.hospitalmedicine.org/Web/About_SHM/Hospitalist_Definition/About_SHM/Industry/Hospital_Medicine_Hospital_Definition.aspx?hkey=fb083d78-95b8-4539-9c5b-58d4424877aa

Society of Hospital Medicine. (2014c). *The BOOST TOOLS®, Project BOOST® Implementation Toolkit* [Society of Hospital Medicine Website]. Retrieved November 8, 2014, from http://www.hospitalmedicine.org/Web/Quality_Innovation/Implementation_Toolkits/Project_BOOST/Web/Quality___Innovation/Implementation_Toolkit/Boost/BOOST_Intervention/BOOST_Tools.aspx

Society of Hospital Medicine. (2014d). *Project BOOST® Implementation Toolkit, Touch Points: Admission, During Hospitalization and Discharge*. Retrieved November 8, 2014, from http://www.hospitalmedicine.org/Web/Quality_Innovation/Implementation_Toolkits/Project_BOOST/Web/Quality___Innovation/Implementation_Toolkit/Boost/BOOST_Intervention/Tools/Risk_Assessment.aspx

Tahan, H. A. (2008). The case management process. In S. K. Powell & H. A. Tahan. (Eds.), *CMSA core curriculum for case management* (2nd ed., pp. 177-189). Philadelphia, PA: Lippincott Williams & Wilkins.

Treiger T. (2011). Case management: Prospects in definition, education, and settings of practice. *The Remington Report, 19*(1), 46–48.

Treiger, T., & Fink-Samnick, E. (2014). COLLABORATE©: A universal, competency-based paradigm for professional case management practice, Part 3. *Professional case management, 19*(1), 4–15.

Watson, D. (2006). The impact of accurate patient assessment on quality of care. *Nursing Times.Net. 102*(6), 34. Retrieved October 8, 2014, from http://www.nursingtimes.net/home/specialisms/nutrition/the-impact-of-accurate-patient-assessment-on-quality-of-care/203387.article

World Health Organization. (2014). *Mental health*. Retrieved November 8, 2014, from http://www.who.int/topics/mental_health/en/

Yildirim, B., & Özkahraman, S. (2011). Critical thinking in the nursing process and education. *International Journal of Humanities and Social Science, 1*(13), 257–262.

14 ORGANIZED

OBJECTIVES

After studying this chapter, you will be able to:

1. Define identified terminology.
2. Distinguish efficiency from effectiveness of practice.
3. Describe a model which contributes to organized case management practice.
4. Identify technology impacts on case management efficiency.
5. Describe the implications of efficiency and effectiveness on case management practice.
6. Describe research comparing the effectiveness of case management intervention.

KEY TERMS

Case Management Roles and Functions Study
Collective accountability
Comparative effectiveness
Covey's Maturity Continuum
Effective
Efficient
Habit
High-functioning work team
Interdisciplinary health care team
Interprofessional education
Organized
TeamSTEPPS

Formed in June 1998 at the Institutes of Medicine (IOM), the Quality of Health Care in America Committee developed a blueprint for quality improvement in the delivery of health care. *To Err Is Human: Building a Safer Heath System* set the stage for addressing systemic shortcomings. In its subsequent report, *Crossing the Quality Chasm: A New Health System for the 21st Century*, the committee described the state of health care delivery, citing seven aims for care in the 21st century as safe, **effective**, patient-centered, timely, **efficient**, and equitable (IOM, 2001). The IOM also outlined four contributors of health care quality problems as the growing complexity of science and technology, the increase in chronic conditions, a poorly organized delivery system, and constraints on exploiting the revolution in information technology. These factors continue to apply in today's health care continuum; having an organized approach to case management (CM) practice is essential for progress toward health care delivery excellence. To the point of practice competency, it is essential to agree with the premise that where an individual is concerned, key elements to being organized include a combination of efficiency and effectiveness. This chapter focuses on the points of impact where the organized practice contributes to defining CM competence.

DEFINITION

Key elements important to the organized competency include efficiency and effectiveness. These concepts are discussed later in the chapter. So, what does it mean to be organized? What contributes to building organizational skills? Applying context by defining common terminology enhances understanding of the competency.

HABIT

Habit is a usual way of behaving or something a person does often in a regular or repeated manner (Merriam-Webster.com., 2014a). Habit is an important preceding concept to organization. Habit is the intersection (and internalization) of knowledge, skill, and desire (Covey, 1989). Covey's seven habits which provide strategies for building personal effectiveness include:

1. Be proactive
2. Begin with the end in mind
3. Put first things first
4. Think win/win
5. Seek first to understand, then to be understood
6. Synergize
7. Sharpen the saw

In Covey's approach, knowledge is a theoretical paradigm (the what-to-do and the why). Skill includes the process mechanics (the how-to-do). Desire is the motivation supporting the action (the want-to-do). In order to make something a habit, all three of these ingredients must be present.

Consider this triad applied to CM practice in Box 14-1. These two depictions of approaching CM assessment demonstrate a significant quality variance. The missing element in Nonny's approach is a desire for assessment practice excellence. Nonny simply looks at the assessment as a task to be completed. The delta between Suzie's and Nonny's approaches to assessment is the habit of excellence, the desire from within to practice CM excellence. This transforms the triad to a quadrant approach, as depicted in Figure 14-1, as the Case Management Practice sQuad. The driver for pursuit of excellence emanates from within the individual who is committed to professional practice, not one who simply goes through the motions of a task because it is a requirement of her or his job.

COLLECTIVE ACCOUNTABILITY

Collective accountability is a concept in which every individual within a defined group (e.g., work team, department) is responsible for the decisions and actions taken by the group. Everyone has a defined role in the group and accepts

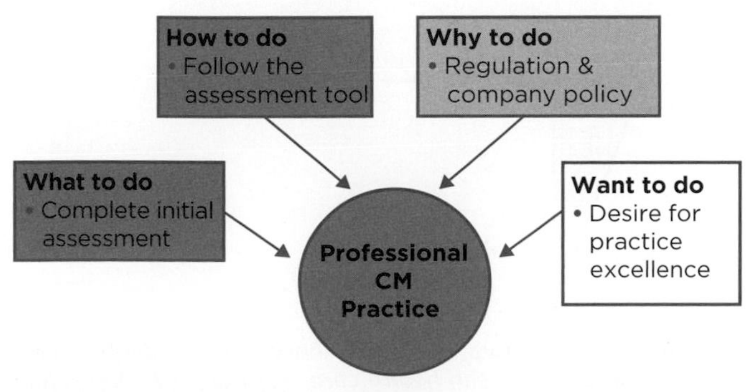

Figure 14-1. The CM Practice sQuad

BOX 14-1 Covey's Triad Applied to Case Management

When conducting a comprehensive assessment, case manager usually relies on a questionnaire to cover all pertinent areas of inquiry. A tremendous amount of information exchanges between the client and the case manager. The following scenario presents two very different approaches to CM assessment.

Sam Smith is a 72-year-old gentleman with a history of emphysema, type 2 diabetes mellitus, and coronary artery disease. It has been 10 years since he underwent two-vessel coronary artery bypass surgery and he recently experienced the onset of peripheral vascular disease.

Suzie is a seasoned case manager with 15 years of complex medical CM experience. She works for an insurance company. In the course of assessment, Suzie interviews Mr. Smith, his partner Joe, his primary care provider, office nurses in endocrine and cardiology, his adult daughter, and his minister. Suzie also reviews his claims history, pharmacy history, and recent laboratory results. She compiles an opportunities list throughout the completion of her initial assessment. She shares her findings with Mr. Smith to confirm details of her investigation. Together, they identify priorities and secondary opportunities on which to work and assemble the CM plan.

Nonny is also a seasoned case manager with 15 years of experience in managed care, currently working at an acute rehabilitation hospital. She relies on Mr. Smith, transfer documentation from the acute hospital, and previous rehabilitation admission medical records as the sources of information in conducting her initial assessment. She completes the assessment tool and identifies transition needs for his eventual discharge to home. She does not discuss priorities with Mr. Smith and files the admission assessment record and CM plan in his medical record.

Over many career years, both of these case managers have performed hundreds of assessments within timeliness constraints imposed by regulation and organizational policy. Both consider repetition and meeting completion requirements to be a demonstration of their organizational skill. However, completing a questionnaire within a certain amount of time is not indicative of organizational skill or the assessment's quality. It is only one aspect of CM's process. A thorough assessment involves gathering information from many sources, as demonstrated by Suzie. However, it is possible to simply interview the client and forego these other resources, as evidenced by Nonny.

There is an immense difference in these two approaches to completing a task. Although knowing what to do, why one is doing it, and how to do it is important, the habit of assessment excellence is missing in the absence of a motivating desire to perform in a comprehensive, consistent, and quality-driven manner.

Adapted from Covey, S. R. (1989). The seven habits of highly effective people (1st ed.). New York, NY: Simon & Schuster.

the responsibility of their position on the team with the understanding that the whole is greater than the sum of its parts. An example of this concept in the health care setting is the multidisciplinary transition team in which all team members accept responsibility for safe care transitions. If one member of the team fails to complete a task required in a client transition, there is no finger pointing or blame affixed to that individual. Instead, other members of the care team step up to complete the task because all team members commit to safe transitions of care.

Collective accountability does not remove the onus of individual responsibility. In fact, the opposite must be embraced by all team members because one person's act or failure to act carries an impact across the entire team. Thus, the standard to which one is held must be a common one across the team within the constraints of one's scope of practice and regulatory boundaries.

THE INTERDISCIPLINARY HEALTH CARE TEAM

The concept of collective accountability extends to interdisciplinary health care teams. The term **interdisciplinary health care team** (IHCT), as well as other terminology applied to teams, is often misunderstood. Case managers are integral members of many teams emanating from affiliation within employer, professional organizations, and familial structures. Regarding IHCT, Drinka and Clark (2000) offer an applicable definition, a group of individuals with diverse training and backgrounds who work together as an identified unit or system. Additional elements include the following:

- Consistent collaboration to solve patient problems,
- Create formal and informal structures that encourage collaborative problem solving,
- Determine mission and common goals to capitalize on disciplinary differences, power differential, and overlapping roles,
- Shared leadership appropriate to problem, and
- Leverage opinion differences to evaluate teamwork and development.

Fostering a culture of interdisciplinary collaboration requires precedent attributes, including leadership support, shared vision, effective communication, trust, mutual respect, shared accountability, individual ownership, expertise, focus on quality, cohesiveness, and stakeholder involvement (Freshman, Rubino, & Chassiakos, 2010). Figure 14-2 depicts converging team and environmental factors associated which may influence the effectiveness of interdisciplinary collaboratives.

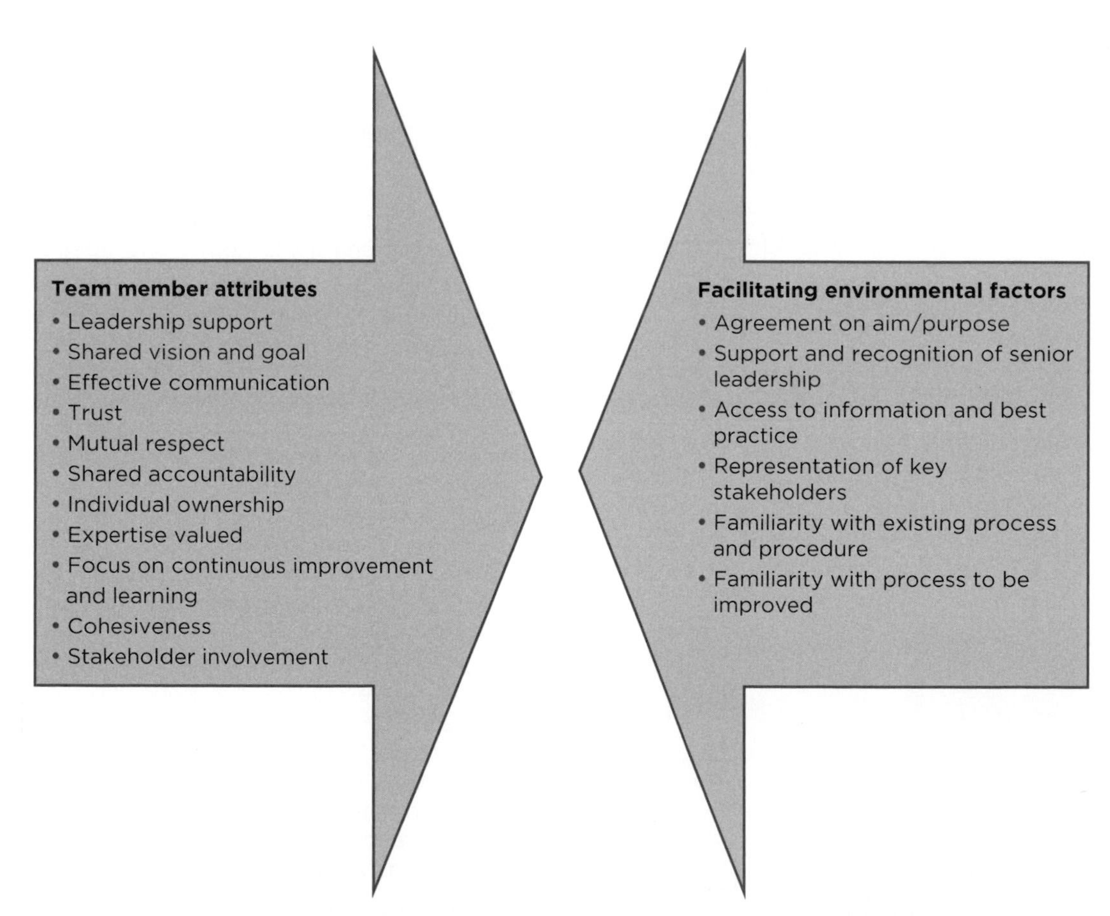

Figure 14-2. Converging attributes and environmental factors associated with effective interdisciplinary team. (Adapted from Freshman, B., Rubino, L., & Chassiakos, Y. R. (2010). *Collaboration across the disciplines in health care*. Sudbury, MA: Jones and Bartlett.)

THE HIGH-FUNCTIONING WORK TEAM

High-functioning work team (HFWT) is an expansion on the IHCT in that the HFWT includes the consideration of the social capital, or relationships among team members, enabling cross-team coordination of function (Gittell, 2009). HFWTs carry the potential to achieve high-performance health care. In measuring high performance, index ratings with specific areas of focus start provide a clearer understanding of work practice and correct performance of tasks and activities. The definition process begins with general interviews followed by clarification sessions which are helpful for identifying variance in task performance and nailing down the standard expectations for performance. A detailed report card of these indexes and practices supports understanding of current function and sources of dysfunction which require investigation (Gittell, 2009). Figure 14-3 depicts how a high-performance health care environment may influence CM performance and satisfaction.

However progressive this path sounds, an environmental shift of this magnitude requires significant pre-implementation effort. An organization is well-served by performing a thorough assessment to identify weaknesses and address those issue(s) to optimize conditions for success.

TeamSTEPPS is an evidence-based approach to building stronger health care teams. The program was co-developed by Agency for Healthcare Research and Quality (AHRQ) (2014a) and the Department of Defense and is based on over 20 years of research and experience. The TeamSTEPPS methodology provides a structured framework for assessing, establishing, and maintaining a cohesive health care team focused on higher quality, safer patient care. The desired outcome is to create and maintain high-performing health care teams.

The three phases of TeamSTEPPS are based on lessons learned, existing master trainer or change agent experience, the literature of quality and patient safety, and culture change. A successful TeamSTEPPS initiative requires a thorough assessment of the organization and its processes and a carefully developed implementation and sustainment plan. The phases of TeamSTEPPS are shown in Figure 14-4. Through a pretraining site-readiness assessment, train-the-trainer and staff education, and an implementation/maintenance phase, the teamwork system is a solution for patient safety improvement–based communication and teamwork skills. The downloadable curriculum and guides are designed to allow integration of the teamwork principles throughout an entire health care system. Training sites are located at major academic institutions across the United States.

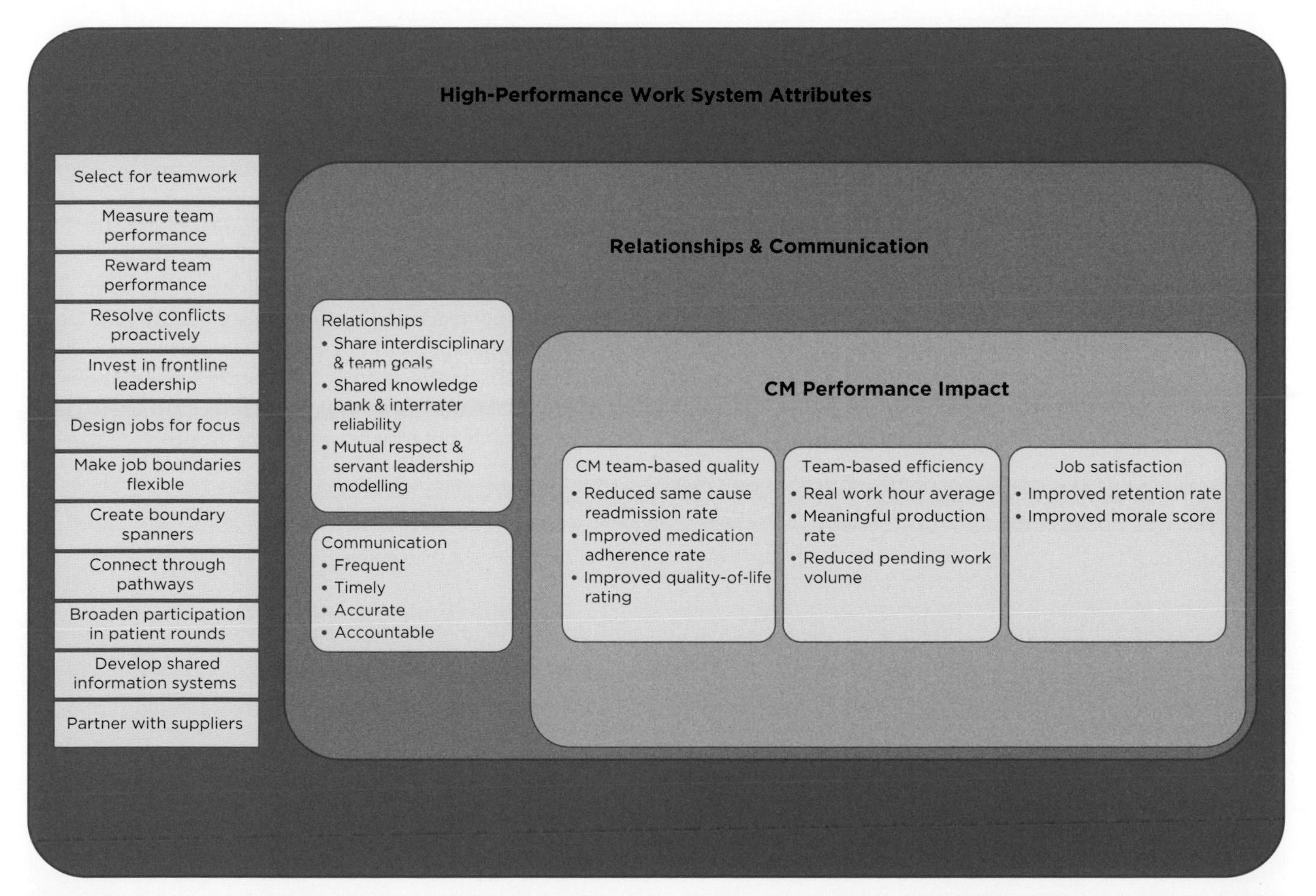

Figure 14-3. High-performance health care with CM modifications. (Adapted from Gittell, J. H. (2009). *High Performance Healthcare: Using the power of relationships to achieve quality, efficiency, and resilience*. New York, NY: McGraw Hill.)

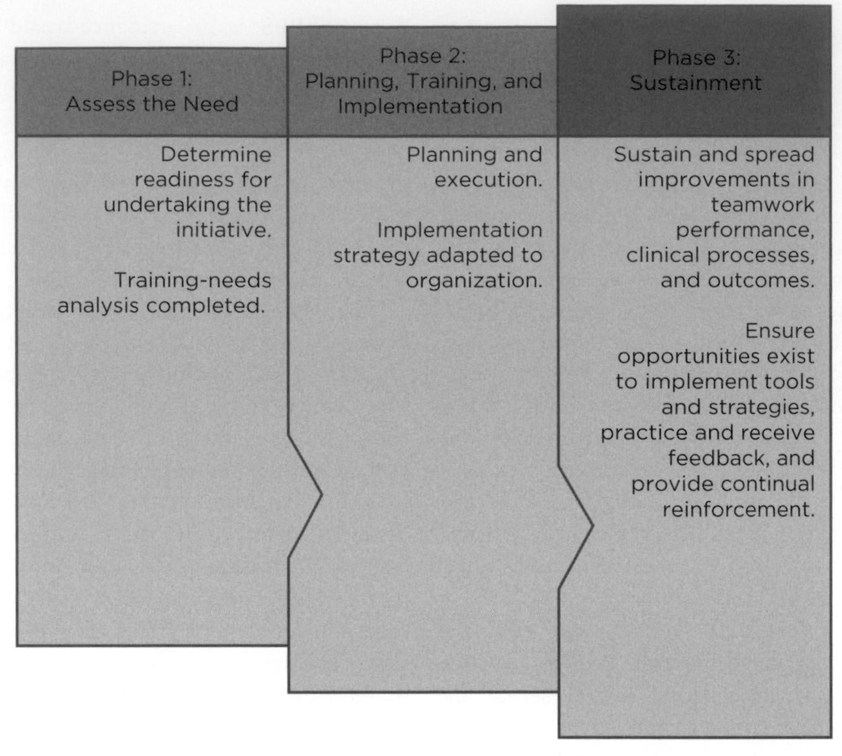

Figure 14-4. TeamSTEPPS implementation approach. (Adapted from Agency for Healthcare Research and Quality. (2014a). *TeamSTEPPS® national implementation*. Retrieved August 7, 2014, from http://teamstepps.ahrq.gov/about-2cl_3.htm)

INTERPROFESSIONAL EDUCATION

Although discussed extensively in chapter 5, **interprofessional education** needs to be mentioned as it pertains to collective accountability because of the role it plays in team member preparation. The World Health Organization (WHO) (2013) defines IPE as the process by which students from different professional backgrounds learn together during certain periods of their education with a view to enhancing collaboration and teamwork, and ultimately improving patient-centered care. IOM (2013) points out that educating both formal and informal leaders with regard to the value of IPE may be a way in which to garner leadership support for the concept itself. The New York Academy of Medicine (NYAM, 2013) recognizes important interprofessional competencies that are essential to effective care coordination. These competencies highlight mutual respect and leveraging strengths from other professions to improve care coordination, clearly reflective of the IOM recommendations for 21st century care (see Table 14-1).

There are published examples highlighting the point that well-functioning teams deliver better care quality (Campbell et al., 2001; Mukamel et al., 2006; Stevenson et al., 2001). Intersecting this is the shifting health care consumer demographic (e.g., expansion, aging). These forces are set to clash with chronic and potentially worsening health care worker

TABLE 14-1 NYAM Interprofessional Care Coordination Competencies

Values/Ethics	Work with individuals of other professions to maintain a climate of mutual respect and shared values.
Roles and responsibilities	Use the knowledge of one's own role and those of other professions to appropriately assess and address the health care needs of patients and populations served.
Interprofessional communication	Communicate with patients, families, and other health professionals in a responsive and responsible manner that supports a team approach to the maintenance of health and treatment of disease.
Interprofessional teamwork and team-based care	Apply relationship-building values and the principles of team dynamics to perform effectively in different team roles to plan and deliver patient and population-centered care that is safe, timely, efficient, effective, and equitable.

From The New York Academy of Medicine. (2013). Interprofessional care coordination: Looking to the future. Retrieved August 4, 2013, from http://www.nyam.org/news/nyam-news/interprofessional-care-may-24-2011.html

shortages (Coppard, Jensen, Cochran, & Goulet, 2009; Humphris & Hean, 2004). Requirements for defusing this critical mass include foundational change in interprofessional education and training opportunities for health care professionals. However, the issues relating to IPE include the fact that there is a lack of outcome evidence relating to IPE effectiveness and disagreement as to how best to measure IPE outcomes (Coppard et al., 2009).

ORGANIZED

As a word, **organized** is defined as something/someone arranged or planned in a particular way. Being organized is an aspect of one's state of existence. The synonyms of organized include neat, orderly, methodical, and systematic. Antonyms include haphazard, irregular, patternless, planless, and unsystematic (Merriam-Webster.com., 2014b). Although many have experienced interruptions of normal patterns during one's workday, the approach to conducting CM remains consistent. To demonstrate the importance of being organized has to a case manager, Figures 14-5 and 14-6 provide a snapshot of a day in a case manager's life in two different care settings. These figures are not step-by-step flow charts. Their purpose is to depict the random variation of concurrent activities that are encountered at any given time of a case manager's day.

The state of being organized requires mindset, process, and flexibility, enabling one to accommodate the unpredictability and high demand common to all health care environments. As applies to CM, organized means being purposeful, nonjudgmental, and consistent in thought, word, and action. Within the paradigm, it necessitates the ability to consider actual and potential influencers, elimination of personal bias, and consideration of benefits and risks concurrently while disregarding convenience or expediency as overriding concerns. This cross-continuum model considers the attribute of being organized to extend beyond workspace clutter into the larger concepts of efficiency and effectiveness of effort. Excellence in these spheres feeds high-quality CM practice. Effective CM must work within a framework demonstrating quality improvements and simultaneously taking the patient's perceptions, values, and expectations into

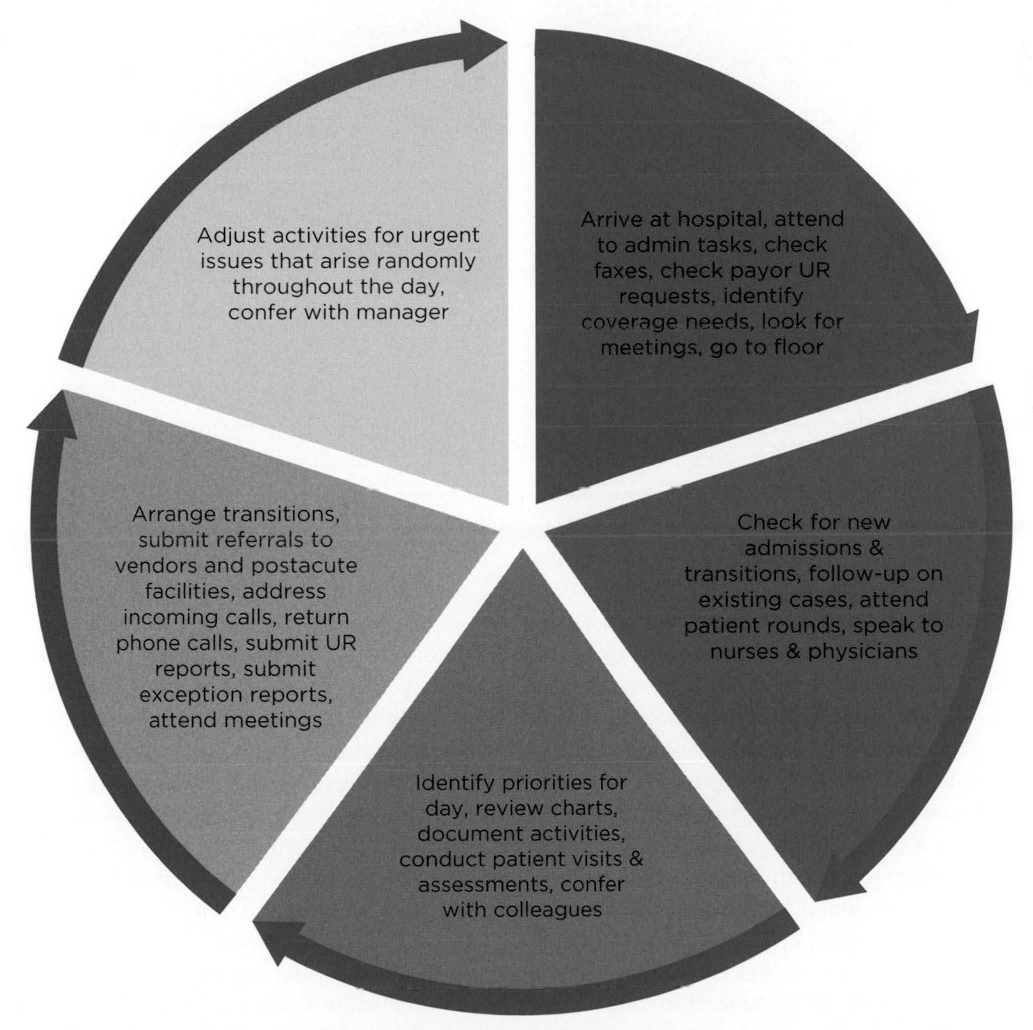

Figure 14-5. A day in the life of a hospital case manager. This is a simplified depiction of general activities, which a hospital case manager completes in the course of her or his day. It is not intended to capture the order in which activities are completed nor the subtasks or time required for completion. This figure demonstrates the iterative nature of activities in the course of a day.

Arrive to office, review calendar & prioritize work queue, check incoming fax, voicemail & email, follow up open requests
Make outgoing calls/ leave messages, review received information, initiate authorizations/ coverage determinations, refer to higher level review, request additional information
Consult with physician advisor, supervisor, attending physicians, specialist providers, ombudsman, provider representatives, vendors, colleagues, refer to special programs
Research evidence/clinical guidelines/standard of care/literature, organizational policy, coverage, & benefit level
Attend team meetings, committee meetings, patient care conferences (may require transportation), conduct client visits/calls
Document work process, prepare & send letters/emails/faxes, send educational material, complete activity reports

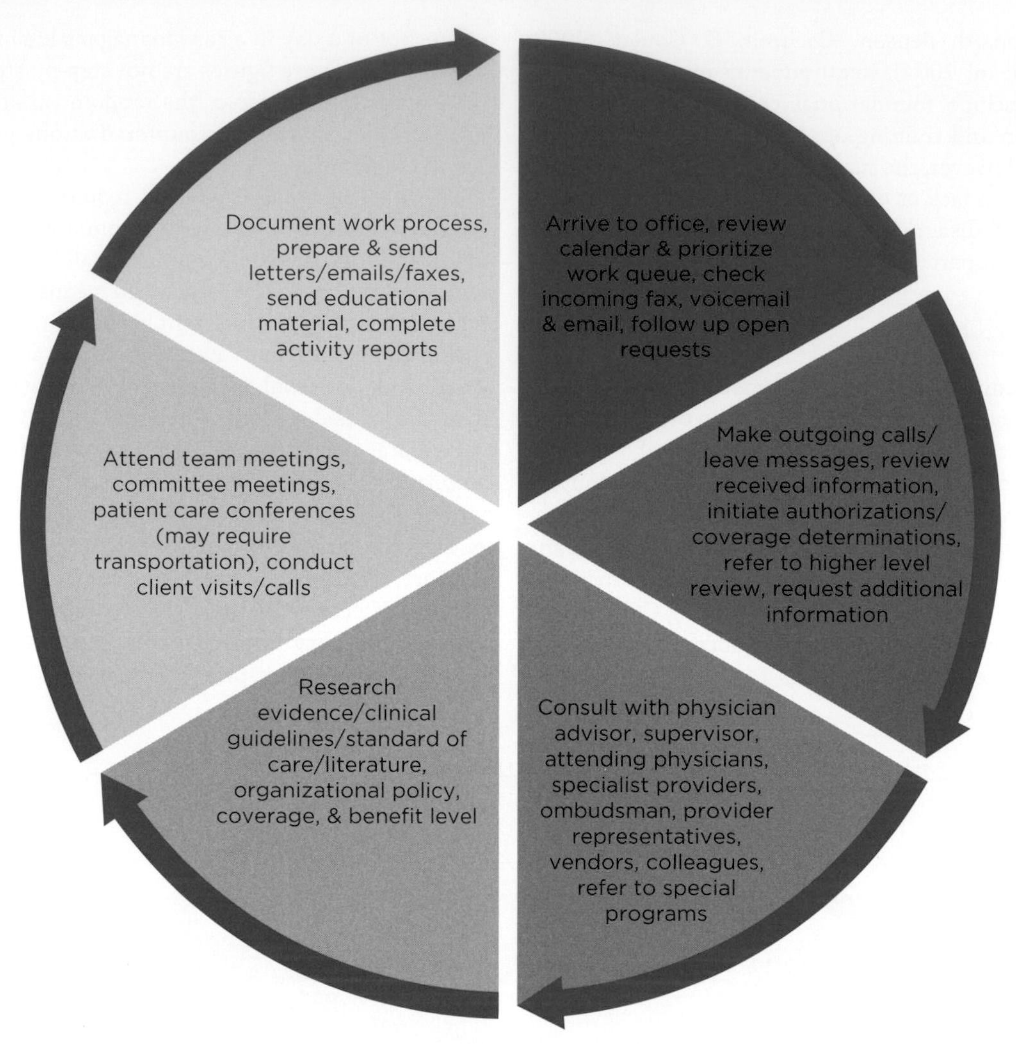

Figure 14-6. A day in the life of a managed care case manager.

account (Cesta & Tahan, 2003). This requires a tremendous reserve of patience and flexibility.

Being organized does not happen by some magical spell; influences of environment, education, intellect, and behavioral development come into play. Exposure to a highly organized household may help build organizational skills through environment. For many people, finding an organizational model requires dedicated effort to learn and maintain a systematic approach, not only to CM practice, but also to life in general. This is where Covey's approach adds value to the case manager's toolbox. The habits of effectiveness lend themselves to creating an organized approach to work.

There are situations in which someone working under the job title of case manager without proper education or training is doing so in a disorganized manner lacking accountability. On the other hand, an experienced professional case manager is notoriously organized and paid to be in control of what many regard as sheer chaos (Cesta & Tahan, 2003).

How is this advanced level of organization quantified or achieved? Figure 14-7 depicts a combination of process, knowledge, experience, and skills that contribute to maintaining an organized practice. However, an accurate determination of whether that person is organized is judged based on organizational priorities, success metrics, and interpretation of results (e.g., relative value as compared to peers).

IMPLICATIONS FOR MANAGERIAL-LEVEL CASE MANAGERS

Being organized is also essential for success in the roles and functions associated with managerial positions. A supervisor's day becomes even more complicated by the addition of resolving interpersonal and departmental issues brought forward by frontline case managers, fielding questions from multiple directions, completing reports, attending meetings, etc. Individuals in supervisory positions must maintain an organized approach to management responsibilities in order to achieve departmental objectives.

Management behaviors include decision making, communication, planning and organizing, managing change, and motivating subordinates (Huber, 2010). Additionally, O'Neil Morjikian, Cherner, Herschkorn, & West (2008) point out that individuals in management positions must develop skills in the areas of effective team building, translating vision to strategy,

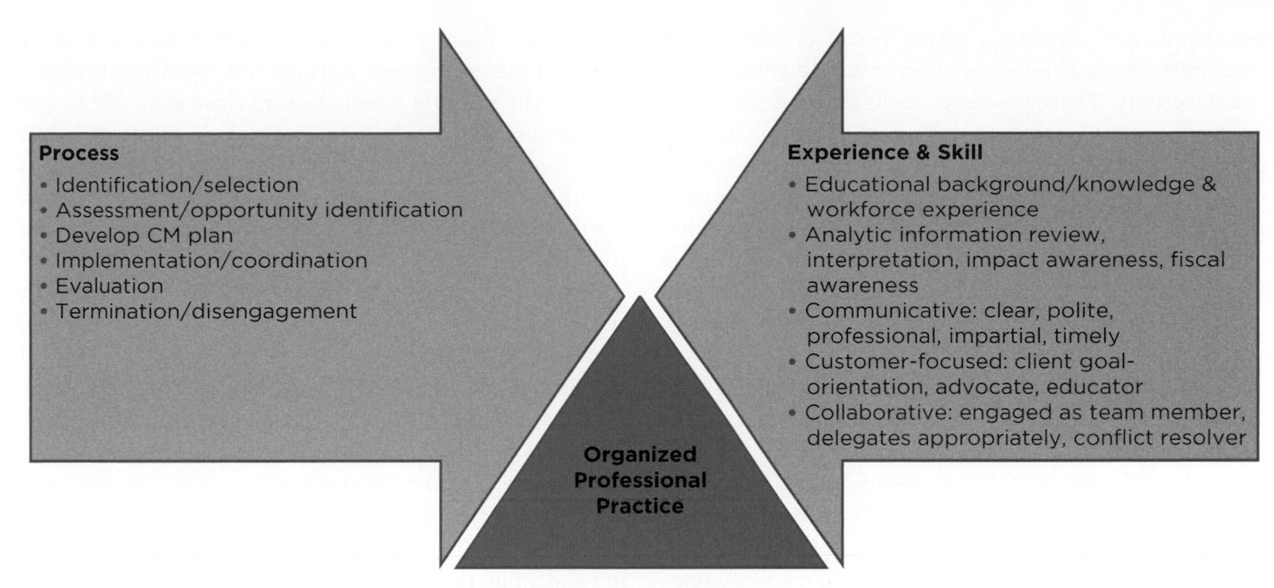

Figure 14-7. Combination of process, knowledge, experience, and skill.

internal communication of organization vision and strategy, conflict management, and managing the focus on the client.

As previously discussed, the difference between leadership and management is significant. Leadership attributes are discussed in the chapter on leadership competency. Although not exclusively applicable, management skills are on point to the discussion of a supervisory organization. The four-step management process of planning, organizing, directing, and controlling make up the major categories associated with managerial effort (Fayol, 1949). In addition to having established one's practice organization, those rising to supervisory positions must develop an organized approach to management in order to maximize staff effort and bring desired business outcomes to fruition.

CONTEXT FOR COLLABORATE APPLICATION

In a random review of Internet job postings for CM positions, virtually every one of them included "strong organizational skill" (or a variation of that phrase) as a desired candidate attribute. It was also clear that organizations seek educated, experienced individuals to fill clinical staff positions as evidenced by requirements attached to both the level of education and years of experience. In addition, there may be regulatory requirements to be addressed in the hiring process. However, it is not clearly known whether there is a connection between any of these requirements, an individual's ability to make responsible health care service determinations, and maintaining an organized approach to practice. In addition to an individual's background, there are situational factors, organizational policies, legal, and regulatory influencers involved in making each determination unique. The best an employer can hope for is that the job description and hiring process meaningfully contribute to the selection process, resulting in the best available candidate being hired.

With these numerous influences at play, one must consider whether imposing a bean counting, transaction-based productivity framework to performance management demonstrates a foundational misunderstanding and/or lack of genuine acceptance as to the value of CM. Hiring and performance management practices will not change overnight. However, messaging as to CM value, clarification around practice effectiveness, and appropriate measures of quality and outcomes is a task that must be assumed by all stakeholders.

There are a number of current practices that compound the lack of clarity around what CM is and what it is not. The slippery slope running between utilization management (UM) and CM create confusion for many people. Repeated medical management department re-organizations shift role functions without relabeling job titles. Because of the identification with and perceived value of the case manager job title, it is difficult for someone to give it up based on a company's changing business priorities. So is often the case, despite clear role function change, the job title root continues to include "case manager." This elastic border does a disservice to authentic CM as well as the health care industry because of the blurring of role/function boundaries. That notwithstanding, in the absence of a clear declaration in the form of regulation or policy as to the edges of the CM sandbox, there is no reason to believe that the practice will end. To this point, the number of "cases" touched in any given day is often tracked and used in performance ratings. However, although transaction volume may be an applicable measure for utilization review, it is not indicative of efficiency or effectiveness in CM practice.

Another practice is that of quality monitoring, also referred to as QC. This task is performed by supervisory staff utilizing a manual, random case file selection process, which requires hours of time to complete. The general process includes case selection and retrieval, review of data entry and narrative notes, review of procedure adherence, review of determination, and affixing a rating based on data entry and timeliness. It is a cumbersome process influenced by reviewer subjectivity. These processes focus on production and technical accuracy according to the organization's quality program and policy in the absence of industry-wide benchmarks. Unfortunately, this makes cross-continuum comparison quite difficult. This practice dominates the CM's quality assurance domain. However, these administrative metrics are not reflective of skill level or directly relatable to CM outcomes. These verify that an organization has met policies, procedures, and timeliness requirements.

When addressing being organized, it is important to distinguish between the flow of a daily schedule and the manner of conducting the CM process. These are very different concepts. As noted in the previous figures, each case manager's daily schedule is fraught with constant change in the form of unexpected events (e.g., family objection to a transition plan) and interruptions to primary work (e.g., staff meeting). Events that suddenly arise in the course of a day affecting the completion of planned activities inject the element of disarray. However, activities such as team meetings and mentoring new staff are not usually unexpected, although the result is a reduction in time available to address primary job responsibilities. Both of these are disruptive to task completion and may contribute to the sense of being disorganized. However, the process by which the case manager approaches each client's case is firmly rooted in organized behaviors that are part of the formal CM process.

From a departmental and organizational perspective, a number of criteria may be used to assess organizational skill. Just as it is challenging to reach agreement on a definition of department and overall organizational success, selecting demonstrative criteria proves to be as daunting (Robbins, 1990). As health care continues down a path balancing competition and business success with quality, access, and cost of care priorities, closer tracking of variations on traditional business measures may prove more helpful to demonstrating CM value than those associated strictly with utilization and production. Examples of potential effectiveness criteria, measures, and CM applicability are provided in Table 14-2.

TABLE 14-2 Criteria and Measures of Effectiveness and Efficiency

Criteria	Measure	CM Application
Productivity	Quantity or volume of major product or service measured at the individual, group, and/or organization level.	Focuses on utilization review functions as a part of CM, the volume of determinations, volume of referrals to physician advisor
Efficiency	Ratio reflecting unit performance to cost incurred for accomplishment	Turnaround time for determinations, appointments, or other priority measure as determined by organization
Profit	Revenue after cost obligation met	One way of looking at profit is the medical loss ratio, the ratio of premium revenues spent on clinical services and quality improvement versus the cost of business (e.g., administrative cost, salaries).
Quality	Worth of the primary service or product based on efficacy, effectiveness, efficiency, optimality, acceptability, legitimacy, and/or equity (Donabedian, 2003)	Number of same or similar cause readmissions or length of stay directly attributable to CM action or failure to take action
Accidents	Frequency of on-the-job accidents	Personal injury sustained in the course of performing CM (e.g., car accidents while driving to face-to-face visits, patient violence toward CM)
Growth	Increase in predetermined variables (e.g., workforce, members)	Number of covered lives receiving CM services
Absenteeism	Excused or unexcused absences from work	Individual and collective absence from regular work
Turnover	Measure of voluntary terminations in a given period	Number of resignations and/or job changes within workforce
Satisfaction	Affective component of individual's attitude toward their work or care	Measurement of patient satisfaction with CM service. This subjective measure must be conducted with a valid and reliable instrument. Often more meaningful when trended.
Morale	Group phenomenon involving communality, commitment, and feeling of belonging	Esprit de corps measures may be reflected in lower turnover or instances of voluntarily assisting fellow team members

Criteria	Measure	CM Application
Flexibility/ adaptation	Level of organizational agility to respond to environmental changes	Departmental shift from procedure-driven UM to needs-driven care coordination
Planning and goal setting	Degree to which organization conducts systematic planning and goal setting for future	Top-down organizational planning where strategic executive goals reflect into tactical and operational goals of divisions, departments, and individual performance objectives
Managerial interpersonal skills	Skill with which management staff deal with subordinates and peers	Subjective impressions of management staff actions and interactions
Utilization of environment	Effective utilization of scarce resources which contributes to goal achievement	Shift from office-based work to work-from-home in order to spread out CM workforce into communities
Stability	Maintenance of structure, function, and resources over time, especially in periods of stress	Consistency of excellent results and satisfaction scores despite in face of shifting health care industry priorities
Value of human resources	Total value or worth of individual members or parts to the organization	Cumulative measure of CM contribution to organizational goals (e.g., member satisfaction with access to care directly attributable to CM activity)

Adapted from Cesta, T. C., & Tahan, H. A. (2003). The case manager's survival guide: Winning strategies for clinical practice (2nd ed.). St. Louis, MO: Mosby; Donabedian, A. (2003). An introduction to quality assurance in health care. New York, NY: Oxford University Press; Robbins, S. P. (1990). Organization theory: Structure, design, and applications (3rd ed.). Englewood Cliffs, NJ: Prentice-Hall.

For further information, refer to the chapter specific to the outcomes competency.

Each of these influencers forms the backdrop argument for fostering better organization in work and practice. The manner in which one goes from theory to practical application varies according to their environment and experience. Whichever approach is utilized, the framework should be consistent. Consider how one takes a desk piled high with papers and begins to categorize the disarray into labeled file folders for easy retrieval. Similarly, the organized case manager uses consistent principles in order to develop and sustain a personal organized practice approach.

AN ORGANIZATIONAL MODEL

In *Organize Your Mind, Organize Your Life* (Hammerness & Moore with Hanc, 2012), the six principles onto which more advanced organizational abilities and skills grow are discussed (Figure 14-8). In CM practice, these may seem impossible at first glance. However, if the individual allows external influences to dictate work habits (or lack thereof) and does not take charge of their own internal well-being and make a mindful effort toward better organization, work output quality and quantity will suffer. Each principle can be depicted in common situations in a case manager's workday.

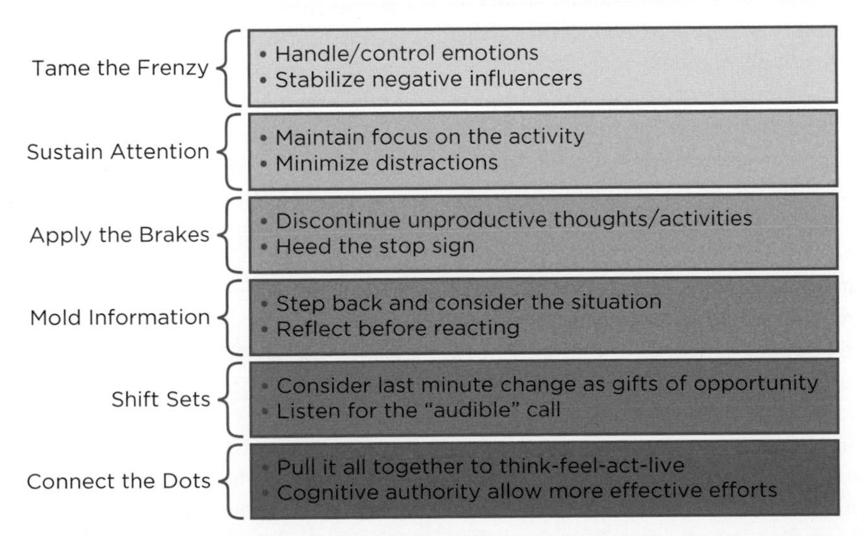

Figure 14-8. Organize your mind, organize your life rules of order. (From Hammerness, P., & Moore, M., with Hanc, J. (2012). *Organize your mind, organize your life*. Ontario, Canada: Harlequin.)

Tame the Frenzy—The start of a Monday day shift at an acute care facility where the case manager is faced with competing priorities of managed care reviews, transition planning, staff meeting, overdue productivity reports, and the breakdown of a child's car on the way to school. Effort must be put forth to filter out the "noise" in order to identify and categorize priorities and deal with them effectively rather than less productive multitasking. What are the next steps to identifying priority activities?

Sustain Attention—The managed care case manager is preparing to have a critical conversation with a client regarding reoccurring nonadherence to medication and an emergency department visit. A review of case notes, claims, and other historical information must precede the client call in order to decide on key talking points and possible educational needs and resources. Where does he find the time and privacy to review the appropriate documentation and conduct the client call?

Apply the Brakes—A department supervisor is responsible for preparing the work schedule for the entire CM staff. This requires concentration in order to account for time-off requests, meeting obligations, education/training time, and off-shift rotations. Just as she lays out all of the variables and requests on the conference room table, three staff members enter in the midst of a debate regarding who was at fault for a delayed discharge and her cellphone rings with a call from her spouse who has to work late and is no longer able to pick up one of their children from school or to bring him to a soccer game. How does she apply the brakes to regain some semblance of control over her environment?

Mold Information—A worker's compensation case manager is looking over a newly referred case file. The 45-year-old gentleman sustained a head injury after falling 25 feet in a worksite scaffolding collapse. The current case file includes medical records, legal documents, company forms, specialist consultations, and referral evaluations for three rehabilitation hospitals. How does this case manager synthesize information from many inputs in order to prepare for an initial conversation with the client and his caregiver?

Shift Sets—A case manager at a rehabilitation facility is leading the weekly patient round meeting when a cardiac arrest alarm is sounded. Although not all attendees at the meeting are on the code team, some individuals excuse themselves to see if they can assist with other activities on the unit. Should the round meeting continue or be postponed until another time?

Connect the Dots—A director of CM is faced with balancing staffing levels to align with accreditation, legal, and regulatory demands and a finite spending budget against the increased number of admissions at a three-campus acute medical center. Her Friday kicked off with a divisional meeting outlining a new round of budget cuts for the coming year, followed by a staff meeting, an educational session she delivered, and a vendor appointment to look at a software solution for recent transition of care delays. Throughout the day, her cellphone chimed with staff questions and email poured into her mailbox. At 4:30 P.M., she sits back wondering where the day went, wraps up email responses, and shuts down her computer.

TECHNOLOGY TO SUPPORT CASE MANAGER ORGANIZATION

Health care has made great strides with regard to developing and implementing technology since the passage of the Health Information Technology for Economic and Clinical Health (HITECH) Act which is part of the American Recovery and Reinvestment Act (ARRA) of 2009. This legislation and subsequent regulations created financial incentives for providers to expand infrastructure as well as technology, which focused on meaningful use of health care technology. In order to qualify for incentives, the Centers for Medicare and Medicaid Services defined meaningful use as being the use of certified electronic health records (EHR) to achieve health and efficiency goals. The three main components of meaningful use included the use of:

- certified EHR in a meaningful manner (e.g., e-prescribing),
- certified EHR technology for electronic exchange of health information to improve quality of health care, and
- certified EHR technology to submit clinical quality information and other measures.

(Centers for Medicare and Medicaid, 2012)

Where CM is concerned, the importance of EHRs to documentation clearly comes to the forefront where adherence management is concerned. The ability to quickly retrieve and aggregate data from various sources (e.g., claims history, interviews, validated assessment results) in order to gauge individual adherence to treatment is an important CM function. Prior to technological advances, data was extracted through visual claims and medical record review with weeks passing between utilization and access to medical records and claims.

Another way adherence management has benefited from technology is the tools available to track and assess adherence, motivation, and readiness to make behavioral changes. The explosion of smartphone applications places the power of adherence tracking at the individual's fingertips and with a single click. All tracked information may be uploaded to a central repository (e.g., EHR) for review and intervention. The efficiencies relating to no longer having to transcribe handwritten notes into a medical record (paper or electronic) are clear. As tools continue to be created for online documentation and receptivity for using patient-generated contributions to the EHR-gained popularity, it is anticipated that the definition of meaningful use of technology will likely need to be updated.

KEY ELEMENTS OF THE ORGANIZED COMPETENCY

Working in an organized manner requires the coveted key elements of both efficiency and effectiveness. For example, consider strong organizational skill is an attribute frequently included in job descriptions. Now, overlay the points that this skill is difficult to define, quantify, and not a distinct topic of formal education, let alone training. What does an employer mean by "strong organizational skill" and how does one prove competence with it at a job interview? One simply needs to state that she or he is organized or provide a scenario in which one worked in a methodical manner.

The objective measurement of organizational skill is not a routine part of pre-employment screening and process performance measures lack direct correlation to actual effective CM performance. It is easy to claim to be organized and to rattle off examples of working according to urgency. However, the demonstration of such an assertion with any degree of certainty in terms of traditional process metrics is difficult.

EFFICIENCY

An organized case manager balances practice standards, regulatory and legal mandates, and organization-specific administrative constructs to provide services in a manner where effort expended results in optimal outcomes without unnecessary waste (e.g., expense, resource, time). COLLABORATE focuses on the development of meaningful CM metrics that contribute to strategic goals and are incorporated into a wide variety of documentation (e.g., job description, performance management program, department goals). These measures focus on individual, team, and department outcomes using peer-to-peer comparison in an effort to create an equitable compensation and rewards system that values performance over longevity.

Identification and agreement upon activities, which are common to CM is an initial step toward development of appropriate efficiency models. For example, case finding and intake are essential activities quantified in the **Case Management Roles and Functions Study** (Tahan & Campagna, 2010). Within this domain, there are functions, which require a variety of skills and experience as well as specific knowledge. How these functions fit together under any given activity provides the foundation for identification of qualitative and quantitative evaluation.

An example is the activity of assessing an individual's ability to participate in CM. This may include direct questions of the client and caregiver as well as evaluating their readiness, activation, health literacy, and general literacy levels. Failure to conduct a sufficiently detailed evaluation or to properly administer these tools contributes to poor enrollment selection and ultimately to poor CM outcomes. The importance of evaluating individual case manager proficiency with each tool requires some form of inter-rater reliability and/or other objective evaluation process, which may include timing of tasks associated with each activity. This level of examination focuses on essential CM activities performed in an expert manner to yield best possible outcomes. When an individual executes essential activities competently and within standard timeframes, the "efficient" label is clearly applicable for that activity. In instances when a case manager is unable to meet defined expectations and when the problem is not directly attributable to process defect, then performance management planning may address the deficiency to the point it returns to an acceptable level.

TECHNOLOGY AND EFFICIENCY

The use of technology to improve case manager efficiency has been a growing influence over the past 30 years. From the early use of computer systems with very basic text entry fields to current CM information systems (CMIS) that build CM plans automatically from responses provided during an assessment to accessing patient-generated health tracking results (e.g., exercise log, blood glucose meter readings, daily weigh-in) to researching claims data within minutes rather than days in order to determine medication adherence information, the case manager has her or his fingertips on many tools that support more effective practice. In addition to patient-specific data, case managers may electronically access regulatory requirements, care-related guidelines, and evidence-based practice recommendations, online journals, patient assessment tools, patient education materials, availability of local support groups, and health care statistics in order to plan a CM intervention strategy (Mastrian, McGonigle, & Pavlekovsky, 2007a).

A well-designed CMIS facilitates practice by supporting the information needs of case managers. Through collection, processing, transition, and dissemination of information, CMIS enables informed case manager analysis and decision making. Elements which should be part of a CMIS include electronic record-keeping system, reminders/alerts, the ability to summarize information, business process analyses, caseload monitoring functionality, report generation, and integrated quality assurance initiatives (McGonigle, Mastrian, & Pavlekovsky, 2007b). Other useful functionality includes transition of care module, condition-specific modules, caseload calculation, supervisory functions (e.g., work queue balancing), and the ability to securely intake, transfer, and refer files attached to an episode of care.

By eliminating the manual, paper-based documentation process, the CMIS supports, but does not overtake, the case manager's intellectual CM process. An automated CMIS carries the potential to positively impact CM practice in three areas: case manager workflow, patient care, and organizational outcomes (McGonigle & Mastrian, 2007). At an organizational level, all of the data entered may be aggregated into return-on-investment and intensity-of-effort analyses which may ultimately demonstrate CM value in an objective manner (McGonigle et al., 2007b). As technology and experience advance the methods used to quantify CM, effectiveness will expand according to system capability and capacity. The case manager's ability to deftly and accurately manipulate and fully utilize data and information systems determines the impact on her or his level of efficiency. One such study is underway which hopes to determine the impact of technology-assisted CM in type 2 diabetes (National Institutes of Health Clinical Trials Registry identifier NCT01373489).

EFFECTIVENESS

Powell (2000) recognized the importance of Covey's work as foundational to case manager's health and well-being, as well as its applicability to professional practice. The seven habits are those of effectiveness and based on principles enabling the development of internal roadmaps and facilitating the integration of learning and growth (Covey, 1989). The case manager ultimately benefits in improved practice by fostering good habits that lay the groundwork for both internal (e.g., private) and external (e.g., public, outward) success. As Covey points out, internal groundwork comes before external recognition. This goes back to the point of internal motivation, also known as the desire for excellence.

The progression of effectiveness, based on **Covey's Maturity Continuum**, follows the natural laws of growth as being incremental, sequential, and integrative (see Figure 14-9). To understand this general concept, consider the following:

- As individuals, we begin our lives as dependent beings reliant on others for survival (the "you" paradigm).
- As years pass, we seek ways in which to establish independence through stages of development (e.g., physiologic, psychological) (the "me" paradigm).
- Eventually, we realize that life and living is based on interdependence (the "we" paradigm).

To place this in the CM paradigm, today's case manager optimally functions in a "we" environment as a member of collaborative health care management in which a team's ethos is based on collective accountability through independent practice excellence. To reach this pinnacle of teamwork excellence, a team and each of its members must adopt and ingrain the principle of collective accountability.

An effective case manager uses evidence-based interventions and tools as integral to CM planning and performance, but remains flexible in order to accommodate the unexpected demands of day-to-day events to achieve desired outcomes (e.g., client objectives, program goals). For instance, an effective case manager is knowledgeable of best practices and utilizes interventions that have been shown to contribute to positive results, sharing this knowledge with his or her peers to improve team performance consistency.

COMPARATIVE EFFECTIVENESS OF CASE MANAGEMENT

In an effort to determine the effectiveness of CM in an outpatient setting, the Effective Health Care Program supported the study of Outpatient Case Management for Adults With Medical Illness and Complex Care Needs (Contract No. 290-2007-10057-I). **Comparative effectiveness** research seeks to identify strengths and weaknesses of current findings relating to specific key questions. Comparative effectiveness research is designed to inform health care decisions by providing evidence on the effectiveness, benefits, and harms of different treatment options. The evidence is generated from research studies that compare drugs, medical devices, tests, surgeries, or ways to deliver health care (AHRQ, 2014b). The report, prepared by the Oregon Evidence-based Practice Center sought clarity around key questions pertaining to CM intervention effectiveness (see Figure 14-10).

The results of this research were underwhelming due to a number of factors identified as limiters to sample size, including small sample size, failure to compare more than one CM model, and the lack of complete descriptive information regarding the content of CM intervention delivered as part of the study. The search for studies to include in this research yielded 5,645 citations, of which only 153 articles pertaining to 109 studies were judged to be relevant (Hickam et al., 2013). The review summary rated the strength of evidence for the conclusions often as only low or moderate with few exceptions for studies of larger sample size. Although the findings of this comparative effectiveness research are disappointing (refer to summary in Table 14-3), a lesson learned highlights a lack of consistent structure and organization of CM research. This point alone is instructive for producing more reliable and informative CM research in the future.

COLLABORATE encourages the use of evidence-based guidelines to develop measurable CM interventions and improve consistency of team-wide service delivery and outcomes (e.g., adherence rate, biometric measures, utilization). These results should be incorporated into CM-specific documentation (e.g., performance expectations, job description)

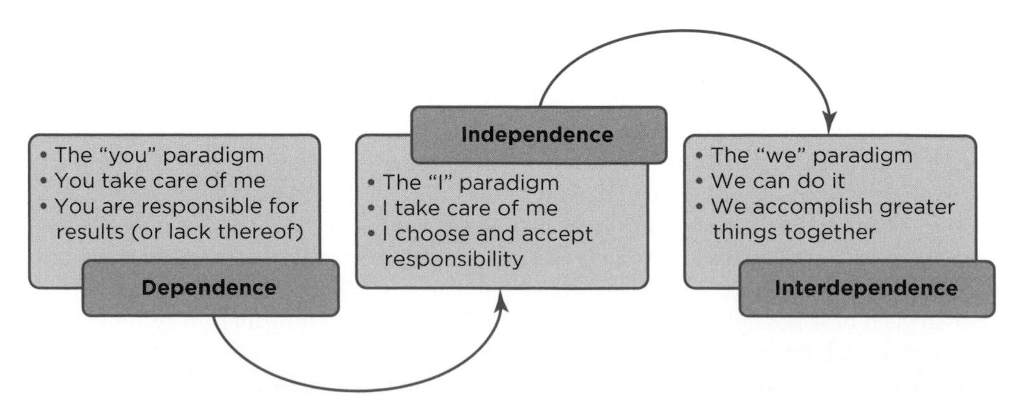

Figure 14-9. Covey's Maturity Continuum. (Adapted from Covey, S. R. (1989). *The seven habits of highly effective people* (1st ed.). New York, NY: Simon & Schuster.)

Key Question #1	Key Question #2	Key Question #3
• In adults with chronic medical illness and complex care needs, is case management effective in improving: • Patient-centered outcomes, including mortality, quality of life, disease-specific health outcomes, avoidance of nursing home placement, and patient satisfaction with care? • Quality of care, as indicated by disease-specific process measures, receipt of recommended health care services, adherence to therapy, missed appointments, patient self-management, and changes in health behavior? • Resource utilization, including overall financial cost, hospitalization rates, days in the hospital, emergency department use, and number of clinic visits (including primary care and other provider visits)?	• Does the effectiveness of case management differ according to patient characteristics, including, but not limited to: particular medical conditions, number or type of comorbidities, patient age and socioeconomic status, social support, and/or level of formally assessed health risk?	• Does the effectiveness of case management differ according to intervention characteristics, including, but not limited to: practice or health care system setting; case manager experience, training, or skills; case management intensity, duration, and integration with other care providers; and the specific functions performed by case managers?

Figure 14-10. EHCP key questions pertaining to outpatient CM. (Adapted from Hickam, D. H., Weiss, J. W., Guise, J-M., Buckley, D., Motu'apuaka, M., Graham, E., ... Saha, S. (2013, January). *Outpatient case management for adults with medical illness and complex care needs*. Rockville, MD: Agency for Healthcare Research and Quality. Retrieved from www.effectivehealthcare.ahrq.gov/reports/final.cfm)

TABLE 14-3 EHCP Comparative Effectiveness Study Results

Key Question	Results
1a. In adults with chronic medical illness and complex care needs, is case effective in improving patient-centered outcomes?	**Mortality** Patients provided CM did not experience lower mortality in general populations of patients with chronic illness, in the frail elderly, those with HIV infection, or in patients with specific diseases such as cancer, congestive heart failure, or dementia. **Quality of Life and Functional Status** CM interventions produced mixed results in terms of improving patients' quality of life (QOL) and functional status. In general, CM was frequently successful in improving aspects of functioning and QOL that were directly targeted by the interventions. For instance, CM was successful in improving caregiver stress among persons caring for patients with dementia and CHF-related QOL among patients with CHF. The measures used to evaluate QOL and functional status varied across studies, and overall, the improvements in QOL and functional status achieved by CM were either small or of unclear clinical significance. CM was less successful in improving overall QOL and functioning, as indicated by global measures not specific to a particular condition. **Ability to Remain at Home** One measure of the clinical significance of improvements in functioning for elderly patients is the ability to remain at home and avoid nursing home placement. This outcome was often the primary objective of CM programs for patients with dementia. In most studies of the frail elderly and of patients with dementia, CM was not effective in maintaining patients' ability to live at home. Evidence from one study suggests that a high-intensity CM intervention sustained over a period of several years can produce a substantial delay in nursing home placement for patients with dementia.
	Disease-Specific Health Outcomes The effect of CM on disease-specific outcomes was inconsistent. In some studies, CM had a positive impact on specific symptoms, including pain and fatigue in patients with cancer and depressive symptoms among caregivers of patients with dementia. Notably, however, CM had an inconsistent impact on clinical outcomes among patients with diabetes, including glycohemoglobin levels, body weight, and lipids. **Patient Satisfaction With Care** CM interventions were generally associated with improved patient (and caregiver) satisfaction, although satisfaction with CM varied across interventions. Studies measuring patient satisfaction typically reported overall satisfaction with care, rather than satisfaction in specific domains. Satisfaction was most substantially improved in the domain of coordination among health care providers.

(continued)

TABLE 14-3 EHCP Comparative Effectiveness Study Results (*Continued*)

Key Question	Results
1b. In adults with chronic medical illness and complex care needs, is CM effective in improving quality of care?	**Disease-Specific Process Measures and Receipt of Recommended Services** CM was effective in increasing the receipt of recommended health care services when it was an explicit objective of the CM intervention. For instance, CM interventions designed to improve cancer therapy adherence for patients with breast and lung cancer were successful in increasing the receipt of radiation treatment, as recommended in clinical guidelines. The effect of CM on guideline-recommended care in general, however, was less consistent. Studies showed only sporadic effects on elements of quality of care, such as receipt of appropriate medications for patients with CHF or diabetes, or receipt of appropriate preventive services for elderly patients. **Patient Self-Management** CM was effective in improving patient self-management behaviors, including dietary and medication adherence, for specific conditions such as CHF or tuberculosis, when patient education and self-management support were included within CM interventions. **Adherence** Few studies measured the frequency of missed appointments or other adherence measures as an outcome of CM interventions.
1c. In adults with chronic medical illness and complex care needs, is CM effective in improving resource utilization?	**Hospitalization Rates** Although hospitalization rates were often included as an outcome, trials of CM generally did not demonstrate reductions in these rates. **Emergency Department Use** CM had a variable effect on emergency department (ED) use. Several studies found reduced ED use in patients receiving CM, but other studies found no effect. **Clinic Visits** Few studies measured the frequency of clinic visits as an outcome of CM interventions. Those that did generally found varying results, and no conclusions can be drawn about this outcome.
2. Does the effectiveness of CM differ according to patient characteristics?	**Medical Conditions** Individual studies had inconsistent findings on whether CM interventions are more successful for patients with high disease burden. Although it is possible that there is a mid-range of disease burden in which CM is most effective, the evidence base does not permit defining how to identify such patients. **Age** Most studies of CM included mainly elderly patients, making it difficult to determine impact of age on CM effectiveness. **Socioeconomic Status** Studies did not routinely report the effect of CM according to socioeconomic indicators among enrolled patients. Some studies explicitly targeted low-income or homeless populations. There was no apparent pattern to suggest an influence of patients' socioeconomic status on the effectiveness of CM. **Social Support** Few studies explicitly evaluated patients' level of social support. However, studies that targeted patients with limited social support did not tend to find better results. **Formally Assessed Health Risk** Some studies explicitly targeted patients considered to be at high risk of poor outcomes. The methods used to evaluate risk, however, varied substantially across studies. The studies have not defined a specific level of risk for which CM is most effective for improving outcomes.
3. Does the effectiveness of CM differ according to intervention characteristics?	**Setting** Characteristics of the setting in which CM was implemented (e.g., integrated health system, home health agency, outpatient clinic) did not clearly influence the effectiveness of CM.

Key Question	Results
	Case Manager Experience, Training, Skills Studies did not consistently provide details about the experience, training, or skills of case managers. In most studies the case managers were registered nurses, and some had specialized training in caring for patients with the conditions targeted by the CM intervention (e.g., diabetes, cancer). There was low strength of evidence indicating that preintervention training of nurses in providing CM for the targeted conditions, the use of protocols or scripts to guide clinical management, and collaboration between a case manager and a physician (or multidisciplinary team) specializing in the targeted clinical condition, resulted in more successful interventions. **Case Management Intensity, Duration, Integration With Other Care Providers** There was low strength of evidence that more intense CM interventions, as indicated by greater contact time, longer duration, and face-to-face (as opposed to only telephone) visits, produced better outcomes, including functional outcomes and lower hospitalization rates. **Case Manager Functions** Case managers typically performed multiple functions. These included, but were not limited to, assessment and planning, patient education, care coordination, and clinical monitoring. In general, emphasis on specific functions varied according to patients' conditions and the primary objectives of specific CM interventions. For example, interventions among patients with cancer typically focused on coordination and navigation, while interventions for patients with diabetes and CHF focused more on patient education (for self-management) and clinical monitoring. Most studies did not carefully measure the amount of effort case managers devoted to different functions, making it difficult to discern the degree to which emphasis on different case manager functions impacted CM effectiveness.

CHF: chronic heart failure.

Adapted from Hickam, D. H., Weiss, J. W., Guise, J-M., Buckley, D., Motu'apuaka, M., Graham, E., ... Saha, S. (2013, January). Outpatient case management for adults with medical illness and complex care needs. *Rockville, MD: Agency for Healthcare Research and Quality. Retrieved from www.effectivehealthcare.ahrq.gov/reports/final.cfmww.effectivehealthcare.ahrq.gov/reports/final.cfm*

in order to align research-proven results with day-to-day practice. As more studies findings are published, the evidential foundation of effective CM interventions will expand and should become a more centralized and reliable industry resource to improve consistent delivery of high-quality CM customer service.

CASE MANAGEMENT PRACTICE IMPLICATIONS

As Fetterolf, Holt, Tucker, & Khan (2010) noted, "Case management programs are materially different from standard medical management or disease management programs in a number of ways. The patients have complex medical conditions combined with many other variables that tend to increase their costs and patterns of utilization." The article goes on to highlight that the variations encountered in CM practice setting, population served, and experience level make it difficult to define the value of CM at both individual and program levels. It is the lack of specificity that contributes to the difficulties in determining meaningful performance measures for CM on the whole, let alone achieving a degree of consensus as to how CM impacts the populations served in clinical and economic terms. In summarizing findings, it was stated that "measures should include those of central tendency and statistical significance to avoid later accusations of misleading information and to further underscore the difficult nature of evaluating widely varying populations. It is important to create a dialogue between providers and purchasers of these services that the inherent variation in complex CM patients requires alternate methods to estimate the value delivered by these programs. Specific needs of the client might be targeted (e.g., better use of hospice, placement in best practice hospitals, preferred network use, return-to-work times) rather than simplistic return on investment calculations. Understanding the complexity of this issue will reduce frustration by all parties and lead to improved relations between suppliers and purchasers of these services (Fetterolf et al., 2010).

This brings up the job title dilemma again. Going forward it is strongly recommended that all research pertaining to the value and/or outcomes associated with CM interventions contain detailed information as to the studied participants' job (e.g., title, position description, scope of responsibilities, education level, qualifications, activities not included in the scope of research). An example of this is found in the study protocol for examination of CM and self-management support for frequent users with chronic disease in primary care (Chouinard et al., 2013). Box 14-2 is an excerpt of a clear description of CM services to be studied, including definition and service scope as it applies in the study. Failure to address the fundamental issue of title control dilutes efficiency and effectiveness research.

BOX 14-2 Study Description Including Case Management Definition and Scope of Services

DESCRIPTION

The first component of the intervention is the follow-up offered under the CM process, which is seen as a collaborative, dynamic, and systematic approach to ensure and coordinate care and services for a defined clientele based on interdisciplinary practice. Here the nurse evaluates, plans, implements, coordinates, and prioritizes options and services according to patient health needs, in close collaboration with the involved partners.

STUDY SCOPE

The intervention focuses on four main components: (1) A thorough evaluation of patient's needs and resources; (2) Establishment and maintenance of a patient-centered, individualized service plan (ISP); (3) Coordination of services among partners; and (4) Self-management support for patients and families.

CASE MANAGEMENT MAIN DUTIES AND RESPONSIBILITIES

Nurses in CM will (1) Evaluate the patient's situation and needs and involve the family with the patient's consent; (2) Identify which partners of the Centre de santé et de services sociaux and of the community network to involve; (3) Jointly plan patient follow-up by establishing an ISP with the partners and with the active participation of the patients and family—minimum of two ISP per patient: one to initiate the intervention and the other approximately 3 months later; (4) Negotiate the services and defend the rights and interests of the individual; (5) Coordinate care and services; (6) Monitor the ISP application; and (7) Educate and support the person. The ISP formulation stage will be oriented toward a self-management support approach that will emphasize the following: the patient's potential; setting objectives according to his or her perspective; developing problem-solving skills; and using the patient's usual support system. Home visits by the nurse may be required, when justified—as in the case of reduced mobility or if a home assessment is needed—while avoiding overlap with home support services already offered.

Adapted from Chouinard, M., Hudon, C., Dubois, M, Roberge, P., Loignon, C., Tchouaket, E., ... Sasseville, M. (2013). Case management and self-management support for frequent users with chronic disease in primary care: A pragmatic randomized controlled trial. BMC Health Services Research, 13, 49. Retrieved August 24, 2014, from http://www.biomedcentral.com/1472-6963/13/49

SUMMARY

This chapter addressed the importance of raising the skill of being organized to the level of practice competency. CM practice incorporates the IOM's six aims for care in the 21st century—safe, effective, patient-centered, timely, efficient, and equitable. Failure to deliver CM in an effective and efficient manner belies its true worth to health care and creates difficulties in evaluating its success. As health care continues to become more complex, the system will collapse under the weight of poorly organized delivery systems without the use of well-designed, evidence-based tools (e.g., CMIS). These factors apply across the health care continuum of today as well as into tomorrow. Establishing and maintaining an organized approach to practice pushes CM to the forefront of accountable and measurable health care delivery excellence.

References

Agency for Healthcare Research and Quality. (2014a). *TeamSTEPPS® national implementation*. Retrieved August 7, 2014, from http://teamstepps.ahrq.gov/about-2cl_3.htm

Agency for Healthcare Research and Quality. (2014b). *What is comparative effectiveness research?* Retrieved August 20, 2014, from http://effectivehealthcare.ahrq.gov/index.cfm/what-is-comparative-effectiveness-research

Campbell, S. M., Hann, M., Hacker, J., Burns, C., Oliver, D., Thapar, A., ... Roland, M. O. (2001). Identifying predictors of high quality care in English general practice: Observational study. *British Medical Journal, 323*, 1–6. Retrieved August 7, 2014, from http://bmj.com

Centers for Medicare & Medicaid Services. (2012). *EHR Incentive Programs*. Retrieved August 12, 2014, from https://www.cms.gov/Regulations-and-guidance/Legislation/EHRIncentivePrograms/index.html?redirect=/EHRIncentivePrograms/30_Meaningful_Use.asp

Cesta, T. C., & Tahan, H. A. (2003). *The case manager's survival guide: Winning strategies for clinical practice* (2nd ed.). St. Louis, MO: Mosby.

Chouinard, M., Hudon, C., Dubois, M, Roberge, P., Loignon, C., Tchouaket, E., ... Sasseville, M. (2013). Case management and self-management support for frequent users with chronic disease in primary care: A pragmatic randomized controlled trial. *BMC Health Services Research, 13*, 49. Retrieved August 24, 2014, from http://www.biomedcentral.com/1472-6963/13/49

Coppard, B. M., Jensen, G. M., Cochran, T. M., & Goulet, C. (2009). Issues relaing to interprofessional assessment. In C. B. Royeen, G. M. Jensen, & R. A. Harvan (Eds.), *Leadership in interprofessional health education and practice* (pp. 63–75). Sudbury, MA: Jones and Bartlett.

Covey, S. R. (1989). *The seven habits of highly effective people* (1st ed.). New York, NY: Simon & Schuster.

Donabedian, A. (2003). *An introduction to quality assurance in health care*. New York, NY: Oxford University Press.

Drinka, T. J. K., & Clark, P. G. (2000). *Health care teamwork: Interdisciplinary practice and teaching*. Westport, CT: Auburn House.

Fayol, H. (1949). *General and industrial management*. London, England: Pitman & Sons.

Fetterolf, D., Holt, A. E., Tucker, T., & Khan, N. (2010). Estimating clinical and economic impact in case management programs. *Population Health Management, 13*(2), 73–82.

Freshman, B., Rubino, L., & Chassiakos, Y. R. (2010). *Collaboration across the disciplines in health care*. Sudbury, MA: Jones and Bartlett.

Gittell, J. H. (2009). *High performance healthcare: Using the power of relationships to achieve quality, efficiency, and resilience*. New York, NY: McGraw Hill.

Hammerness, P., & Moore, M. with Hanc, J. (2012). *Organize your mind, organize your life*. Ontario, Canada: Harlequin.

Hickam, D. H., Weiss, J. W., Guise, J-M., Buckley, D., Motu'apuaka, M., Graham, E., ... Saha, S. (2013, January). *Outpatient case management for adults with medical illness and complex care needs*. Rockville, MD: Agency for Healthcare Research and Quality. Retrieved from www.effective healthcare.ahrq.gov/reports/final.cfm

Huber, D. L. (Ed.). (2010). *Leadership and nursing care management* (4th ed.). Maryland Heights, MO: Saunders Elsevier.

Humphris, D., & Hean, S. (2004). Educating the future workforce: Building the evidence about interprofessional learning. *Journal of Health Services Research & Policy*, *9*(Suppl. 1), 24–27. Retrieved August 7, 2014, from Proquest database

Institute of Medicine. (2001). *Crossing the quality chasm: A new health system for the 21st century*. Washington, DC: The National Academies Press.

Institute of Medicine. (2013). *Interprofessional education for collaboration: Learning how to improve health from interprofessional models across the continuum of education to practice: Workshop summary*. Washington, DC: The National Academies Press.

McGonigle, D., & Mastrian, K. (2007). Information systems in case management. In S. Powell & H. Tahan (Eds.), *CMSA core curriculum for case management*. Philadelphia, PA: Wolters Kluwer Lippincott Williams & Wilkins.

McGonigle, D., Mastrian, K., & Pavlekovsky, K. (2007a). Information systems and case management practice series part I (I (of III): Introduction to information systems and case management information system. *Professional Case Management*, *12*(3), 181–183.

McGonigle, D., Mastrian, K., & Pavlekovsky, K. (2007b). Information systems and case management practice series part II (of III): Case management information systems goals, benefits, and system selection or development. *Professional Case Management*, *12*(4), 239–241.

Merriam-Webster.com. (2014a). Habit. Retrieved July 20, 2014, from http://www.merriam-webster.com/dictionary/habit

Merriam-Webster.com. (2014b). Organized. Retrieved July 20, 2014, from http://www.merriam-webster.com/dictionary/organized

Mukamel, D. B., Temkin-Greener, H., Delavan, R., Peterson, D. R., Gross, D., Kunitz, S., & Williams, T. F. (2006). Team performance and risk-adjusted health outcomes in the Program of All-Inclusive Care for the Elderly (PACE). *The Gerontologist*, *46*(2), 227–237. Retrieved August 7, 2014, from Proquest database

The New York Academy of Medicine. (2013). *Interprofessional care coordination: Looking to the future*. Retrieved August 4, 2013, from http://www.nyam.org/news/nyam-news/interprofessional-care-may-24-2011.html

O'Neil, E., Morjikian, R. L., Cherner, D., Herschkorn, C., & West, T. (2008). Developing nursing leaders: An overview of trends and programs. *Journal of Nursing Administration*, *38*(4), 178–183.

Powell, S. K. (2000). *Advanced case management: Outcomes and beyond*. Philadelphia, PA: Lippincott Williams & Wilkins.

Robbins, S. P. (1990). *Organization theory: Structure, design, and applications* (3rd ed.). Englewood Cliffs, NJ: Prentice-Hall.

Stevenson, K., Baker, R., Farooqi, A., Sorrie, R., & Khunti K. (2001). Features of primary health care teams associated with successful quality improvement of diabetes care: A qualitative study. *Family Practice*, *18*(1), 21–26.

Tahan, H. A., & Campagna, V. (2010). Case management roles and functions study across various settings and professional disciplines. *Professional Case Management*, *15*(5), 245–277.

World Health Organization. (2013). *Transforming and scaling up health professionals' education and training: World health organization guidelines 2013*. Retrieved August 4, 2014, from http://www.who.int/iris/bitstream/10665/93635/1/9789241506502_eng.pdf

15 RESOURCE AWARENESS

OBJECTIVES

After studying this chapter, you will be able to:

1. Define resource awareness and resource management in the case management context.
2. Differentiate utilization review types and the implication of medical loss ratio to payer-based case management.
3. Discuss the progress of utilization management and its implications to case management.
4. Articulate the role of Quality Improvement Organizations and where the 11th Scope of Work intersects with case management.
5. Discuss the key elements of resource awareness and how to implement them into case management practice.

KEY TERMS

Avoidable cost
Concurrent review
Cost–benefit analysis
Covered benefits
Medical loss ratio
Outcomes management
Prospective review
Quality Improvement Organizations
Resource awareness
Resource management
Retrospective review
Utilization management
Utilization review

America has developed a habit of taking all actions necessary in attempting to cure illness and injury. The reality is, the well from which these resources are drawn is not bottomless. For the overwhelming majority of health care consumers, resources are limited. In spite of that fact, health care resources continue to be spent on interventions that are of little benefit or are even harmful (Sirovich, Gottlieb, Welch, & Fisher, 2006). There has been wide variation in the utilization of health care resources across the United States as proven by studies which clearly demonstrate that quality of care, access to care, and patient satisfaction are not better in regions where more resources are expended (Fisher, Wennberg, Stukel, Gottlieb, & Lucas, 2003; Sirovich et al., 2006). Case management, resource management, and quality management are inextricably bonded to ensuring the delivery of appropriate, high-quality health care. As a consequence, it is essential for the professional case manager to have knowledge fluency regarding evidence-based criteria, utilization patterns, and available resources, as well as the skills to find new resource channels in order to optimize resource allocation. This chapter discusses the importance of the resource awareness competence because of the influence case management exerts on the decision making associated with health care delivery.

RESOURCE AWARENESS

For the purpose of this text, **resource awareness** encompasses possessing the knowledge of the existing resources applied during a case management engagement as well as the decision-making and networking skills associated with acquiring resources to address health care needs. It is inadequate simply to negotiate a criteria framework in order to flip a yes or no lever regarding the appropriateness of a health care service or product for a complex, multimorbid patient. The professional case manager applies critical thinking skills to factors such as patient safety, quality, outcome potential, access to care, organizational resources, and the cost of procuring the health care service or product (and/or alternatives) in order to reach a well-considered resource allocation determination.

COVERED BENEFITS

Appropriate resource management is predicated on having a working knowledge about an individual's **covered benefits**. Covered benefits (or services) are those services specified in a payer's contract which specify the services and supplies for which the payer will provide reimbursement. Usually the services outlined in a contract are a combination of mandatory and optional services (Dasco & Dasco, 1999). Benefit descriptions are legal documents which provide the details of covered benefits of a given plan. Detailed benefit descriptions, also referred to as summary descriptions, are provided by the payer at the time which coverage by the plan is being considered or has been adopted. It is important for individuals to understand what benefits their health plan or insurance provides. Unfortunately, benefit description documents are not the most compelling reading and the terminology used is formal and sufficiently abstract so as to make it incomprehensible to some readers. It is often when a benefit is accessed that the specifics of coverage, as well as its limitations, become clear to the consumer. Many of the following benefit categories are included in many coverage description documents:

- Eligibility for coverage requirements
- Administrative information regarding changes in status and life events
- Deductibles, coinsurance, and co-payment structure
- In- and out-of-network benefit levels
- Out-of-pocket expense limitations
- Hospital care
- Medical care
- Prescription drug
- Special high-cost care (e.g., organ transplantation)
- Emergency care, including transportation
- Maternity care
- Extended care (e.g., skilled nursing, home, hospice care)
- Wellness visits
- Healthy lifestyle benefits (e.g., gym membership, smoking cessation)
- Behavioral health and substance dependency care
- Preventive dental care
- Durable medical equipment
- Physical, occupational, and speech therapies
- Vision care
- Hearing care

It is important to note that this is not an exhaustive list of possible benefits. The case manager must examine the plan document specific to the patient in order to fully understand the available resources covered by their client's health plan.

RESOURCE MANAGEMENT

Resource management encompasses a diverse set of activities designed to influence the efficient and appropriate use of services. It represents the vehicle with which case managers attempt to match an individual's health care needs with the right level of care (Daniels & Ramey, 2005). Appropriate resource management is so essential to professional practice that it is included in several practice standards, the most common of which are outlined in Figure 15-1.

The four components of the resource management process are appropriateness of requested service/product, efficiency of delivery, effectiveness of service/product, and documentation of outcome. These components are discussed in Figure 15-2. Each component plays a part in ensuring that individual receive the right care, at the right time, in the right place, and in the right amount.

AVOIDABLE COST

Avoidable cost may be considered in two ways. The first is as the cost that occurs as a result of things done wrong or when unnecessary steps are applied in a process. This is as opposed to necessary costs which are needed to sustain a certain care standard (Cesta & Tahan, 2003). For example, an individual is readmitted to an acute hospital for congestive heart failure 10 days after discharge because prescriptions were not filled or not taken as prescribed. The cost generated by the second admission may be considered avoidable due to the failure in medication adherence.

A second way in which cost avoidance may viewed is the savings generated that are attributed to case manager intervention. For example, an 89-year-old patient is getting ready for discharge after a prolonged hospital stay following a stroke and hip fracture. The managed care case manager takes into account the deconditioned state of the individual and realizes he will not be able to tolerate an intense rehabilitation program, so recommends a stay at a skilled nursing facility versus an acute rehabilitation hospital. The avoided cost is the difference between the skilled facility and rehabilitation hospital daily charge. In this example, it is the case manager's understanding of the individual's current state of health, ability to withstand rigorous rehabilitation, authorization criteria, and existing benefits which leads to the recommendation, not that something necessarily was wrong with their health care.

COST-BENEFIT ANALYSIS

In order to justify or compare financial impact of goods and/or services, case managers are asked to provide documentation and rationale for various alternatives of care. This

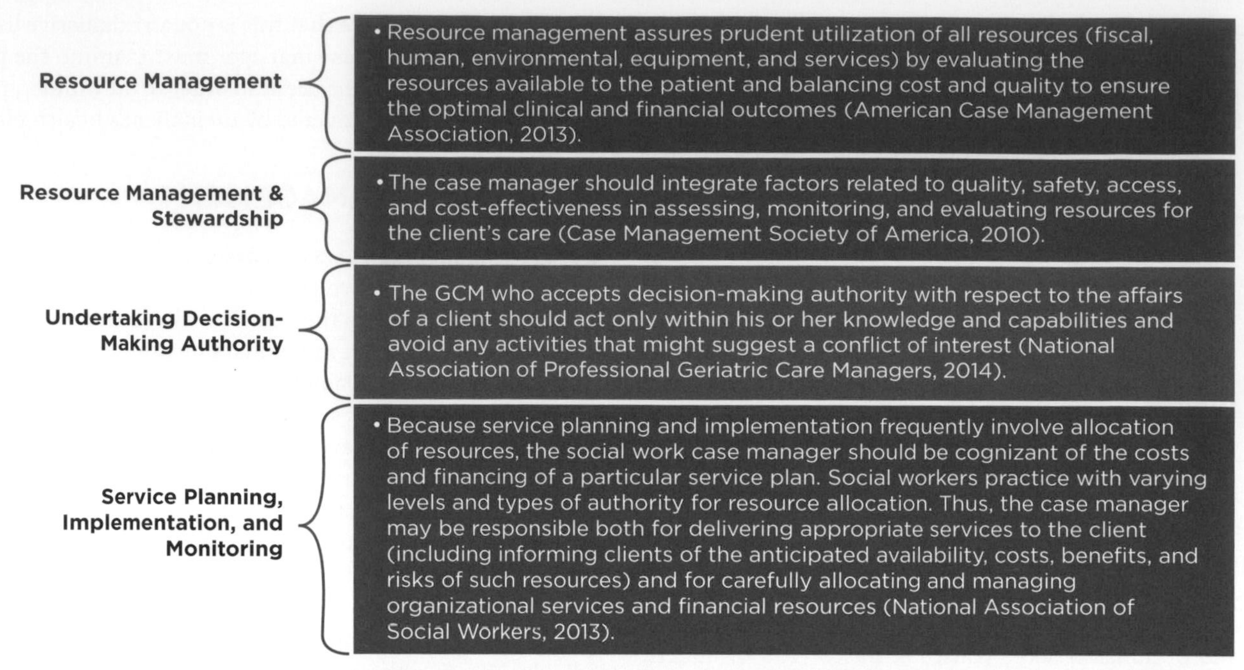

Figure 15-1. Resource management included in case management practice standards. (Adapted from American Case Management Association. (2013). *Standards of practice and scope of services for healthcare delivery system case management and transition of care professionals*. Retrieved April 25, 2013, from www.acmaweb.org/Standards; Case Management Society of America. (2010). *CMSA standards of practice for case management* (Rev.). Retrieved April 25, 2013, from http://www.cmsa.org/portals/0/pdf/memberonly/StandardsOfPractice.pdf; National Association of Professional Geriatric Care Managers. (2013). *Standards of practice*. Retrieved April 29, 2013, from http://www.caremanager.org/about/standards-of-practice; National Association of Social Workers. (2013). *NASW standards for social work case management*. Retrieved April 25, 2013, from http://www.socialworkers.org/practice/naswstandards/CaseManagementStandards2013.pdf)

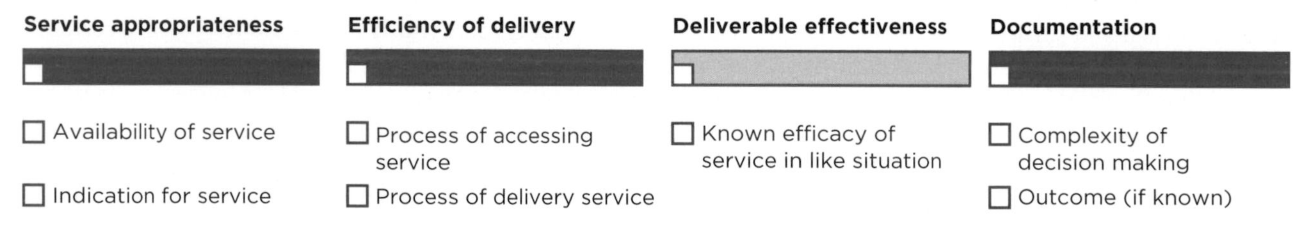

Figure 15-2. Resource management components. (Adapted from Daniels, S., & Ramey, M. (2005). *The leader's guide to hospital case management*. Sudbury, MA: Jones and Bartlett Learning.)

comparative analysis is often referred to as a **cost–benefit analysis** (Daniels & Ramey, 2005; Powell, 2000; Powell & Tahan, 2010). This approach is also used to quantify the benefit of case management services, or its return on investment, in organizations that continue to view case management as an expense versus an investment (Daniels & Ramey, 2005). Simply put, cost–benefit analysis answers the question—Is the program or service or product worth the expenditure (in dollars)?

If case management was solely about financial impact, cost–benefit analyses would focus strictly on dollars spent versus saved. However, case management has the potential to impact much more than the bottom line, so it is essential for each program to define itself by more than financial indicators. Calculation methodology and reporting should be built into the case management information system. In the absence of (or to verify) system-generated reports, the professional case manager must understand how to prepare clear and straightforward reports that demonstrate how a benefit to the individual justifies the expenditure. The following elements are standard inclusions in a cost–benefit statement, which applies to overall case management of an individual's care:

- Case identifier
- Summary of case management intervention
- Statement of case management fees (when applicable)
- Actual charges for health care products and services
- Itemization of all areas of case management intervention
- Areas in which case management intervention resulted in savings broken down by savings type (e.g., avoided cost, discounts, negotiated savings, reduced cost)
- Gross savings total
- Net savings total
- Case status and anticipated activity

Although case managers working in some care settings are not directly responsible for preparing cost–benefit reports, there may be situations in which a product or service expense is more than a particular benefit coverage or outside of benefit coverage altogether, also known as extra-contractual. In those situations, case managers may find it helpful to prepare a cost–benefit analysis comparing the various alternatives for care in order to demonstrate the value potential of the alternatives. Although a product may seems to cost more on face value, when other factors of importance are considered, the expenditure may be justified in order to reap longer-termed benefits. Box 15-1 provides examples of cost–benefit analyses.

BOX 15-1 Examples of Cost-Benefit Analysis

Request for Noncovered Benefit	Extending Length of Stay
Maynon is a 64-year-old widow who lives alone. Although generally healthy, her diagnosis profile includes type 2 diabetes, atrial fibrillation, rheumatoid arthritis, and significant osteoporosis. She experienced two falls in the bathroom over the past year while getting in and out of her shower, one resulting in compression fractures of lumbar vertebrae. Functionally independent and cognitively intact, Maynon refused transition to assisted living, preferring to remain in her two-bedroom ranch-style home of over 50 years. A home safety evaluation identified the benefit of having safety bars installed in the bathroom. Although a noncovered benefit, the medical home-based case manager submits an authorization request for strategically placed grab bars using the rationale that the expenditure is justified in order to allow Maynon to continue safe independent living and mitigate the risk of a catastrophic injury likely to require acute hospitalization, possible surgical intervention, long-term rehabilitation.	Carl is a 39-year-old married man diagnosed with acute myeloid leukemia who is ready for discharge home after undergoing a successful stem cell transplant. Although medically stable, one of his children was recently diagnosed with varicella, the other two are not yet symptomatic. Rather than expose him to this risk and possible implications of viral infection, the medical center case manager requests an extension of his length of stay until it is determined that his home environment is safe and family is clinically cleared as an infection risk.

Request	Benefit exception for installation of safety grab bars	**Request**	Length-of-stay extension
Benefit available	None	**Benefit available**	Per diem rate
Rationale	Risk mitigation, home safety	**Rationale**	Infection risk status post stem cell transplant
Cost of installation	$750 for safety bars and proper installation	**Cost of extension**	Range between $7,500–$15,000
Cost of potential injury	$45,000 for acute hospitalization and subsequent rehabilitation	**Cost of transplant failure**	Range between $100,000–$250,000

Justification for case management intervention:	There are situations in which the cost of case management intervention itself requires justification. When such is the case, all aspects of care being overseen by the case manager must be quantified and reported. The point is to clearly identify where case manager intervention resulted in an impact on the cost of care. The following is an example of such documentation.
File #:	Unique identifier of the individual
Employer/Group ID	Unique identifier of the group, if applicable
Case open date	Date on which case was opened
Case closure date	Date on which case was formally closed
Total case management time	Days of active case management
Rationale for case management	Brief synopsis regarding request for case management intervention
Diagnoses	List of active diagnoses
Cumulative case management fees	Accounting for case management fees broken down by time

(continued)

BOX 15-1 Examples of Cost-Benefit Analysis (*Continued*)

Summary of case facts	Client history pertinent to case management
Services in place at initiation of case management intervention	List of all services that were in place at the time the case management intervention was initiated
Products in place at initiation of case management intervention	List of all products that were in place at the time the case management intervention was initiated
Total cost of services & products in place at initiation of case management intervention	Total cost associated with all services and products in place at the time the case management intervention was initiated
Alternative services negotiated by case manager	List of all services which were negotiated to replace preexisting services
Alternative products negotiated by case manager	List of all products which were negotiated to replace preexisting products
New services negotiated by case manager	List of new services procured by case management, including negotiated savings
New products negotiated by case manager	List of new products procured by case management, including negotiated savings
Other avoided costs	Charges not previously accounted for that were avoided due to case management intervention
Total charges for "as is" products & services without case management intervention	The total cost of care, real or anticipated, without case management. Anticipated costs may include charges for patterns of care which were established prior to case management intervention. For instance, if the individual frequented the emergency department due to medication nonadherence, the projected cost of each visit could be included here.
Total charges for case manager-negotiated products and services	The total cost of care as negotiated or influenced by case management
Case management fees	The dollar total for case management fees
Net savings	Total charges for "as is" care minus total charges for case manager-negotiated care
Actual savings	Net savings minus case management fees
Summary of case management intervention	

UTILIZATION MANAGEMENT

There does not appear to be a universally agreed-upon definition of **utilization management** (UM). However, there are similarities across commonly accepted definitions. UM is used as an umbrella term most often applied to describe the combined activities of a payer to reduce the cost of medical utilization by decreasing the amount of unnecessary utilization and by managing the cost of utilization (Kongstvedt, 2013). It is a general term describing the entire process—including preadmission certification, concurrent review, and retrospective review used to evaluate health care on the basis of appropriateness, necessity, and quality (Dasco & Dasco, 1999). Although **utilization review** (UR) is a central element of UM, the activities of provider profiling, adoption of clinical practice guidelines, referral management, case management, and pharmaceutical access may be included within an organization's overall approach to UM. It is applied when describing the entirety of processes and techniques employed, not simply a particular review functions associated with administrative authorization processes. Although frequently associated with insurers and managed care organizations, aspects of UM are practiced in all care settings (Powell & Tahan, 2010) and include:

- Prospective and concurrent medical record review
- Medical necessity criteria application
- Resource utilization monitoring for appropriateness
- Transition planning
- Denial management
- Communication with members of the care team, including the consumer and her or his caregiver

UTILIZATION REVIEW

UR falls under the auspices of UM. It is a process in which medical review determinations are made based on clinical guidelines and structured processes. UR modalities use established criteria to evaluate medical services for necessity, level of care, quality, and timeliness (Sederer, 1987). UR is the process used by health insurers and health maintenance organizations (HMOs) to determine if coverage of a particular product or service is appropriate given the status and needs of the individual and based on a determination of medical necessity for the treatment and availability of effective alternatives (Kongstvedt, 2013).

The degree to which a case manager participates in various types of UR is driven by each organization and its use of job titles and job descriptions. However, in the payer sector, changes in the calculation methodology of the **medical loss ratio** (MLR) appear to have a direct impact on the responsibilities associated with job titles. This is discussed later in this chapter.

Types of UR activity include prospective review, concurrent review, and retrospective review.

Prospective review is conducted prior to service delivery. This includes preadmission certification in which the provider notifies the payer source of a proposed treatment and/or admission. Additional information required as part of the request process includes patient demographics, diagnosis, and proposed treatment (Dasco & Dasco, 1999). The payer's representative, usually a UR nurse or other health care professional with specific knowledge relating to the request, applies evidence-based medical necessity criteria to the provided information in order to determine if patient-specific situation meets medical necessity criteria. Precertification review is applied in situations of planned or anticipated admissions and when a high-cost medication, treatment, or piece of medical equipment is prescribed on a nonemergent basis. Examples of prospective review decision-making process is shown in Figures 15-3 and 15-4.

Concurrent review is part of monitoring that is performed during the course of treatment delivery. It involves evaluating whether the care being delivered continues to be medically necessary based on the individual's needs (Dasco & Dasco, 1999). A payer representative, usually a UR nurse, obtains a verbal or written report of care at specific intervals in order to apply criteria and determine the necessity of care at the requested level of service. When care is deemed unnecessary at the requested level, the payer issues a denial of payment. In the case of a hospital admission, the contractual arrangement between payer and institution defines the terms of concurrent review. In the situation where an acute facility is paid on a per diem basis, the severity of illness and intensity of treatment is evaluated each day to ensure

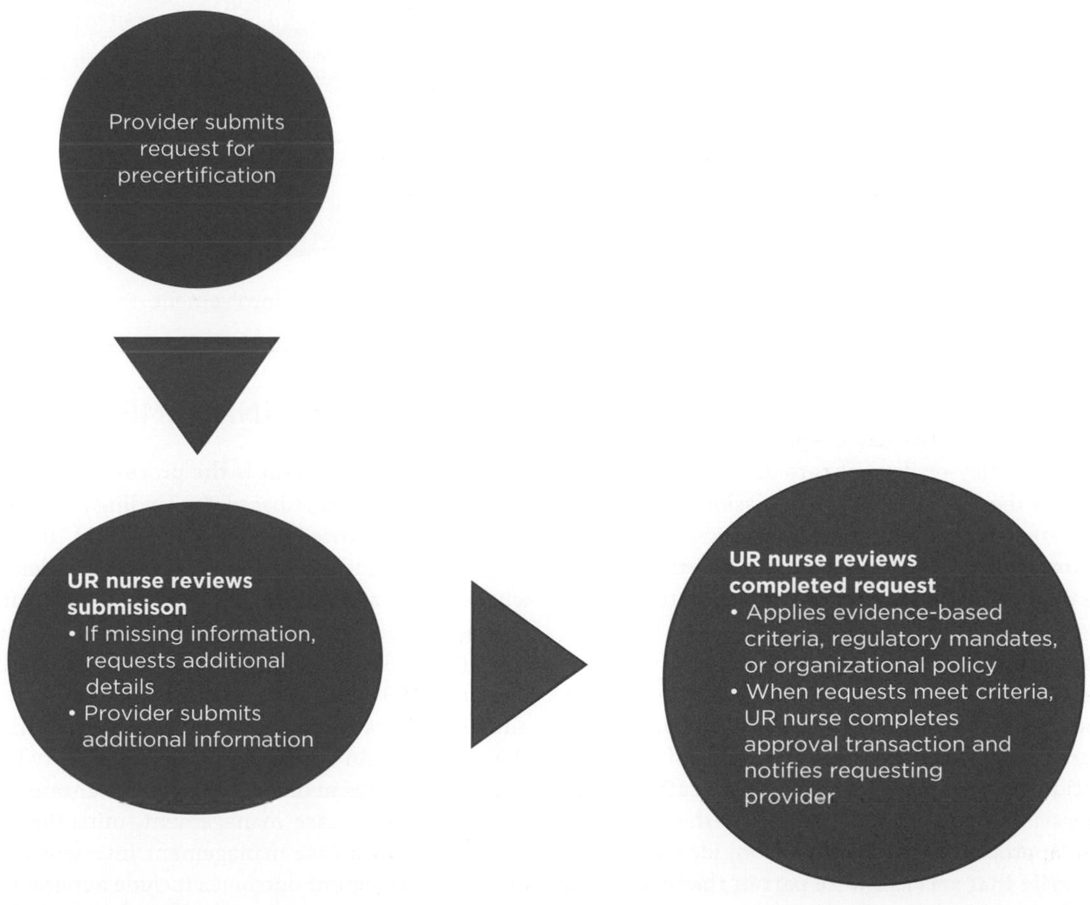

Figure 15-3. Prospective utilization review process flow—approval.

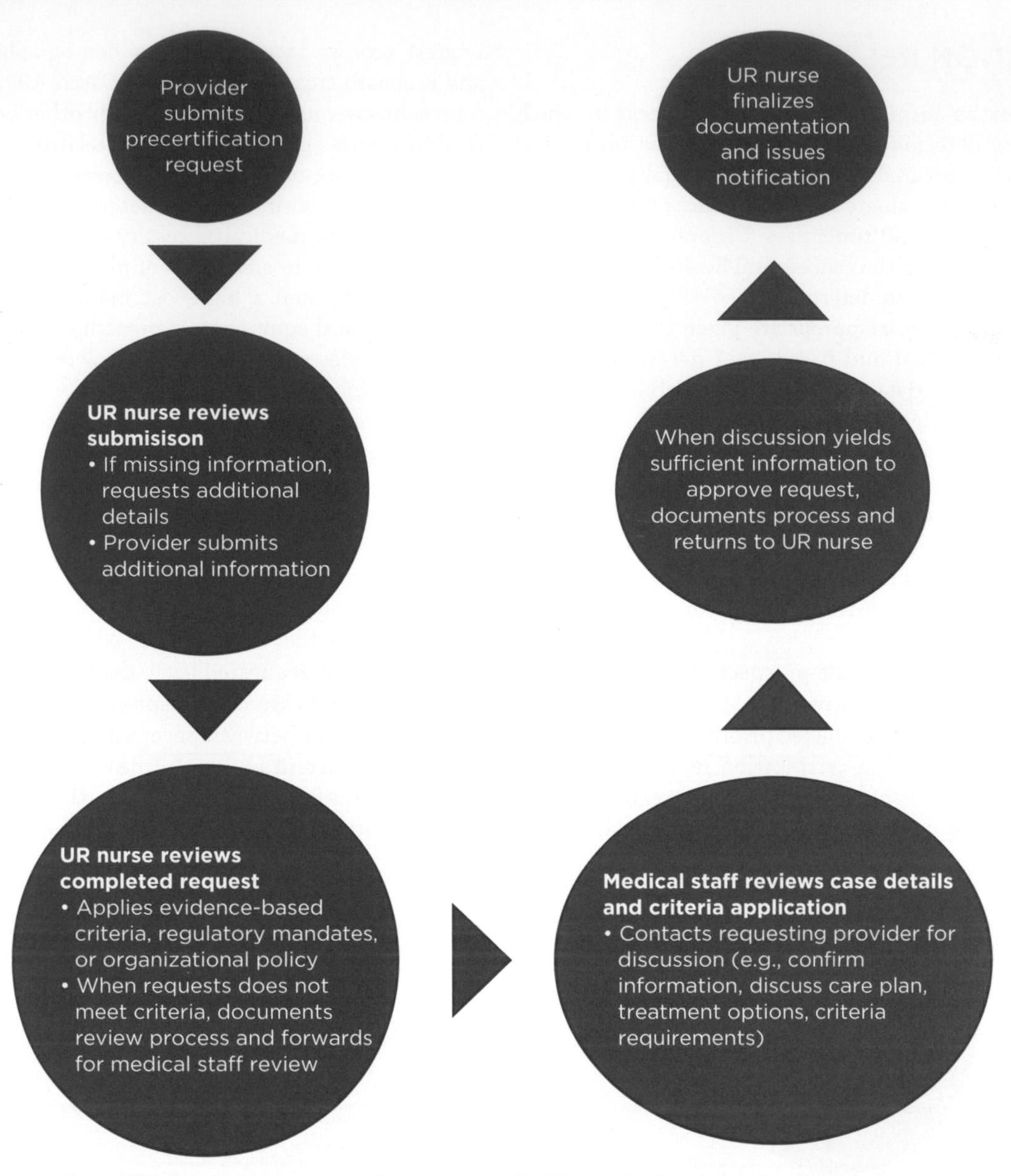

Figure 15-4. Prospective utilization review process flow—approval with medical reviewer involvement.

it meets established evidence-based criteria. When the level of service meets criteria, the day is approved. When it does not meet criteria, a day or days of care are denied and payment withheld at the time of claims submission. An example of when concurrent review technique is applied is in the case of emergent or urgent admissions when precertification is not possible due to the unexpected or sudden nature of the precipitating event. Figures 15-5 and 15-6 depict examples of a per diem concurrent review process.

Retrospective review involves analysis of data on hospital admissions, patterns of treatment, and utilization of certain procedures. It is often used to identify areas of over- and underutilization and/or cost (Dasco & Dasco, 1999). This review process is applied to determine whether provided services were appropriate to the admission, identify delays in care, and verify that services were part of the individual's covered benefit (Daniels & Ramey, 2005).

OUTCOMES MANAGEMENT

Outcomes management is the process of actively changing health care practices based on findings obtained through measurement procedures (Wojner, 2001). It has also been defined as a multidisciplinary health care delivery process whose goals are to provide quality health care, decrease fragmentation, enhance patient outcomes, and constrain costs (Moss & O'Connor, 1993). However, as pointed out by Nadzam (1997), it is not possible to manage an outcome in and of itself, rather one manages the process used to obtain the outcome and applies continuously quality improvement (CQI) techniques in order to obtain better outcomes.

As applies to case management, outcomes are measurable results of a case management intervention. Examples of case management outcomes include adherence to medication, improvement in quality of life, or satisfaction with case

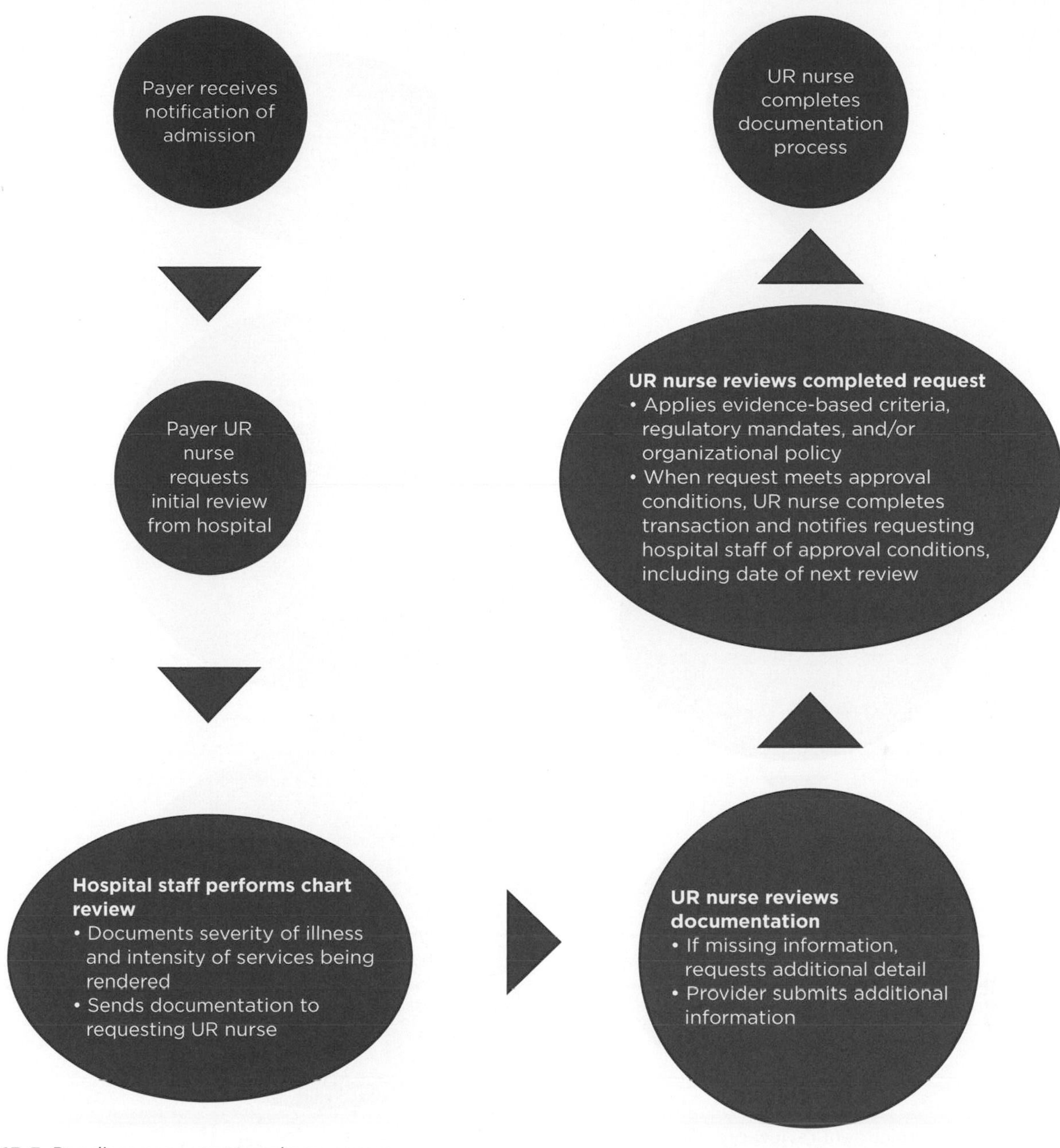

Figure 15-5. Per diem concurrent review process.

management services (Case Management Society of America [CMSA], 2010). Outcomes are discussed more in chapter 14.

Where this enters the equation of resource management and stewardship is in the process of service delivery, the case manager applies CQI principles to demonstrate adherence to the case management process in carrying out interventions, which are best suited to meet the client's health care needs. In the patient Maynon scenario, the case manager used evidence-based guidelines and medical appropriateness criteria to ensure the intensity of service met the severity of illness, thus promoted the best use of available resources. This lead to a better outcome for Maynon in that she was able to regain strength and endurance within the limitations of her physical abilities during the early part of her rehabilitation, contributing to a more robust recovery. As her physical tolerance improved she was able to more actively participate in subsequent therapy and avoid feeling defeated by having been placed in a program which had a more rigorous schedule than she was able to withstand. By managing the rehabilitation process, the case manager contributed toward better outcomes for the patient.

POPULATION HEALTH MANAGEMENT

A lookback at disease management is helpful for establishing the context of current population health management initiatives as they relate to case management. Originally referred to as disease management, the definition of population health management is consistent with the original definition of disease management offered by the Disease Management

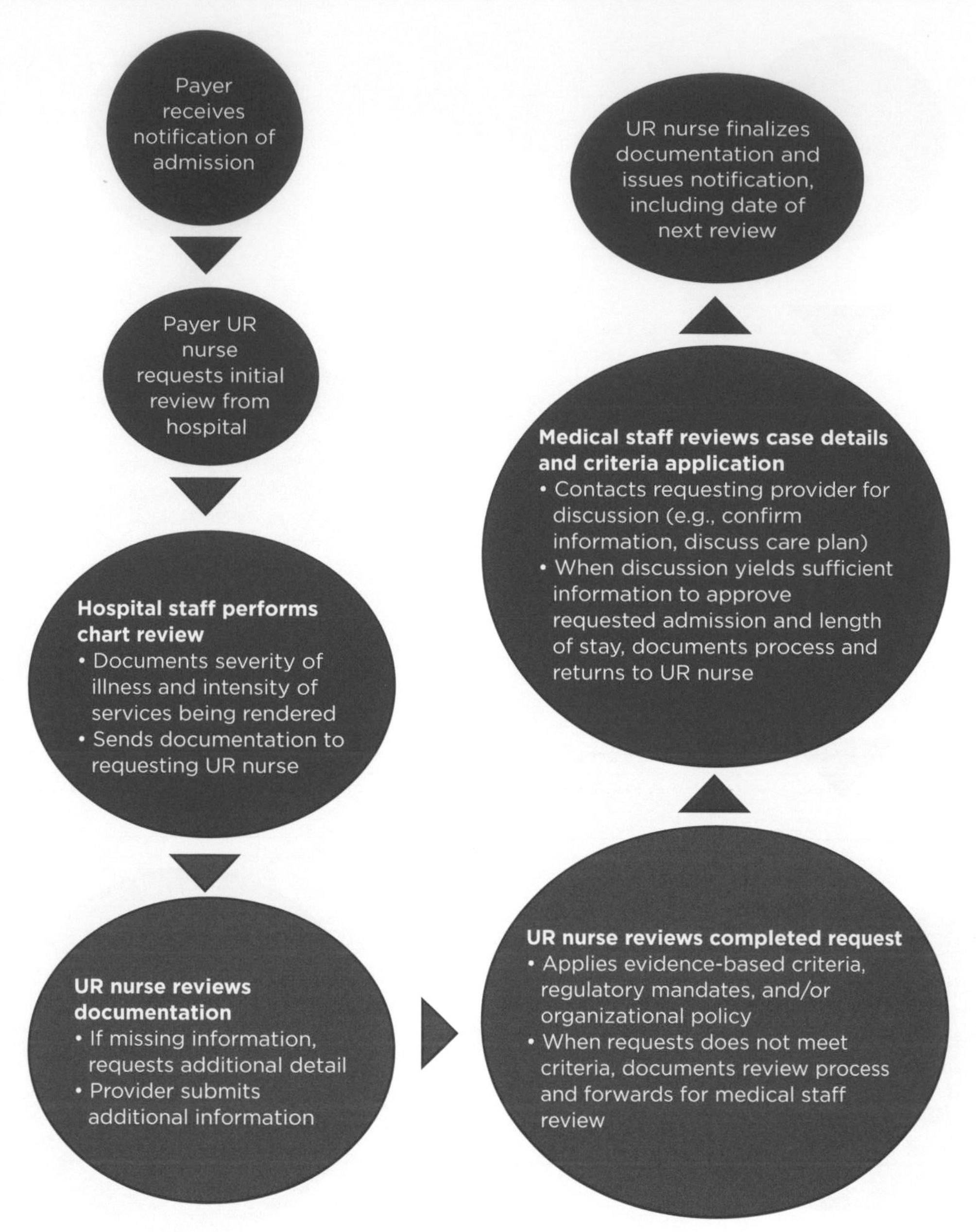

Figure 15-6. Per diem concurrent review process with medical reviewer involvement.

Association of America as "a system of coordinated health care interventions and communications for populations with conditions in which patient self-care efforts are significant." According to Population Health Alliance (2014) disease management supports the following:

- Supports the physician or practitioner–patient relationship and plan of care,
- Emphasizes prevention of exacerbations and complications using evidence-based practice guidelines and patient empowerment strategies, and
- Evaluates clinical, humanistic, and economic outcomes on an ongoing basis with the goal of improving overall health.

This definition has remained the same through the transformation from DMAA to the Care Continuum Alliance to the present-day Population Health Alliance.

The defined components of a disease management program (Population Health Alliance, 2014) also remain consistent as previously defined:

- Population identification processes;
- Evidence-based practice guidelines;
- Collaborative practice models to include physician and support-service providers;
- Patient self-management education (may include primary prevention, behavior modification programs, compliance/surveillance);
- Process and outcomes measurement, evaluation, and management; and
- Routine reporting/feedback loop (may include communication with patient, physician, health plan and ancillary providers, and practice profiling).

Although both case management and population health management seek the outcome of improved health status of the individual, case management involves an intensive focus on the individual relative to her or his overall health condition complexity, whereas population health management focuses on a particular disease or condition in context of an entire population versus an individual client (Huber, 2005). However, both interventions are important along the entire continuum of care.

The implication to a practicing case manager is mostly applicable to those working in or with managed care and third-party organizations offering condition-specific management programs (e.g., Health Dialogue, Healthways). Because of the difference in program purpose and previously identified confusion pertaining to job titles, the case manager should verify the responsibilities when working with someone in a population health management program. Understanding the scope of work and potential overlap in functions of all individuals involved in coordinating aspects of care for an individual will help avoid duplication of effort and potentially disadvantageous work situations.

CONTEXT FOR COLLABORATE RESOURCE AWARENESS

Understanding the shifting sand that underlays UM requires a lookback at the history of how health care finance has changed over the decades. Making the case for UM appears straightforward albeit a somewhat crooked path. Noted in the National Health Expenditures 2012 Highlights, in the fourth consecutive year of slow growth, health care spending in the United States has increased 3.7% to reach $2.8 trillion, or $8,915 per person. In 2012, the share of the economy devoted to health spending was 17.2% (Centers for Medicare and Medicaid, 2014a). In examining expenditure as a percentage of gross domestic product (GDP), in 1960 health care spending was 5.2%, in 1970 this rose to 7.2%, in 1980 it increased to 9.2%, in 1990 to 12.5%, and in 2000 health care costs were 13.8% of GDP (Figure 15-7).

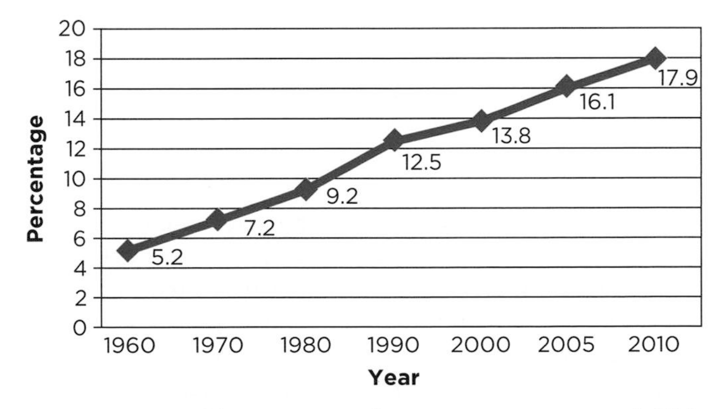

Figure 15-7. Health care expenditure as a percentage of GDP. (Adapted from data provided by the Centers for Medicare and Medicaid Services. (2014a). *National health expenditure highlights 2012*. Retrieved August 27, 2014, from http://www.cms.gov/Research-Statistics-Data-and-Systems/Statistics-Trends-and-Reports/NationalHealthExpendData/NationalHealthAccountsHistorical.html)

THE PROGRESSION OF UTILIZATION MANAGEMENT

The steady increase in health care spending made the case for risk mitigation strategies aimed at ensuring reasonable and appropriate resource allocation. Neither the practice nor the success of utilization control was uniform throughout the payer sector. However, the growth explosion of various payment models and the subsequent backlash created by inconsistency and overly restrictive policies made working conditions for clinical professionals who occupied utilization and case management positions more challenging.

Prior to the 1970s

Although all case managers are involved with the activities of UM, the degree to which this is true is outlined within each plan's case management program and job descriptions. The forebears of present-day UM go as far back as the 1800s when workers in charitable societies began validating the equitable distribution of services to avoid duplication, fraud, and misuse of limited resources (see chapter 1). This confirmation process continued as new areas of case management began to open up (e.g., Worker's Compensation, veteran's services, insurance companies). The importance of controlling expenditure of finite resources increased along with the cost of those resources.

In the 1960s, the creation of Medicare and Medicaid included requirements to monitor and control service distribution through the creation of hospital-based committees for the purpose of reviewing service appropriateness. This self-policing mandate was not regulated and each hospital was allowed to take a different approach to determinations of appropriateness (Starr, 1982). There were no consequences for discovery of inconsistencies, so the Social Security Amendments of 1972 introduced measures enacted to protect against utilization fraud and abuse, including the following:

1. Establishment of a peer review system through the use of organizations representing a substantial number of practicing physicians in local areas to be called Professional Standards Review Organizations (PSROs) (these organizations would assume responsibility for comprehensive and ongoing review of services provided under Medicare and Medicaid);
2. Establishment of an Office of Inspector General for Health Administration within the Department of Health, Education, and Welfare having the responsibility to review and audit Medicare and other health programs on a continuing and comprehensive basis and the authority to suspend any regulation, practice, or procedure employed in the administration of such programs, if he determines that the suspension will promote efficiency and economy of administration or that the regulation, practice, or procedure involved is contrary to or does not carry out the objectives and purposes of applicable provisions of law;

3. Provisions of conforming requirements for participation under Medicare and Medicaid of extended care facilities and skilled nursing homes;
4. Broadening of penalty provisions relating to the making of a false statement of representation of a material fact in any application for Medicare payments to include the soliciting, offering, or acceptance of kickbacks or bribes by providers of health care services; and
5. Establishment of a Provider Reimbursement Appeals Board to resolve disputes between providers and fiscal intermediaries concerning the amount of reasonable cost reimbursement (Ball, 1973).

Although the effectiveness of the PSRO structure was undecided, the end result was the institution of reliable infrastructure and data capacity (Kongstvedt, 2013). The PSROs transitioned to Peer Review Organizations (PROs) and subsequently came to be known as Quality Review Organizations (QROs) or **Quality Improvement Organizations** (QIOs). This progression and recognition of QIOs' work is discussed further in this chapter.

The 1970s to 1980s

The explosion of managed care in response to passage of the HMO Act of 1973 resulted in payment realignment from a fee-for-service (FFS) payment system, encouraging billing of more services to a capitation model, which paid a flat rate to primary care providers for each enrolled member regardless of the number of services rendered. UR processes required precertification for elective hospital admissions and concurrent review made an impact on reducing the length of inpatient stays. Procedures that were previously performed as inpatient admissions moved to the outpatient setting, thus reducing the cost of care. However, consumers and providers were increasingly concerned that quality of care was being compromised in favor of cost control (Sultz & Young, 2014).

By the early 1980s, Congress authorized Medicare to pay HMOs on a capitated payment basis with the passage of the Tax Equity and Fiscal Responsibility Act. In addition, Medicaid began transitioning from FFS to capitation with granting of the Arizona waiver, allowing capitation as the sole means of provider reimbursement rather than in addition to FFS methodology (Kongstvedt, 2013).

HMOs became a popular alternative to traditional, indemnity health plans because of the lower cost and perception of better benefits (e.g., preventative care, prescription drug coverage). This spurred carriers of traditional insurance and the Blues plans to begin including preventative services coverage in non-HMO products. These changes brought expanding job opportunities for nurses, social workers, and other health care professionals beyond the hospital and provider office settings. The advantages of working in the business environment included having a job that leveraged years of clinical knowledge and experience, the ability to positively impact health care beyond an individual patient-level, consistency in work days and hours (e.g., Monday through Friday, 9:00 a.m. to 5:00 p.m.), the absence of having to work weekends and holidays, and the reduction of physical stress relating to patient care. Nurses were especially employable in both UR and case management job types in both medical and behavioral health areas, social workers found more opportunities in behavioral health and social service plans, and physical/occupational therapists found opportunities in areas focusing on outpatient therapies and durable medical equipment.

An offshoot of the HMO, referred to as a Preferred Provider Organization (PPO), came about as a means of offering lower costs because of rate discounts offered to entities considered to be in-network. Initially a hospital discount, PPOs expanded to include providers and other vendors/suppliers. Generally, PPOs did not require assignment of a primary care provider and fee discounts applied as long as services were obtained through a provider within the established network. Consumers incurred a higher out-of-pocket expense when services were obtained from out-of-network providers, except in emergencies. PPOs continued precertification and concurrent review requirements to monitor inpatient admissions (Kongstvedt, 2013). Jobs similar to those found in HMOs became available; however, when PPOs were offered by the same payers who marketed HMO products, the same UM departments processed those requests. It was up to the individual worker to identify the insured's product type and manually modify the authorization processing rules applied to the request.

For all payer types, management of complex and catastrophically ill/injured individuals focused on utilization control and coordination of necessary services. Trigger diagnosis lists and claims analysis identified high-cost/high-utilization illnesses and injuries, prompting contact by a plan representative to screen eligibility for inclusion in case management. Conditions often included on trigger lists were certain cancers, premature births, strokes, and neuromuscular diseases. If screening demonstrated the possibility that an individual might benefit from case management, a comprehensive interview took place followed by development and implementation of a case management plan. Ostensibly, once the plan's objectives were met, individuals were transitioned out of case management. However, recurrence or exacerbation of serious illness could trigger another case management engagement.

Other forms of cost control undertaken by payers included institution of case rates and fixed reimbursement for services/admissions based on diagnostic groupings. In these situations, the onus of cost control shifted to the provider who was incented to reduce the length of stay in order to maximize the fixed payment amount. For example, a hospital was paid for an organ transplant admission at the same rate regardless of the length of stay. However, some contract terms often included situational modifiers affecting payment level when applicable. Consumers who qualified for case management often found themselves bouncing between a UR nurse and case manager depending on their condition and/or hospitalization status. In situations where the individual had behavioral health issues, the ping-pong effect became even more pronounced because the nature of the prevailing condition dictated which part of the insurance benefit was primarily responsible for monitoring. This constant change of payer staff challenged the formation of a solid, trusting relationship between payer case manager and consumer. It also resulted in frustration for case managers working on the provider side of care delivery because it was never clear they would be talking to the same case manager regarding a consumer's care.

The 1980s to 2000s

Managed care continued to expand with new product variants. The point-of-service plans resembled PPOs but with the added twist of naming a primary care provider who made in-plan referrals paid at full reimbursement rates. Cost-sharing responsibility arose when the individual sought care outside of the network or by seeking unauthorized care. This and other new plan types added to the administrative burden of benefit monitoring performed by those on the frontline of UM. Archaic computer systems, not designed for complex benefit manipulation or automation of utilization rules, necessitated development of manual workarounds and created pages of hard copy reference sheets. Unfortunately, this contributed to inconsistency and delays in the processing time for authorization requests.

Because of the cost-shift resulting from transition of inpatient to outpatient care, UM techniques were increasingly applied to care delivered in outpatient setting as well as to prescription medication, diagnostic testing, and specialty care (Kongstvedt, 2013). In addition, disease management programs rose in popularity. The rationale behind initial disease management initiatives was that many individuals with chronic conditions would become the uber-utilizers of tomorrow unless significant education and severity control measures were put into place earlier in the disease process. These new work areas resulted in hiring booms for health plans but also pulled existing human resources out of areas focusing on utilization and case management; some organizations added disease management functions to existing jobs. Although disease management mainly focused on education, workers also maintained knowledge of benefits and available resources in order to facilitate access to needed care and services.

Another development during this period was the passage of the Health Insurance Portability and Accountability Act (HIPAA) of 1996. This legislation was intended to place some controls on the growing uninsured population by extending health coverage beyond job loss or change, limiting preexisting condition clauses, and creating special enrollment clauses for specific changes in family composition or employment status (Sultz & Young, 2014). In addition, other parts of this legislation required transition to electronic/computerized medical records intended to reduce both cost and administrative burden. Ultimately, this requirement was not met. HIPAA also placed demands on institutions in maintaining the security of patient information, referred to as protected health information. The resulting regulations had a stifling effect not only on the sharing of patient information but also on the consistency of interpretation as to the requirements of regulations as to how information was protected and shared. Each provider defined their own internal process often within the boundaries of the technology that was in place and/or the type of information requests it most frequently received. Although simplification of administrative burden was a desired outcome of HIPAA, in many ways it overcomplicated the process of transferring medically necessary information needed to conduct the business of health care delivery. Many organizations used HIPAA as an excuse for not sharing information needed to perform review functions, causing further delays in UM processes.

2000 to the Present

The Medicare Modernization Act of 2001 added the significant benefit expansion of drug coverage in the form of Medicare Part D. Managed Medicare became known as Medicare Advantage, and reimbursement for services to managed plan enrollees increased over that which were made for services to Medicare FFS beneficiaries. Medicaid programs shifted to private management companies in order to close state budget gaps.

Employers dropped health coverage benefits or shifted the cost-sharing load to more out-of-pocket expense for the consumer through higher co-payments, tiered benefit structures, higher deductibles, and higher coinsurance. In response, there was a growing problem associated with the uninsured and underinsured shortfall accumulated by institutional providers. Public health care resources were dwindling which pushed social service responsibility toward private sector funding and faith-based charitable efforts. Case managers sought resources from a wider variety of sources, often building personal contact networks to reach out to when needed goods and services were not provided within the terms of an individual's coverage or that which were needed on a charitable basis. In some situations, case managers negotiated extra-contractual benefits in order to reduce the financial burden on their client. Although these arrangements were extremely valuable on a case-by-case basis, the practice of individual negotiation created greater variances in procured services. If an individual was fortunate to have a professional case manager skilled in negotiation, she or he reaped an additional benefit of receiving products or services, which a fellow enrollee-in-need may not obtain.

In addition, there were other influencers of health care cost, which included an aging multi-morbid population, increasingly expensive technology-based diagnostic and treatment options, the desire for more physically active longevity, the demand for treatment regardless of cost, less rigorous payor utilization control, and the rising administrative cost of care delivery (e.g., information technology, skilled labor force). Insurance coverage costs continued to rise and a larger proportion shifted to the employee. By 2013, the average annual worker contribution to health care had risen from $2,412 in 2003 to $4,565 (Kaiser Family Foundation, Health Research & Educational Trust, 2013).

Another development in the array of health care coverage options has been consumer-driven health care (CDHC). This iteration of health care financing is characterized by its defined contribution, as opposed to defined benefit, orientation. Employers contribute a specific dollar amount to an employee health account, often a personal health care account. The employee takes an active role in determining how these dollars are spent by understanding the cost of care at various providers. Common CDHC insurance products offer personal health care accounts, flexible benefit design, decision-support tools, plan options, and tiered coverage based on choice of provider. The case manager should consider these variances in health care coverage before making care recommendations because the consequences of out–of-pocket cost to the consumer can be substantial.

QUALITY IMPROVEMENT ORGANIZATIONS

QIOs are organizations staffed by doctors and other health care professionals who are trained to review medical care and help beneficiaries with complaints about the quality of care. In addition, QIOs are charged with implementing improvements in the quality of care (Steinman, 2014). Most often, QIOs are private, not-for-profit organizations.

As defined in Section 1152 of 42 U.S.C. 1320c–1, a QIO is an entity meeting the following requirements:

- Is able, as determined by the Secretary, to perform its functions under this part in a manner consistent with the efficient and effective administration of this part and title XVIII;
- Has at least one individual who is a representative of health care providers on its governing body; and
- Has at least one individual who is a representative of consumers on its governing body.

This amendment eliminated the previous titles of utilization and quality-control peer review, changing it to quality improvement organization for contracts entered into or renewed on or after January 1, 2012 (Social Security Administration, 2011).

The QIO program is one of the largest federal programs committed to improving health quality for Medicare beneficiaries. It is an essential ingredient of the U.S. Department of Health and Human Services' National Quality Strategy. The QIO mission is "to improve the effectiveness, efficiency, economy, and quality of services delivered to Medicare beneficiaries." QIO core functions are defined by statute as:

- Improving quality of care for beneficiaries;
- Protecting the integrity of the Medicare Trust Fund by ensuring that Medicare pays only for services and goods that are reasonable and necessary and that are provided in the most appropriate setting; and
- Protecting beneficiaries by expeditiously addressing individual complaints, such as beneficiary complaints; provider-based notice appeals; violations of the Emergency Medical Treatment and Labor Act; and other related responsibilities as articulated in QIO-related law.

(Centers for Medicare and Medicaid, 2014b)

In August 2014, the QIO program began a functional framework transformation, essentially splitting into two distinct areas. One group is slated to handle quality-of-care complaints, referred to as Beneficiary and Family Centered Care (BFCC)-QIOs. The first phase of the restructuring allows two BFCC-QIOs to perform the program's case review and monitoring activities. The contractors selected are Livanta LLC and KePRO. Their review scope is to ensure consistency in the review process with consideration of local factors of importance to beneficiaries.

The second group, referred to as Quality Innovation Network (QIN)-QIOs, will focus on working with providers and stakeholders to improve the quality of health care for targeted health conditions according to the 11th Statement of Work issued for comment in August 2014 (Centers for Medicare and Medicaid, 2014c). Table 15-1 identifies organizations selected as QIN-QIOs. The following are identified as QIN-QIO focus areas in this Statement of Work applicable from August 1, 2014 to July 31, 2019:

- Improving Cardiac Health and Reducing Cardiac Healthcare Disparities
- Reducing Disparities in Diabetes Care: Everyone With Diabetes Counts
- Improving Prevention Coordination Through Meaningful Use of HIT and Collaborating With Regional Extension Centers
- Reducing Healthcare-Associated Infections in Hospitals
- Reducing Healthcare-Acquired Conditions in Nursing Homes
- Coordination of Care
- Quality Improvement Through Value-Based Payment, Quality Reporting, and the Physician Feedback Reporting Program
- QIN-QIO-Proposed Projects That Advance Efforts for Better Care at Lower Cost
- Quality Improvement Initiatives

(Centers for Medicare and Medicaid, 2014d)

QIOs offer a variety of services including support with quality improvement, health information technology and electronic health records, patient-centered medical home, adult education, long-term care, patient safety, and health care quality reporting. A case manager may interact with a QIO when employed by a company doing business with or undergoing a review by the QIO. It may also be a career step for a case manager with quality improvement experience may qualify for quality or project coordination positions.

TABLE 15-1 QIN-QIOs and Coverage Areas

Organization	Coverage Area
Great Plains Quality Innovation Network	KS, ND, NE, SD
TMF	AR, MO, OK, TX
Lake Superior/Stratis	MN, WI, MI
Telligen	CO, IA, IL
HealthInsight	NM, NV, OR, UT
Georgia Medical Care Foundation	GA, NC
Qsource	AL, KY, MS, TN
Mountain-Pacific Quality Health Foundation	AK, HI, MT, WY
IPRO	DC, NY, SC
WVMI Quality Insights	DE, LA, NJ, PA, WV
VHQC	MD, VA
Qualis	ID, WA
Health Services Advisory Group	AZ, CA, FL, OH
HealthCentric Advisors	CT, MA, ME, NH, RI, VT
Contracts which are yet to be identified (as of July 18, 2104)	IN, Puerto Rico, and U.S. Virgin Islands

MEDICAL LOSS RATIO

There are implications to health plans for having case managers significantly involved in concurrent and retrospective review activities. This is related to the redefinition of MLR calculation in regulations issued subsequent to the Patient Protection and Affordable Care Act. MLR calculation is a health plan requirement in which each plan must submit data on the proportion of premium revenues spent on clinical and quality improvement activities versus administrative functions. Regulations require plans to spend at least 80% or 85% of collected premium dollars (dependent on group enrollment) on health care and quality improvement. If a plan fails to meet these standards, it is required to provide a rebate to their customers beginning in 2012 (Centers for Medicare and Medicaid, 2014e).

For purposes of MLR calculation, effective case management was identified as a patient-centered intervention, inclusive of activities including, but not limited to:

- Making/verifying appointments,
- Medication and care compliance activities,
- Arranging and managing care transitions from one setting to another (e.g., hospital to home),
- Programs supporting shared decision making, and
- Activities aimed to improve adherence with attending physician appointment, completing lab tests, or other appropriate contact with specific providers.

On the other end of the spectrum are activities classified as administrative functions which were excluded from being calculated as a health promotion or quality expense:

- All retrospective and concurrent utilization review,
- Some fraud prevention activities,
- Expenses relating to the development and execution of provider contracts,
- Fees associated with establishing or managing a provider network,
- Provider credentialing,
- Marketing expenses,
- Accreditation fees that are not directly related to specified activities,
- Costs associated with calculating and administering individual enrollee or employee incentives, and
- Functions or activities not expressly defined as included.

(National Association of Insurance Commissioners, 2011)

The case management implication concerns alignment of responsibilities within job descriptions. Jobs using the case manager title must be predominantly focused on the activities within the regulations recognized as health promotion and quality improvement in nature. The activities of concurrent and retrospective review are clearly excluded from this category. Therefore, positions focused on concurrent and retrospective review activities should not be described or titled as case management positions, especially within the payer sector.

DISCUSSION OF KEY ELEMENTS

Utilization Management

The resource-aware case manager considers all aspects of a situation when developing recommendations for accessing of available resources. Factors including quality, safety, access to care, and cost-effectiveness weigh into the assessment, implementation, monitoring, and evaluation of resources utilized in health care (CMSA, 2010). This is accomplished through consulting with the client and relevant care team members, understanding the medical necessity criteria being applied, and understanding the benefits offered by their client's health plan. In addition, the pros and cons associated with available options are evaluated prior to offering proposals for case management interventions.

The mindfulness of available resources and advocacy for their appropriate use focuses on what is in the best interest of the client in addressing her or his individual need rather than convenience or expedience. A case manager is expected to advocate for the patient while balancing the responsibility of stewardship for their organization and, in general, the judicial management of resources by using a defined review methodology and work collaboratively with colleagues in applicable practice settings (e.g., managed care, acute hospital, postacute facilities, community-level practices) to ensure appropriate utilization of resource (American Case Management Association [ACMA], 2013). The case manager's effort is on proactive avoidance of service denial through meticulous assessment and documentation of findings in order to meet or exceed criteria requirements. If a service denial occurs, the case manager conducts follow-up review to provide the clinical and circumstantial documentation to support a favorable outcome during the appeal process.

Effective UM takes a variety of factors into consideration. Figure 15-8 depicts the UM course of an inpatient admission. The approach of a professional case manager should be to interact with all other case managers across the care continuum as colleague rather than adversary. A case manager's overriding concern should be what is in the best interest of the client, based on her or his unique circumstances regardless of care setting. This is a unifying principle of practice and a cause to collaborate instead of to act in an obstructive or hostile manner. Boxes 15-2 and 15-3 provide glimpses into productive and unproductive interactions between hospital and managed care case managers. The tone of each encounters contributes to the respective outcomes, as well as to future interactions at the individual and organizational level.

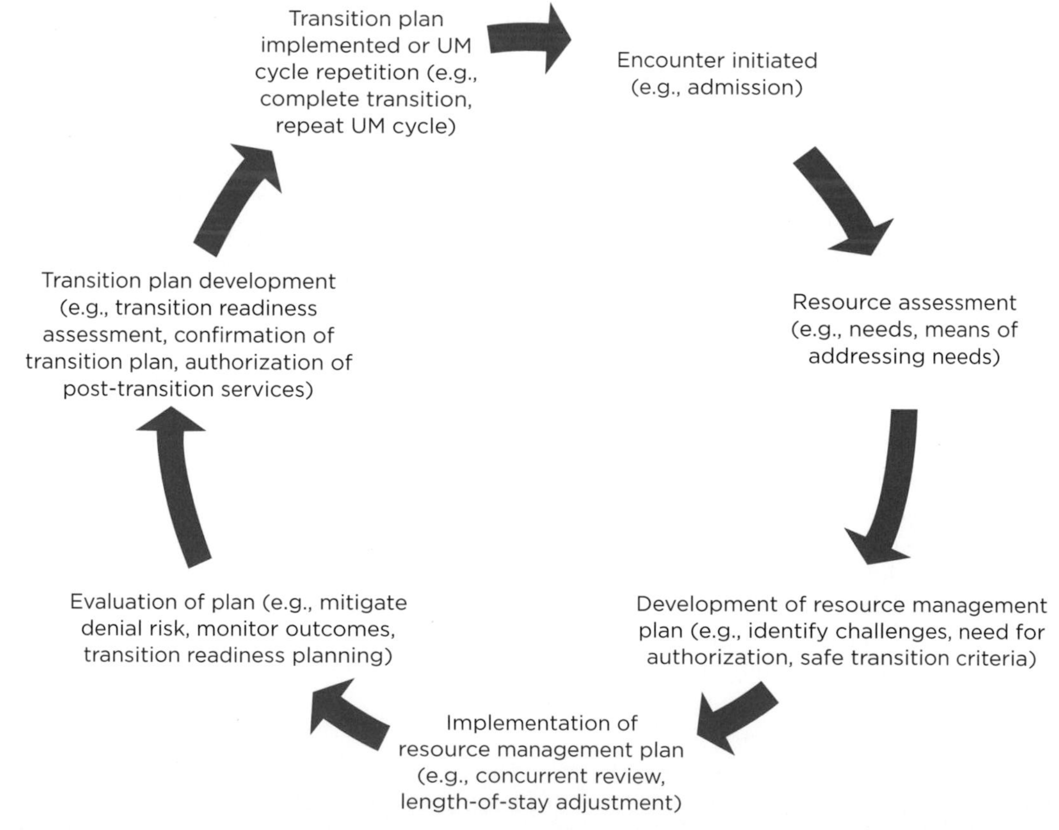

Figure 15-8. Utilization management considerations—inpatient admission scenario. (Adapted from Cesta, T. C., & Tahan, H. A. (2003). *The case manager's survival guide: Winning strategies for clinical practice* (2nd ed.). St. Louis, MO: Mosby.)

BOX 15-2 Productive Acute Care and Managed Care Case Manager Interaction

Maureen is a case manager at a large urban medical center. She has 15 years of experience in her current position after working in the community hospital as a staff nurse. She arrives to find that she must cover for a colleague who will not be in due to an elder parent's sudden illness. She collects information about the reviews that are due on her colleague's floor, a 30-bed surgical unit, and then heads off to her usual 45-bed medical floor.

She attends patient rounds and learns of three new admissions from the previous night, adding those to her growing list of reviews. She completes and submits concurrent reviews for those that are due, including illness intensity details (e.g., vital signs, test results, mental status) and treatment intensity information (e.g., diagnostic tests, treatments) for each day of stay. She also notes anticipated discharge dates and service needs. Of the five patients anticipated to be going home, four do not need services, but later that day it was decided that one would benefit from short-term visiting nurse services due to her difficulty with dressing changes and lack of consistent caregiver support. Maureen checks in with the patient to see if she has a preferred agency. Before leaving for her colleague's unit, she reaches out to the payer case manager to let him know of the change in plan, noting that the requested postacute services will help avoid a delay in discharge and possible readmission due to the patient's difficulty following the dressing change procedure.

The payer case manager, Ben, begins his day by validating receipt of concurrent reviews, completing updates in the information system and triggering extension of stay communication back to the facility. He includes the date of next review for each individual, adding a note on one patient who is stabilizing and appears to be ready for discharge tomorrow. Because he is responsible for all types of authorizations, he also lets Maureen know that the visiting nurse authorization was approved.

Maureen is now completing reviews on her colleague's unit when she receives Ben's voicemail regarding the approval for visiting nurse services. She calls the patient's nurse who notifies the patient that her return home is taking place as planned.

Maureen returns to completing concurrent reviews and transition plans. She notes that two patients require transfer to other facilities for short-term rehabilitation and that both appear to qualify for acute rehabilitation placement. However, one lives quite a distance from either of the available rehabilitation hospitals, so she visits with him to see if there are facilities closer to home that he prefers. On calling the patient's wife, it is agreed that it would better for him to be closer to home, so address and contact information for three facilities is given to the patient's wife who agrees to tour each and let Maureen know of her preference the next day.

She initiates evaluations with the three skilled nursing facilities and includes the facilities by name in her concurrent review updates. Maureen includes her contact information with each review, noting that her colleague is off for the day. She also checks and responds to messages left on her colleague's voicemail throughout the day.

BOX 15-3 Unproductive Acute Care and Managed Care Case Manager Interaction

Cheryl works at a 250-bed community hospital outside of Sacramento. She is responsible for utilization review on three medical-surgical units with a total bed capacity of 76. On Tuesday, she notes that 25 concurrent updates and 10 new admission reviews are needed. She knows that the main payers use two different criteria sets for medical necessity reviews.

She begins to review new patients and jots down the pertinent clinical history for each including vital signs on admission and each patient's current condition. She notes the services being provided (e.g., intravenous fluids, oxygen, medications) as well as anticipated disposition. She also gathers information for updates on previously admitted patients. In the afternoon, she transfers her notations to the clinical documentation system and submits each to the appropriate payer for review. Some reports are required to be faxed manually which the administrative office staff are responsible for sending.

Reviews are received and reviewed at the various payer offices. Of the 25 concurrent reviews, 15 receive continued approval but 10 are returned requesting information pertinent to each day of stay. Cheryl returns to the respective medical records to gather the details, reenter these into the clinical documentation system. She must fax additional review details to two payers because administrative staff leave at 3:00 P.M.

Cheryl grows increasingly frustrated with the administrative burden of review work. She "thinks" that she sent sufficient information for continued approvals. Unfortunately, she did not verify the criteria being applied by each payer to clearly understand the information required to demonstrate medical necessity. She did not provide anticipated transition plans on every patient nor details regarding their clinical status (e.g., vital signs, laboratory results) or treatment intensity for each day of stay as required by the hospital's contract with the payer.

Over time, she comes to believe that one particular managed care organization is being purposefully adversarial toward her because they do not authorize admissions or continued stays for at least half of her reviews. Instead of calling the reviewer directly to communicate details, she continues to send what she believes to be sufficient review details which ultimately result in denials due to lack of information. This has a downstream impact because of the additional expense relating to retrieval and copying medical records for appeal submissions.

The professional case manager focuses on communication and collaboration with all payers to conduct administrative tasks, such as medical necessity reviews, in the most efficient and business-like manner. The importance of this approach is validated in various practice standards including those issued by the CMSA and the ACMA.

Condition/Population Specific

The resource-aware case manager maintains current knowledge of health conditions, cultural influences, and community resources in order to prepare a realistic and responsible case management plan that meets the client's individual needs. Participation and/or coordination with population health management programs (also referred to as disease management) is of extreme importance due to the considerable overlap potential relating to the interest of both interventions in improving care coordination, access to necessary services, and better health outcomes for the client (Huber, 2005).

The COLLABORATE perspective is highlighted when a client diagnosed with chronic obstructive pulmonary disease is ready for hospital discharge following an acute exacerbation. The client's primary care provider prefers that his patient returns home and returns to her outpatient pulmonary clinic, which includes condition-specific educational sessions and clinic-based case management services. Although the condition-specific education sessions would not start for a few weeks after returning home, in discussing options with the client, the hospital case manager learns that there is a challenge with reliable transportation resources and a concern that once back to work, he would not be able to get time off to attend clinic sessions. Further conversation with care team members reveal that education sessions are offered in both day and evening sessions. In addition, transportation is available through a number of resources, which simply require a little advance planning for the patient in order to arrange. Through the effort of a couple extra telephone calls, the case manager addresses the patient's condition-specific education needs as well as a transportation barrier to care access.

In the COLLABORATE paradigm, population-specific care also encompasses practicing with cultural and linguistic competence. As pointed out by Lipson and Dibble (2005), health care providers cannot provide good care without assessing both cultural group patterns and individual variations within a cultural group. This requires partnering in trust-based, respectful, and responsible ways between providers, patients, families, and communities.

Definition of culturally competent care is often related to one's professional credential and/or certification. The National Association of Social Workers (NASW) issued standalone practice standards for cultural competence in 2001. The American Nurses Association addresses cultural issues throughout their Code of Ethics statement (2001), and guidelines for culturally competent nursing care have been published in the Journal of Transcultural Nursing (refer to Table 15-2). As applies to case management, CMSA highlights the importance of cultural competence as a standalone practice standard of cultural competence, the NASW's (2013) standards for case management practice highlight cultural and linguistic competence in Standard 4, and the ACMA embeds the topic within their advocacy standard. Regardless of the standard or position statement one follows, the professional case manager explores relevant cultural education in order to understand important issues relating to her or his client and includes an assessment of linguistic preferences and resources available to optimize communication and educational efforts in all health care matters. Although organizations develop internal assessment tools, Box 15-4 contains sample questions developed by the University of Michigan Medical School to assess cultural and linguistic issues which may arise during an health care encounter. The important point is to provide evidence in the form of documentation that cultural and linguistic needs were assessed, identified, and taken into account as part of the case management engagement.

Management of Expectations (per Setting of Care)

The resource-aware case manager understands that setting and managing client expectations from the point of initial contact facilitates subsequent interactions. It also contributes to building a trust-based relationship relative to over-promising to deliver something when it is unclear whether or not the individual qualifies for it. The best way in which the professional case management accomplishes expectation management is through ensuring her or his own understanding of situational complexity and the reasonably anticipated factors involved. By framing expectations within what is known, the dynamic establishes clear, accurate, and objective communication.

When the case manager fails to manage expectations, she or he risks a poor outcome, including, but not limited to, low client satisfaction and avoidable delays in care. An example of this is transition of care situations where the level of care that a patient qualifies for is in question. Box 15-5 provides a scenario where failure to set a reasonable expectations resulted in unnecessary frustration and a delay in transfer date. Ultimately, a poor match, which does not balance the patient's condition and abilities to the receiving facility's level of care, sets the stage of forcing a suboptimal choice for location of care. This places the patient at risk for deterioration of her or his health condition and possible readmission.

It is inappropriate for a case manager to foster client expectations that health insurance covers all products and services, but rather he or she should take the time to assess the client's understanding of their health care coverage as part of the assessment of health literacy. Where gaps in knowledge is existing, explaining health plan benefits and reassessing understanding is helpful. In addition, the professional case manager should critically analyze individual situations in order to identify available alternatives. This analysis supports

TABLE 15-2 Guidelines for the Practice of Culturally Competent Nursing Care

Guideline	Description
1. Knowledge of Cultures	Nurses shall gain an understanding of the perspectives, traditions, values, practices, and family systems of culturally diverse individuals, families, communities, and populations they care for, as well as knowledge of the complex variables that affect the achievement of health and well-being.
2. Education and Training in Culturally Competent Care	Nurses shall be educationally prepared to provide culturally congruent health care. Knowledge and skills necessary for assuring that nursing care is culturally congruent shall be included in global health care agendas that mandate formal education and clinical training, as well as required ongoing, continuing education for all practicing nurses.
3. Critical Reflection	Nurses shall engage in critical reflection of their own values, beliefs, and cultural heritage in order to have an awareness of how these qualities and issues can impact culturally congruent nursing care.
4. Cross-Cultural Communication	Nurses shall use culturally competent verbal and nonverbal communication skills to identify client's values, beliefs, practices, perceptions, and unique health care needs.
5. Culturally Competent Practice	Nurses shall utilize cross-cultural knowledge and culturally sensitive skills in implementing culturally congruent nursing care.
6. Cultural Competence in Health Care Systems and Organizations	Health care organizations should provide the structure and resources necessary to evaluate and meet the cultural and language needs of their diverse clients.
7. Patient Advocacy and Empowerment	Nurses shall recognize the effect of health care policies, delivery systems, and resources on their patient populations, and shall empower and advocate for their patients as indicated. Nurses shall advocate for the inclusion of their patient's cultural beliefs and practices in all dimensions of their health care.
8. Multicultural Workforce	Nurses shall actively engage in the effort to ensure a multicultural workforce in health care settings. One measure to achieve a multicultural workforce is through strengthening of recruitment and retention efforts in the hospitals, clinics, and academic settings.
9. Cross-Cultural Leadership	Nurses shall have the ability to influence individuals, groups, and systems to achieve outcomes of culturally competent care for diverse populations. Nurses shall have the knowledge and skills to work with public and private organizations, professional associations, and communities to establish policies and guidelines for comprehensive implementation and evaluation of culturally competent care.
10. Evidence-Based Practice and Research	Nurses shall base their practice on interventions that have been systematically tested and shown to be the most effective for the culturally diverse populations that they serve. In areas where there is a lack of evidence of efficacy, nurse researchers shall investigate and test interventions that may be the most effective in reducing the disparities in health outcomes.

Adapted from Douglas, M. K., Rosenkoetter, M., Pacquiao, D. F., Callister, L. C., Hattar-Pollara, M., Lauderdale, J., ... Purnell, L. (2014). Guidelines for implementing culturally competent nursing care. Journal of Transcultural Nursing, 25(2), 109–121. doi:10.1177/1043659614520998. Retrieved September 2, 2014 from tcn.sagepub.com at Apollo Group – UOP.

effective advocacy. Failure to take a methodical approach often leads to a number of unnecessary and unproductive dynamics in care transitions such as the following:

- Client disappointment and frustration
- Perception of good versus bad care providers
- Pitting the client and requesting case managers against the health plan case manager

Advocacy, on behalf of a client, for a product or service that is not covered by health insurance is a function of case management. However, this is best approached by the case manager who is knowledgeable about the patient, understands the desired product or service, considers the available evidence to support using the desired product or service, and able to articulate the benefit(s) and risk(s) clearly and concisely as part of her or his benefit exception request.

CASE MANAGEMENT PRACTICE IMPLICATIONS

It is within the case manager's sphere of responsibility to request, review, authorize, and coordinate resources as part of their overall of addressing an individual's comprehensive

BOX 15-4 Examples of Cultural Assessment Questions

So that I might be aware of and respect your cultural beliefs,

Can you tell me what languages are spoken in your home and the languages that you understand and speak?

Please describe your usual diet. Also, are there times during the year when you change your diet in celebration of religious and other ethnic holidays?

Can you tell me about beliefs and practices including special events such as birth, marriage, and death that you feel I should know?

Can you tell me about your experiences with health care providers in your native country?

How often each year did you see a health care provider before you arrived in the United States?

Have you noticed any differences between the type of care you received in your native country and the type you receive here? If yes, could you tell me about those differences?

Is there anything else you would like to know?

Do you have any questions for me? (Encourage two-way communication.)

Do you use any traditional health remedies to improve your health?

Is there someone, in addition to yourself, with whom you want us to discuss your medical condition?

Are there certain health care procedures and tests which your culture prohibits?

Are there any other cultural considerations I should know about to serve your health needs?

Adapted from University of Michigan Medical School's Cultural Competence for Clinicians. http://www.med.umich.edu/pteducation/cultcomp.htm

BOX 15-5 Expectation Setting Leading to an Effective, Collaborative Care Transition

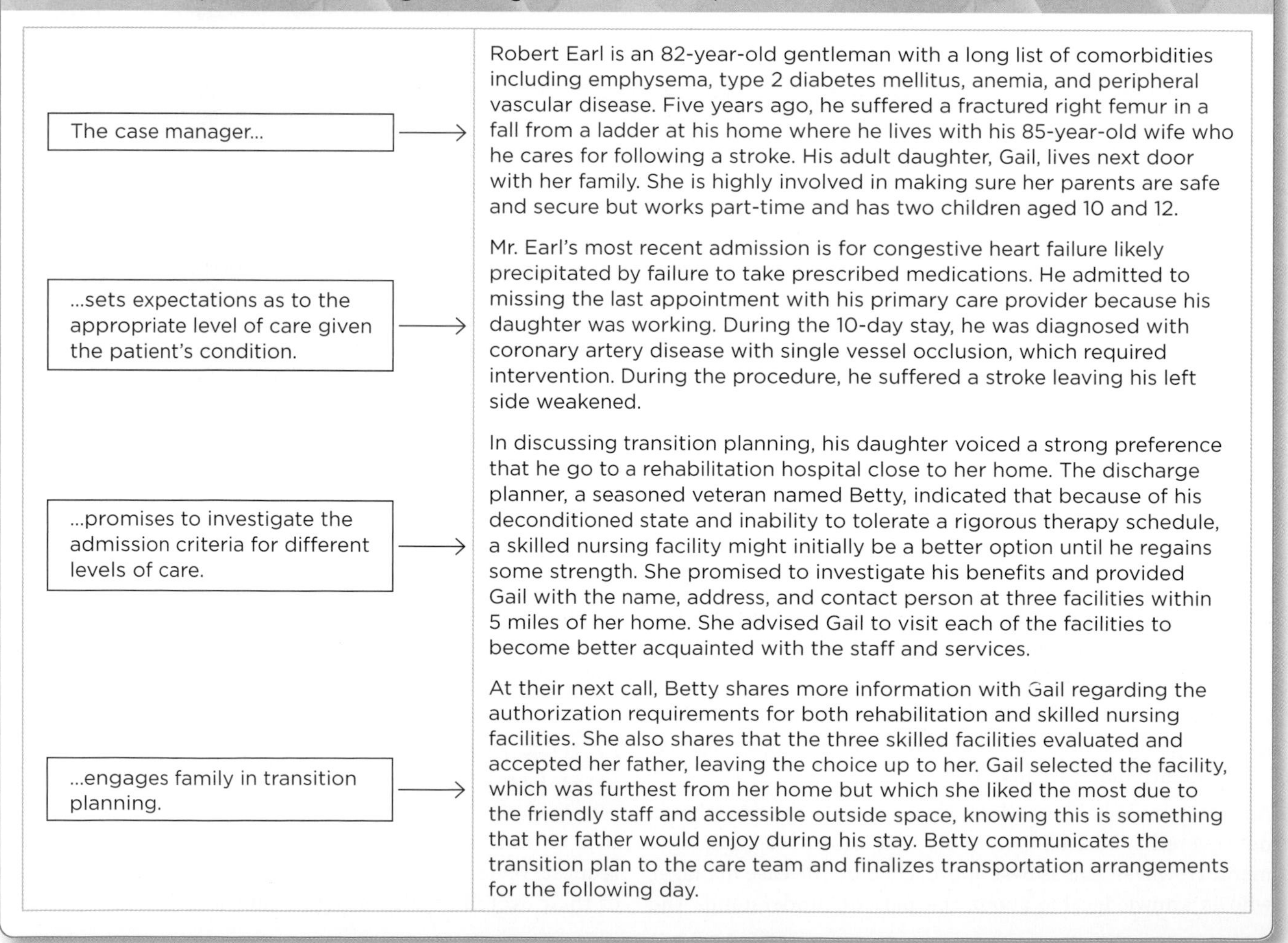

The case manager... →	Robert Earl is an 82-year-old gentleman with a long list of comorbidities including emphysema, type 2 diabetes mellitus, anemia, and peripheral vascular disease. Five years ago, he suffered a fractured right femur in a fall from a ladder at his home where he lives with his 85-year-old wife who he cares for following a stroke. His adult daughter, Gail, lives next door with her family. She is highly involved in making sure her parents are safe and secure but works part-time and has two children aged 10 and 12.
...sets expectations as to the appropriate level of care given the patient's condition. →	Mr. Earl's most recent admission is for congestive heart failure likely precipitated by failure to take prescribed medications. He admitted to missing the last appointment with his primary care provider because his daughter was working. During the 10-day stay, he was diagnosed with coronary artery disease with single vessel occlusion, which required intervention. During the procedure, he suffered a stroke leaving his left side weakened.
...promises to investigate the admission criteria for different levels of care. →	In discussing transition planning, his daughter voiced a strong preference that he go to a rehabilitation hospital close to her home. The discharge planner, a seasoned veteran named Betty, indicated that because of his deconditioned state and inability to tolerate a rigorous therapy schedule, a skilled nursing facility might initially be a better option until he regains some strength. She promised to investigate his benefits and provided Gail with the name, address, and contact person at three facilities within 5 miles of her home. She advised Gail to visit each of the facilities to become better acquainted with the staff and services.
...engages family in transition planning. →	At their next call, Betty shares more information with Gail regarding the authorization requirements for both rehabilitation and skilled nursing facilities. She also shares that the three skilled facilities evaluated and accepted her father, leaving the choice up to her. Gail selected the facility, which was furthest from her home but which she liked the most due to the friendly staff and accessible outside space, knowing this is something that her father would enjoy during his stay. Betty communicates the transition plan to the care team and finalizes transportation arrangements for the following day.

needs to achieving maximum health and wellness. Without fluent knowledge about resources and how best to access and manage them, the case manager fails in providing quality health care service to her or his client.

The professional case manager must document her or his effort regarding appropriate resource management. This includes noting the evaluation of quality, options, safety, risks, and benefits while aligning evidence-based findings with the client's desired goals. When resources are scarce, the case manager brings value to the care team through sharing knowledge of available resources. This skill is especially helpful when working with emotionally fragile caregivers who are coming to grips with a loved one's condition. Their interpretation of the situation often contributes to unrealistic demands. The case manager takes a thoughtful, sensitive approach to communication, incorporating a culturally and linguistically appropriate manner to support the client and caregiver through a challenging period.

As important as it is for each case manager to pursue personal knowledge, it is critically important that the experienced case manager takes the time to share knowledge regarding resources with individuals new to the workforce. Hoarding information or acting as if one has been inconvenienced by a peer inquiry perpetuates a perception that case managers are difficult to work with or lack the desire to mentor those newer to the role.

SUMMARY

Effective resource management is inextricably bonded case management practice. Understanding evidence-based criteria, health plan benefits, client and caregiver strengths, and community resources requires ongoing investigation and validation of previous knowledge. The professional case manager promotes evidence-based care through responsible use of health care services and financial resources to meet the client's needs in order to support the achievement of optimal health and wellness.

References

American Case Management Association. (2013). *Standards of practice and scope of services for healthcare delivery system case management and transition of care professionals*. Retrieved April 25, 2013, from www.acmaweb.org/Standards

Ball, R. M. (1973). Social security amendments of 1972: Summary and legislative history. *Social Security Bulletin, 36*(3), 3–25.

Case Management Society of America. (2010). *CMSA standards of practice for case management* (Rev.). Retrieved April 25, 2013, from http://www.cmsa.org/portals/0/pdf/memberonly/StandardsOfPractice.pdf

Centers for Medicare and Medicaid. (2014a). *National health expenditure highlights 2012*. Retrieved August 27, 2014, from http://www.cms.gov/Research-Statistics-Data-and-Systems/Statistics-Trends-and-Reports/NationalHealthExpendData/NationalHealthAccountsHistorical.html

Centers for Medicare and Medicaid. (2014b). *Quality improvement organizations*. Retrieved August 29, 2014, from http://www.cms.gov/Medicare/Quality-Initiatives-Patient-Assessment-Instruments/QualityImprove mentOrgs/index.html?redirect=/qualityimprovementorgs

Centers for Medicare and Medicaid Services. (2014c). *QIO news special focus on QIO program transformation*. Retrieved August 29, 2014, from http://www.qionews.org/sites/default/files/pdf/QIONews_JULY2014_508.pdf

Centers for Medicare and Medicaid Services. (2014d). *Quality innovation network quality improvement organization scope of work. task order no. 001: Excellence in operations and quality improvement*. Retrieved August 31, 2014, from www.nahc.org/assets/1/7/QIN-QIO_Task_Order_001.docx

Centers for Medicare and Medicaid. (2014e). *Medical loss ratio*. Retrieved August 31, 2014, from http://www.cms.gov/CCIIO/Programs-and-Initiatives/Health-Insurance-Market-Reforms/Medical-Loss-Ratio.html

Cesta, T. C., & Tahan, H. A. (2003). *The case manager's survival guide: Winning strategies for clinical practice* (2nd ed.). St. Louis, MO: Mosby.

Daniels, S., & Ramey, M. (2005). *The leader's guide to hospital case management*. Sudbury, MA: Jones and Bartlett Learning.

Dasco, S. T., & Dasco, C. C. (1999). *Managed care answer book* (3rd ed.). Gaithersburg, NY: Aspen.

Fisher, E. S., Wennberg, D. E., Stukel, T. A., Gottlieb, D. J., & Lucas, F. L. (2003). The implications of regional variations in Medicare spending. Part 2: Health outcomes and satisfaction with care. *Annals of Internal Medicine, 18*(138), 288–298.

Huber, D. L. (2005). *Disease management: A guide for case managers*. St. Louis, MO: Elsevier Saunders.

Kaiser Family Foundation, & Health Research & Educational Trust. (2013). *Survey of employer-sponsored health benefits*. Retrieved August 20, 2014, from http://kaiserfamilyfoundation.files.wordpress.com/2013/08/8465-employer-health-benefits-20132.pdf

Kongstvedt, P. R. (2013). *Essentials of managed health care* (6th ed.). Sudbury, MA: Jones and Bartlett.

Lipson, J. G., & Dibble, S. L. (2005). *Culture & clinical care* (8th ed.). San Francisco, CA: UCSF Nursing Press.

Moss, M. T., and O'Connor, S. (1993). Outcomes management in perioperative services. *Nursing Economics, 11*(6), 364–369.

Nadzam, D. M. (1997). *Nurses and the measurement of health care: An overview. In Nursing practice and outcomes management*. Oakbrook Terrace, IL: The Joint Commission.

National Association of Insurance Commissioners. (2011). *Recommendations to DHHS Secretary Sebelius regarding adoption of medical loss ratio calculation methodology*. Retrieved August 29, 2014, from http://www.naic.org/documents/committees_ex_mlr_reg_asadopted.pdf

National Association of Social Workers. (2013). *NASW standards for social work case management*. Retrieved April 25, 2013, from http://www.socialworkers.org/practice/naswstandards/CaseManagementStandards2013.pdf

Population Health Alliance. (2014). *Definition of disease management*. Retrieved August 31, 2014, from http://www.populationhealthalliance.org/research/phm-glossary/d.html

Powell, S. K. (2000). *Case management: A practical guide to success in managed care* (2nd ed.). Philadelphia, PA: Wolters Kluwer, Lippincott Williams & Wilkins.

Powell, S. K., & Tahan, H. A. (2010). *Case management A practical guide for education and practice* (3rd ed.). Philadelphia, PA: Wolters Kluwer, Lippincott Williams & Wilkins.

Sederer, L. I. (1987). Utilization review and quality assurance: Staying in the black and working with the blues. *General Hospital Psychiatry, 9*(3), 210–219.

Sirovich, B. E., Gottlieb, D. J., Welch, H. G., & Fisher, E. S. (2006). Regional variations in health care intensity and physician perceptions of quality of care. *Annals of Internal Medicine, 144*, 641–649.

Social Security Administration. (2011). *Quality improvement organizations*. Retrieved August 29, 2014, from http://www.cms.gov/Medicare/Quality-Initiatives-Patient-Assessment-Instruments/QualityImprove mentOrgs/index.html?redirect=/qualityimprovementorgs

Starr, P. (1982). *The social transformation of American medicine*. New York, NY: Basic Books.

Steinman, A. (2014). *CMS announcement next phase of the QIO program*. Retrieved August 28, 2014 from http://www.qioprogram.org/cms-announces-next-phase-qio-program

Sultz, H. A., & Young, K. M. (2014). *Health care USA: Understanding its organization and delivery* (8th ed.). Sudbury, MA: Jones and Bartlett Learning.

Wojner, A. W. (2001). *Outcomes management: Applications to clinical practice*. St. Louis, MO: Mosby.

16 ANTICIPATORY

OBJECTIVES

After studying this chapter, you will be able to:

1. Discuss anticipatory and/or proactive case management.
2. Discuss how proactive case management is depicted in various practice standards.
3. Discuss the key elements of anticipatory practice and implications to case management practice.
4. Identify impacts of an anticipatory approach on case management practice.
5. Discuss impacts of failing to engage in proactive advocacy on organizational policy.

KEY TERMS

Anticipate
Anticipatory care
Clinical practice guidelines
National Guideline Clearinghouse
Practice act
Proactive
Risk management
Risk mitigation
Stereotype

Case management has long-sought recognition for addressing existing care challenges, for proactive identification of care barriers, and for creating and activating plans that mitigate, if not prevent, their furtherance (Treiger & Fink-Samnick, 2013). Anticipatory interventions have been a part of the case management value equation for decades; however, sparse evidence is found in literature of case management's impact in this realm. The skill of practicing from an anticipatory position extends beyond one's client-specific approach. It requires the individual to be proactive in all things pertaining to professional practice. This chapter examines the concepts associated with proactive and anticipatory care and career management, the key part that proactive competence plays in the COLLABORATE model, and the implications to current and future case management practice.

DEFINITIONS

Anticipate

To **anticipate** means that one gives advance thought, discussion, or treatment or foresees and deals with something in advance (Merriam-Webster.com., 2014a). For the experienced case manager, to anticipate client needs includes the ability to identify risks in addition to actual barriers to care. Applying the case management process, one leverages critical thinking and clinical experience to identify foreseeable risks and enact strategies to reduce or prevent their occurrence. This is accomplished through problem identification in tandem with taking measures to reduce possible harms. Relative to the COLLABORATE paradigm, to anticipate includes the careful consideration of client-specific circumstances and the provision of educated, evidence-based, and well-informed recommendations to optimize a positive result or minimize a downside impact or outcome as a result of risk associated with a care barrier (Treiger & Fink-Samnick, 2013).

Anticipatory Care

Anticipatory care is defined as working with clients to identify any circumstances that may have a negative impact on their mental, physical, and social health and to put in place proactive strategies to avert those impacts (Kennedy, Harbison, Mahoney, Jarvis, & Veitch, 2011; Kralik, 2011). This approach to care focuses on early identification and prevention of health problems before they actually occur and cause difficulty for an individual. This is an increasingly important approach to care delivery in the United Kingdom and other European countries from where a majority of literature on the topic emanates.

Proactive

Proactive is defined as controlling a situation by making things happen or by preparing for possible future problems or acting in anticipation of future problems, needs, or changes (Merriam-Webster.com., 2014b). The importance of assuming a proactive stance in case management practice is evident in the following practice standards:

- Transition management, utilization management, and care coordination (American Case Management Association [ACMA], 2013)
- Facilitation, coordination, and collaboration (Case Management Society of America [CMSA], 2010)
- Cultural and linguistic competence (National Association of Social Workers [NASW], 2013)

Table 16-1 highlights specific passage excerpts from the aforementioned practice standards.

Risk Management

Risk management (RM), as applied to a health plan's operations, refers to taking steps to reduce the risk of litigation or regulatory sanctions (Kongstvedt, 2013). Pertaining to health care delivery, RM is frequently viewed as a damage control intervention, activated after-the-fact in an attempt to minimize the impact of an untoward event. Because of the post-event nature of RM activation, this is often considered to be a reactive strategy with the purpose of minimizing the consequences of events which may be perceived as public-relations nightmares outside of the organization. Ideally, RM should focus more on identification of risk potential and the actions required to reduce risk and improve patient safety (Powell & Tahan, 2010).

Although RM and case management are separate and distinct, a case manager identifies and addresses client-specific risks throughout the case management engagement. In addition, the case manager works with their organization's legal, quality, and/or RM departments to define and implement strategies to minimize or eliminate potential harms. This is accomplished by identifying and addressing client care problems, maintaining solid working knowledge of organizational, legal, and regulatory factors affecting care delivery and management, assessment and engagement of appropriate resources to meet each client's needs, and educating care team members and others with regard to case management's roles in health care delivery (Cohen & Cesta, 2005).

Risk Mitigation

Risk mitigation refers to a proactive strategy of identifying potential risks and implementing preventative strategies to reduce or eliminate them from occurring (Powell & Tahan, 2010). As stated by the Committee on Quality of Health Care in America, "care must be delivered by systems that are carefully and consciously designed to provide care that is safe, effective, patient-centered, timely, efficient, and equitable. Such systems must be designed to serve the needs of patients, and to ensure that they are fully informed, retain control and participate in care delivery whenever possible" (Institute of Medicine [IOM], 2001). To this end, the fourth recommendation from *Crossing the Quality Chasm* charged the entire health care system with working together to redesign health care systems according to 10 principles

TABLE 16-1 Proactive Focus in Case Management Practice Standards

Organization	Proactive-Focused Practice Standard
American Case Management Association (2013)	**Transition Management** "For those patients at risk for readmission, case management will apply interventions to *proactively* prevent readmissions and evaluate those who are readmitted to identify and implement strategies for improvement." **Utilization Management** "Case management will *proactively* prevent medical necessity denials by providing education to physicians, staff and patients, interfacing with payers and documenting relevant information." **Care Coordination** "*Proactively* identifies, communicates and resolves barriers that impede the progression of care."
Case Management Society of America (2010)	**Standard: Facilitation, Coordination, and Collaboration** "Development and maintenance of *proactive*, client-centered relationships and communication with the client, and other necessary stakeholders to maximize outcomes."
National Association of Social Workers (2013)	**Standard 4: Cultural and Linguistic Competence** "Given the complexity of cultural identity, the social work case manager needs to approach every interaction with clients and colleagues as a cross-cultural exchange, recognizing the potential for value conflicts and being *proactive* to ensure that such conflicts do not undermine practice."

(Table 16-2). Anticipation of needs is articulated as the eighth rule focusing on proactive versus reactive health care according to patient need.

Arguably, case management has begun to cross a quality threshold of needs anticipation through its use of predictive modeling, geographic profiling, and risk stratification for the identification and selection of individuals most in need of case management services. This is captured in practice standards issued by ACMA and CMSA (Table 16-3). The reasons why proactive practice is not a widespread reality include the definition and scope of some case management programs, the use of screening and assessment tools which focus more on existing barriers and needs, and the lack of emphasis on proactive/anticipatory practice in practice acts and standards of practice documentation. When risk mitigation is undertaken as a case management intervention, it is often a secondary gain subsequent to addressing the more pressing issues facing the client. However, the case manager assumes

TABLE 16-2 IOM's Rules of Redesigning Health Care Processes

Rule	Detail
1. Care based on continuous healing relationships	Patients should receive care whenever they need it and in many forms, not just face-to-face visits. This rule implies that the health care system should be responsive at all times (24 hours a day, every day) and that access to care should be provided over the Internet, by telephone, and by other means in addition to face-to-face visits.
2. Customization based on patient needs and values	The system of care should be designed to meet the most common types of needs, but have the capability to respond to individual patient choices and preferences.
3. The patient as the source of control	Patients should be given the necessary information and the opportunity to exercise the degree of control they choose over health care decisions that affect them. The health system should be able to accommodate differences in patient preferences and encourage shared decision making.
4. Shared knowledge and the free flow of information	Patients should have unfettered access to their own medical information and to clinical knowledge. Clinicians and patients should communicate effectively and share information.
5. Evidence-based decision making	Patients should receive care based on the best available scientific knowledge. Care should not vary illogically from clinician to clinician or from place to place.
6. Safety as a system property	Patients should be safe from injury caused by the care system. Reducing risk and ensuring safety require greater attention to systems that help prevent and mitigate errors.
7. The need for transparency	The health care system should make information available to patients and their families which allows them to make informed decisions when selecting a health plan, hospital, or clinical practice, or choosing among alternative treatments. This should include information describing the system's performance on safety, evidence-based practice, and patient satisfaction.
8. Anticipation of needs	The health system should anticipate patient needs, rather than simply reacting to events.
9. Continuous decrease in waste	The health system should not waste resources or patient time.
10. Cooperation among clinicians	Clinicians and institutions should actively collaborate and communicate to ensure an appropriate exchange of information and coordination of care.

Adapted from Institute of Medicine. (2001). Crossing the quality chasm: A new health system for the 21st century. Washington, DC: National Academy Press.

TABLE 16-3 Identification of Need for Case Management Service Recognized in Practice Standards

Organization	Standard
ACMA (2013)	Case management will screen all patients for clinical, psychosocial, financial, and operational factors that may affect the progression of care and through the use of identification criteria stratify patients at risk/barriers/strengths or in need of case management services.
CMSA (2010)	The case manager should identify and select clients who can most benefit from case management services available in a particular practice setting.

a more proactive approach when employing an engagement strategy inclusive of the identification of potential risks associated with an individual's bio-psycho-social-spiritual states.

APPROACHES TO ANTICIPATORY CASE MANAGEMENT

A case manager undertakes activities of an anticipatory nature as part of their individual and ongoing pursuit of knowledge and professional education. While these are mandated as part of licensure and/or certification requirements, the true professional strives to maintain current knowledge regarding influences on clinical practice, including legal and regulatory developments, evidence based care, and case management best practices regardless of whether or not it is a benefit of their employment. The importance of continuous education is emphasized throughout the COLLABORATE paradigm and highlighted within the chapter devoted to the lifelong learning competency.

Knowledge of Legal, Regulatory, and Professional Credential Developments

The case manager's knowledge of legal and regulatory developments is guided by a number of factors, including the following:

- Primary licensure or certification (e.g., nursing, social work, physical therapy) and professional practice act(s)
- Place of employment (e.g., worker's compensation, managed care)
- Individual credential (e.g., certification)

The implication to anticipatory practice is that the lack of knowledge regarding applicable laws, regulations, and policies on one's practice usurps the ability to be proactive with regard to the implications of such influencers on direct patient care and health care delivery.

Licensure and Professional Practice Acts

Licensure is required to practice nursing within the United States; however, not all states require licensure for social workers. In instances where licensure is not required, states provide other recognition criteria (e.g., endorsement). The purpose of these requirements is to protect the public from harm by setting minimal qualifications and competencies for safe entry-level practitioners. Nursing is regulated because "it is one of the health professions that poses a risk of harm to the public if practiced by someone who is unprepared and/or incompetent" (National Council of State Boards of Nursing [NCSBN], 2011).

Regardless of one's educational background, it is a case manager's responsibility to pursue and maintain knowledge of applicable laws and regulations governing professional practice. When one finds variance in the interpretation of a particular law or regulation, it is essential to seek further clarification from reliable and objective sources. The excuse of "I did not know" or relying on one's employer's legal department for personal advice is insufficient in light of the fact that licensure and/or endorsement is held on an individual, as opposed to an organizational, basis. The story in Box 16-1 provides amplification of how organizational operations intersect with individual licensure.

BOX 16-1 The Intersection of Individual Licensure and Company Operations

The Scenario

Mavis is a registered nurse, licensed to practice in Massachusetts. She works as a case manager at RWB Health Plan, a regional health insurer with indemnity and managed care products. RWB was recently awarded a contract with XLant, a technology company with employees residing across the United States. At a staff meeting, Mavis raises the concerns about working with members who do not reside in Massachusetts, where she is licensed to practice. Her supervisor brings the matter to the attention of the department director, human resources, and the legal department. Within the week, the response is handed down that Mavis has nothing to be concerned about because she is not working as a nurse.

The Facts

Mavis researches nursing licensure at the Massachusetts Board of Registration in Nursing (MABoR), the National Council of State Boards of Nursing (NCSBN), and a professional case management association websites seeking clarification on whether case management is considered a nursing function. She obtains the following information:

MABoR

"All nurses who practice within Massachusetts are required to have a current Massachusetts license. Massachusetts is not a member of the Nurse Licensure Compact (NLC)" (Health and Human Services, 2014).

NCSBN (2014)

"Licensure is the process by which boards of nursing grant permission to an individual to engage in nursing practice after determining that the applicant has attained the competency necessary to perform a unique scope of practice. Licensure is necessary when the regulated activities are complex, require specialized knowledge and skill and independent decision making. The licensure process determines if the applicant has the necessary skills to safely perform a specified scope of practice by predetermining the criteria needed and to evaluate licensure applicants to determine if they meet the criteria. Licensure provides that:

- A specified scope of practice may only be performed legally by licensed individuals
- Title protection
- Authority to take disciplinary action should the licensee violate the law or rules in order to assure that the public is protected

(continued)

BOX 16-1 The Intersection of Individual Licensure and Company Operations (*Continued*)

Professional Association

"Case managers should adhere to applicable local, state, and federal laws, as well as employer policies, governing all aspects of case management practice. It is the responsibility of the case manager to work within the scope of his/her licensure" (CMSA, 2010).

Additional Actions

Mavis also reviews the job qualifications and requirements of her current position at RWB Health Plan, noting that a requirement of the position is holding an active, unrestricted registered nurse license. She goes on to note that the position description and performance management program specifically mention her nursing licensure, clinical knowledge, and ability to make sound decisions guided by clinical information, evidence-based guidelines, and organizational policy.

Follow-Up

Upon bringing the above information to the attention of RWB Health Plan administration, the organization revamps its case management assignment policy, aligning the assignment of individual members to case managers holding a license in the member's state of residence.

Once licensed, an individual's practice is governed by her or his respective practice act(s). The purpose of a **practice act** is to lay out the edges of one's professional practice by defining its scope and restricting practice to properly qualified individuals. Professional practice acts are specific to the issuing jurisdiction as well as the practice specialty, meaning all states and territories have legislated practice acts for various licensed professions (e.g., nursing, social work).

Nursing. A Nurse Practice Act establishes a Board of Nursing (BON) which may also be known as a Board of Registration. The BON has the authority to administer rules or regulations which clarify the laws governing nursing practice. BONs cannot enact rules or regulations that extend beyond the legal scope of these laws and the resulting rules and regulations undergo close scrutiny and public comment before becoming active. Once enacted, rules and regulations are considered administrative law.

Founded in 1978, the NCSBN is an independent not-for-profit organization whose mission is to address issues of common interest across the collective boards of nursing and to act together on these matters. Part of the NCSBN mission is to reduce administrative burden on state boards of nursing through the following activities:

- Developing the NCLEX-RN, NCLEX-PN, NNAAP, and MACE examinations
- Monitoring trends in public policy, nursing practice, and education
- Promoting uniformity in relationship to the regulation of nursing practice
- Disseminating data related to the licensure of nurses
- Conducting research on nursing practice issues
- Serving as a forum for information exchange for members
- Providing opportunities for collaboration among its members and other nursing and health care organizations
- Maintaining the Nursys database, which coordinates national publicly available nurse licensure information

(NCSBN, 2014)

As of September 2014, there are 60 member boards and 21 associate members of NCSBN. The NCSBN has taken a leadership role in advocating for adoption of the Nurse Licensure Compact. To learn more about a particular state's BON, search the official state or territory government website using terms such as "board of nursing," "board of registration of nursing," or see the interactive map for links for all member boards of nursing at the NCSBN website at https://www.ncsbn.org/contactbon.htm.

Social Work. Social work is a profession which impacts public health, safety, and welfare. All 50 states, the District of Columbia, the U.S. Virgin Islands, and all 10 Canadian provinces regulate the practice of social work; however, not all states require licensure for social workers, and the levels of recognition for social work licensure and practice vary state to state.

The Association of Social Work Boards (ASWB) is the nonprofit organization composed of the social work regulatory boards and colleges of 49 U.S. states, the District of Columbia, the U.S. Virgin Islands, and all 10 Canadian provinces. It is a nonprofit organization focusing on social work regulation and promoting uniformity of regulation across its membership. Its mission is to strengthen public protection through support and services to its member boards. In addition, the ASWB (2014) oversees the following:

- Owns and maintains the social work licensing examinations used to assess competence to practice ethically and safely
- Maintains the social work model practice act
- Approves Continuing Education Program for approved continuing education
- Offers continuing education audit contract services
- Offers licensure services (e.g., application, issuance)
- Maintains the Public Protection Database
- Maintains the Look Up a License Database

For additional discussion of ASWB, refer chapter 2.

To learn more about a particular state's Board of Social Work, search the official state or territory government's website using terms such as "board of social work," "board of registration in social work," or see the listing of links for member boards provided on the ASWB website.

Knowledge of Evidence-Based Clinical Practice Guidelines

Clinical practice guidelines are statements that include recommendations intended to optimize patient care. They are informed by a systematic review of evidence and an assessment of the benefits and harms of alternative care options

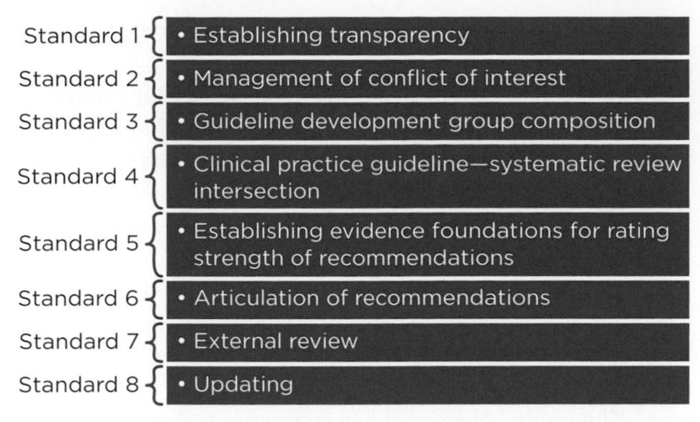

Figure 16-1. IOM standards for developing trustworthy clinical practice guidelines. (Adapted from Institute of Medicine. (2011). *Clinical practice guidelines we can trust*. Retrieved September 4, 2014, from http://www.iom.edu/reports/2011/clinical-practice-guidelines-we-can-trust.aspx)

(IOM, 2011). The Medicare Improvements for Patients and Providers Act of 2008 put forth a request for definition of the best methodology to develop clinical practice guidelines. The IOM returned eight standards for developing guidelines that were scientifically rigorous and reliable. These IOM standards are presented in Figure 16-1.

The Agency for Healthcare Research and Quality (AHRQ) notes the importance of evaluating the strength of evidence underlying clinical guidelines. Many organizations have adopted systematic approaches to rating the strength of evidence supporting their guidelines. Because a wide variety of grading systems are available for this purpose and different organizations weigh elements of a body of evidence differently, it is important for a case manager to have a working knowledge of research types and strength-rating scales.

When looking at practice guidelines, a case manager must be able to evaluate the information presented in an organized and methodical manner. It is especially important for a case manager to accurately interpret the evidence supporting clinical guidelines. In light of the acknowledged variation in research approaches, the prudent case manager is mindful of the specific methodology strength used in evidence rating when considering incorporation of findings into his or her practice and when making recommendations relating to treatment or practice to others. For evidence to be of high quality, the rigor of research and testing must also be held to a high standard. The strength of evidence may be classified as minimal, moderate, and strong. Table 16-4 aligns study type to strength of evidence. Knowing where to look for evidence and clinical guidelines is also important. Table 16-5 identifies common databases, which aid in efficient literature searches. Also, refer chapter 9 which covers evidence-based practice and the outcomes-driven competency.

In addition to databases, AHRQ maintains the **National Guideline Clearinghouse** (NGC), a repository for clinical practice guidelines from around the world. NGC was originally created by AHRQ in collaboration with the American

TABLE 16-4 Study Type and Evidence Strength

Strength of Evidence		
Minimal	**Moderate**	**Strong**
Review articles	Cohort studies	Randomized-controlled trials
	Case-control studies	Systematic reviews
	Clinical practice guidelines	Metaanalyses

TABLE 16-5 Helpful Databases for Evidence Search

Resource	Description
CINAHL	The Cumulative Index to Nursing and Allied Health Literature is a database dedicated to nursing and allied health research.
The Cochrane Library	The Cochrane Library contains systematic reviews of primary research in human health care and health policy. Systematic review is considered the highest level of evidence.
DynaMed	DynaMed is a clinical reference tool created for physicians and other health care professionals. It contains summaries on more than 3,000 health care topics.
PubMed and MEDLINE	PubMed provides free access to MEDLINE. PubMed includes more than 24 million citations for biomedical literature, life science journals, and online books. MEDLINE contains journal citations and abstracts for biomedical literature.

Medical Association (AMA) and the American Association of Health Plans (now America's Health Insurance Plans). For ease of reference, the guidelines are classified by disease/condition, treatment/intervention, health services administration, and originating organization.

Knowledge of Case Management Evidence

Focusing in on case management evidence that is applicable to a specific care setting or specialty is more difficult than one might expect. This is caused by a number of factors including lack of specificity as to the term case management, resulting in highly diluted search results, lack of clear description relating to studied groups, case management scope of practice that differs by employer, and high variability of interventions applied from study to study. There is also the phenomenon of organization-based projects not being considered as study-worthy. This results in a failure to organize these projects as actual studies. This also leads to lack of publishable results.

As noted by Hickam et al., prior to the AHRQ Comparative Effectiveness Review of Outpatient Case Management for Adults With Medical Illness and Complex Care Needs in 2013, there were no systematic reviews that evaluated studies of case management across multiple disease categories and those that existed used definitions of case management that differed from AHRQ's definition (Hickam et al., 2013). The case management definition adopted for the AHRQ review was "a process in which a person (alone or in conjunction with a team) manages multiple aspects of a patient's care." The study considered key component of case management as being planning and assessment, coordination of services, patient education, and clinical monitoring. Of the 5,645 citations identified, AHRQ screened and reviewed over 1,000, including 153 articles representing 109 studies. A list of studies included in the AHRQ comparative review is found in Box 16-2.

BOX 16-2 Included Studies in AHRQ Comparative Effectiveness Review, No. 99 Outpatient Case Management for Adults with Medical Illness and Complex Care Needs

Allen, K. R., Hazelett, S., Jarjoura, D., et al. (2002). Effectiveness of a postdischarge care management model for stroke and transient ischemic attack: A randomized trial. *Journal of Stroke and Cerebrovascular Diseases*, *11*(2), 88–98.

Andersen, M., Hockman, E., Smereck, G., et al. (2007, May–June). Retaining women in HIV medical care. *The Journal of the Association of Nurses in AIDS Care*, *18*(3), 33–41.

Applebaum, R., Straker, J., Mehdizadeh, S., et al. (2002, Spring). Using high-intensity care management to integrate acute and long-term care services: Substitute for large scale system reform? *Care Management Journals*, *3*(3), 113–119.

Babamoto, K. S., Sey, K. A., Camilleri, A. J., et al. (2009, February). Improving diabetes care and health measures among hispanics using community health workers: Results from a randomized controlled trial. *Health Education & Behavior*, *36*(1), 113–126.

Bernabei, R., Landi, F., Gambassi, G., et al. (1998, May). Randomised trial of impact of model of integrated care and case management for older people living in the community. *BMJ*, *316*(7141), 1348–1351.

Berra, K., Ma, J., Klieman, L., et al. (2007 December). Implementing cardiac risk-factor case management: Lessons learned in a county health system. *Critical Pathways in Cardiology*, *6*(4), 173–179.

Bird, S., Noronha, M., Sinnott, H. (2010). An integrated care facilitation model improves quality of life and reduces use of hospital resources by patients with chronic obstructive pulmonary disease and chronic heart failure. *Australian Journal of Primary Health*, *16*(4), 326–333.

Bird, S. R., Kurowski, W., Dickman, G. K., et al. (2007, August). Integrated care facilitation for older patients with complex health care needs reduces hospital demand. *Australian Health Review*, *31*(3), 451–61. discussion 49–50.

Bouey, P. D., Druan, B. E. (2000). The Ahalaya case-management program for HIV-infected American Indians, Alaska Natives, and Native Hawaiians: Quantitative and qualitative evaluation of impacts. *American Indian and Alaska Native Mental Health Research*, *9*(2), 36–52.

Boult, C., Reider, L., Frey, K., et al. (2008, March). Early effects of "Guided Care" on the quality of health care for multimorbid older persons: A cluster-randomized controlled trial. *The Journals of Gerontology. Series A, Biological Sciences and Medical Sciences*, *63*(3), 321–327.

Boult, C., Reider, L., Leff, B., et al. (2011, March 14). The effect of guided care teams on the use of health services: Results from a cluster-randomized controlled trial. *Archives of Internal Medicine*, *171*(5), 460–466.

Bourbeau, J., Collet, J. P., Schwartzman, K., et al. (2006, December). Economic benefits of self-management education in COPD. *Chest*, *130*(6), 1704–1711.

Bourbeau, J., Julien, M., Maltais, F., et al. (2003, March 10). Reduction of hospital utilization in patients with chronic obstructive pulmonary disease: A disease-specific self-management intervention. *Archives of Internal Medicine*, *163*(5), 585–591.

Boyd, C. M., Reider, L., Frey, K., et al. (2010, March). The effects of guided care on the perceived quality of health care for multi-morbid older persons: 18-month outcomes from a cluster-randomized controlled trial. *Journal of General Internal Medicine*, *25*(3), 235–242.

Brodaty, H., Mittelman, M., Gibson, L., et al. (2009, September). The effects of counseling spouse caregivers of people with Alzheimer disease taking donepezil and of country of residence on rates of admission to nursing homes and mortality. *The American Journal of Geriatric Psychiatry*, *17*(9), 734–743.

Brown, S. A., Garcia, A. A., Winter, M., et al. (2011). Integrating education, group support, and case management for diabetic Hispanics. *Ethnicity & Disease*, *21*(1), 20–26.

California Medi-Cal Type 2 Diabetes Study Group. (2004, January). Closing the gap: Effect of diabetes case management on glycemic control among low-income ethnic minority populations: The California Medi-Cal type 2 diabetes study. *Diabetes Care*, *27*(1), 95–103.

Callahan, C. M., Boustani, M. A., Unverzagt, F. W., et al. (2006, May 10). Effectiveness of collaborative care for older adults with Alzheimer disease in primary care: A randomized controlled trial. *JAMA*, *295*(18), 2148–2157.

Challis, D., von Abendorff, R., Brown, P., et al. (2002, April). Care management, dementia care and specialist mental health services: An evaluation. *International Journal of Geriatric Psychiatry*, *17*(4), 315–325.

Chi, Y. C., Chuang, K. Y., Wu, S. C., et al. (2004, December). The assessment of a hospital-based care management model for long-term care services. *The Journal of Nursing Research*, *12*(4), 317–326.

Chien, W. T., Lee, Y. M. (2008). A disease management program for families of persons in Hong Kong with dementia. *Psychiatric Servics*, *59*(4), 433–436.

Chow, S. K. Y., Wong, F. K. (2010). Health-related quality of life in patients undergoing peritoneal dialysis: Effects of a nurse-led case management programme. *Journal of Advanced Nursing*, *66*(8), 1780–1792.

Chu, P., Edwards, J., Levin, R., et al. (2000). The use of clinical case management for early stage Alzheimer's patients and their families. *American Journal of Alzheimers Disease*, *15*(5), 284–90.

Claiborne, N. (2006). Efficiency of a care coordination model: A randomized study with stroke patients. *Research on Social Work Practice*, *16*(1), 57–66.

Clark, P., Bass, D. M., Looman, W. J., et al. (2004). Outcomes for patients with dementia from the Cleveland Alzheimer's Managed Care Demonstration. *Aging & Mental Health*, *8*(1), 40–51.

Creason, H. (2001, July–August). Congestive heart failure telemanagement clinic. *Lippincott's Case Management*, *6*(4), 146–156.

Curtis, J., Lipke, S., Effland, S., et al. (2009, Sep–Oct). Effectiveness and safety of medication adjustments by nurse case managers to control hyperglycemia. *The Diabetes Educator*, *35*(5), 851–856.

DeBusk, R. F., Miller, N. H., Parker, K. M., et al. (2004, October 19). Care management for low-risk patients with heart failure: A randomized, controlled trial. *Annals of Internal Medicine*, *141*(8), 606–613.

Dewan, N. A., Rice, K. L., Caldwell, M., et al. (2011, Junuary). Economic evaluation of a disease management program for chronic obstructive pulmonary disease. *COPD*, *8*(3), 153–159.

Dorr, D. A., Wilcox, A. B., Brunker, C. P., et al. (2008, December). The effect of technology-supported, multidisease care management on the mortality and hospitalization of seniors. *Journal of the American Geriatrics Society*, *56*(12), 2195–2202.

Dorr, D. A., Wilcox, A., Donnelly, S. M., et al. (2005, October). Impact of generalist care managers on patients with diabetes. *Health Services Research*, *40*(5, Pt. 1), 1400–1421.

Dorr, D. A., Wilcox, A., Jones, S., et al. (2007, January). Care management dosage. *Journal of General Internal Medicine*, *22*(6), 736–741.

Duke, C. (2005, March–April). The frail elderly community-based case management project. *Geriatric Nursing*, *26*(2), 122–127.

Duru, O. K., Ettner, S. L., Vassar, S. D., et al. (2009). Cost evaluation of a coordinated care management intervention for dementia. *The American Journal of Managed Care*, *15*(8), 521–528.

Eggert, G. M., Zimmer, J. G., Hall, W. J., et al. (1991, October). Case management: A randomized controlled study comparing a neighborhood team and a centralized individual model. *Health Services Research*, *26*(4), 471–507.

Eloniemi-Sulkava, U., Notkola, I. L., Hentinen, M., et al. (2001). Effects of supporting community-living demented patients and their caregivers: A randomized trial. *Journal of the American Geriatrics Society*, *49*(10), 1282–1287.

Eloniemi-Sulkava, U., Saarenheimo, M., Laakkonen, M., et al. (2009). Family care as collaboration: Effectiveness of a multicomponent support program for elderly couples with dementia. Randomized controlled intervention study. *Journal of the American Geriatrics Society*, *57*(12), 2200–2208.

(continued)

BOX 16-2 Included Studies in AHRQ Comparative Effectiveness Review, No. 99 Outpatient Case Management for Adults with Medical Illness and Complex Care Needs (*Continued*)

Engelhardt, J. B., McClive-Reed, K. P., Toseland, R. W., et al. (2006, February). Effects of a program for coordinated care of advanced illness on patients, surrogates, and healthcare costs: A randomized trial. *The American Journal of Managed Care*, *12*(2), 93–100.

Fan, V. S., Gaziano, J. M., Lew, R., et al. (2012, May 15). A comprehensive care management program to prevent chronic obstructive pulmonary disease hospitalizations: A randomized, controlled trial. *Annals of Internal Medicine*, *156*(10), 673–683.

Fitzgerald, J. F., Smith, D. M., Martin, D. K., et al. (1994, August 8). A case manager intervention to reduce readmissions. *Archives of Internal Medicine*, *154*(15), 1721–1729.

Fleishman, J. A., Mor, V., Piette, J. (1991, October). AIDS case management: The client's perspective. *Health Services Research*, *26*(4), 447–470.

Fletcher, K., Mant, J. A. (2009, April). A Before and after study of the impact of Specialist Workers for Older People. *Journal of Evaluation in Clinical Practice*, *15*(2), 335–340.

Gagnon, A. J., Schein, C., McVey L, et al. (1999, September). Randomized controlled trial of nurse case management of frail older people. *Journal of the American Geriatrics Society*, *47*(9), 1118–1124.

Gary, T. L., Batts-Turner, M., Bone, L. R., et al. (2004, February). A randomized controlled trial of the effects of nurse case manager and community health worker team interventions in urban African-Americans with type 2 diabetes. *Controlled Clinical Trials*, *25*(1), 53–66.

Gary, T. L., Batts-Turner, M., Yeh, H. C., et al. (2009, October). The effects of a nurse case manager and a community health worker team on diabetic control, emergency department visits, and hospitalizations among urban African Americans with type 2 diabetes mellitus: A randomized controlled trial. *Archives of Internal Medicine*, *169*(19), 1788–1794

Gary, T. L., Bone, L. R., Hill, M. N., et al. (2003, July). Randomized controlled trial of the effects of nurse case manager and community health worker interventions on risk factors for diabetes-related complications in urban African Americans. *Preventive Medicine*, *37*(1), 23–32.

Gary, T. L., Hill-Briggs, F., Batts-Turner, M., et al. (2005). Translational research principles of an effectiveness trial for diabetes care in an urban African American population. *The Diabetes Educator*, *31*(6), 880–889.

Goodwin, J. S., Satish, S., Anderson, E. T., et al. (2003, September). Effect of nurse case management on the treatment of older women with breast cancer. *Journal of the American Geriatrics Society*, *51*(9), 1252–1259.

Gravelle, H., Dusheiko, M., Sheaff, R., et al. (2007, January 6). Impact of case management (Evercare) on frail elderly patients: Controlled before and after analysis of quantitative outcome data. *BMJ*, *334*(7583), 31.

Hammer, B. J. (2001, September–October). Community-based case management for positive outcomes. *Geriatric Nursing*, *22*(5), 271–275.

Hebert, R., Durand, P. J., Dubuc, N., et al. (2003, August). Frail elderly patients. New model for integrated service delivery. *Canadian Family Physician*, *49*, 992–997.

Hsieh, C. J., Lin, L. C., Kuo, B. I., et al. (2008, April). Exploring the efficacy of a case management model using DOTS in the adherence of patients with pulmonary tuberculosis. *Journal of Clinical Nursing*, *17*(7), 869–875.

Husbands, W., Browne, G., Caswell, J., et al. (2007, September). Case management community care for people living with HIV/AIDS (PLHAs). *AIDS Care*, *19*(8), 1065–1072.

Huws, D. W., Cashmore, D., Newcombe, R. G., et al. (2008). Impact of case management by advanced practice nurses in primary care on unplanned hospital admissions: A controlled intervention study. *BMC Health Services Research*, *8*, 115.

Ishani, A., Greer, N., Taylor, B. C., et al. (2011, August). Effect of nurse case management compared with usual care on controlling cardiovascular risk factors in patients with diabetes: A randomized controlled trial. *Diabetes Care*, *34*(8), 1689–1694.

Izquierdo, R., Meyer, S., Starren, J., et al. (2007, June). Detection and remediation of medically urgent situations using telemedicine case management for older patients with diabetes mellitus. *Therapeutics and Clinical Risk Management*, *3*(3), 485–489.

Jaarsma, T., van der Wal, M. H., Lesman-Leegte, I., et al. (2008, February 11). Effect of moderate or intensive disease management program on outcome in patients with heart failure: Coordinating Study Evaluating Outcomes of Advising and Counseling in Heart Failure (COACH). *Archives of Internal Medicine*, *168*(3), 316–324.

Jansen, A. P., van Hout, H. P., van Marwijk, H. W., et al. (2005). (Cost)-effectiveness of case-management by district nurses among primary informal caregivers of older adults with dementia symptoms and the older adults who receive informal care: Design of a randomized controlled trial [ISCRTN83135728]. *BMC Public Health*, *5*, 133.

Jansen, A. P., van Hout, H., Nijpels, G., et al. (2011). Effectiveness of case management among older adults with early symptoms of dementia and their primary informal caregivers: A randomized clinical trial. *International Journal of Nursing Studies*, *48*(8), 933–943.

Jennings-Sanders, A., Anderson, E. T. (2003, May–June). Older women with breast cancer: Perceptions of the effectiveness of nurse case managers. *Nursing Outlook*, *51*(3), 108–114.

Jennings-Sanders, A., Kuo, Y. F., Anderson, E. T., et al. (2005, May). How do nurse case managers care for older women with breast cancer? *Oncology Nursing Forum*, *32*(3), 625–632.

Jowers, J., Corsello, P., Shafer, A., et al. (2000). Partnering specialist care with nurse case management: A pilot project for asthma. *Journal of Clinical Outcomes Management*, *7*(5), 17–22.

Kasper, E. K., Gerstenblith, G., Hefter, G., et al. (2002, Febryary 6). A randomized trial of the efficacy of multidisciplinary care in heart failure outpatients at high risk of hospital readmission. *Journal of the American College of Cardiology*, *39*(3), 471–480.

Keating, P., Sealy, A., Dempsey, L., et al. (2008). Reducing unplanned hospital admissions and hospital bed days in the over 65 age group: Results from a pilot study. *Journal of Integrated Care*, *16*(1), 3–8.

Krein, S. L., Klamerus, M. L., Vijan, S., et al. (2004, June 1). Case management for patients with poorly controlled diabetes: A randomized trial. *The American Journal of Medicine*, *116*(11), 732–739.

Kristensson, J., Ekwall, A. K., Jakobsson, U., et al. (2010, December). Case managers for frail older people: A randomised controlled pilot study. *Scandinavian Journal of Caring Sciences*, *24*(4), 755–763.

Kruse, R. L., Zweig, S. C., Nikodim, B., et al. (2010). Nurse care coordination of older patients in an academic family medicine clinic: 5-year outcomes. *Journal of Clinical Outcomes Management*, *17*(5), 209–215.

Kushel, M. B., Colfax, G., Ragland, K., et al. (2006, July 15). Case management is associated with improved antiretroviral adherence and CD4+ cell counts in homeless and marginally housed individuals with HIV infection. *Clinical Infectious Disease*, *43*(2), 234–242.

Lam, L. C., Lee, J. S., Chung, J. C., et al. (2010, April). A randomized controlled trial to examine the effectiveness of case management model for community dwelling older persons with mild dementia in Hong Kong. *International Journal of Geriatric Psychiatry*, *25*(4), 395–402.

Laramee, A. S., Levinsky, S. K., Sargent, J., et al. (2003, April). Case management in a heterogeneous congestive heart failure population: A randomized controlled trial. *Archives of Internal Medicine*, *163*(7), 809–817.

Latour, C. H., de Vos, R., Huyse, F. J., et al. (2006, September–October). Effectiveness of post-discharge case management in general-medical outpatients: A randomized, controlled trial. *Psychosomatics*, *47*(5), 421–429.

Latour, C. H., Bosmans, J. E., van Tulder, M. W., et al. (2007, March). Cost-effectiveness of a nurse-led case management intervention in general medical outpatients compared with usual care: An economic evaluation alongside a randomized controlled trial. *Journal of Psychosomatic Research*, *62*(3), 363–370.

Lehrman, S. E., Gentry, D., Yurchak, B. B., et al. (2001, August). Outcomes of HIV/AIDS case management in New York. *AIDS Care*, *13*(4), 481–92.

Leung, A. C., Yau, D. C., Liu, C. P., et al. (2004). Reducing utilisation of hospital services by case management: A randomised controlled trial. *Australian Health Review*, *28*(1), 79–86.

Leung, A. C., Liu, C. P., Chow, N. S., et al. (2004). Cost-benefit analysis of a case management project for the community-dwelling frail elderly in Hong Kong. *Journal of Applied Gerontology*, *23*(1), 70–85.

Lin, R. L., Lin, F. J., Wu, C. L., et al. (2006, August). Effect of a hospital-based case management approach on treatment outcome of patients with tuberculosis. *Journal of the Formosan Medical Association*, *105*(8), 636–644.

Long, M. J. (2002, June). Case management model or case manager type? That is the question. *Health Care Manager*, *20*(4), 53–65.

Long, M. J., Marshall, B. S. (2000, August). What price an additional day of life? A cost-effectiveness study of case management. *The American Journal of Managed Care*, *6*(8), 881–886.

Lu, K. Y., Lin, P. L., Tzeng, L. C., et al. (2006, November). Effectiveness of case management for community elderly with hypertension, diabetes mellitus, and hypercholesterolemia in Taiwan: A record review. *International Journal of Nursing Studies*, *43*(8), 1001–1010.

Luzinski, C. H., Stockbridge, E., Craighead, J., et al. (2008, May–June). The community case management program: For 12 years, caring at its best. *Geriatric Nursing*, *29*(3), 207–215.

Ma, J., Berra, K., Haskell, W. L., et al. (2009, November). Case management to reduce risk of cardiovascular disease in a county health care system. *Archives of Internal Medicine*, *169*(21), 1988–1995.

Ma, J., Lee, K. V., Berra, K., et al. (2006). Implementation of case management to reduce cardiovascular disease risk in the Stanford and San Mateo Heart to Heart randomized controlled trial: Study protocol and baseline characteristics. *Implementation Science*, *1,* 21.

(*continued*)

BOX 16-2 Included Studies in AHRQ Comparative Effectiveness Review, No. 99 Outpatient Case Management for Adults with Medical Illness and Complex Care Needs (*Continued*)

Mangura, B., Napolitano, E., Passannante, M., et al. (2002, August). Directly observed therapy (DOT) is not the entire answer: An operational cohort analysis. *The International Journal of Tuberculosis and Lung Disease*, *6*(8), 654–661.

Marshall, B. S., Long, M. J., Voss, J., et al. (1999, November-December). Case management of the elderly in a health maintenance organization: The implications for program administration under managed care. *Journal of Healthcare Management*, *44*(6), 477–91. discussion 92–93.

Martin, D. C., Berger, M. L., Anstatt, D. T., et al. (2004, October). A randomized controlled open trial of population-based disease and case management in a Medicare Plus Choice health maintenance organization. *Preventing Chronic Disease*, *1*(4), A05.

Mayo, N. E., Nadeau, L., Ahmed, S., et al. (2008). Bridging the gap: The effectiveness of teaming a stroke coordinator with patient's personal physician on the outcome of stroke. *Age and Ageing*, *37*(1), 32–38.

McCorkle, R., Benoliel, J. Q., Donaldson, G., et al. (1989, September 15). A randomized clinical trial of home nursing care for lung cancer patients. *Cancer 64*(6), 1375–1382.

McCoy, H. V., Dodds, S., Rivers, J. E., et al. (1992). Case management services for HIV-seropositive IDUs. *NIDA Research Monograph*, *127*, 181–207.

Miller, R., Newcomer, R., Fox, P. (1999, August). Effects of the Medicare Alzheimer's Disease Demonstration on nursing home entry. *Health Services Research*, *34*(3), 691–714.

Mittelman, M. S., Roth, D., Haley, W., et al. (2004). Effects of a caregiver intervention on negative caregiver appraisals of behavior problems in patients with Alzheimer's Disease: Results of a randomized trial. *The Journals of Gerontology. Series B, Psychological Sciences and Social Sciences*, *59*(1), 27–34.

Mittelman, M. S., Roth, D., Coon, D., et al. (2004). Sustained benefit of supportive intervention for depressive symptoms in Alzheimer's caregivers. *The American Journal of Psychiatry*, *161*, 850–856

Mittelman, M. S., Brodaty, H., Wallen, A. S., et al. (2008). A Three-country randomized controlled trial of a psychosocial intervention for caregivers combined with pharmacological treatment for patients with Alzheimer disease: Effects on caregiver depression. *The American Journal of Geriatric Psychiatry*, *16*(11), 893–904.

Mittelman, M. S., Haley, W. E., Clay, O. J., et al. (2006). Improving caregiver well-being delays nursing home placement of patients with Alzheimer disease. *Neurology*, *67*(9), 1592–1599.

Moore, S., Corner, J., Haviland, J., et al. (2002, November 16). Nurse led follow up and conventional medical follow up in management of patients with lung cancer: Randomised trial. *BMJ*, *325*(7373), 1145.

Morales-Asencio, J. M., Gonzalo-Jimenez, E., Martin-Santos, F. J., et al. (2008). Effectiveness of a nurse-led case management home care model in Primary Health Care. A quasi-experimental, controlled, multi-centre study. *BMC Health Services Research*, *8*, 193.

Moran, G., Coleman, V., Heaney, S., et al. (2008, May). An alternative model for case management in Flintshire. *Br J Community Nurs*. *13*(5), 227–231.

Mor, V., Wool, M., Guadagnoli, E., et al. (1995). The impact of short term case management on cancer patients' concrete needs and quality of life. *Advances in Medical Sociology*, *6*, 269–294.

Newcomer, R., Maravilla, V., Faculjak, P., et al. (2004, December). Outcomes of preventive case management among high-risk elderly in three medical groups: A randomized clinical trial. *Eval Health Prof*. *27*(4), 323–348.

Newcomer, R., Miller, R., Clay, T., et al. (1999). Effects of the Medicare Alzheimer's Disease Demonstration on Medicare expenditures. *Health Care Financing Review*, *20*(4), 45–65.

Newcomer, R., Spitalny, M., Fox, P., et al. (1999, August). Effects of the Medicare Alzheimer's Disease Demonstration on the use of community-based services. *Health Services Research*, *34*(3), 645–667.

Newcomer, R., Yordi, C., DuNah R, et al. (1999, August). Effects of the Medicare Alzheimer's Disease Demonstration on caregiver burden and depression. *Health Services Research*, *34*(3), 669–689.

Nickel, J. T., Salsberry, P. J., Caswell, R. J., et al. (1996, April). Quality of life in nurse case management of persons with AIDS receiving home care. *Res Nurs Health*. *19*(2), 91–99.

Nyamathi, A. M., Christiani, A., Nahid, P., et al. (2006, July). A randomized controlled trial of two treatment programs for homeless adults with latent tuberculosis infection. *Int J Tuberc Lung Dis*. *10*(7), 775–782.

Nyamathi, A., Stein, J. A., Schumann, A., et al. (2007, January). Latent variable assessment of outcomes in a nurse-managed intervention to increase latent tuberculosis treatment completion in homeless adults. *Health Psychology*, *26*(1), 68–76.

Okin, R. L., Boccellari, A., Azocar, F., et al. (2000, September). The effects of clinical case management on hospital service use among ED frequent users. *The American Journal of Emergency Medicine*, *18*(5), 603–608.

Oliva, N. L. (2010, March–April). A closer look at nurse case management of community-dwelling older adults: Observations from a longitudinal study of care coordination in the chronically ill. *Professional Case Management*, *15*(2), 90–100.

Onder, G., Liperoti, R., Bernabei, R., et al. (2008, June). Case management, preventive strategies, and caregiver attitudes among older adults in home care: Results of the ADHOC study. *Journal of the American Medical Directors Association*, *9*(5), 337–341

Onder, G., Liperoti, R., Soldato, M., et al. (2007, March). Case management and risk of nursing home admission for older adults in home care: Results of the AgeD in HOme Care Study. *Journal of the American Geriatrics Society*, *55*(3), 439–444.

Palmas, W., Shea, S., Starren, J., et al. (2010, March–April). Medicare payments, healthcare service use, and telemedicine implementation costs in a randomized trial comparing telemedicine case management with usual care in medically underserved participants with diabetes mellitus (IDEATel). *Journal of the American Medical Informatics Association*, *17*(2), 196–202.

Peikes, D., Chen, A., Schore, J., et al. (2009, February 11). Effects of care coordination on hospitalization, quality of care, and health care expenditures among Medicare beneficiaries. *JAMA*, *301*(6), 603–618.

Peters-Klimm, F., Campbell, S., Hermann, K., et al. (2010). Case management for patients with chronic systolic heart failure in primary care: The HICMan exploratory randomised controlled trial. *Trials.*, *11*, 56.

Pettitt, D. J., Okada Wollitzer, A., Jovanovic, L., et al. (2005, December). Decreasing the risk of diabetic retinopathy in a study of case management: The California Medi-Cal Type 2 Diabetes Study. *Diabetes Care*, *28*(12), 2819–2822.

Picariello, G., Hanson, C., Futterman, R., et al. (2008, August). Impact of a geriatric case management program on health plan costs. *Population Health Management*, *11*(4), 209–215.

Poole, P. J., Chase, B., Frankel, A., et al. (2001, March). Case management may reduce length of hospital stay in patients with recurrent admissions for chronic obstructive pulmonary disease. *Respirology*, *6*(1), 37–42.

Pugh, G. L. (2009). Exploring HIV/AIDS case management and client quality of life. *Journal of HIV/AIDS and Social Services*, *8*(2), 202–218.

Pugh, L. C., Havens, D. S., Xie, S., et al. (2001). Case management for elderly persons with heart failure: The quality of life and cost outcomes. *MEDSURG Nursing*. *10*(2), 71–8.

Rice, K. L., Dewan, N., Bloomfield, H. E., et al. (2010, October 1). Disease management program for chronic obstructive pulmonary disease: A randomized controlled trial. *American Journal of Respiratory and Critical Care Medicine*, *182*(7), 890–6.

Rich, M. W., Beckham, V., Wittenberg, C., et al. (1995, November 2). A multidisciplinary intervention to prevent the readmission of elderly patients with congestive heart failure. *The New England Journal of Medicine*, *333*(18), 1190–1195.

Rich, M. W., Vinson, J. M., Sperry, J. C., et al. (1993, November). Prevention of readmission in elderly patients with congestive heart failure: Results of a prospective, randomized pilot study. *Journal of General Internal Medicine*, *8*(11), 585–590.

Riegel, B., Carlson, B., Glaser, D., et al. (2006, April). Randomized controlled trial of telephone case management in Hispanics of Mexican origin with heart failure. *J Card Fail*. *12*(3), 211–219.

Riegel, B., Carlson, B., Kopp, Z., et al. (2002, March 25). Effect of a standardized nurse case-management telephone intervention on resource use in patients with chronic heart failure. *Archives of Internal Medicine*, *162*(6), 705–712.

Ritz, L. J., Nissen, M. J., Swenson, K. K., et al. (2000, July). Effects of advanced nursing care on quality of life and cost outcomes of women diagnosed with breast cancer. *Oncol Nurs Forum*. *27*(6), 923–932.

Roth, D. L., Mittelman, M. S., Clay, O. J., et al. (2005, December). Changes in social support as mediators of the impact of a psychosocial intervention for spouse caregivers of persons with Alzheimer's disease. *Psychol Aging*. *20*(4), 634–644.

Rubenstein, L. Z., Alessi, C. A., Josephson, K. R., et al. (2007, February). A randomized trial of a screening, case finding, and referral system for older veterans in primary care. *Journal of the American Geriatrics Society*, *55*(2), 166–174.

Sadowski, L. S., Kee, R. A., VanderWeele, T. J., et al. (2009, May 6). Effect of a housing and case management program on emergency department visits and hospitalizations among chronically ill homeless adults: A randomized trial. *JAMA*, *301*(17), 1771–1778.

Sansom, S. L., Anthony, M. N., Garland, W. H., et al. (2008). The costs of HIV antiretroviral therapy adherence programs and impact on health care utilization. *AIDS Patient Care STDs*, *22*(2), 131–138.

Schein, C., Gagnon, A. J., Chan, L., et al. (2005, April). The association between specific nurse case management interventions and elder health. *Journal of the American Geriatrics Society*, *53*(4), 597–602.

(*continued*)

BOX 16-2 Included Studies in AHRQ Comparative Effectiveness Review, No. 99 Outpatient Case Management for Adults with Medical Illness and Complex Care Needs (*Continued*)

Schifalacqua, M., Hook, M., O'Hearn P., et al. (2000, Spring). Coordinating the care of the chronically ill in a world of managed care. *Nursing Administration Quarterly*, *24*(3), 12–20.

Schifalacqua, M. M., Ulch, P. O., Schmidt, M. (2004, January–March). How to make a difference in the health care of a population. One person at a time. *Nursing Administration Quarterly*, *28*(1), 29–35.

Schore, J., Brown, R., Cheh, V., et al. (1997). *Costs and consequences of case management for medicare beneficiaries.* Report prepared for the Health Care Financing Administration. Princeton, NJ: Mathematica Policy Research.

Schore, J. L., Brown, R. S., Cheh, V. A. (1999, Summer). Case management for high-cost Medicare beneficiaries. *Health Care Financing Review*, *20*(4), 87–101.

Schore, J., Peikes, D., Peterson, G., et al. (2011, March). *Fourth report to congress on the evaluation of the medicare coordinated care demonstration*. Baltimore, MD: Centers for Medicare & Medicaid Services.

Schraeder, C., Fraser, C., Clark, I., et al. (2008). Evaluation of a primary care nurse case management intervention for chronically ill community dwelling older people. *Journal of Nursing and Healthcare of Chronic Illnesses*, *17*, 407–417.

Shah, R., Chen, C., O'Rourke S, et al. (2011, February). Evaluation of care management for the uninsured. *Medical Care*, *49*(2), 166–171.

Shea, S. (2007). IDEATel Consortium. The Informatics for Diabetes and Education Telemedicine (IDEATel) project. *Transactions of the American Clinical and Climatology Association*, *118*, 289–304.

Shea, S., Starren, J., Weinstock, R. S., et al. (2002, January–February). Columbia University's Informatics for Diabetes Education and Telemedicine (IDEATel) Project: Rationale and design. *Journal of the American Medical Informatics Association*, *9*(1), 49–62.

Shea, S., Weinstock, R. S., Starren, J., et al. (2006, January–February). A randomized trial comparing telemedicine case management with usual care in older, ethnically diverse, medically underserved patients with diabetes mellitus. *Journal of the American Medical Informatics Association*, *13*(1), 40–51.

Shea, S., Weinstock, R. S., Teresi, J. A., et al. (2009, July–August). A randomized trial comparing telemedicine case management with usual care in older, ethnically diverse, medically underserved patients with diabetes mellitus: 5 year results of the IDEATel study. *Journal of the American Medical Informatics Association*, *16*(4), 446–456.

Shelton, P., Schraeder, C., Dworak, D., et al. (2001, December). Caregivers' utilization of health services: Results from the Medicare Alzheimer's Disease Demonstration, Illinois site. *Journal of the American Geriatrics Society*, *49*(12), 1600–1605.

Sisk, J. E., Hebert, P. L., Horowitz, C. R., et al. (2006). Improving patient care. Effects of nurse management on the quality of heart failure care in minority communities: A randomized trial. *Annals of Internal Medicine*, *145*(4), 273.

Sorensen, J. L., Dilley, J., London, J., et al. (2003). Case management for substance abusers with HIV/AIDS: A randomized clinical trial. *The American Journal of Drug and Alcohol Abuse*, *29*(1), 133–150.

Specht, J., Bossen, A., Hall, G. R., et al. (2009, June–July). The effects of a dementia nurse care manager on improving caregiver outcomes. *American Journal of Alzheimer's Disease and Other Dementias*, *24*(3), 193–207.

Tatum, W. O., Al-Saadi, S., Orth, T. L. (2008, December). Outpatient case management in low-income epilepsy patients. *Epilepsy Research*, *82*(2–3), 156–161.

Trief, P. M., Morin, P. C., Izquierdo, R., et al. (2006, April). Depression and glycemic control in elderly ethnically diverse patients with diabetes: The IDEATel project. *Diabetes Care*, *29*(4), 830–835.

Trief, P. M., Teresi, J. A., Izquierdo, R., et al. (2007, May). Psychosocial outcomes of telemedicine case management for elderly patients with diabetes: The randomized IDEATel trial. *Diabetes Care*, *30*(5), 1266–1268.

Vickrey, B. G., Mittman, B. S., Connor, K. I., et al. (2006, November 21). The effect of a disease management intervention on quality and outcomes of dementia care. *Annals of Internal Medicine*, *145*(10), 713–726.

Wetta-Hall, R. (2007). Impact of a collaborative community case management program on a low-income uninsured population in Sedgwick County, KS. *Applied Nursing Research*, *20*(4), 188–194.

Wilson, C., Curtis, J., Lipke, S., et al. (2005, August). Nurse case manager effectiveness and case load in a large clinical practice: Implications for workforce development. *Diabetic Medicine*, *22*(8), 1116–1120.

Wohl, A. R., Garland, W. H., Valencia, R., et al. (2006, June). A randomized trial of directly administered antiretroviral therapy and adherence case management intervention. *Clinical Infectious Diseases*, *42*(11), 1619–1627.

Wolf, A. M., Conaway, M. R., Crowther, J. Q., et al. (2004). Translating lifestyle intervention to practice in obese patients with type 2 diabetes: Improving Control with Activity and Nutrition (ICAN) study. *Diabetes Care*, *27*(7), 1570–1576.

Wolf, A. M., Siadaty, M., Yaeger, B., et al. (2007, August). Effects of lifestyle intervention on health care costs: Improving Control with Activity and Nutrition (ICAN). *Journal of the American Dietetic Association, 107*(8), 1365–1373.

Wolff, J. L., Giovannetti, E. R., Boyd, C. M., et al. (2010, August). Effects of guided care on family caregivers. *Gerontologist, 50*(4), 459–470.

Zimmer, J. G., Eggert, G. M., Chiverton, P. (1990, August). Individual versus team case management in optimizing community care for chronically ill patients with dementia. *Journal of Aging and Health, 2*(3), 357–372.

Adapted from Hickam, D. H., Weiss, J. W., & Guise, J. M., Buckley, D., Motuapuaka, M., Graham, E. ... Saha, S. (2013, January). Outpatient case management for adults with medical illness and complex care needs [Internet]. Rockville, MD: Agency for Healthcare Research and Quality. Retrieved from http://www.ncbi.nlm.nih.gov/books/NBK116482/

The findings of the AHRQ study serves as a bellwether to case management stakeholders that consistent, coordinated, and concerted effort must be focused on the adoption of universally accepted terminology and definitions, formal protection of the job title, acceptable education and training paths, and continuous support and production of evidence on which to base safe, effective, and efficient case management practice. At the individual level, the professional case manager must adopt a methodical approach to knowledge-seeking behavior, remain abreast of evidence-based developments influencing practice, and promote effective case management practices across organizations and among colleagues in order to enhance the overall quality and perception of case management.

CONTEMPORARY WORK IN ANTICIPATORY CARE

The knowledge and ability to expect and intervene on the impact of health conditions has been an assumed strength of case management practice. Generally speaking, it has not been the focus of specific research or development as a formal strategy in the past. For example, understanding the progressive effect of emphysema on an individual's ability to participate in self-care activities allows the case manager to facilitate home care service arrangements in advance of the patient's worsening condition. This proactive approach improves the ability of an individual to continue living independently and contributes to reducing the risk of acute hospitalization or placement in an inpatient facility (e.g., assisted living, long-term care). Although not possible in every case, the intersection of disease process knowledge and familiarity with available services allows a case manager to act in advance of crisis development rather than react to a decline in health status to engage in care.

INTERNATIONAL HEALTH CARE DELIVERY

Since the early 2000s, the topic of anticipatory care has been a recurring one in nursing and health care literature emanating from the United Kingdom and other European nations. In this context, anticipatory care has been defined as working with clients to identify circumstances that may have a negative impact on their mental, physical, and social health and to put in place proactive strategies to avert those impacts (Kennedy, Harbison, Mahoney, Jarvis, & Veitch, 2011; Kralik, 2011). However, in reviewing literature regarding anticipatory care, there was no acknowledgment of case management as an anticipatory or proactive component of health care delivery, leaving one to wonder why anticipatory care appeared to be a new concept to some and why was case management not acknowledged as an influence? Could it have been

- a matter of semantics that authors defined care as being specific to hands-on direct patient care that did not include case management?
- a health system characterization that did not include case management practice in the same way as it is within the United States?
- the authors who did not consider case management to be a nursing or care function?
- an indicator that case management had not articulated its proactive approach clearly in literature or proven it with actual outcomes?

As noted by Baker et al. (2012), anticipatory care fits into the equation of community-based case management in that it provides patients the opportunity to express their wishes for care prior to a sudden deterioration in their health. Beginning with the identification of individuals at high risk prior to the need for hospitalization, patients and families are supported in making care choices which provides a higher level of autonomy and more opportunities to participate in the decision making regarding their own health care. Through community-based efforts, the care team focuses on preventing hospitalization rather than reacting to worsening needs following a hospital admission. In this way, anticipatory care seeks to achieve patient-centered, cost-effective care to individuals with complex health conditions who are most likely to consume increasing resources over a longer period of time.

The anticipatory approach to health care management outside of the United States appears to align case management's focus on promoting quality, cost-effective outcomes with the IOM aims for health care improvement (safe, effective, patient-centered, timely, efficient, and equitable). The references to anticipatory care raise questions as to whether case management theory and practice should be more specific with regard to documenting the function of anticipating situational risks and mitigation strategies associated with client care (Treiger & Fink-Samnick, 2013).

DISCUSSION OF KEY ELEMENTS

In the COLLABORATE paradigm, a case manager demonstrates the key elements of this competency through forward-thinking, proactive care strategy, and self-directed practice.

Forward-Thinking (Professionalism)

The forward-thinking case manager considers the immediate and future implications of her or his interactions across the entire health care continuum and understands the importance of contributing to the positive perception of all working case managers.

The Impact of Stereotype

When an individual identifies herself or himself as a case manager, the manner in which one handles interpersonal interactions (e.g., verbal, written) can have significant influence on the perception of all subsequent case managers. Regardless of whether either party to the interaction was simply having an off day, the impression left by an interaction colors other people's perceptions and helps create personal biases both positive and negative in nature. When an individual shares their personal experience with others, that personal bias adds momentum to the development of stereotypes.

Stereotypes have been classified into three general headings as being aids to explanation (e.g., helping to explain a situation), energy-saving devices (e.g., reducing the effort of an individual), and shared group beliefs (e.g., formed in alignment with views or norms that are accepted to one's social group) (McGarty, Yzerbyt, & Spears, 2002).

- As an aid to explanation, a stereotype is one way in which an individual makes sense of a situation by considering new information within the context of existing knowledge. Hence, in an input-rich environment, such as a hospital, an individual distills the multiple inputs into manageable chunks in order to process at least some of the information in a way that makes most sense.
- As an energy-saving device, rather than recognizing individuals and their differences, stereotypes allow an individual to treat a person as a homogeneous group and ignore the diversity and information detail that actually exists.
- As a shared group belief, stereotypes may be formed and shared through coincidence of experience, existence of shared knowledge, or coordination of behavior.

When groups of health care consumers stereotype case managers based on a less-than-positive personal experience (or the experience of someone from their social group), they assume that those identifying themselves as case managers are of equal quality and competence. Consider the emergence of stereotyping in reaction to an unsatisfactory interaction with someone identified as a case manager. In light of the inconsistent practice of case management across the continuum of care, in combination with the effects of disease process, injury, or other cognitive challenge, the belief that all case managers are the same will undoubtedly contribute to challenging relationships with subsequent case managers.

A forward-thinking case management professional interacts in a positive and productive manner in all facets of practice. Communication and interpersonal skills are critical in all aspects of practice. (See discussion of professional communication in chapter 11.) Incompetence in these skills results in tasks becoming even more challenging. For example, as case managers delve into personal history, assessment questions quickly touch on highly sensitive topics. When entering into a new relationship, the case manager is often a stranger to the health care consumer, one of many people asking the same (or similar) questions. Not unexpectedly, an individual may resort to providing incomplete, misleading, or untruthful information, when trust has not yet developed or in a situation where a stereotype may have been applied to case managers. The implication of communication competence across the ranks of case managers practicing in every health care setting, is considerable.

The Impact of Advocacy

As a competency, advocacy is discussed in chapter 12. For the purpose of this chapter, advocacy bears specific mention with regard to a case manager's awareness and action pertaining to legislation and regulation. From practice acts to resource allocation policy, the forward-thinking case manager understands that maintaining awareness of and advocating with regard to the frameworks that govern practice is essential. Informed individuals articulate the boots-on-the-ground reality that legislative and regulatory actions have on day-to-day practice. A case manager participating in these forums has the potential to influence the outcome of these debates in a way that is positive and beneficial to all practitioners. Again, consider the scenario in Box 16-3, which returns to the issue of multistate nursing licensure. In this case, failure to participate in advocacy affects organizational policy in a different way.

Proactive (vs. Reactive) Care Strategy

The professional case manager embodies proactivity by developing and implementing client-centered interventions that address existing barriers to care as well as includes mitigation strategies that address reasonably foreseeable risks. Where care facilitation is concerned, taking a proactive-anticipatory approach is mentioned within the practice standards issued by CMSA, ACMA, and NASW.

COLLABORATE's proactive approach is a hallmark of professional case management which showcases the case

BOX 16-3 Impact of Not Participating in Advocacy

Total Health Care Plan (THCP) is a managed care organization having large employer contracts covering a workforce across the United States. Over the past 10 years, the case managers at THCP raised concerns about working with members from states in which they are not licensed. The issue was raised in a staff meeting, resulting in human resources seeking feedback from the legal department. The organization's legal counsel responded that because case management was not hands-on clinical practice, state-based licensure did not apply and the case managers should continue to work with members regardless of geographic location. The last time this issue came up was 5 years ago.

Dan is a case manager working at THCP for the past 3 years. Over the past 2 years, he heard about the local case management chapter's informational campaign pertaining to the importance of multistate licensure. The chapter pleaded with members to contact legislators with regard to a bill proposing adoption of the Nurse Licensure Compact (NLC). Previous attempts at passing this bill failed because of the vocal opposition of a collective bargaining unit representing nurses working at hospitals within the state. The argument presented illustrated a worst-case scenario in which nurses from other states flooded in to assume positions left vacant due to a work stoppage. Unfortunately, no testimony was given on behalf of those working in case management to describe the concerns relating to working with out-of-state members at their place of employment. The bill never got beyond subcommittee hearing.

The failure of working case managers to advocate for passage of this bill contributed to its demise. However, the heightened awareness of multistate licensure resulted in THCP's legal counsel to advise a policy change. Although a case manager was previously assigned new clients based on her or his clinical expertise, THCP now maintains an assignment process based on which state a case manager maintains licensure. In addition, a new team of multistate case managers was established. New case managers holding licensure in Compact states are assigned members residing in those states. This assignment change affected many members who had established trusting relationships with their case manager. It also affects case managers unfamiliar with the rarer conditions and treatments as these members had previously been assigned to colleagues having specific clinical experience.

manager's value to the health care team. Discovering conflicts in information is reason for actively probing of the incongruity. Failure to investigate situations in which conflicting information presents itself, will likely result in subsequent challenges. While overlooking an issue may simplify one's tasks at that moment, failure to address an inconsistency neither facilitates the care team's effort nor improves the patient's condition.

Consider the situation in which a client mentions that the sister who drives him to all health care appointments is moving out of state next month. Instead of waiting for the client to miss an appointment or fail to fill a prescription, the proactive case manager works with the individual to identify and engage other transportation resources, facilitates arrangements for upcoming appointments, and initiates home delivery of prescriptions and groceries to alleviate additional transportation demands (Treiger & Fink-Samnick, 2013). This is one example illustrating how a case manager identifies and addresses additional impact areas (e.g., medication, food) resulting from a known problem (e.g., lost means of transportation).

Self-Directed Practice (Professional Autonomy)

COLLABORATE defines self-directed practice in terms of functional autonomy to practice independently within the scope of one's professional practice act and/or other imposed limitations (e.g., legislation, regulation, certification, organization). The self-directed case manager maintains a collaborative yet independent approach to practice. The case manager demonstrates self-directed practice through performance of responsibilities, without being prompted or directly supervised by another person.

Defining self-directed practice for case management requires attention. Meaningful discussion and research are needed to ensure the identification and acceptance of self-directed practice as well as the adoption of defined standards into legislation and/or regulation. Case management's continued professional development must be undertaken as a collaborative effort involving representation and endorsement of primary stakeholders (e.g., academia, professional organizations, certification agencies) across the health care continuum, complementary sectors (e.g., regulation, accreditation), as well as individual practitioners and large employer groups.

Within nursing and social work, autonomy and control over practice have been developed and debated for years. Key issues in the discussion of nursing were identified by Weston (2008) who sought to clarify and delineate the definition of control over nursing practice versus autonomy and Skår (2008) who focused on the defining concepts of nurse autonomy (e.g., authority of total patient care, the power to make decisions, the freedom to make clinical judgments). Within the social work realm, the issues of licensure, education level, and scope of practice are also matters of ongoing concern. The topic of case management certification adds another layer of complexity to the discussion, specifically with regard to the levels of recognition and licensure, which vary state to state.

Educational Preparation

Another barrier to establishing professional autonomy is the formal declaration and acceptance of the mandatory minimum educational degree required to begin practice, as well as the need for advanced degrees for specialty and advancement to administrative positions. This effort is challenged by the fact that case managers come from various professional affiliations, nursing and social work being the predominant forces. The lack of regulatory consensus on degree minimums within each of these professional affiliations does not help the effort to define it specifically for case management practice.

Nursing. The American Nurses Association (ANA) issued its position statement in 1965 as a Board of Directors adopted a committee recommendation that a minimum preparation for beginning professional nursing practice should be baccalaureate degree education in nursing. Also included was a concept of three-tiered nursing education which included baccalaureate education for beginning nursing practice, associate degree education for beginning technical nursing practice, and vocational education for assistants in the health service occupations. This statement was reaffirmed in 1978 by the ANA House of Delegates resolution, which included a recommendation that by 1985 the minimum preparation for entry into professional nursing practice would be the baccalaureate degree. A two-tiered nursing practice, professional and technical, was also affirmed at that time (ANA, 2013).

In a position statement issued by the American Association of Colleges of Nursing (AACN), first issued in 1996, the need for mandatory minimum educational preparation included specific mention of case management,

Rapidly expanding clinical knowledge and mounting complexities in health care mandate that professional nurses possess educational preparation commensurate with the diversified responsibilities required of them. As health care shifts from hospital-centered, inpatient care to more primary and preventive care throughout the community, the health system requires registered nurses who not only can practice across multiple settings—both within and beyond hospitals—but also can function with more independence in clinical decision making, case management, provision of direct bedside care, supervision of unlicensed aides and other support personnel, guiding patients through the maze of health care resources, and educating patients on treatment regimens and adoption of healthy lifestyles. In particular, preparation of the entry-level professional nurse requires a greater orientation to community-based primary health care, and an emphasis on health promotion, maintenance, and cost-effective coordinated care.

Accordingly, the AACN recognizes the bachelor of science degree in nursing as the minimum educational requirement for professional nursing practice. Since 2005, legislation requiring a baccalaureate degree in nursing within 10 years of initial licensure has been introduced in three states (New York, New Jersey, and Rhode Island), none of which passed (ANA, 2013). A 2012 National League of Nursing newsletter highlighted the New York state "BSN in 10" initiative. Despite bipartisan support in both chambers, the New York legislation failed to get past the committee. The bill's advocates stated that in addition to improving patient care, the law improved the opportunity for nurses wishing to advance to administrative positions, specialty care (e.g., oncology), and also addressed issues relating to the projected shortfall in nursing school faculty due to the average age of instructors being 53 years.

Social Work. Although there is no universally accepted minimum education level for social workers, the Council on Social Work Education (2008) sets the bar for generalist practice as requiring a baccalaureate degree. Refer to chapter 4 for more discussion on this point.

Case Management. There is a lack of cohesion among professional case management-specific organizations as to minimum degree requirement. The following is how these organizations address education within their respective practice standards:

- The ACMA practice standards for case management in health systems offer no guidance as to the practitioner's minimum education level but does support attaining its own credential within a specific time frame on 2 years of health system case management experience.
- The CMSA (2011) qualification standard is the most specific of the case management-specific practice standards. It highlights the need for having one of the following: "Current, active, and unrestricted licensure or certification in a health or human services discipline that allows the professional to conduct an assessment discipline independently within the scope of practice of that discipline, or in the case of a state that does not require licensure or certification, the individual must have a baccalaureate or graduate degree in social work or another health or human service field that promotes the physical, psychosocial and/or vocational well-being of the persons being served. The degree must be from an institution that is fully accredited by a nationally recognized educational accreditation organization, and the individual must have completed a supervised field experience in case management, health, or behavioral health as part of the degree requirements." This section of the 2010 CMSA practice standards is noted to have been updated for clarification in October, 2011.
- The National Association of Professional Geriatric Care Managers does not address educational degree minimums directly, although it does mention the issues of continuing education and certification.
- The NASW (2013) case management practice standards specify that "The social work case manager shall possess a baccalaureate or advanced degree in social work from a school or program accredited by the Council on Social Work Education."

The minimum educational standard is a significant barrier to overcome as part establishing professional autonomy. Because of the numerous issues that need to be incorporated in a productive discussion, coupled with consumer confidence and protection concerns, COLLABORATE supports defining the baccalaureate degree as the minimum requirement for generalist case management practice, and higher

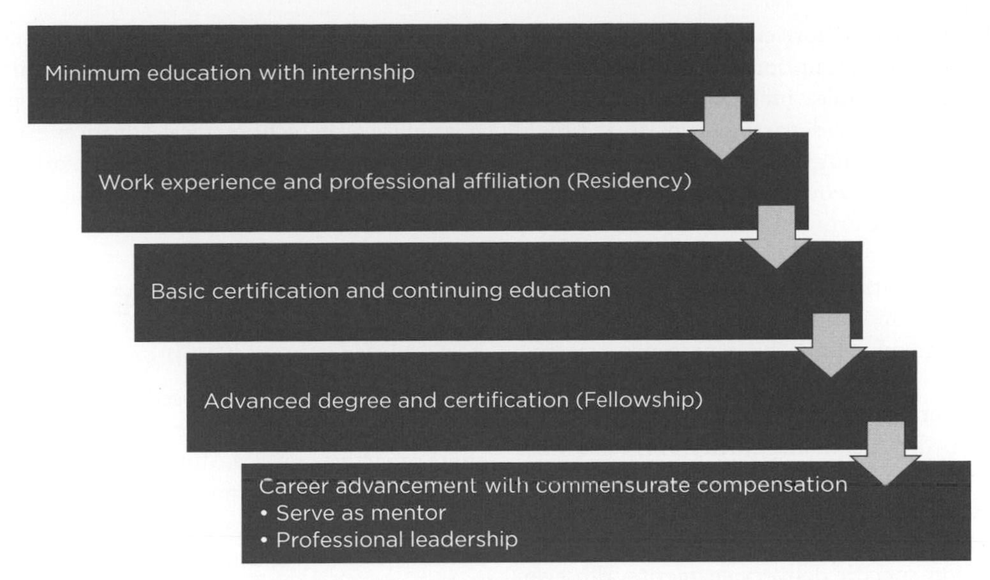

Figure 16-2. Greater emphasis on a professional development path, which includes defined educational and experiential components.

degree achievement for specialty practice and administrative positions. This undertaking must utilize a unified approach with the development of consensus statements regarding case management definition, professional autonomy, and educational expectations. These position statements will help drive needed change in degree requirements, licensure, accreditation, and certification. Figure 16-2 depicts a professional path which values professional development through higher education and defined experiential components.

CASE MANAGEMENT PRACTICE IMPLICATIONS

The implications of moving to an anticipatory case management approach extend beyond the identification of risk. Proactive case management must include strategies to address risk prior to actual development of care barriers and other challenges contributing to health complexity.

Case Finding Methodology

Currently, the strategies relied on for the identification of individuals who may benefit from case management intervention include looking at the population according to risk using the following:

- Screening tools
- Trigger event (e.g., diagnosis, procedure, admission)
- Utilization (e.g., frequent emergency department visits, polypharmacy)
- Age
- Social issue (e.g., elder or child neglect)
- Predictive modeling
- Stratification
- Referral (e.g., request by provider, intradepartment, self)

These are all reactive strategies to various degrees. The use of existing mechanisms will continue; however, there needs to be movement toward more proactive case finding methodologies. Enter the use of financial profiling to identify high-risk characteristics via consumer habits. For example, looking at spending trends on items such as cigarettes and alcohol or the absence of spending on necessary items (e.g., food, prescription medication) allows for identification of high-risk characteristics, which may benefit from a closer look and earlier intervention.

Other sources of information, such as electronic documentation systems, personal health tracking devices (e.g., personal health records, smartphone applications, electronic pill dispensers, weight scales), health risk appraisals, and patient satisfaction surveys, collect a tremendous amount of data, including geographic location of the user. Once harvested and combined with purchase transactions and demographic details (e.g., socioeconomic status, ethnicity), the results could be used to identify barriers to care and health problems much earlier in their development cycle.

As intriguing as this possibility may sound, these are clearly more aggressive and invasive means for leveraging technology as an investigative tool for health care purposes. The potential benefits of identifying health and lifestyle risks must be weighed against expectations of privacy, freedom of choice, and self-determination. The ethics and legal implications of these approaches require substantial further discussion and agreement on limitations prior to widespread use.

Use of Case Management Intervention Beyond the Top 1% to 3% in Payer-Based Practice Settings

Although there are limitations to validity of claims data, health plans utilize it to produce utilization and costs reports, often breaking this information down to a per-member, per-month statistic. A cut-off of the top 1% to –3% of high-cost members is frequently used to identify individuals who might benefit from case management. This is generally representative of individuals whose claims include high-cost products and services or consumption of large quantities of products and services. Examples include frequent hospital admissions and/or emergency department visits and high-cost treatment (e.g., transplantation, premature birth). The belief is that these members would potentially benefit from the intervention of a clinical professional who is able to apply the case management process and provide direction regarding the appropriate utilization of health care resources. Unfortunately, by the time an individual is classified in the top percentile of a plan's membership, this represents a reactive intervention.

In an effort to intervene more proactively in the chronic disease progression, disease management programs were launched. These initiatives provided individuals with information, tools, and education in order to help them become more informed health care consumers. Programs were often divided into condition-specific delivery segments. However, this approach presented challenges with regard to managing multimorbid members (e.g., program prioritization) and often resulted in shuffling members between disease management, case management, and utilization review departments depending on the individual's location within the care continuum. What disease management programs did not routinely address were the social influencers contributing to progressive worsening of health status and barriers to care (e.g., transportation, nutrition support, family issues).

When considering the involvement of case management in an individual's care, a compromise should be struck to balance an increasing level of health complexity and the administrative burden associated with delivering an intensive management program. The introduction of case management earlier on the path of developing health complexity is worthy of further study. The use of social or barrier triggers alone or in conjunction with utilization indicators may provide richer opportunities on which to intervene, thus supporting medical interventions to slow or reverse the trend of worsening health and fostering a higher level of responsible health choices and self-determination through education.

Change in Case Management Assessment Tools

Existing case management assessment tools focus on a comprehensive approach to the evaluation of bio-psycho-social-spiritual aspects affecting an individual's health. Areas of focus include, but are not limited to, an individual's health and bio-psycho-social-spiritual history. This information feeds into subsequent case manager activities, such as case management planning, care facilitation, monitoring, and evaluation of interventional impact. When assessment tools are automated within an information system, the responses often trigger a list of opportunities and interventions for the case manager to consider as part of her or his case management plan. These results are reactive in nature relative to the information provided by the interviewee. But consider the value of a case management tool that employed background risk calculation algorithms and correlated individual responses with evidence-based databases which compared and predicted individual results with similar populations? The possibilities of technological advances for continuous improvement of risk predictors and tailoring proactive interventions to the individual client over the course of time are staggering.

EMPHASIS ON PROFESSIONAL ACTION

Although advocacy is discussed as part of the specific competency, it bears mention here as an element of establishing a more proactive practice. Shifting the health care industry perspective from the case manager being an employee with a job to that of being a clinical professional following a career path requires transformation in both education and professional realms. The importance of participation in professional organizations as a means of influencing health care policy and professional recognition cannot be overemphasized.

The case management professional maintains awareness of and lobbies for health care policy at federal, state, local, and organizational levels to improve clinical practice, patient care, and health care quality. In addition, the case manager raises awareness of disparities in health care and facilitates access to appropriate care. This is undertaken with the understanding that resource availability and benefit limitations may affect the ability to obtain certain products and services. In those situations, the case manager carefully documents all factors taken into consideration in making recommendations or coverage decisions (CMSA, 2010).

SUMMARY

As case management continues to fight for recognition as a proactive health care intervention, the emphasis on anticipatory practice needs to be cultivated. This will require the case manager to assume a proactive stance in all aspects of practice and advocacy. This chapter examines some of the ideas relating to proactive case management and career development. Competence in this realm holds significant impact on both contemporary and future case management practice.

References

Agency for Healthcare Research and Quality. (2002). *Systems to rate the strength of scientific evidence* [Summary, Evidence Report/Technology Assessment: Number 47. Publication No. 02-E015]. Retrieved September 4, 2014, from http://hstat.nlm.nih.gov/hq/Hquest/screen/DirectAccess/db/strensum

American Association of Colleges of Nursing. (1996). *The baccalaureate degree in nursing as minimal preparation for professional practice*. Retrieved September 14, 2014, from http://www.aacn.nche.edu/publications/position/bacc-degree-prep

American Case Management Association. (2013). *Standards of practice and scope of services for healthcare delivery system case management and transition of care professionals*. Retrieved April 25, 2013, from www.acmaweb.org/Standards

American Nurses Association. (2013). *Nursing education*. Retrieved September 16, 2014, from http://www.nursingworld.org/MainMenu Categories/Policy-Advocacy/State/Legislative-Agenda-Reports/NursingEducation

Association of Social Work Boards. (2014). *About ASWB*. Retrieved September 4, 2014, from http://www.aswb.org/about

Case Management Society of America. (2010). *CMSA standards of practice for case management* (Rev. 2010) Retrieved April 25, 2013, from http://www.cmsa.org/portals/0/pdf/memberonly/StandardsOfPractice.pdf

Case Management Society of America. (2011). *CMSA standards of practice for case management* (Rev. 2010) and updated 2011. Retrieved April 25, 2013, from http://www.cmsa.org/portals/0/pdf/memberonly/StandardsOfPractice.pdf

Cohen, E. L., & Cesta, T. G. (2005). *Nursing case management from essentials to advanced practice applications*. Philadelphia, PA: Elsevier.

Council on Social Work Education. (2008). *Educational policy and accreditation standards*. Retrieved September 16, 2014, from http://www.cswe.org/File.aspx?id=13780

Health and Human Services. (2014). *Massachusetts board of registration in nursing licensing*. Retrieved September 4, 2014, from http://www.mass.gov/eohhs/gov/departments/dph/programs/hcq/dhpl/nursing/licensing

Hickam, D. H., Weiss, J. W., Guise, J. M., Buckley, D., Motuapuaka, M., Graham, E. ... Saha, S. (2013, January). *Outpatient case management for adults with medical illness and complex care needs* [Internet]. Rockville, MD: Agency for Healthcare Research and Quality. Retrieved from http://www.ncbi.nlm.nih.gov/books/NBK116482/

Institute of Medicine. (2001). *Crossing the quality chasm: A new health system for the 21st century*. Washington, DC: National Academy Press.

Institute of Medicine. (2011). *Clinical practice guidelines we can trust*. Retrieved September 4, 2014, from http://www.iom.edu/reports/2011/clinical-practice-guidelines-we-can-trust.aspx

Kennedy, C., Harbison, C. J., Mahoney, C., Jarvis, A., & Veitch, L. (2011). Investigating the contribution of community nurses to anticipatory care: A qualitative exploratory study. *Journal of Advanced Nursing*, *67*(7), 1558–1567. doi:10.1111/j.1365-2648.2010.05589.x

Kongstvedt, P. R. (2013). *Essentials of managed health care* (6th ed.). Sudbury, MA: Jones and Bartlett.

Kralik, D. (2011). Is anticipatory care fundamental to nursing? *Journal of Advanced Nursing*, *67*(7), 1407–1408.

McGarty, C., Yzerbyt, V. Y., & Spears, R. (2002). *Stereotypes as explanations: the formation of meaningful beliefs about social groups*. Cambridge, England: Cambridge University Press.

Medicare Improvements for Patients and Providers Act of 2008. *Public Law 110–275*. Retrieved September 16, 2014, from http://www.gpo.gov/fdsys/pkg/PLAW-110publ275/pdf/PLAW-110publ275.pdf

Merriam-Webster.com. (2014a). Anticipate. Retrieved August 20, 2014, from http://www.merriam-webster.com/dictionary/anticipate

Merriam-Webster.com. (2014b). Proactive. Retrieved August 20, 2014, from http://www.merriam-webster.com/dictionary/proactive

National Association of Professional Geriatric Care Managers. (2013). *NAPGCM standards of practice*. Retrieved September 16, 2014 from http://www.caremanager.org/about/standards-of-practice

National Association of Social Workers. (2013). *NASW standards for social work case management*. Retrieved April 25, 2013, from http://www.socialworkers.org/practice/naswstandards/CaseManagementStandards2013.pdf

National Council of State Boards of Nursing. (2011). *Nursing licensure*. Retrieved September 4, 2014, from https://www.ncsbn.org/Nursing_Licensure.pdf

National Council of State Boards of Nursing. (2014). *About NCSBN*. Retrieved September 4, 2014, from https://www.ncsbn.org/about.htm

National League of Nursing. (2012). NY "BSN in 10" initiative. *National Education Policy Newsletter*, *9*(1). Retrieved September 16, 2014, from http://www.nln.org/publicpolicy/newsletter/vol9_issue1_blast.htm

Powell, S.K., & Tahan, H.A. (2010). *Case management a practical guide for education and practice* (3rd ed.). Philadelphia, PA: Wolters Kluwer | Lippincott Williams & Wilkins.

Skår, R. (2008). The meaning of autonomy in nursing practice. *Journal of Clinical Nursing*, *19*, 2226–2234. doi:10.1111/j.1365–2702.2009.02804.x

Treiger, T. M. and Fink-Samnick, E. (2013). COLLABORATE: A universal, competency-based paradigm for professional case management practice, Part II. *Professional Case Management*, *18*(5), 219–243.

Weston, M. J. (2008). Defining control over nursing practice and autonomy. *Journal of Nursing Administration*, *38*(9), 404–408.

17 TRANSDISCIPLINARY

OBJECTIVES

After studying this chapter, you will be able to:

1. Define terms relevant to health care teams.
2. Compare and contrast the four types of health care teams.
3. Identify the professional standards specific to transdisciplinary practice.
4. Discuss the five stages of Tuckman and Jensen's Group Development Model.
5. Understand the key elements of the Transdisciplinary Competency.

KEY TERMS

Care Coordination
Discipline
Health care consumer
Interdisciplinary
Interprofessional
Medical Model
Multidisciplinary
Professional Diversity
Stakeholder
Transdisciplinary
Team

Amid the spirited industry dialogue about quality health care delivery that subsumes this era of patient-centered care, exists the often tumultuous topic of health care teams. There is most likely a team in place at every practice setting across all transitions of care; one that has been recently formed, re-formed, or refocused based on the latest, greatest industry trend.

The discussion of teams and team structure has been a dominant dialogue in health care for well over five decades. Emphasis on teamwork in health care increased after the publication of two reports from the Institute of Medicine (IOM) which illustrated a quality chasm in U.S. health care and called for vastly improved teamwork to help stem the tide of medical errors and preventable conditions (IOM, 2001).

Teams, teamwork, and the manifesting dynamics and dysfunction can easily impact the outcomes of an organization. Case managers are front and center in facilitating and often leading these efforts. The growth, evolution, transition, value, and continued need to advance teams to a transdisciplinary mind-set, is the focus of this chapter.

DEFINITIONS

Countless articles have been written over the past several decades to address the value of diverse professional expertise comprising the health care team. Those with longevity in our case management industry have most likely experienced a continuum of teams. Each one of these stems from the basic definition of a **team**, a number of persons associated together in work or activity (*Merriam-Webster's Online Dictionary*, 2014d). There are a variety of teams with people often aligned with a particular sports team, such as those for football or baseball. There are work teams for new projects, and those to assess whether or not an organization should pursue a grant request for proposals. For the purposes of this chapter, the focus is on the teams that appear across health and behavioral care organizations.

A **discipline** is defined as a field of study, or training that corrects, molds, or perfects the mental faculties or moral character (*Merriam-Webster's Online Dictionary*, 2014a). The health care industry has many disciplines that comprise the workforce (e.g., medicine, nursing, pharmacy, and social work are disciplines). All serve a valuable role in the patient care process and the efforts of health care teams.

Team work brings the disciplines together in a purposeful effort. Xyrichis and Ream (2008) defined team work as a dynamic process involving two or more health professionals with complementary backgrounds and skills, sharing common health goals and exercising concerted physical and mental effort in assessing, planning, or evaluating patient care. They focused on the importance of interdependent collaboration, open communication, and shared decision making (SDM), which in turn generate value-added patient, organizational, and staff outcomes. These are clear indicators of return on investment for most, if not all, organizations (Xyrichis & Ream, 2008).

SDM refers to a collaborative process that allows patients and their providers to make health care decisions together, taking into account the best scientific evidence available as well as the patient's values and preferences (Informed Medical Decisions Foundations, 2014). Both parties share information: the involved practitioner offers options and describes their risks and benefits, and the patient expresses his or her preferences and values. In this way, each involved participant is armed with a better understanding of the relevant factors and shares responsibility in the decision about how to proceed (Barry & Edgman-Levitan, 2012).

In the event that there is more than one treatment option being discussed, the practitioner can engage SDM by encouraging patients to discuss what they care about and by providing decision aids that raise the patient's awareness and understanding of treatment options and possible outcomes (Barry & Edgman-Levitan, 2012). SDM honors both the treatment practitioner's expert knowledge and the patient's right to be fully informed of all care options and the potential harms and benefits. This process provides patients with the support they need to make the best individualized care decisions, while allowing providers to feel confident in the care they prescribe (Informed Medical Decisions Foundations, 2014). SDM affords all involved are strategic partners in the health care effort, particularly with patients and their family members taking a more active role of the patient care team.

The cultural change to a more concerted and collective team endeavor across the health care industry has contributed to the evolution of a new generation of **health care consumers**. This term refers to any actual or potential recipients of health care, such as a patient in a hospital, a client in a community mental health center, or a member of a prepaid health maintenance organization (Mosby's Medical Dictionary, 2009). Health care consumers are active and interested in the care process.

Working with this new generation of health care consumers can be challenging for case managers. Today's health care consumer can be seen as more aggressive than assertive, due to their increased efforts to ask questions and communicate about their care, if not the care of a family member. The increased modes of communication available to consumers are a blessing and curse as well, as many utilize mobile devices, as well as traditional means such as office visits, to obtain information. Though consider your own stance when you or a family member has a medical and/or behavioral health episode that warrants intervention. Few case managers would take a stance that was anything less than direct and assertive in their efforts to obtain information about and advocate for those loved ones who are patients.

Health care consumers are often viewed as **stakeholders**. These are persons who have a stake in an enterprise or are involved in or affected by a course of action (*Merriam-Webster's Online Dictionary*, 2014c). There can be an exhaustive list of stakeholders, including, but not limited to, members of the treatment team, other treatment providers, health care administrators, community agencies who provide resources (e.g., medical devices and equipment, certified home health care, transportations), contracted managed care providers, and other insurers, attorneys, case managers, and so on.

Care coordination has attracted national attention as an important component of service delivery to achieve quality, efficient, and efficacy goals (Fink-Samnick, 2011a). The literature identifies a range of definitions, several of which appear in Box 17-1. Amid the distinct meanings for care coordination across the globe, there exists a common thread, reference to a concerted, effective, if not organized, effort by professionals from across the health care team to deliberately work together toward the purpose of a treatment plan that is client and/or patient-centered. "Effective" care coordination brings the essential dimension of cost into the definition (National Coalition on Care Coordination, 2009).

With care coordination models, the patient or consumer's needs are coordinated with the assistance of a primary point of contact. This may be the case manager in many instances, or the physician. The latter is based on the approval the CMS 2015 Physician Fee Schedule, and allows for physicians to bill Medicare for "nonface to face" chronic care management under CPT code 99490 (Wicklund, 2014). The amount is designated as 46 dollars and 20 cents per patient for 20 minutes of care.

PAST AND CURRENT THINKING

The internet is ripe with articles about health care teams. There is an array of terms for team-based care, which populate the literature, some of them hybrids of each other. For the purposes of this chapter, the focus is on the most common team structures, interdisciplinary, multidisciplinary, transdisciplinary, and interprofessional.

Independent of the type of team, every profession had laid claim to at least one, if not more, models of team interaction. Most, if not all, professional health care disciplines include language in their professional standards and codes of ethics that speak to collaboration with other colleagues and providers from diverse backgrounds and professionals and the public in promoting community, national, and international

BOX 17-1 Care Coordination Definitions

Deliberately organizing patient care activities and sharing information among all of the participants concerned with a patient's care to achieve safer and more effective care.

Agency for Healthcare Research and Quality, 2014

"Care coordination" is a client-centered, assessment-based interdisciplinary approach to integrating health care and social support services in which an individual's needs and preferences are assessed, a comprehensive care plan is developed, and services are managed and monitored by an identified care coordinator following evidence-based standards of care.

National Care Coordination Coalition, 2009

Components of care coordination:

- Working with an individual and his/her carer(s) to ensure that a high-level, integrated, and personalised care plan is implemented;
- Monitoring services to ensure they are delivered effectively on time and achieve their objectives;
- Facilitating communication between multiple agencies and professionals, and overseeing discussions/meetings as appropriate;
- Maintaining contact with the individual during hospital stay and arranging for discharge; and
- Ensuring that reviews of care are undertaken

Segen's Medical Dictionary, 2012

Practice-based care coordination within the medical home is a direct, family/youth-centered, team-oriented, outcomes-focused process designed to:

- Facilitate the provision of comprehensive health promotion and chronic condition care;
- Ensure a locus of ongoing, proactive, planned care activities;
- Build and use effective communication strategies among family, the medical home, schools, specialists, and community professionals and community connections; and
- Help improve, measure, monitor, and sustain quality outcomes (clinical, functional, satisfaction, and cost).

McAllister et al., 2007

efforts to meet health needs (American Nurses Association [ANA], 2010, 2001; National Association of Social Workers [NASW], 2013). With every new generation of health care culture comes a series of innovative team-based care delivery models and new standards of practice.

Most case managers who work in the health care industry have engaged in a wide variety of teams. There are dynamics which both enhance and impede the team's quality of efforts, such as patterns of communication, leadership, adaptability, collective, and SDM, to name a few. In order to have a better grasp of the important role these dynamics can play in the context of patient care, case managers must have a preliminary understanding of the various types of teams that can appear at their respective organizations.

MULTIDISCIPLINARY TEAMS

Multidisciplinary teams refer to a group composed of members with varied but complimentary experience, qualifications, and skills that contribute to the achievement of the organization's specific objectives (BusinessDictionary.com, 2014a). This approach consists of various disciplines working with a patient, but staff members function independently of each other (Gordon et al., 2013). They are not considered to overlap, with their skill sets geared to complement each other, and ultimately improve patient care.

However, a number of challenges manifest with multidisciplinary teams. One concern lies in their structures, in that they are hierarchically organized. This translates to there being a designated program "chief" usually with the highest-ranking profession (commonly an MD) (Zeiss & Steffer, 1996). Although this power structure can be beneficial to assure oversight of the flow of the meeting and resolve conflicts, there is a downside. The other team members will only feel a responsibility for the clinical work of their discipline. As a result they do not share a sense of responsibility for program function and effectiveness (1996). This is far from conducive for the high level of team interaction and communication that case managers rely on.

Multidisciplinary team members can be somewhat siloed as each professional focuses on a situation from their unique scope of care. This approach can lead to different or contradictory expectations and goals from various members of the treatment team that can be confusing for patients and their families (Linder, 1983). It could also present that a multidisciplinary effort does not allow for or promote communication among each member.

Imagine the situation where a patient with a complex medical condition is being followed by a multidisciplinary team. Each individual professional is consulted and all diligently document their impressions and treatment plans. However, the consults may or may not take into account the multiple views presented, which becomes challenging when the consults conflict with each other. There may be no formal mechanism to pull the common parties together. There may be a patient and family conference scheduled; however, it is not an expectation for all participating treatment providers to attend. Although there may be perspectives/consults of multiple disciplines, there is no formal process in place for those consulted to actually confer with and speak to each other.

The team functions as its name implies: as multiple disciplines who have been asked to consult on a particular patient and/or situation. Despite the newer generation of health care teams to follow, multidisciplinary teams continue to be discussed in the literature as acknowledging the complexities of modern critical care and the important role of communication between health care providers in delivering comprehensive care (Lowry, 2010).

INTERDISCIPLINARY TEAMS

Interdisciplinary teams are defined as a coordinated group of experts from several different fields who work together toward a common business goal (BusinessDictionary.com, 2014b). These teams saw a major emergence in the health care industry following the appearance of diagnostic-related groups (DRGs) that appeared in the 1980s, as well as managed care organizations.

The terms of interdisciplinary and multidisciplinary can be viewed by some as interchangeable, yet they are quite distinct. Interdisciplinary teams have increased communication and collaboration among team members, which occurs over the entire process of work together. The term "inter" marks the distinction from 'multi', meaning the team is driven by what occurs between or among members (*Merriam-Webster's Online Dictionary*, 2014b).

The process that interdisciplinary team members go through is as important, if not more so, as the end goal. It is common to see professionals assigned to an interdisciplinary team who share the primary assignment of a particular program, unit, or population. There is defined expertise that is shared among, with this expertise as important as any treatment recommended.

However, despite the merits of interdisciplinary teams, with their increased attention to communication, gaps in care continue to appear. The challenges of the interdisciplinary model include the need for them have more open, flexible, collaborative, and respectful communication among the various disciplines in resolving conflicts, priorities, negotiating roles, and developing common goal (Butt & Caplan, 2010).

The popularity of interdisciplinary teams occurred as the result of several factors.

Hall and Weaver (2001) identified the influence of the pursuit of continuity of care within the move of continuous quality improvement. In fact, it presented during these days that all health care organizations created mechanisms for team members of various disciplines to discuss patients and define more focused and strategic treatment plans. These dialogues were far clearer and more defined, always documented and often signed off on by all who attended. A high level of accountability for implementation of the plan accompanied these efforts.

Other factors to drive interdisciplinary team work over the past 20 years included are the following (Hall & Weaver in Nancarrow et al., 2013):

1. An aging population with frail older people and larger numbers of patients with more complex needs associated with chronic diseases;
2. The increasing complexity of skills and knowledge required to provide comprehensive care to patients;
3. Increasing specialization within health professions and a corresponding fragmentation of disciplinary knowledge, resulting in no one health care professional being able to meet all the complex needs of their patients;
4. The emphasis in many countries' policy documents on multiprofessional team work and development of shared learning.

Despite the increasing focus on interdisciplinary team work over the past two decades, there is still no clear synthesis of the "essence" of what makes a good interdisciplinary team and there is a limited amount of empirical research to define what such a team might look like (Nancarrow et al., 2013). It has also been suggested that a broad set of competencies to guide interdisciplinary team work would enhance the sustainability of this type of team in the industry.

Ten competencies were developed by Nancarrow et al. (2013) and appear in the Team Competency Comparison, Table 17-1. It was also identified that teams must regularly invest time in the processes of team development and maintenance of team functioning to ensure the competencies become entrenched and enacted as a part of one's daily practice (Nancarrow et al., 2013).

The Big Five Teamwork Behaviors (Salas et al., 2005) also yield competencies applicable to health care teams. Included in Table 17-1, they are aligned with the related competencies developed by Nancarrow et al. (2013). Although Salas's work has been associated with the more advanced transdisciplinary and interprofessional teams (Leasure et al., 2013), it is interesting to compare and contrast these two competency-based models within the industry.

Despite the lack of tangible research to denote the refutable characteristics of the interdisciplinary team, they appear across the industry. Case managers engage with interdisciplinary teams in a variety of ways. Examples include reorganization initiatives, quality teams focused on sentinel events and manifesting root cause analyses, as well as leadership teams who strive to implement the new generation of electronic health record systems.

TRANSDISCIPLINARY TEAMS

Transdisciplinary teams are defined as those composed of members of a number of different professions cooperating across disciplines to improve patient care through practice or research (Miller-Keane, 2003). Clinicians are enabled to implement a unified, holistic, and integrated treatment plan, with all members of the team responsible for the same patient-centered goals (Gordon et al., 2013). This is a fluid model that is driven by those directly involved in the care of the patient. Mutual respect and trust are hallmarks of this approach, with special attention to the value of each discipline's unique knowledge, skills, and expertise. This results in more consistent communication, interaction, and cooperation among team members (Gordon et al., 2013). Examples of programs to engage transdisciplinary practice, exist across hospice and palliative care, pain management, and the

TABLE 17-1 Comparison of Team Competency Models

Ten Competencies of an Interdisciplinary Team (Nancarrow et al., 2013)	The "Big Five" Teamwork Behaviors (Salas et al., 2005)
1. Identifies a leader who establishes a clear direction and vision for the team while listening and providing support and supervision to the team members	1. Leadership The ability to coordinate team members' activities, ensure that tasks are distributed appropriately, evaluate performance, provide feedback, enhance the team's ability to perform, inspire the drive for high-level performance
2. Incorporates a set of values that clearly provide direction for the team's service provision; these values should be visible and consistently portrayed	2. Mutual performance monitoring The ability to develop a shared understanding among team members regarding one another's intentions, roles, and responsibilities so that members can accurately monitor one another's performance for the purpose of collective success
3. Demonstrates a team culture and interdisciplinary atmosphere of trust where contributions are valued and consensus is fostered	
4. Ensures appropriate processes and infrastructures are in place to uphold the vision of the service (e.g., referral criteria, communications infrastructure)	
5. Provides quality patient-focused services with documented outcomes; utilizes feedback to improve the quality of care	3. Backup behavior The ability to anticipate the needs of other team members and shift tasks in real time to achieve and maintain balance during times of variable workload or increased pressure
6. Utilizes communication strategies that promote intrateam communication, collaborative decision making, and effective team processes	
7. Provides sufficient team staffing to integrate an appropriate mix of skills, competencies, and personalities to meet the needs of patients and enhance smooth functioning	
8. Facilitates recruitment of staff who demonstrate interdisciplinary competencies including team functioning, collaborative leadership, communication, and sufficient professional knowledge and experience	4. Adaptability The capability of team members to adjust their strategies for completing task on the basis of feedback from the work environment. Each team member must be able to redistribute team resources or alter a course of action in response to changing conditions, allowing the team to meet mutually defined goals including: • Recognizing that a change has occurred and • Identifying the potential negative impact if course present for care quality outcomes
9. Promotes role interdependence while respecting individual roles and autonomy	5. Team or collective orientation • The tendency to prioritize team goals over individual goals • To encourage different viewpoints and perspectives, and • To show respect and regard for each team member by evaluating and integrating his or her input in an interdependent manner
10. Facilitates personal development through appropriate training, rewards, recognition, and opportunities for career development	

rehabilitation continuum (e.g., inpatient, residential and day treatment, and outpatient), as well as the patient-centered medical home (Gordon et al., 2013, Leasure et al., 2013). The unique features of a transdisciplinary team include the following:

1. Integrated goal setting that can be shared by each discipline (i.e., the same goal can be carried out by more than one discipline),
2. Co-treatment when clinically indicated,
3. Assessment that is performed together by a number of disciplines,
4. An emphasis of mutual learning and the flexible exchange of discipline-specific interventions, and
5. The importance of consistent communication provided to patients and their families/support systems.

The latest reports on care coordination highlight the importance of a transdisciplinary team approach, particularly to address the increasingly complex needs of patients. As a result, no one profession can be expected to meet them all. By working together in a transdisciplinary environment, members of the health care team bring the best of their practices to improve the delivery of care to patients. This is the essence of care coordination (Fink-Samnick, 2011a).

Amid the promise of transdisciplinary teams, there have been series of pitfalls, which have been identified. Several experts note the importance of the cultural transformation, which must first occur for the successful implementation of this approach (Gordon et al., 2013; Leasure et al., 2013). The concept of cultural change has been discussed in previous chapters of this book and can be a cumbersome obstacle to manage. Despite the freedom which can stem from developing shared goals, team members can become easily frustrated from what often presents as role overlap, due to the presence of fluid professional boundaries (Gordon et al., 2013). Amid the fast pace and pressure at which health care delivery happens, it can feel easier for professionals to simply develop the goals from a single perspective, whether a nurse, pharmacist, or a respiratory therapist.

Conflict may also emerge as team members vie for ownership of information or particular treatment goal as opposed to being viewed as a contributor. Therefore, time and openness to ongoing dialogues that recognize and respect the potential for competition are required for ease of sharing and for trust to develop (Gordon et al., 2013).

INTERPROFESSIONAL TEAMS

Interprofessional practice is among the more recent additions to the spectrum of teams in the industry, as shown in Figure 17-1. As discussed in chapter 5, the concept of interprofessional practice was rooted in the educational realm and emerged with support of the global work of a series of experts and organizations, including the IOM, the Canadian Interprofessional Health Care Collaborative (CIHC), and

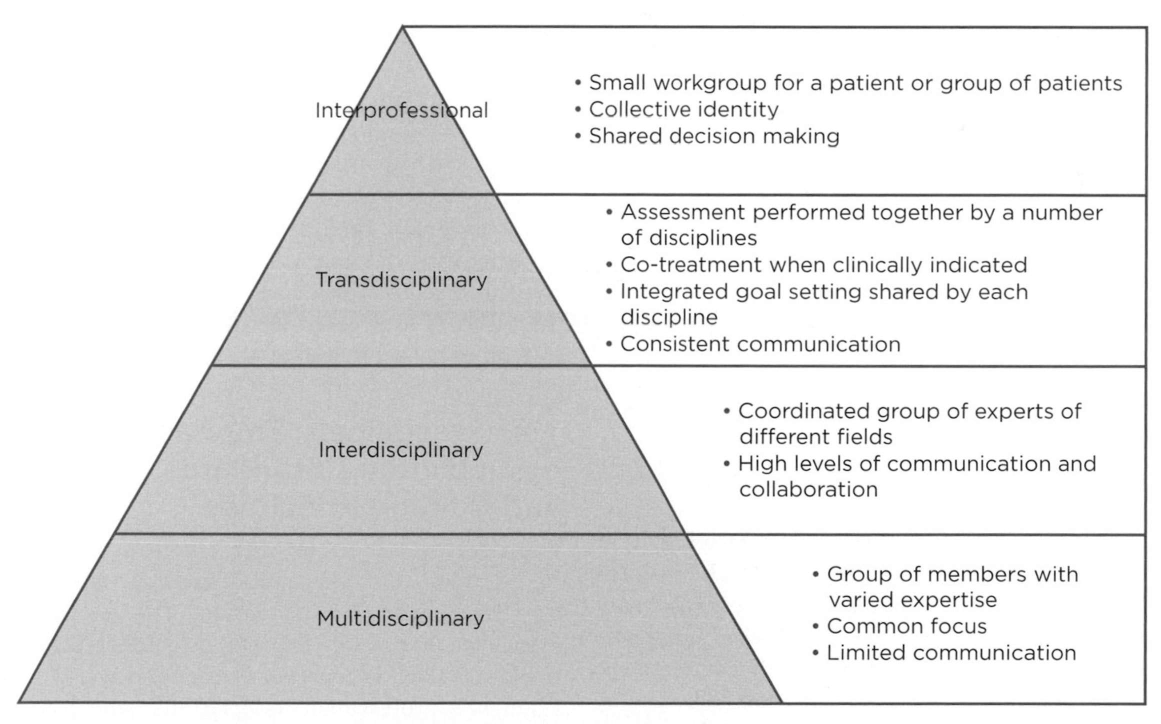

Figure 17-1. Spectrum of teams. (Data compiled from Interprofessional Education Collaborative. (2011). *Core competencies for interprofessional collaborative practice: Report of an expert panel*. Washington, DC: Author. Retrieved April 30, 2014, from http://www.aacn.nche.edu/news/articles/2011/ipec; Merriam-Webster. (2014a). *Team*. Retrieved November 17, 2014, from http://www.merriam-webster.com/dictionary/team; Merriam-Webster. (2014b). *Discipline*. Retrieved November 13, 2014, from http://www.merriam-webster.com/dictionary/discipline; Gordon, R. M., Corcoran, J. R., Bartley-Daniele, P., Sklener, D., Sutton, P., & Cartwright, F., (2013). A transdisciplinary team approach to pain management in inpatient health care settings. *Pain Management Nursing*, *15*(1), 426–435.)

the Interprofessional Education Collaboration (IPEC). The IOM's five competency model (2003) included the distinct domain, "Work in Inter-Professional Teams." This competency framed that professionals must cooperate, collaborate, communicate, and integrate care (IOM, 2003).

The interprofessional identity does not replace the individual identity and pride of each distinct professional discipline. This approach is about students in professional schools learning together in a way that allows them to ultimately improve the health and the safety of patient (IOM, 2013). Interprofessional education is different from multidisciplinary learning, where students from different professions learn or even work in a group, a way that many case managers were educated. To be truly interprofessional, there needs to be purposeful integration and collaboration among the disciplines, whether in an educational or practice environment (IOM, 2013).

Interprofessional practice is becoming increasingly popular, with outcomes rapidly emerging to validate the value of this approach. These emerging models are marked by high levels of cooperation, coordination, and collaboration characterizing the relationships between professions in delivering patient-centered care (IPEC, 2011). Grant funding through a number of entities, including the IOM and IPEC, is awarded annually. All involved entities publish reports to present the creative and innovative initiatives occurring which are listed among the references for this text (IOM, 2013; IPEC, 2011).

The definition of the **interprofessional** team-based care is as follows:

> Care delivered by intentionally created, usually relatively small work groups in health care, who are recognized by others as well as by themselves as having a collective identity and shared responsibility for a patient or group of patients. (e.g., rapid response team, palliative care team, primary care team, operating room team).
>
> *IPEC, 2011*

Interprofessional practice sets a new tone for the health care workplace, one where practitioner cohesion rather than continued fragmentation and competition between disciplines is allowed to flourish (Fink-Samnick, 2014).

CASE MANAGEMENT'S PERSPECTIVE

The topic of transdisciplinary practice is not new to case management and has taken assorted forms. There has been robust discussion regarding the diverse professional disciplines that comprise the case management workforce—which discipline owns case management and who makes the best case manager. There have been equally spirited discourses regarding the scope, diversity, and interactional dynamics of the treatment teams that deliver care. These topics have been addressed by case management experts and professional associations, with all providing solid food for transdisciplinary thought.

Disciplinary Versus Interdisciplinary

Case management has been referred to as disciplinary and interdisciplinary in scope (Huber, 2002). The literature yields a vast number of articles to promote discipline-specific models and roles across practice settings (e.g., nursing case management, social work case manager), though no one discipline "owns" case management; multiple disciplines are involved (Huber, 2002).

Providers who are schooled in their own discipline or origin, often yield a more siloed approach to practice, for they tend to be familiar with, or at the least accept only their requisite professional discipline's definition, model, and case management practice paradigms (Huber, 2002). Over the years, this philosophy has led to drastic staffing changes in case management departments, often as a result of restructuring and reorganization initiatives, and usually based on professional discipline alone. One must wonder about the benefits of disciplinary titles in an interdisciplinary and interprofessional industry. Confusion and misinterpretations can and do occur when discipline-focused providers do not recognize the diversity inherent in case management, nor understand the other disciplines' perspectives when collaborating on multidisciplinary teams and projects (Huber, 2002).

The rich professional perspectives valued by health care's involved disciplines have been referenced to throughout this text. The complex needs of the patients whom case managers encounter in the scope of their role, mandate a transdisciplinary approach to case management itself. There are emerging care coordination models defined by evidence-based initiatives; each promotes interprofessional practice as a means to achieve quality patient-centered care. This focus on interprofessional teamwork is now fused into higher education as the means to provide education at the gateway of workplace entry (Owen et al., 2014).

In order to respond to the expanding number of complex, multifaceted cases, there must be true diversity of competency in the field (Fink-Samnick, 2011b). In this era of cross-continuum care management, those following a path of segregating case management into separate camps based not only on educational background but also on practice setting, level of experience, or any other artificial divider, are misguided at best (Owen et al., 2014).

Transdisciplinary Emphasis by Definitions, Standards, and Guiding Principles

The assorted definitions of case management set the tone for the vital role case management serves to the health care industry and its stakeholder. The very nature of case management practice begs for a concerted effort by the workforce to work together. Although several of case management's professional associations and accrediting entities may promote a disciplinary (Llewellyn & Leonard, 2009; NASW, 2013) versus interdisciplinary focus (ACMA, 2013; CMSA, 2010), their mutual definitions for case management practice speak to the importance of combined efforts to achieve goals. One entity's definition has evolved over time, though continues to begin with the words, "Case management is a collaborative process" (CMSA, 2010). Another association presents the definition as a description of how the role appears in the hospitals and health care systems (ACMA, 2013).

Considerable emphasis is placed by professional associations on the industry goal of minimizing fragmentation of care within the health care delivery system (CMSA, 2010). The composition and vital role of the interdisciplinary team are also seen as integral to advancing case management credibility and complement the current trends in health care (CMSA, 2010).

A series of distinct, yet related, standards have been developed which emphasize the importance of shared accountability (ACMA, 2013), the concepts of coordination, communication, and collaboration across the transitions of care (ACMA, 2013; CMSA, 2010; NASW, 2013), plus interdisciplinary and interorganizational collaboration (NASW, 2013). Guiding principles have been established which speak to collaborative partnership and teamwork (CMSA, 2010; NASW, 2013). One entity includes collaborative communication under its scope of services (ACMA, 2013). Table 17-2 shows the professional associations, which have case management practice standards focused on transdisciplinary practice and related concepts. Table 17-3 shows those associations with additional case management-specific definitions and guiding principles.

GENERAL PERSPECTIVES

Tuckman's Stages of Group Development

Bruce Tuckman is a psychologist who focused his research on the concept of teamwork. In his 1965 article, *Developmental Sequence in Small Groups*, he proposed a developmental model for four stages of group development. Often referred to as the forming, storming, norming, and performing model (Tuckman, 1965), it posed a developmental life cycle of four phases of dynamics that groups experience in their work together. The four stages foster the group's ability to grow, face challenges, tackle problems, find solutions, plan work, and ultimately deliver results. In 1977, Tuckman joined with Jensen and completed a retrospective review of the model. In doing so, a fifth developmental stage was added. The five stages of the model appear in Figure 17-2, with the each of the stages explained in Table 17-4.

There have been adjustments and revisions to the stages proposed by experts over the years. Rickards and Moger (2000) proposed an extension to the Tuckman model when a group breaks out of its norms, through a process of creative problem solving. Few have achieved the global level of recognition, or universal application of Tuckman and Jensen's model. In terms of the health care industry, consider the robust application that this model has for teams across the care continuum, particularly given the current industry emphasis on team-based work.

National Coalition on Care Coordination

A number of organizations have formed in recent years to reflect the transdisciplinary focus of the health care industry. The IOM, CIHC, and IPEC have been discussed considerably throughout this book, and again in this chapter. The National Transitions of Care Coalition was discussed in chapter 13. Each of these entities shares a vision that provides ongoing attention to the unique transdisciplinary perspective that health care is embracing as it moves forward.

Another player to join those discussed is the National Coalition on Care Coordination (N3C), formed in 2008 by leading social, health care, family caregiver, and professional organizations (N3C, 2009). The goal of this coalition is to promote better coordinated health and social services for older adults with multiple chronic conditions. The group began as a partnership between the Social Work Leadership Institute, The American Society on Aging, and Rush University Medical Center, and is now composed of over 114 individual members organizations representing consumer, aging, social service, health care, family caregiver, and professional organizations.

N3C's purpose is to advocate for enactment of public policies that support care coordination. The coalition's goal is to effectively link health and long-term care on behalf of vulnerable populations—with particular focus on older adults. The coalition believes that care coordination should:

- be patient-centered
- be supportive of family and informal caregivers
- be accessible
- take an interdisciplinary approach
- focus on chronic care and health care transitions
- bridge health and social services
- employ a comprehensive assessment; and
- implement and monitor a flexible care plan.

(Social Work Leadership Institute, 2014a)

The list of recent actions and initiatives provided on the N3C website is inspirational and exciting to review. From an extensive list of research awards from the Patient-Centered Outcomes Research Institute, to demonstration projects and workforce alliances, N3C is on the cutting edge of transdisciplinary program development. Given the extensive and evolving information on the website, those interested should explore the content as interest and time allow.

CONTEXT FOR COLLABORATE TRANSDISCIPLINARY

The value of how a competency approach serves to ground health care's distinct professional disciplines is discussed in chapter 5. It is through this grounding that the cornerstones for a case manager's individual professional practice foundation are set. These cornerstones are then reinforced at the various stages of a case manager's professional journey, as he or she advanced through formal education, on-the-job training, licensure, and other regulatory efforts, plus organizational initiatives.

TABLE 17-2 Professional Association Case Management Transdisciplinary-Focused Practice Standards

American Case Management Association (2013)	Case Management Society of America (2010)	National Association of Social Workers (2013)
Standard I. Accountability Accountability is ownership for the achievement of optimal outcomes within their standards of practice. The case manager: • Recognizes and demonstrates shared accountability, both at the individual and the team levels, that joint responsibility and joint accountability is inherent in collaborative practice • Follows through on his or her own commitments and expects/prompts others to follow through on their commitments • Contributes to decision making and decision support as a member of the interdisciplinary team • Ensures timely sequencing through the case management encounter **Standard III.** Collaboration Collaboration is working with patients, families, caregivers, and health care team to jointly communicate, problem solve, and share accountability for optimal outcomes. These outcomes respect patient preferences and their available resources.	**Standard H:** Facilitation, Coordination, and Collaboration The case manager should facilitate coordination, communication, and collaboration with the client and other stakeholders in order to achieve goals and maximize positive client outcomes How demonstrated: Recognition of the case manager's professional role and practice setting in relation to that of other providers and organizations caring for the client Development and maintenance of proactive, client-centered relationships and communication with the client, and other necessary stakeholders to maximize outcomes. Evidence of transitions of care, including: • A transfer to the most appropriate health care provider/setting • The transfer is appropriate, timely, and complete • Documentation of collaboration and communication with other health care professionals, especially during each transition to another level of care within or outside of the client's current setting	**Standard 8:** Interdisciplinary and Interorganizational Collaboration The social work case manager shall promote collaboration among colleagues and organizations to enhance service delivery and facilitate client goal attainment The social work case manager plays an integral role in fostering, maintaining, and strengthening collaborative partnerships on behalf of clients and shall demonstrate the following abilities: • Differentiate social work perspectives, values, and interventions from those of other disciplines • Describe and support the roles of other disciplines and organizations involved in supporting case management clients • Articulate and fulfill the missions and functions of their employing organizations, with consideration of social work ethics and values • Communicate effectively with all professionals, paraprofessionals, and volunteers involved in supporting case management clientele • Advocate for clients' integral role in team communications and service planning, delivery, and monitoring

American Case Management Association (2013)	Case Management Society of America (2010)	National Association of Social Workers (2013)
The case manager: • Respects and values the contribution of all disciplines • Communicates and collaborates with patients, families, caregivers, and members of the health care team • Builds and maintains relationships that foster trust and confidence	Adherence to client privacy and confidentiality mandates during collaboration Use of mediation and negotiation to improve communication and relationships • Use of problem-solving skills and techniques to reconcile potentially differing points of view • Evidence of collaborative efforts to optimize client outcomes: this may include working with community, local and state resources, primary care physician or other primary provider, other members of the health care team, the payer, and other relevant health care stakeholders • Evidence of collaborative efforts to maximize regulatory adherence within the case manager's practice setting	• Communicate client and family information in a respectful, objective manner while protecting confidentiality and privacy • Promote the strengths, and advocate for the goals, of case management clients • Facilitate communication between clients and providers/organizations • Share team leadership in planning and providing services to case management clients • Foster an organizational culture that promotes effective, coordinated services for case management clients • Develop and maintain partnerships across disciplines, organizations, and the service spectrum to enhance access to and continuity of services for case management clientele • Integrate a strengths perspective in program and organizational administration to maximize and sustain human and fiscal resources on behalf of case management clients • Manage personal and interpersonal processes at the intraorganizational, interorganizational, and community levels to optimize services for case management clientele
Standard IV. Care Coordination A case manager facilitates the progression of care by advancing the care plan to achieve desired outcomes and integrates the work of the health care team by coordinating resources and services necessary to accomplish agreed-upon goals. The case manager: • Ensures the development of a safe and effective plan of care through early identification and thorough assessment of the patient's needs and the resources available • Assures the designation of primary responsibility among the team members for each aspect of the plan, avoiding duplication and fragmentation • Carries out individual responsibilities according to the plan • Monitors progress toward the goals of the plan and ensures revisions in response to changes in patient needs and condition • Proactively identifies, communicates, and resolves barriers that impede the progression of care • Utilizes an organizationally defined escalation process to refer facets of the care plan beyond the control or influence of the team • Evaluates the patient's/caregiver's level of understanding and comfort with the progress toward goals and incorporates findings into the plan of care • Arranges services among community agencies, physicians, patient/family/caregivers, and others involved in the plan of care • Ensures timely sequencing of interventions for optimal results and smooth transition along the continuum • Identifies clinical, psychosocial, and/or spiritual needs and addresses/refers to attain expected outcomes • Elicits and incorporates the realistic expectations of patients/family/caregiver health care team members and payers in the planning process • Identifies barriers to achieving recommended goals identified in the plan of care		

TABLE 17-3 Case Management Professional Association Transdisciplinary Definitions and Guiding Principles

American Case Management Association (2013)	Case Management Society of America (2010)	National Association of Social Workers (2013)	American Nurses Credentialing Center (Llewellyn and Leonard, 2009)

Scope of Services:
• Care Coordination:
  • Communication
  • Communication both verbal and written is the foundation on which knowledge transfers, and collaboration and relationship building is based
	Guiding Principle: Case managers:
	• Use a client-centric, collaborative partnership approach
	• Use a comprehensive, holistic approach
		Guiding Principle: Collaborative teamwork
		
		Collaborative teamwork. The social work case manager does not work in isolation. Collaboration with other social workers, other disciplines, and other organizations is integral to the case management process.	

Description: Case Management in hospital and health care systems is a collaborative practice model including patients, nurses, social workers, physicians, other practitioners, caregivers, and the community. The case management process encompasses communication and facilitates care along a continuum through effective resource coordination. The goals of case management include the achievement of optimal health, access to care, and appropriate utilization of resources, balanced with the patient's right to self-determination."	**Definition for Case Management:** Case management is a collaborative process of assessment, planning, facilitation, care coordination, evaluation, and advocacy for options and services to meet an individual's and family's comprehensive health needs through communication and available resources to promote quality cost-effective outcomes.	**Definition for Social Work Case Management:** A process to plan, seek, advocate for, and monitor services from different social services or health care organizations and staff on behalf of a client. The process enables social workers in an organization, or in different organizations, to coordinate their efforts to serve a given client through professional teamwork, thus expanding the range of needed services offered. Case management limits problems arising from fragmentation of services, staff turnover, and inadequate coordination among providers. Case management can occur within a single, large organization or within a community program that coordinates services among settings.	**Definition for Nursing Case Management:** A dynamic and systematic collaborative approach to providing and coordinating health care services to a defined population. It is a participative process to identify and facilitate options and services for meeting individuals' health needs, while decreasing fragmentation and duplication of care and enhancing quality, cost-effective clinical outcomes. The framework for nursing case management includes five components: assessment, planning, implementation, evaluation, and interaction.

From the COLLABORATE perspective, case managers must do more than accept the notion of engaging in treatment teams with other professionals. They must adapt the habit of a transdisciplinary competency. Teams have been a part of the industry long enough that they are an expectation of any practice setting, whether that team functions as one which is multidisciplinary (hopefully not), interdisciplinary (better but not there yet), or potentially interprofessional (now we're talking!).

In the scope of rapidly changing and increasingly complex patient populations, most case managers know the importance of the mantra, "it takes a village." Most by now have

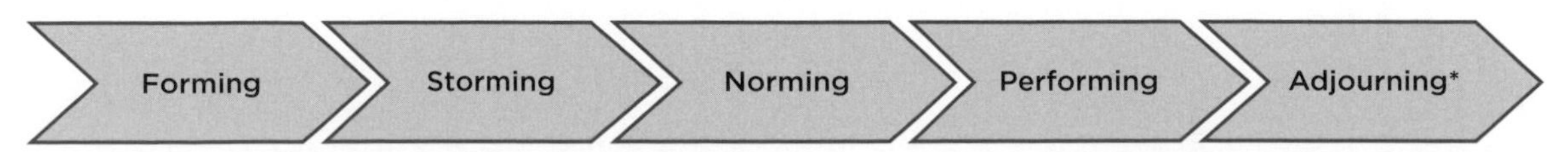

Figure 17-2. Tuckman's model of team development. (Adapted from Tuckman, B. W. (1965). Developmental sequence in small groups. *Psychological Bulletin*, *63*(6), 384–399; Tuckman, B. W., & Jensen, M. A. C. (1977). Stages of small group development revisited. *Group and Organization Studies*, *2*(4), 419–427.)

TABLE 17-4 Tuckman and Jensen's Group Developmental Stages

Stage	Explanation
1. Forming	Begins with the group being formed. Members are oriented to the group, with testing often manifesting between group members. Each individual member strives to be accepted by the others in the group. As a result, all are usually on their best behavior. The tasks are defined, as is the group structure.
2. Storming	Intragroup conflict emerges and members begin to trust each other, yet become resistant to group influence and task requirements. This can be an especially challenging stage for members to go through due to constant testing of each other. There can be emotional reactions to demands for task completion.
3. Norming	Ingroup feeling and cohesiveness begin to develop with new standards evolving, plus new roles adopted by members. There is a more open exchange of perspectives, interpretations, and personal opinions as trust develops among members.
4. Performing	Constructive action begins with group member roles becoming flexible and functional. Structural issues are resolved with the focus on the group performance. The interpersonal structure becomes the tool of task activities; group energy is channeled into the task; solutions can now emerge. This is a high-performing term which functions as a unit. Despite achieving this level of performance, teams may cycle through earlier stages as new members and/or tasks are introduced.
5. Adjournment	This is the final stage where anxiety about separation and termination emerge. It is also referred to as the "mourning" stage. The team breaks up, with self-evaluation the main task. The group works to resolve feelings about the completion of its work together.

Adapted from Tuckman, B. W. (1965). Developmental sequence in small groups. Psychological Bulletin, 63(6), 384–399; Tuckman, B. W., & Jensen, M. A. C. (1977). Stages of small group development revisited. Group and Organization Studies, 2(4), 419–427.

also heard the phrase, "there is no I in teamwork." These are all powerful themes to embrace in the current team-based culture of health care practice.

However, it is not enough for case managers to simply talk about the importance of greater collegiality, mutual respect, and cooperation among the professionals rendering care. Case managers must engage in their professional practice from a transdisciplinary stance, which presumes that case management is a practice built on skills and knowledge from various health practitioners (Owen et al., 2014). One profession is not above, one is not below, and working together exemplified the value and expertise necessary to work through the complexities of case management and health care today (Owen et al., 2014). It is not about the development of yet another type or generation of health care team that will yield success in the next wave of health care programming. Instead, the focus should be on an innovative shift in perspective by all of the team members, one that promotes the messaging of the sum of all efforts that yields the best outcome for health care consumers.

KEY ELEMENTS OF TRANSDISCIPLINARY COMPETENCY

Health care quality is a comprehensive and consolidated team effort, which is interprofessional, and thus transdisciplinary in scope (Treiger & Fink-Samnick, 2013).

Taking this premise into account, the transdisciplinary competency is viewed as transcending across the key elements of:

- Professional disciplines
- Teams, and
- The continuum

The expectation for this high level of professional behavior occurs at every turn of a case manager's work. It exists in the treatment team at a case manager's practice setting, and is equally expected across those areas where case managers intervene on behalf of patients. This extends to when case managers speak with any and all colleagues with whom they share mutual patients across the transitions of care. The transdisciplinary competency transcends meetings that case managers have with community treatment providers, when advocating on behalf of patients. In this way all professionals can respectfully share perspectives about the needs of rapidly changing and increasingly complex patient populations. This is how the true essence of quality-driven patient-centered care coordination is achieved. This is how health care consumers and stakeholders effectively partner with health care teams.

Case managers must first accept a mind-set of **Professional Diversity**, which is detailed in Table 17-5. Through this concept, every case manager and treatment team member's input is valuable and respected, even amid the vast disagreement that often manifests. Moving forward from those points defined by the IOM and IPEC initiatives discussed in section 1 of COLLABORATE, Professional Diversity sets a context and minimum standard by which health care teams should function. The focus is not nursing or social work centric, with case managers viewed as professional case managers. The **medical model** has no place for communication is unilateral and not top-down.

COLLABORATE speaks to implementation of a transdisciplinary perspective, which is powered by the consolidated expertise and energy of all individual team members of the distinct professional disciplines. It is an approach that mandates a high standard for professional behavior, especially communicating openly, honestly, and respectfully with any and all colleagues across disciplines. Consider the case scenario in Box 17-2, which demonstrates the transdisciplinary competency in action.

IMPLICATIONS FOR PRACTICE

The Changing Nature of Communication Challenges

Communication challenges across the continuum of care are another compelling reason for health care organizations, and especially case management, to embrace the

TABLE 17-5 Professional Diversity

Definition	The collective synergy of health and human service discipline-specific competencies utilized to enhance care coordination
The Concept is	A foundation of all case management practice Transdisciplinary in application Transcends traditional professional boundaries Patient-centered in scope Applicable across transitions of care (Fink-Samnick, 2012b)
The Concept promotes	Approaching patient situations by involved team members orienting to the needs of the person as opposed to the context of a specific discipline or expertise The ability of the entire team to develop workable solutions by reaching across perceived boundaries of respective professional disciplines to: • Communicate openly • Share insight • Form strategic partnerships, and • Identify resources through open dialogues Mutual respect as an underlying theme (Fink-Samnick, 2010)

From Treiger, T. M., & Fink-Samnick, E. (2013). COLLABORATE©: A universal, competency-based paradigm for professional case management practice, part I. Professional Case Management, 18(3), 122–135.

BOX 17-2 Transdisciplinary Competency: Case Scenario

Mr. Matus is a 56-year-old married man admitted from his home for the third hospitalization in as many months for pneumonia and respiratory failure. With a diagnosis of amyotrophic lateral sclerosis (ALS) Mr. Matus is alert, fully oriented, and deemed competent to make his own medical decisions. He communicates by mouthing words and a picture board. Mr. Matus is totally dependent for activities of daily living, on continuous oxygen at 40% via trach collar, as well as parenteral nutrition. He has advanced directives in place, which detail his "do not resuscitate" status. Mrs. Matus has durable power of attorney for her husband and is supportive of his request for no life-sustaining care.

During a meeting with the treatment team, Mrs. and Mrs. Matus request the treatment team coordinate a discharge plan to safely transition Mr. Matus to his apartment in Florida. He is aware being at the end stage of his disease process and wants to "die looking out at the ocean." Mrs. Matus tells the team she will drive the couple's van to the destination, some 10 hours away from the hospital.

Gail is the case manager at the managed care organization, who recommends Mr. Matus be discharged to a nursing home with hospice, over the next 48 hours. "They can set everything up from there," she tells Donna, the hospital case manager for Mr. Matus.

Donna has a solid working relationship with the team members involved in Mr. Matus's care. She asks them to define what would need to be in place to implement a safe plan. At first, Mr. Matus's nurse reacts strongly to the exercise, telling Donna "this is a waste of time." Donna responds: "What do we lose by spending a few minutes discussing what must be in place? We each know Mr. Matus well and it won't take long to define each piece of this puzzle. If we identify objectives which make the plan unsafe and unviable, then we convey that to Mr. Matus. We also need to know we can implement it within the next 72 hours. Gail has given us that much time before we need to transfer him. At least we know the plan will be given fair consideration by all, and everyone's perspective will be heard."

The team discussed the situation, and presented the following necessary components for the safe transition of Mr. and Mrs. Matus to Florida:

1. Private hire of a nurse capable of rendering respiratory care including suctioning, monitoring of parenteral feedings, and all identified activities of daily living. This nurse will demonstrate competence to render care to the team's patient care coordinator.
2. Coordinate with a durable medical equipment (DME) provider for appropriate oxygen and supplies for the trip, plus to secure the tanks in the vehicle. A list will be provided of all DME and supplies, with assurance of delivery and setup of all items prior to patient's discharge.
3. A dialogue will occur between the patient's current attending physician at the hospital and his physician in Florida, to assure care needs are discussed. Gail will fax the discharge summary to the attending physician on the day of his discharge.
4. All medications will be called into the pharmacy in Florida. The pharmacy will coordinate delivery of all meds and supplies with a family friend, so the items are present in the home upon the patient's arrival. This includes nutritional supplements as recommended.
5. The patient's physician in Florida will complete a referral to hospice and coordinate with that team directly to assure all orders are completed.
6. Maximum implementation time frame: 72 hours

Everyone is notified and approves the plan, which is implemented within 48 hours. Mrs. Matus contacted Gail and Donna upon the couple's arrival in Florida. She called again 2 weeks later and left the following message. "Please thank the entire team for helping make my husband's last few weeks so peaceful. Mr. Matus died over the weekend, but his last view was of the ocean and the sunset, as he had requested."

transdisciplinary competency as a way of practice. Poor communication processes manifesting across care settings with their often fragmented and siloed approaches to care have a negative impact on the quality of care (Treiger & Lattimer, 2011).

Focus on the nature, quality, and frequency of team communication has become even more heightened in our global society. Patients now access care across settings regionally, nationally, and internationally. Communication about patients occurs through a variety of modes from the traditional in-person, telephone, and email to more complex encrypted electronic health records and patient portals. The Health Information and Patient Protection Act Final Rule mandated that by January 2014, all covered entities were required to have end-user devices encrypt by default, with hospitals and physicians providing patients with access to their health records through portals (Office of the Federal Register, 2013).

Telehealth, telemedicine, and remote health monitoring continue their popularity and expansion. At the time of this writing, the National Council of State Legislatures (NCSL) website shows 43 states providing some form of Medicaid reimbursement for telehealth services. Nineteen states have private insurance requirements in place (NCSL, 2014), with the number continuing to expand. Licensure portability challenges and the inconsistency of professional regulations continue to serve as further obstacles to the maximum utilization of these new modes of health care intervention. Regulations being out of sync with practice reality negate the ability of professionals to consistently and appropriately render intervention across state lines and cyberspace (Fink-Samnick, 2012).

Accountable Care Organizations and a New Generation of Teams

Transdisciplinary expertise within teams presents as the optimal means to address the scope of obstacles that have emerged on health care's horizon. The increased number of facilities seeking Magnet accreditation is cited specifically as a key motivator for evidence-based transdisciplinary team expertise (Satterfield et al., 2009).

The emergence of accountable care organizations (ACOs) under Patient Protection and Affordable Care Act (PPACA) offers further incentive and motivation for the development of transdisciplinary teams. An ACO calls for a group of providers and suppliers of services (e.g., hospitals, nurses, physicians, and others involved in patient care) to work together to coordinate care for the Medicare beneficiaries they serve. Collaboration is mandated for the hospitals, physicians, and others involved in coordinating care for the patients they serve with original Medicare (ANA, 2014). All providers and patients are to be true partners in care decisions (Healthcare.gov, 2013).

There have been early naysayers of ACOs, who pondered why any level of legislative mandate was necessary to assure care be rendered in an accountable manner. One would expect both the organizations and its professionals who are tasked with providing care should be accountable for the highest quality of practice by virtue of regulations, licensure, and the like. Let us not cloud the issue with logic (Treiger & Fink-Samnick, 2013).

Perhaps a question to consider is whether or not ACOs serve a greater purpose, as incentive for the population's need for a transdisciplinary perspective of practice.

Bullying in the Health Care Workplace

The appearance of bullying within the treatment team has gross potential to hamper the quality-of-patient care processes. Bullying manifests as an act perpetrated by an individual in a higher level of authority toward others. They could be covert or overt acts of verbal or nonverbal aggression (Dellasega, 2009 on ANA, 2014b).

Bullying behavior has both intensified and escalated over the past decade with the current industry figures staggering (Fink-Samnick, 2014). A survey of more than 4,500 health care workers yielded that 77% reported disruptive behavior by doctors, 65% reported the same presentation among nurses, and 99% indicated these behaviors led to impaired nurse–physician relationships (Rosenstein & O'Daniel, 2008). Case managers easily find themselves wasting valuable time and effort mediating and negotiating these less-than-optimal circumstances in their workplace. These interactions also grossly interfere with the implementation of the transdisciplinary competency.

A study by the Workplace Bullying Institute found 35% of workers have been bullied in the workplace. The actions detailed included verbal abuse, job sabotage, misuse of authority, intimidation and humiliation, and deliberate destroying of relationships. Other pivotal outcomes note that bullying is four times more common than either sexual harassment or racial discrimination on the job, though not yet illegal (Drexler, 2013). Again, these issues do nothing to enhance mutual team respect or collaborative practice.

The Joint Commission (JC) identified how intimidating and disruptive behaviors fuel medical errors and lead to preventable adverse outcomes (The JC, 2008). Another study found that more than 75% of those surveyed identified how disruptive behaviors led to medical errors with nearly 30% contributing to patient deaths (Painter, 2013). Other reports cite the number at potentially as high as 200,000 deaths a year (Brown, 2011). These reports are evidence of the dangerous culture of silence that has been permitted to invade the health care workplace, environments tasked with assuring the highest attention to quality and safe delivery of health care for so very many consumers (Fink-Samnick, 2014). This pattern of behavior cannot be allowed to continue, and begs for the insertion of a transdisciplinary perspective as a means to promote a sense of mutual respect among those providing care.

The High Cost of Health Care

The increased cost of health care continues as a fiscal priority for all stakeholders, serving as yet another factor that begs for a transdisciplinary perspective that promotes coordinated and collaborative communication across the health care continuum. Health expenditures in the United States alone neared $3.4 trillion in 2012 (Munro, 2014). This amount is well over 10 times the $256 billion spent in 1980. About 75% of these national health expenditures alone have been related to chronic disease treatment (KaiserEDU.org, 2013).

This information adds further fuel to the fire for the industry's need to engage all optimal means to appropriately manage health care's processes, treatments, and accompanying interventions (Treiger & Fink-Samnick, 2013). This includes the more strategic development and purposeful implementation of transdisciplinary perspectives to care.

Care Coordination as the Impetus for Transdisciplinary Teams

The latest reports on care coordination highlight the global importance of a transdisciplinary approach for the health care industry. Care among many different providers must be well-coordinated to avoid waste, over-, under-, or misuse of prescribed medications, and conflicting plans of care (National Quality Forum, 2010). This is in step with continuing to address the gross system problems within health care, highlighted by the IOM back in 2001. It is well over a decade since the seminal work, *Crossing the Quality Chasm: A New Health System for the 21st Century* (2001) was released. Yet, the problems identified continue to challenge the workforce and compromise the quality and safety of patient care: lack of coordination within the delivery system, fragmentation that slows care and undermines accountability, poor communication and use of information technology, and failure of health care professionals to work together to ensure that care is appropriate, timely, and safe (IOM, 2001).

Care coordination can reduce hospitalizations and Medicare costs and improve quality of care for chronically ill older adults—provided the programs: promote direct engagement of teams of primary care physicians, nurses, and social workers; create close communication among all providers involved in a patient's care; and empower patients to help manage their own care (N3C, 2009).

The PPACA) has elevated care coordination as an important means to serve a wide variety of patients with particular needs, such as the frail elderly and those with preexisting and chronic conditions, including many who until now did not have access to health care coverage (Fink-Samnick, 2011a). Not only does a transdisciplinary approach bring together a variety of disciplines to meet the overall needs of these patients, but it also allows for those disciplines to bring the best of their practices forward to improve the delivery of care (Fink-Samnick, 2011a).

Care coordination models continue to increase across the industry from expanded reimbursement and the advancing body of outcomes to denote both fiscal incentives and quality improvement. These models set the stage for the further expansion and integration of transdisciplinary teams for years to come.

SUMMARY

As Henry Ford is quoted to have said, "Coming together is a beginning. Keeping together is progress. Working together is a success." Amid all the change that is occurring in the health care industry, applying a transdisciplinary competency to the industry itself, as well as the case management process, is a necessary constant. A team orientation must replace individualistic notions within all aspects of health professions training, and curricular content, policies, pedagogy, and assessment must align *inter*dependence—not *in*dependence—with success (Leasure et al., 2013). In this way case managers foster the ability of any team to render the right care, through the right communications in the right setting, in the right way, at the right cost, and at the right time.

References

Agency for Healthcare Research and Quality. (2014). *Care coordination*. Retrieved November 13, 2014, from http://www.ahrq.gov/professionals/prevention-chronic-care/improve/coordination/

American Case Management Association. (2013). *Standards of practice and scope of services for health care delivery system case management and transitions of care professionals*. Little Rock, AK: Author.

American Nurses Association. (2001). *Code of ethics for nurses with interpretive statements*. Silver Spring, MD: Author.

American Nurses Association. (2010). *Scope and standards of practice: Nursing* (2nd ed.). Silver Spring, MD: Author.

American Nurses Association. (2014a). *Accountable care organizations*. Retrieved November 22, 2014, from http://www.nursingworld.org/ACOs

American Nurses Association. (2014b). *Bullying and workplace violence*. http://www.nursingworld.org/MainMenuCategories/WorkplaceSafety/Healthy-Nurse/bullyingworkplaceviolence

Barry, M. J., & Edgman-Levitan, S. (2012). Shared decision making-the pinnacle of patient-centered care. *The New England Journal of Medicine*, *366*, 780–781.

Brown, T. (2011). Physician heel thyself [The Opinion Pages]. *The New York Times*. Retrieved from http://www.nytimes.com/2011/05/08/opinion/08Brown.html?partner=rss&emc=rss&_r=0

Business Dictionary.com. (2014a). *Multidisciplinary team*. Retrieved November 15, 2014, from http://www.businessdictionary.com/definition/multidisciplinary-team.html

Business Dictionary.com. (2014b). *Interdisciplinary team*. Retrieved November 17, 2014, from http://www.businessdictionary.com/definition/interdisciplinary-team.html

Butt, L., & Caplan. (2010). The rehabilitation team. In R. G. Frank (Ed.), *Handbook of rehabilitation psychology* (2nd ed., pp. 451–457). Washington, DC: American Psychological Association.

Case Management Society of America. (2010). *CMSA standards of practice for case management* (Rev). Retrieved April 25, 2013, from http://www.cmsa.org/portals/0/pdf/memberonly/StandardsOfPractice.pdf

Commission for Case Manager Certification. (2009). *Code of professional conduct for case managers*. Retrieved October 31, 2014, from http://ccmcertification.org/content/ccm-exam-portal/code-professional-conductcase-managers

Drexler, P. (2013). Are workplace bullies rewarded for their behavior? *Forbes*. Retrieved April 25, 2014 from http://www.forbes.com/sites/peggydrexler/2013/07/10/are-workplace-bullies-rewarded-for-their-behavior/

Fink-Samnick, E. (2011a, Summer). Understanding care coordination: Emerging opportunities for social workers. *The New Social Worker Online Magazine*. Retrieved November 22, 2014, from http://www.socialworker.com/feature-articles/practice/Understanding_Care_Coordination%3A_Emerging_Opportunities_for_Social_Workers/

Fink-Samnick, E. (2011b). Providing patient centered care demands professional diversity in case management. *Professional Case Management*, *16*(1), 3–5.

Fink-Samnick, E. (2012). Aligning professional ethics with innovation: Licensure portability's predicament. *CMSA Today*, *2*, 10–13.

Fink-Samnick, E. (2014). The dangerous culture of silence: Ethical implications for bullying in the health care workplace. *N21: Nursing in the Twenty-First Century: A Mobile Journal* (HudsonWhitman/Excelsior College Press), Vol. 3.

Gordon, R. M., Corcoran, J. R., Bartley-Daniele, P., Sklener, D., Sutton, P., & Cartwright, F., (2013). A transdisciplinary team approach to pain management in inpatient health care settings. *Pain Management Nursing*, *15*(1), 426–435.

Hall, P., & Weaver, L. (2001). Interdisciplinary education and teamwork: A long and winding road. *Medical Education*, *35*(9), 867–875.

Healthcare.gov. (2013). *Accountable care organization fact sheet*. Retrieved November 18, 2014, from http://www.healthcare.gov/news/factsheets/2011/03/accountablecare03312011a.html

Huber, D. (2002). The diversity of case management models. *Lippincott's Case Management*, *7*(6), 212–220.

Informed Medical Decisions Foundation. (2014). *What is shared decision making?* Retrieved November 17, 2014, from http://www.informedmedicaldecisions.org/what-is-shared-decision-making/

Institute of Medicine. (2001). *Crossing the quality chasm: A new health system for the 21st century*. Washington, DC: The National Academies Press.

Institute of Medicine. (2003). *Health professions' education: A bridge to quality* (The Quality Chasm Series). Washington, DC: The National Academies Press.

Institute of Medicine. (2013). *Interprofessional education for collaboration: Learning how to improve health from interprofessional models across the continuum of education to practice*. Washington, DC: The National Academies Press.

Interprofessional Education Collaborative. (2011). *Core competencies for interprofessional collaborative practice: Report of an expert panel*. Washington, DC: Author. Retrieved April 30, 2014, from http://www.aacn.nche.edu/news/articles/2011/ipec

The Joint Commission. (2008). *Sentinel event alert, issue 40: Behaviors that undermine a culture of safety*. Retrieved May 17, 2014, from http://www.jointcommission.org/assets/1/18/SEA_40.PDF

KaiserEDU.org. (2013). *Health policy unexplained. U.S. Healthcare costs: Issues, modules, background brief.* Retrieved April 28, 2013, from http://www.kaiseredu.org/issue-modules/us-health-care-costs/background-brief.aspx

Leasure, E., Jones., R. R., Meade, L. B., Sanger, M. I., Thomas, K. G., Tilden, V. P., . . . Warm, E. J. (2013). There is no 'I' in teamwork in the patient-centered medical home: Defining teamwork competencies for academic practice. *Academic Medicine, 88*(5), 584–592.

Linder, T. (1983). *Early childhood special education: Program development and administration*. Baltimore, MD: Brookes Publishing.

Llewellyn, A., & Leonard, M. (2009). *Nursing case management review and resource manual* (3rd ed.). Silver Spring, MD: American Nurses Credentialing Center.

Lowry, F. (2010). Team approaches to hospital care may improve outcomes. *Medscape Medical News*. Retrieved November 23, 2014, from http://www.medscape.com/viewarticle/717448

McAllister, J. W., Presler, E., & Cooley, W. C. (2007, September). Practice-based care coordination: A medical home essential. *Pediatrics, 120*(3), e723–e733.

Merriam-Webster's online dictionary. (2014a). Discipline. Retrieved November 13, 2014, from http://www.merriam-webster.com/dictionary/discipline

Merriam-Webster's online dictionary. (2014b). Inter. Retrieved November 21, 2014, from http://www.merriam-webster.com/medical/inter-

Merriam-Webster's online dictionary. (2014c). Stakeholders. Retrieved November 13, 2014, from http://www.merriam-webster.com/dictionary/stakeholder

Merriam-Webster's online dictionary. (2014d). Team. Retrieved November 17, 2014, from http://www.merriam-webster.com/dictionary/team

Miller-Keane encyclopedia and dictionary of medicine, nursing, and allied health. (2003). Transdisciplinary (7th ed.). Camden, NJ: Saunders/Elsevier.

Mosby's Medical Dictionary. (2009). *Health care consumer*. (8th ed.). Philadelphia, PA: Elsevier.

Munro, D. (2014). U.S. healthcare spending is a stunning $3.4 trillion, says study, *Forbes*. Retrieved November 21, 2014, from http://www.forbes.com/sites/danmunro/2014/11/17/new-deloitte-study-u-s-healthcare-spending-for-2012-was-over-3-4-trillion/

Nancarrow, S. A., Booth, A., Ariss, S., Smith, T., Enderby, P., & Roots, A. (2013). Ten principles of good interdisciplinary team work. *Human Resources for Health*, 11(1), 19.

National Association of Social Workers. (2013). *NASW Standards for Social Work Case Management*. Retrieved November 21, 2014, from http://www.socialworkers.org/practice/naswstandards/CaseManagementStandards2013.pdf

National Coalition on Care Coordination. (2009). *Models that decrease and improve outcomes for medicare beneficiaries with chronic illnesses*. New York, NY: New York Academy of Medicine.

National Conference of State Legislatures. (2014). *State coverage for telehealth services*. Retrieved November 19, 2014, from http://www.ncsl.org/research/health/state-coverage-for-telehealth-services.aspx

National Quality Forum. (2010). *Endorsing preferred practices and performance measures for measuring and reporting care coordination* (Overview). Retrieved November 21, 2014, from http://www.qualityforum.org/Publications/2010/10/Preferred_Practices_and_Performance_Measures_for_Measuring_and_Reporting_Care_Coordination.aspx

Owen, M., Treiger, T., & Fink-Samnick, E. (2014). Time to reflect and celebrate professional case management-you deserve It! *Professional Case Management*, *19*(5) 235–236.

Painter, K. (2013). When doctors are bullies, patient safety may suffer. *USA Today* Retrieved April 25, 2014, from http://www.usatoday.com/story/news/nation/2013/04/20/doctor-bullies-patients/2090995/

Rickards, T., & Moger, S. (2000). Creative leadership processes in project team development: An alternative to Tuckman's stage model. *British Journal of Management*, *11*, 273–283.

Rosenstein, A., & O'Daniel, M. (2008). Professional communication and team collaboration. In R. G. Hughes (Ed.), *Patient safety and quality: An evidenced-based handbook for nurses*. New York, NY: Agency for Healthcare Research and Quality.

Salas, E., Sims, D. E., & Burke, C. S. (2005). Is there a big five in teamwork. *Small Group Research*, *36*, 555–599.

Satterfield, J. M., Spring, B., Brownson, R. C., Mullen, E. J., Newhouse, R. P., Walker, B. B., & Whitlock, E. P. (2009). Toward a transdisciplinary model of evidence-based practice. *Milbank Quarterly*, *87*(2), 368–390.

Segen's Medical Dictionary. (2012). *Care coordination*. Huntingdon Valley, PA: Farlex.

Social Work Leadership Institute. (2014a). *About N3C: National coalition on care coordination*. Retrieved November 21, 2014, from http://www.nyam.org/social-work-leadership-institute-v2/care-coordination/n3c/about-n3c.html

Treiger, T. M., & Fink-Samnick, E. (2013). COLLABORATE©: A universal, competency-based paradigm for professional case management practice—Part I. *Professional Case Management*, *18*(3), 122–135.

Treiger, T. M., & Lattimer, C. (2011). The interdisciplinary team and transitions of care. In P. Dilworth-Anderson, M. H. Palmer, & T. C. Antonucci (Eds.), *Annual review of gerontology and geriatrics* (Vol. 31). New York, NY: Springer.

Tuckman, B. W. (1965). Developmental sequence in small groups. *Psychological Bulletin*, *63*(6), 384–399.

Tuckman, B. W., & Jensen, M. A. C. (1977). Stages of small group development revisited. *Group and Organization Studies*, *2*(4), 419–427.

Wicklund, E. (2014). $46 for 20 Minutes of mHealth is a 'good start' for doctors. *mHealth News*. Retrieved November 21, 2014, from http://www.mhealthnews.com/news/46-20-minutes-mhealth-good-start-doctors

Xyrichis, A., & Ream, E. (2008, January). Teamwork: A concept analysis. *Journal of Advanced Nursing*, *61*(2), 232–241.

Zeiss, A. M., & Steffer, A. M. (1996). Interdisciplinary health care teams: The basic unit of geriatric care. In L. L. Carstensen, B. A. Edelstein, & L. Dornbrand (Eds.), *The practical handbook of clinical gerontology* (pp. 423–449). Thousand Oaks, CA: SAGE.

18 ETHICAL-LEGAL

OBJECTIVES

After studying this chapter, you will be able to:

1. Define terms relevant to the ethical and legal domains in case management.
2. Identify professional standards specific to ethical and legal case management practice.
3. Discuss the Ethical Principles Screen.
4. Discuss the realms of moral distress for case managers.
5. Demonstrate understanding of the key elements of the ethical-legal competency.

KEY TERMS

Autonomy
Beneficence
Bioethics
Conflict of interest
Contract
Dual relationships
Ethics
Ethical Rules Screen
Fidelity
Four-Quadrant Model
Justice
Legal
Liability
Malpractice
Morality
Nonmalfeasance
Professional ethics
Risk management
Subpoena
Tenets
Unprofessional
Values
Veracity

A synergistic relationship exists between ethical and legal practice for case managers. Independent of a case manager's discipline of origin, that professional is beholden to all the legal regulations and ethical codes that underlie his or her primary credential, whether that credential is a license or certification. Equally relevant is how the laws that underlie professional licensure intersect with the reality of a case manager's individual values and beliefs. As a result, any case manager can easily find himself or herself in an ethical–legal tango, with two partners each vying to lead; one partner is objective, rigid and defined by the law, and the other is subjective, free flowing and philosophical.

Although there is an undisputed connection between the ethical and legal realms of practice, they have continued to appear as separate planets orbiting around the professional case management universe. A growing focus of the literature addresses the legal, ethical, and often moral struggle and obligation faced by case managers in addressing the scope of their professional practice (Fink-Samnick, 2012; Moffat, 2014; Muller, 2008; Pronovost & Vohr, 2010). This chapter delves into the aligned relationship of the ethical and legal realms, exploring the bearing they have on professional case management, and providing validation of why the industry mandates a single united ethical–legal competency.

DEFINITIONS

Although this chapter discusses the importance of a combined ethical and legal competency for the health care industry, it is acknowledged that each of the two areas has distinct definitions and aligned concepts. **Ethics** is defined as the analysis of principles, rules, or language that characterize an action or judgment bearing on human welfare as right or good or wrong, harmful, evil, beneficial, burdensome, etc. (Beauchamp & Childress, in Powell & Tahan, 2008). The term is also known as the prepositional statements (standards) used by members of a profession or group to determine what the right course of action in a situation is. This is a cognitive process that relies on logical and rational criteria to reach a decision (Allen, 2012; Congress, 1999; Dolgoff et al., 2009; Reamer, 1995).

All health care professionals, case managers included, face ethical dilemmas. The literature discusses several categories, which include a wide berth of circumstances across personal values and professional ethics to bioethics (Allen, 2012; Dolgoff et al., 2009; Fink-Samnick, 2013b; Muller, 2013). Each of these situations plays a significant role in a case manager's ethical, as well as legal, grounding.

An absolute or pure ethical dilemma occurs when two (or more) ethical standards apply to a situation but are in conflict with each other (Allen, 2012). This is the most common type of ethical dilemma, although far from simple in practicality. For instance, a patient has an advanced directive in place, but the document is not in the person's possession when a medical event occurs. As a result, the patient receives aggressive life-sustaining treatment by the health care providers, who are left little choice in the moment, and is now on a ventilator. The family arrives at the hospital to find out what has occurred and provides the patient's clear and explicit advanced directives to the case manager. However, as the hospital is a faith-based institution, the patient cannot be terminally weaned. The family makes arrangements with a nearby hospice program to transfer the patient in order for the patient's advanced directives to be implemented.

There are also ethical dilemmas that require a decision be made by the involved professional, but involve conflicts between values, laws, and policies for organizations. These situations are specifically referred to as approximate dilemmas (Allen, 2012). An example of this type of dilemma involves how a case manager is legally mandated to report child abuse or domestic violence to the proper authorities but is hesitant to do so because of concern about releasing confidential or private information. The legal requirements are clear across jurisdictions regarding a professional's responsibility to report the situation to law enforcement. However, professionals often engage in serious critical thinking to reconcile the situation with their ethical codes.

Some professionals mistake ethics for **values**, the latter term referring to the core beliefs which guide and motivate a person's attitudes or actions (Ethics Resource Center, 2012). These beliefs may involve cultural or personal values with the potential to impact how each individual, person, and/or profession defines their sense of service, integrity, dignity and worth of the person, importance of human relationships, social justice, and competence (National Association of Social Workers [NASW], 2008). Values often play a vital role in determining whether or not a case manager accepts a promotional opportunity to work for a particular type of organization (e.g., one that is faith-based, profit, or not-for-profit) or a new assignment to intervene with a specialty patient population (e.g., hospice patients in a state that has recently legalized marijuana for medical use).

Professional ethics encompass personal and corporate standards of behavior which are expected (Chadwick, 1998). These appear in the form of principles or rules across the various established resources for case managers (e.g., codes of ethics and professional conduct, standards of practice, and so on).

Bioethics involves the philosophical implications of certain biological and medical procedures, technologies, and treatments as organ transplants, genetic engineering, and care of the terminally ill (Random House Unabridged Dictionary, 2014). Case managers are faced with the bioethics realm when dealing with a variety of situations on behalf of patients and their caregivers, such as those dealing with:

- end-of-life treatment decisions
- whether or not to proceed with experimental treatment protocols
- medication management for severe mental illness

Morality is another term to emerge across the ethical context of a case manager's professional practice, which also has legal implications. It is defined as the degree to which something is right or good, or beliefs one has about what is right behavior and what is wrong behavior (*Merriam-Webster's Online Dictionary*, 2014b). In the health care arena the conduct and behavior of a case manager can be easily scrutinized as morally right or wrong. Let us say the case manager is conducting a family meeting and responds to a patient in a way perceived by the family as rude, disrespectful, and inappropriate. As a result, the family member of the patient questions the morality of the case manager, subsequently filing a complaint with his or her professional board and certification entity. The behavior of the case manager can also be seen as **unprofessional**, which means that it deviates from norms, guidelines, standards, and ethical codes that inform professional behavior (Banja, 2008)

Conflict of interest (COI) is applied across both ethical and legal resources and regulations and refers to a situation that has the potential to undermine the impartiality of a person because of the possibility of a clash between the person's self-interest and professional or public interest. It also involves a circumstance in which a party's responsibility to a second party limits its ability to discharge its responsibility to a third party (BusinessDictionary.com, 2014). These are situations where a case manager may have a competing interest or loyalty that impacts his or her ability to be impartial. Examples include where the case manager:

- Refers patients to agencies for homecare or other services where the case manager is employed and may have direct responsibility or oversight for the unit providing service to those patients.
- Fails to disclose to a potential employer that a patient is a family member or close friend.
- Sits on a professional board for one organization and is asked to work on a product being developed by a competing professional association.

In situations where there is concern for COI, professionals are advised to be transparent and disclose any real or perceived situations to those in positions of authority. This avoids the perception that the professional is trying to deny or hide the situation from others.

Dual relationships are often viewed as a type of COI. These occur when professionals relate to clients in more than one relationship, whether professional, social, or business. Dual or multiple relationships can occur simultaneously or consecutively (NASW, 2008). For example, a case manager is unknowingly assigned to intervene with a family member or friend.

It has been identified across professions and populations, that dual relationships can and will happen at one time or another (NASW, 2008). Take for example the scenario of a case manager who resides in a rural region, and perhaps is the only worker's compensation case manager for that jurisdiction. A referral is made to the case manager for a client who turns out to be a cousin. The appearance of a dual relationship and potentially divided loyalty is clear. As a result, the onus is on the involved case manager to act in accordance with current state laws and professional codes of conduct for their discipline and certification. It could be acceptable for a case manager to intervene with the client, as long as there is a specific contract in place. This could also be a situation not allowed under organizational policies, with the responsibility on the case manager to work with the employer to make sure the client is reassigned.

Case managers hear the term **legal** and their brains embark on a lengthy journey to what is defined as deriving authority from or founded on law, or conforming to or permitted by law or established rules (*Merriam-Webster's Online Dictionary*, 2014a). This includes an expansive list of items from organizational policies and procedures to state and federal laws, including the administrative regulations that underlie a professional case manager's professional licensure and/or certification. Chapter 2 discusses the responsibilities of professional boards and their roles in defining the administrative laws, practice act, and scope of practice for those licensed and/or certified in the state.

Case managers focus on issues involving adherence and compliance. These words are often viewed as synonyms; however, they have distinct meanings and applications. Adherence is defined as the act of doing what is required by a rule, belief, and so on (*Merriam-Webster's Online Dictionary*, 2014c). A patient's medication adherence is an area for attention by the industry, especially case managers. Newer literature suggests that adherence is the preferred term when the discussion is focused on a patient's behavior and patient motivation, and includes the patient in the determination and success of the therapy (Astreja et al., 2005; Gottlieb, 2014). In the context of patient care, adherence is viewed as a partnership, whereas compliance is not (Gould & Mitty, 2010). The use of adherence focuses on empowering patients to take care matters into their own hands, ultimately allowing them to be partners with their assorted treatment providers.

Compliance, on the other hand, is defined as the act or process of doing what one has been asked or ordered to do, or conformity in fulfilling official requirements (*Merriam-Webster's Online Dictionary*, 2014d). Case managers often view compliance as specific to laws, rules, and regulations, such as their compliance with federal rules involving the Health Information Portability and Accountability Act (HIPAA). It has been suggested that viewed compliance is an outdated concept which should be abandoned as a clinical practice/goal in the medical management of patient and illness. It connotes dependence and blame, and does not move the patient forward on a pathway of better clinical outcomes (Gould & Mitty, 2010).

Risk management is a function of administration of a hospital or other health facility directed toward identification, evaluation, and correction of potential risks that could lead to injury to patients, staff members, or visitors and result in property loss or damage (*Mosby's Medical Dictionary*, 2009). Case managers can find themselves involved in risk management incidents when their patients are involved in adverse occurrences, such as falling out of bed at facility, or allegedly given the wrong dosage of a medication. Most organizations have a risk management department or contracted entity involved with oversight of this area.

In the litigious nature of the health care industry, case managers are increasingly concerned about several other terms, which include **contract**, **liability**, **subpoena**, and **malpractice**.

A contract is a set of promises for breach of which the law gives a remedy, or the performance of which the law in some way recognizes as a duty (Garner, 2014). Contracts are the method by which case managers define the terms of their associations and are the simplest and most valuable way of determining business relationships (Muller, 2011b). Case managers develop a variety of contracts with clients; from legal contracts with organizations who employ them to those with clients whom one case manages, which frame the expectations of a professional relationship.

In the context of the HIPAA, case managers are increasingly concerned with business associate contracts. A business associate is defined as a person or entity that performs certain services for a covered entity. For example, this could refer to a case manager contracted to do a series of clinical reviews for a particular insurance company. A covered entity is any organization that directly handles personal health information (PHI) or personal health records (PHR). The most common examples of covered entities are hospitals, doctors' offices, and health insurance providers (Muller, 2011a).

The foremost value of having a written contract is that the expectations of the parties are clearly defined. When people know what the rules are, they have a greater level of comfort and confidence in their interactions (Muller, 2011a). This is a powerful lesson for case managers to include in their tool box.

Liability is the quality or state of being legally obligated or responsible (*Merriam-Webster's Online Dictionary*, 2014e). Case managers are increasingly concerned about their liability in the course of their work, especially when it involves their interactions with clients and caregivers. A variety of questions can run through a case manager's mind to this end, including the following:

- Were promises made by the case manager to the client about the services that could be provided?
- Did the case manager misrepresent himself or herself or his or her credentials in the course of the relationship?
- What are the caregiver's expectations of the case manager and the services which would be provided?

Subpoena is a court order commanding the appearance of a witness, subject to penalty for compliance (Garner, 2014). A case manager may receive a subpoena to provide testimony in court, or to submit his or her documentation about a client for the purpose of an upcoming lawsuit.

Malpractice is negligence or incompetence on the part of a professional (Garner, 2014). Although the literature shows the incidence of case managers as direct defendants in malpractice lawsuits occurs far less than one would imagine, case managers do find themselves in depositions or in courtrooms giving testimony (Muller, 2011b). As a result, malpractice is a topic for case managers to be knowledgeable of and informed about.

PAST AND CURRENT THINKING

A series of established resources set the professional tone and expectation for a case management professional's practice. In the context of ethical and legal intervention, each of these resources serves a valuable role in defining, guiding, and implementing the case management process.

STANDARDS, PRINCIPLES, TENETS, AND CODES

All professions and credentialing bodies have regulations and practice acts that underlie state licensure and certification. The professional associations and certification entities associated with case management are consistent in that a case manager's paramount responsibility for ethical and legal adherence lies with the licensure and/or certification that underlie(s) his or her primary discipline (e.g., nursing, social work, counseling, medicine) (American Nurses Association [ANA], 2001, 2010; CMSA, 2010; NASW, 2008, 2013). Table 18-1 provides examples of the legal standards, principles, and rules.

A number of professional disciplines (e.g., nursing and social work) weave together ethical practice with legal adherence in several provisions and standards. These include but are not limited to the areas of privacy and confidentiality, and duty to warn (ANA, 2001; NASW 2008). As explicitly noted by Muller (2013),

> Whether by Federal Law, state statute, or Code of Professional Ethics, the one-to-one dialogue between a medical professional and his or her patient is confidential. That having been said, there is no doubt that if you are a health care professional and you are aware that someone is in imminent danger, there is no question that you have duty to warn. This simple concept becomes more complicated by your state of licensure and a myriad of laws, rules, and regulations, each with their own purpose.
>
> In the case of duty to warn, it is incumbent upon the case manager to look to his or her state of licensure, certifying body, Standards of Practice from both the Case Management Society of America, and your professional organization, such as the American Nurses Association, National Association of Social Workers, or the American Medical Association, whether you're a member or not.

Case managers often forget, or are unaware, that their codes of ethical and professional conduct plus standards of practice do not dictate a defined course of action or a set of rules to tell the professionals represented how they should act in all situations (Fink-Samnick, 2013b). Instead, these established resources frame a licensed professional:

- Responsibility as paramount in situations where concern is for public safety (Commission for Case Manager Certification [CCMC], 2009)
- A set of values, principles, and standards to guide decision making and conduct when ethical issues arise (NASW, 2008)
- Responsibility to maintain competence in their area of practice through compliance with national and/or local laws and regulations that apply to the jurisdiction(s) and discipline(s) in which the case manager practices (CMSA, 2010)

(Fink-Samnick, 2013b)

A majority of certification entities aligned with case management have a distinct code of ethics or code of professional conduct for their certificants (CCMC, 2009; Certification of Disability Management Specialists [CDMS], 2010; CRCC, 2010). All of these codes are understood to guide rather than prescribe a case manager's actions (CCMC, 2009). Table 18-2 shows examples of the ethical standards, professional codes, and principles for case management.

Ethical Tenets

There are a series of ethical **tenets** which all health care professional adhere to. Tenets are defined as principles, beliefs,

TABLE 18-1 Legal Standards of Practice, Principles, and Rules for Case Management

American Case Management Association: Standards of Practice and Scope of Services for Health Care Delivery System Case Management and Transition of Care Professionals (2013)	Case Management Society of America: Standards of Practice (2010)	Commission for Case Manager Certification: Code of Professional Conduct for Case Managers (2009)	National Association of Social Workers: Standards for Social Work Case Management (2013)
Compliance: Case management will be knowledgeable of and ensure compliance with the federal, state, local hospital, and accreditation requirements that impact their scope of services. • Case management organizational structure and staffing, policies, and procedures must meet the Centers for Medicare & Medicaid Services (CMS) conditions of participation • All disciplines practice within the scope of practice as defined by state licensing regulations	Standard J: Legal The case manager should adhere to applicable local, state, and federal laws, as well as employer policies, governing all aspects of case management practice, including client privacy and confidentiality rights. It is the responsibility of the case manager to work within the scope of his or her licensure. 1. Confidentiality and Client Privacy: The case manager should adhere to applicable local, state, and federal laws, as well as employer policies, governing the client, client privacy, and confidentiality rights and act in a manner consistent with the client's best interest. 2. Consent for Case Management Services: The case manager should obtain appropriate and informed client consent before case management services are implemented.	Principles 2 and 7: Certificants will 2. respect the rights and inherent dignity of all of their clients. 7. obey all laws and regulations. Rules 1-7: A Certificant will not 1. intentionally falsify an application or other documents 2. be convicted of a felony 3. violate the code of ethics governing the profession upon which the individual's eligibility for the CCM designation is based 4. lose the primary professional credential (or licensure) upon which eligibility for the CCM designation is based 5. violate or breach the Standards for Professional Conduct (i.e., professional misconduct) 6. fail to pay required fees to CCMC. 7. violate the rules and regulations governing the taking of the certification examination	Standard 2: Qualifications The social work case manager shall possess a baccalaureate or advanced degree in social work from a school or program accredited by the Council on Social Work Education; shall comply with the licensing and certification requirements of the state(s) or jurisdiction(s) in which she or he practices; and shall possess the skills and professional experience necessary to practice social work case management. Standard 10: Record Keeping The social work case manager shall document all case management activities in the appropriate client record in a timely manner. Social work documentation shall be recorded on paper or electronically and shall be prepared, completed, secured, maintained, and disclosed in accordance with regulatory, legislative, statutory, and organizational requirements.

or doctrines generally held to be true, especially one held in common by members of an organization, movement, or profession (*Merriam-Webster's Online Dictionary*, 2014e). They are often included in codes of ethics, and/or professional conduct, as they are in case management.

Although the tenets for a profession remain fairly constant, the societal trends and constructs shift and change (Fink-Samnick, 2013a). As a result, there are intricacies (e.g., laws) that impact how case managers may interpret and subsequently act with respect to these tenets.

In reviewing a series of health care professions, the tenets that resonate for case managers include the following:

- **Autonomy**
- **Beneficence**
- **Fidelity**
- **Justice**
- **Nonmalfeasance**
- **Veracity**

(CMSA, 2010; Banja, 2008)

TABLE 18-2 Ethical Standards, Professional Codes, and Principles for Case Management

Commission on Rehabilitation Counselor Certification: Code of Conduct (2010)	Case Management Society of America: Standards of Practice (2010)	Commission for Case Manager Certification: Code of Professional Conduct (2009)	National Association of Social Workers, Standards for Social Work Case Management (2013)
Section A: The Counseling Relationship Section B: Confidentiality, Privileged Communication, and Privacy Section C: Advocacy and Accessibility Section D: Professional Responsibility Section E: Relationships With Other Professionals Section F: Forensic and Indirect Services Section G: Evaluation, Assessment, and Interpretation Section H: Teaching, Supervision, and Training Section I: Research and Publication Section J: Technology and Distance Counseling Section K: Business Practices Section L: Resolving Ethical Issues	Standard K: Ethics Case managers should behave and practice ethically, adhering to the tenets of the code of ethics that underlies his or her professional credential (e.g., nursing, social work, rehabilitation. counseling, etc.). How demonstrated: • Awareness of the five basic ethical principles and their application • Recognition that a case manager's primary obligation is to his or her clients • Maintenance of respectful relationships with coworkers, employers, and other professional • Recognition that laws, rules, policies, insurance benefits, and regulations are sometimes in conflict with ethical principles. In such situations, case managers are bound to address such conflicts to the best of their abilities and/or seek appropriate consultation.	Principles 1, 3, 4, 5, 6: Certificants will 1. place the public interest above their own at all times. 3. always maintain objectivity in their relationships with clients 4. act with integrity in dealing with other professionals to facilitate their clients achieving maximum benefits 5. keep their competency at a level that ensures each of their clients will receive the benefit of services that are appropriate and consistent for the client's conditions and circumstances 6. honor the integrity and respect the limitations placed on the use of the CCM designation	Standard 1: Ethics and Values The social work case manager shall adhere to and promote the ethics and values of the social work profession, using the NASW Code of Ethics as a guide to ethical decision making in case management practice.

Table 18-3 displays each tenet, their definitions, and the application to a practice example.

Social Media and Technology

A current industry trend has been toward the development of professional standards and white papers that speak to accountability for social media. These resources are significant in how they align the ethical responsibilities and practice expectations of each professional with their legal adherence to the regulations and laws. It is a constant reminder to the workforce, case managers included, of the powerful interplay of the ethical and legal domains of practice.

A number of entities have developed either a distinct body of standards or practice guidelines specific to technology practice, which speak to ethical and legal parameters (ANA, 2012; NASW & ASWB, 2005). Several of these resources have included definitions for technology within the body of their ethical codes (CDMS, 2010; CRCC, 2010), while others have produced white papers with distinct guidance and recommendations for the workforce (National Council of State Boards of Nursing, 2011).

TABLE 18-3 Case Management's Ethical Tenets and Principles

Tenet	Definition	Example
Autonomy	To respect individuals' rights to make their own decisions	The case manager is assigned a patient who has stage 4 colon cancer and wants no further treatment. Family members of the patient have mixed feelings about the patient's plan of care. The case manager coordinates a meeting for the patient to discuss his advanced directives with his family, so all are aware of his treatment decisions.
Beneficence	To do good	A case manager is intervening with a pediatric patient on a ventilator. It is important to the patient to be able to celebrate his next birthday with his friends. The case manager stays late at work to arrange a birthday party for the patient at the hospital in a meeting room on the unit. She obtains permission from administration for the patient's four close friends to attend the celebration.
Fidelity	To follow through and keep promises	The managed care organization case manager is intervening with a patient who has rheumatoid arthritis. The patient and family members explore a series of experimental protocols and provide the information to the case manager, who agrees to review and further discusses them with the medical director. The case manager agrees to contact the patient by the end of the week. Three days later, the case manager contacts the patient to schedule a videoconference to discuss the approval given by the medical director, and next steps.
Justice	To treat others fairly	The case manager is assigned with patients who have infectious diseases. Because of the heightened awareness of this population courtesy of the recent Ebola scare, there is concern that stigma may impact the quality of care in the organization. Case management co-leads psychoeducation groups with the director of infectious diseases for the organization.
Nonmalfeasance	To do no harm	A patient is admitted to the hospital with a lengthy medical history. The family indicates the presence of advanced directives that clearly designate the patient's desire to have no treatment. In the emergency to get the patient to the hospital, they left the documents at home but have sent another family member to get them. The patient deteriorates and the hospitalist wants to engage in an aggressive treatment regime in lieu of having the patient's code status at the hospital. The case manager remembers the patient had a prior admission at another system facility, and is able to access the documentation courtesy of the new electronic health record (EHR). There is a scanned copy of the patient's advanced directives in the EHR, which the case manager is able to show to the hospitalist.
Veracity	The act of telling the truth, or the truthfulness of one's behavior	The hospital case manager is meeting with the transdisciplinary team and a patient to review the patient's continued treatment needs, among them the pending approval for a specialized wheel chair. The team wonders why the approval for the chair is taking longer than prior approvals of the same type. The hospital case manager reviews the documentation and suddenly remembers that the managed care case manager called earlier in the week, requesting further information about the chair specifications. In the hospital case manager's haste to leave for a personal appointment that day, she forgot to return the call. The hospital case manager apologizes to the team and to the patient, excuses herself from the meeting, and contacts the managed care case manager. Approval for the chair is provided during this phone call and the team and patient are notified.

Adapted from Case Management Society of America. (2010). CMSA standards of practice for case management (Rev.). Retrieved April 25, 2013, from http://www.cmsa.org/portals/0/pdf/memberonly/StandardsOfPractice.pdf; Banja, J. (2008). Ethical issues in case management practice. In S. Powell & H. Tahan (Eds.), CMSA Core Curriculum for Case Management (2nd ed., pp. 594–607). Philadelphia, PA: Lippincott Williams & Wilkins.

Guidelines for telehealth and telemedicine are actively evolving across the industry (American Telemedicine Association, 2014), though as previously noted, each professional must check with his or her licensure board to adhere to the standards and regulations that underlie each requisite primary licensure and/or certification possessed.

Case managers are also reminded of the importance to check the websites for their professional state boards and associations and certification entities for changes and updates to existing standards, codes, and laws which guide their practice. It is recommended that this take place quarterly given how quickly innovation and professional intervention are advancing. Individual state laws impacting distinct areas of practice focus (e.g., telehealth practice and reimbursement, mandated reporting) can be accessed through the National Conference of State Legislatures website (http://www.ncsl.org). With the rate at which technology and innovation continue to progress, there is no conclusive, comprehensive listing of laws that can be developed.

GENERAL PERSPECTIVES

Ethical decision making is a process (NASW, 2014). To that end, a variety of ethical decision-making frameworks with interprofessional application exist across the industry. These frameworks are of particular note for they also include attention to the legal scope of professional practice.

ETHICAL DECISION-MAKING MODELS

Each of the following ethical decision-making models incorporates emphasis on the legal regulations and policies across sectors (e.g., health care, legislative, regulatory). The critical thinking model presented in chapter 8 is also designed for application as an ethical decision-making tool for case managers.

The Ethical Assessment, Rules, and Principles Screens

Dolgoff et al. (2009) developed a series of ethical screens to guide professionals to clarify and integrate the ethical, and usually legal, aspects of decision making in social work practice. All of these have universal application across professional disciplines. The authors are clear that those who are alert to the ethical aspects of practice, will examine and assess the available options and alternatives somewhat differently from colleagues who may not be as attuned with those aspects (Dolgoff et al., 2009).

Case managers are used to working through situations at a rapid pace; the flow of job requirements in the workplace often mandates it. However, a face-paced effort is not the case manager's best friend in ethical and legal situations. Case managers are reminded that especially with respect to ethical and legal decision making, expediency is the enemy of integrity.

The three screens are shown in Box 18-1. Each provide distinct cues to case managers, in order to guide decision making that accounts for ethical and legal considerations. The Ethical Assessment Screen (EAS) offers a series of self-checks or reminders. It takes into account that most professionals can plan rationally what is needed for intervention in human situations. Most strive to minimize the irrational, the impulsive, and the unplanned consequences of their actions (Dolgoff et al., 2009).

The **Ethical Rules Screen** (ERS) is a simple reminder to check the assorted codes of ethics that underlie a case manager's professional licensure. It is not uncommon for case

BOX 18-1 Ethical Assessment, Rules, and Principles Screen

Ethical Assessment Screen

1. Identify relevant professional values and ethics, your own relevant values, and societal values relevant to the ethical decision to be made in relation to the ethical dilemma.
2. What can you do to minimize conflicts between personal, societal, and professional values.
3. Identify alternative ethical options that you may take.
4. Which of the alternative ethical options will minimize conflicts between your client's, others', and society's rights and protect to the greatest extent your client's and others' rights and welfare, and society's rights and interests?
5. Which alternative action will be most efficient, effective, and ethical, as well as result in your doing the "least harm" possible?
6. Have you considered and weighed both short- and long-term ethical consequences?
7. Final check: Is the planned action impartial, generalizable, and justifiable?

Ethical Rules Screen

1. Examine the Codes of Ethics for application of rules.
2. If Code applies, follow Code rules.
3. If Code does not address specific problem or poses conflicting guidance, use the Ethical Principles Screen.

Ethical Principles Screen

The principles of:

1. Protection of life
2. Equality and inequality
3. Autonomy and freedom
4. Least harm
5. Quality of life
6. Privacy and confidentiality
7. Truthfulness and full disclosure

Adapted from Dolgoff, R., Loewenberg, F. M., & Harrington, D. (2009). Ethical decisions for social work practice. (8th ed.). Belmont, CA: Thomson Higher Education.

TABLE 18-4 Ethical Principles Screen With Explanation and Examples

Principle	Explanation
1. Protection of life	The protection of human life applies to all persons, both to the life of a client and to the lives of all others (e.g., treatment providers being aware of state and federal laws regarding futility of care, patient advanced directives).
2. Equality and inequality	All persons of the same circumstances should be treated in the same way (e.g., in the context of abuse, neglect, and/or exploitation, case managers are mandated to refer to appropriate authorities in accordance with the regulations that underlie their state laws and professional licensure).
3. Autonomy and freedom	All practice decisions should foster a person's self-determination, autonomy, independence, and freedom (e.g., case managers do not have the right to harm others or make decisions on behalf of others who are competent to do so).
4. Least harm	When faced with dilemmas that have the potential for causing harm, a case manager should attempt to avoid or prevent such harm. If harm is unavoidable, the professional should always choose the option that will cause the least harm, the least permanent harm, and/or the most easily reversible harm (e.g. case manager should contact legal authorities in the context of abuse, neglect, exploitation, concerns regarding suicidal, and/or homicidal intent).
5. Quality of life	The option should be chosen that promotes the best quality of life for all people, for the client as well as for the community (e.g., there must be attention to current laws guiding treatment decisions, patient's right to self-determination amid safety).
6. Privacy and confidentiality	Practice decisions should be made by professionals that strengthen every client's right to privacy and confidentiality (e.g., professionals have a duty to protect the privacy of clients and groups to the greatest extent possible, though this must be consistent with laws).
7. Truthfulness and full disclosure	Practice decisions must be made by the professional which permit one to fully disclose all relevant information to clients and others (e.g., on the front end of a professional relationship, inform clients about the limits of privacy and confidentiality, particularly when concern regarding the patient's imminent danger to himself herself or others exists).

Adapted from Dolgoff, R., Loewenberg, F. M., & Harrington, D. (2009). Ethical decisions for social work practice. (8th ed.). Thomson, Brooks/Cole Publishing.

managers to find advice to guide their next steps in these assorted documents. Traditionally, most codes of ethics defer to state and federal laws and regulations (ANA, 2001; CCMC, 2009; NASW, 2008). Should a professional not be able to obtain the needed guidance from the ERS, proceeding to the Ethical Principles Screen (EPS) comes next.

The EPS provides a rank-ordering of the ethical principles for consideration when assessing the various alternatives for action. The authors deny that the principles have been put in any specific order (Dolgoff et al., 2009), yet it is not uncommon for health care professionals to refer to the protection of life in many risk assessment models. Table 18-4 provides further elaboration of the EPS with examples of each principle.

The Four-Quadrant Model

The **Four-Quadrant Model** (Jonsen et al., 2010) is used across the health care industry to identify and group all ethically important aspects of the situation at hand. The model does not resolve the situation a health care professional is dealing with nor does it prioritize which of the ethical elements must be addressed or in which order. However, the Four-Quadrant Model does provide those who use it a framework that presents assorted questions and topics for consideration during the ethical decision-making process. The Four Quadrants are shown in Figure 18-1 and include the following:

1. Medical indications
2. Patient preferences
3. Quality of life
4. Contextual features

Of particular notice for this chapter, is how the legal area of focus is included for consideration in the fourth quadrant, contextual features. Jonsen et al. (2010) note how health care providers and their patients are subject to the varying influence of a number of factors in the context of the treatment relationship. These include community and professional standards, legal rules, governmental and institutional policies about financing and access to health care, computerized methods of storage and retrieval of medical information, the relationship between research and practice, and

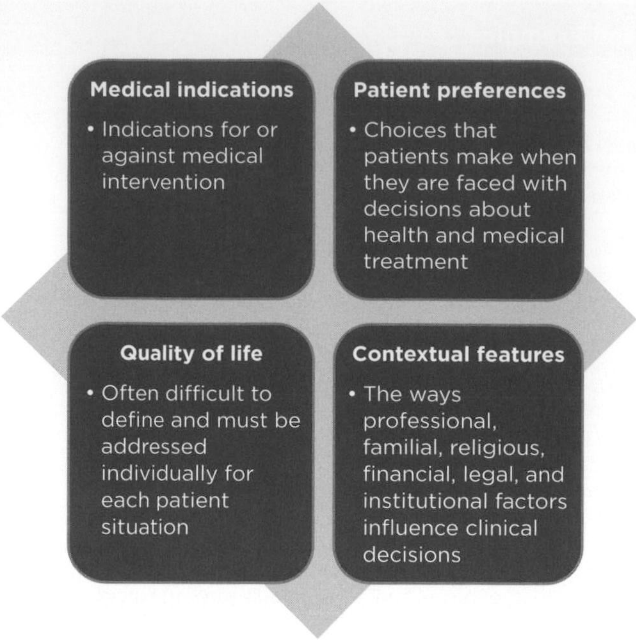

Medical indications
- Indications for or against medical intervention

Patient preferences
- Choices that patients make when they are faced with decisions about health and medical treatment

Quality of life
- Often difficult to define and must be addressed individually for each patient situation

Contextual features
- The ways professional, familial, religious, financial, legal, and institutional factors influence clinical decisions

Figure 18-1. The Four-Quadrant Model. (Adapted from Jonsen, A., Siegler, M., & Winslade, W. (2010). *Clinical ethics: A practical approach to ethical decision-making* (7th ed.). New York, NY: McGraw Hill.)

other factors (Jonsen et al., 2010). The questions for each of the Four Quadrants appear in Table 18-5.

CONTEXT FOR COLLABORATE ETHICAL AND LEGAL

In our litigious society, case managers are concerned with an ethical–legal conflict in which they want to provide quality case management services, obey the law, meet licensing requirements and regulations, please their employers or contractors, and still act as an advocate for their patients (Muller, 2008). Given the wide scope of practice settings where case managers work plus the large number of professional disciplines that comprise case management, there is a great deal for professionals to consider in the context of their ethical and legal practice.

For instance, the laws related to practicing outside of the scope of a professional's license have potential, equally dramatic ethical implications, such as misrepresenting credentials or not advocating appropriately for a patient. These situations may prompt sanction for case managers from two fronts: legal from a warning to revoking of licensure, and potentially equal ethical sanction from a certification entity, resulting in loss of a credential. There are common threads that bind many ethical and legal situations.

It is not uncommon for a case manager to analyze the legal implications of his or her practice, but then ignore the ethical emphasis, and vice versa. Particularly in our litigious society, case managers are concerned with ethical–legal conflict in which they want to provide quality case management services (Muller, 2008). It is for this reason that although the COLLABORATE approach acknowledges the distinct ethical and legal domains that exist in the industry, case managers must view them in tandem. When case managers think ethical impact of a situation, they must consider the legal connection. As case managers ponder how new laws and potential legislation impact their practice, they must in turn consider how their ethical practice will be challenged as a result of the passage of said laws. When a case manager's employer creates new policies and procedures with respect to new industry trends, such as telehealth, there must be attention to the ethical and legal parameters of practice and whether or not they will allow for that practice to occur.

KEY ELEMENTS OF ETHICAL–LEGAL COMPETENCY

The key elements include the following:

- Licensure;
- Certification;
- Administrative and professional standards;
- Organizational policies and procedures; and
- Ethical codes of conduct.

The COLLABORATE perspective focuses on the multifaceted and usually complex ethical–legal relationship that exists in all situations. The ethical–legal competency transcends several key elements, which case managers must consider with respect to their:

- unique professional discipline and the scope of their practice,
- assorted credentials and administrative requirements,
- practice setting with their distinct role and function, organizational policies and procedures, and
- the assorted ethical codes that underlie their credentials, which defer to the laws for their primary licensure and certifications.

To illustrate how to account for each of these key elements in the context of the case manager's role, review the case scenario in Box 18-2. It involves Sam, a case manager, for a large regional managed care organization. Consider how Sam must focus his ethical and legal attention to assure adherence to professional practice across each of the key elements.

IMPLICATIONS FOR PRACTICE

Case Manager Versus Employer: Moral Distress

In an era of multiple accountabilities, (nurse) case managers are constantly faced with situations that demand ethical choices and judgments to coordinate the care of patients who have diverse needs and interests within a health care context that requires reduced cost, increased access, and improved

TABLE 18-5 The Four-Quadrant Model: Questions

Four Quadrants	Ask and Answer the Following to Guide Next Steps
Medical indications	a. What is the client's medical problem and why? b. Diagnosis and prognosis c. Is the problem acute, chronic, critical, emergent, incurable, or reversible? d. What are the goals of treatment? e. What are the probabilities of success? f. What is the plan in case of therapeutic failure? g. How can the client be benefitted and how can harm be prevented?
Patient preferences	a. Is the client mentally capable and legally competent? b. If competent, what are the client's preferences for treatment? c. Has the client been informed of benefits and risks? d. Has he or she given consent? e. If incapacitated, who is the appropriate decision maker? f. Is the client's surrogate or proxy making decisions as the client would wish (which is ethical) or as the surrogate prefers (which is unethical)? g. Has the client expressed prior preferences, such as by an advance directive (e.g., living will, durable power of attorney for health care)? h. Is the client's right to choose being respected to the greatest extent possible in ethics and law?
Quality of life	a. What are the prospects, with or without treatment, for a return to a normal life? b. What physical, mental, and social deficits is the client likely to experience if the treatment succeeds? c. Are there biases that might prejudice the professional's evaluation of the client's quality of life? d. Is the client's present or future consideration such that his or her continued life might be judged undesirable? e. Is there any plan or rationale to forego treatment? f. Are there plans for comfort or palliative care?
Contextual features	a. Are there family issues, financial and economic factors, or religious or cultural factors that might unjustly influence treatment decisions? b. Are there legal issues or clinical trials (research) involvement that might compromise the client's welfare? c. Is there any conflict of interest on the part of the providers or institution?

Adapted from Jonsen, A., Siegler, M., & Winslade, W. (2010). Clinical ethics: A practical approach to ethical decision-making (7th ed.). New York, NY: McGraw Hill.

quality (O'Donnell, 2007a). In addition, case managers face moral distress in the course of their daily decisions, working to interconnect organizational, clinical, and personal ethics (Moffat, 2014).

Moral distress is a human response to conflict, which is created by "on-the-job" ethical conflicts (Moffat, 2014). It is a painful condition experienced by a professional caregiver who knows what is ethically appropriate but is unable to act on it (Jameton, 1984). Case managers experience these ethical conflicts across several realms: organizational, clinical, and personal (Moffat, 2014), which are shown in Figure 18-2. When case manager's values, as well as ethics, are marginalized and authority is lacking, the decision making perceived to be "inferior ethical prioritizing" puts case managers at risk for moral distress (Moffat, 2014).

Case managers are beholden to the licensure regulations for their primary discipline, plus professional standards and ethical codes. However, another dimension of accountability exists for case managers: organizational/employer policies and procedures. This is a slippery slope for many a case manager who strive to assure ethical and legal adherence to professional practice while ascertaining the impact of conflicting organizational policies. As a result, it is here where moral distress can be especially compounded. The case scenarios in Box 18-3 illustrate some of the circumstances case managers face daily that have potential to evoke considerable moral distress.

Moral distress for case managers is further compounded by the addition of the current legal concerns related to professional liability and adherence to laws and regulations (e.g., privacy and confidentiality, scope of practice, licensure portability). These relentless experiences combine to create an environment of conflict and constraint that are common risk factors for moral distress (Moffat, 2014). Table 18-6 provides further expansion of the ethical categories associated with moral distress, also noting the potential legal focus.

BOX 18-2 Ethical-Legal Competency: Case Scenario

Sam is ecstatic to hear that her managed care organization has received a one-million-dollar grant through Substance Abuse and Mental Health Services Administration (SAMHSA) to implement an integrated behavioral health pilot project, one expected to expand nationally. The program will expand telemedicine and telehealth in the region, ensuring patients in rural areas have access to high-quality health and mental health care they might not otherwise receive.

Sam attends a meeting on the new program. All of the patients chosen to participate have been diagnosed with both a mental disorder and a series of chronic medical conditions. Many of the patients reside in the surrounding tri-state area. Sam knows one of these states is a member of the nurse licensure compact, but the other two are not. He raises his hand to ask questions and present his concerns about practicing across state lines. The medical director, Dr. Heath, replies: "Your interactions are not considered assessing, but follow-up contacts, Sam you worry too much about these things." Sam could not disagree more and thinks to himself, "I don't worry enough."

Sam reluctantly agrees to move forward with beginning to call patients. It does not take long for the first phone call to become more convoluted than one could ever imagine. What begins as a simple follow-up, has Sam assessing a patient across state lines in a state where he is not licensed, with the patient potentially at risk of suicidal ideation. Ethical and legal issues are tangled and intertwined. It is tough for Sam to see where one issue ends and the other begins. His journey to unravel this mess begins

Licensure

Sam is a case manager in the know and aware that there is NO mandated duty to report statute in his state. He is surprised but has scoured the administrative practice laws and called the board of nursing to verify it. Sam is confident that the code of ethics that underlies his profession is clear with respect to his duty to report a patient who is at risk of harming himself or others. As a result, he contacts law enforcement immediately.

Certification

Sam contacts the organization that provides his case management certification to request an advisory opinion. They are supportive, guiding Sam to the appropriate place in their code of ethics and to support his decision to adhere with his mandated duty to warn. Sam then takes this opportunity to discuss his new role and whether the situation he just engaged in involved assessment, one of his primary concerns about the role.

It is suggested that he potentially performed an assessment in this situation, though for some states this level of assessment is allowed in emergent situations. As a result, his certification entity recommends that Sam contact the board of nursing in his home state for further guidance and direction. It is also advised that he review his scope of practice with the state board regarding telemedicine and telehealth regulations. New administrative regulations are being developed and revised swiftly to this end and it is best practice to review these updates at least every quarter, if not more frequently. There was further dialogue about exploring how current Sam's organizational policies and procedures reflect the new information on this evolving area of telehealth.

Administrative and Professional Standards

Sam is now on a mission to collect all the evidence he can to discuss this matter further with his corporate director of care coordination, Irene, plus Dr. Heath. Serious advocacy is needed to address the interplay of potentially practicing against ethical codes, as well as illegally. It is his license and case management certification on the line; those hard-earned letters after his name that he is not about to give up. Sam prints out a copy of both the ethics and legal professional standards. All are clear in their language that he is beholden to:

1. Behave and practice ethically, adhering to the tenets of the code of ethics that underlies your professional credential and
2. Adhere to applicable local, state, and federal laws as employer policies, governing all aspects of case management practice, including client privacy and confidentiality rights. It is the responsibility of the case manager to work within the scope of his or her licensure.

(CMSA, 2010)

Organizational Policies and Procedures

Sam's meeting with Irene and Dr. Heath is spirited. He discusses his contact and information with the certification entity and nursing boards. Sam is direct that there must be new policies to reflect the current practice trends. All case managers must know the scope of their practice to minimize liability or at least how to access the information. Sam feels strong that the new policy should include a listing of the online resources and contact information for each state professional board, certification entity, and professional association. The new policy section will be called Ethical and Legal Parameters for Case Management Practice.

(Continued)

BOX 18-2 Ethical-Legal Competency: Case Scenario (*Continued*)

Ethical Codes of Conduct

Sam is appreciative that the ethical codes across the assorted entities he is aligned with are as clear as they are. In fact, Sam sees they are more similar than different. He has renewed appreciation for the important role these documents serve to ground all professionals in their actions. He contacts his professional association to discuss this topic further.

In meeting with his colleagues, Sam discusses how ethics is never black and white, and there is guidance to bring others out to the other side of the gray. Sam downloads the documents for nursing and case management, adding them to his stack of resources for inclusion in those new policies he has been assigned to write.

TODAY'S CASE MANAGEMENT CHALLENGES WILL BE TOMORROW'S EDUCATIONAL OPPORTUNITIES

Health care is a fluid and robust industry amid more changes than anyone could have ever foreseen. COLLABORATE defines competencies necessary for value-driven case management practice. The key elements associated with each competency reinforce the importance of case manager self-awareness. Learning is, after all, a journey of continuous knowledge acquisition, not a destination at which one knows-it-all. This journey is especially true in the context of ethical and legal practice.

As readily as the health care industry will continue to evolve, a rash of new challenges to a case manager's ethical and legal practice will emerge. Case managers must view any limits to their knowledge base as education opportunities. They must actively strive to stay informed through the pursuit of new learning, through whatever form best addresses their style. This process includes exploring journal articles, engaging in online continuing education, aligning with professional associations, and networking with colleagues.

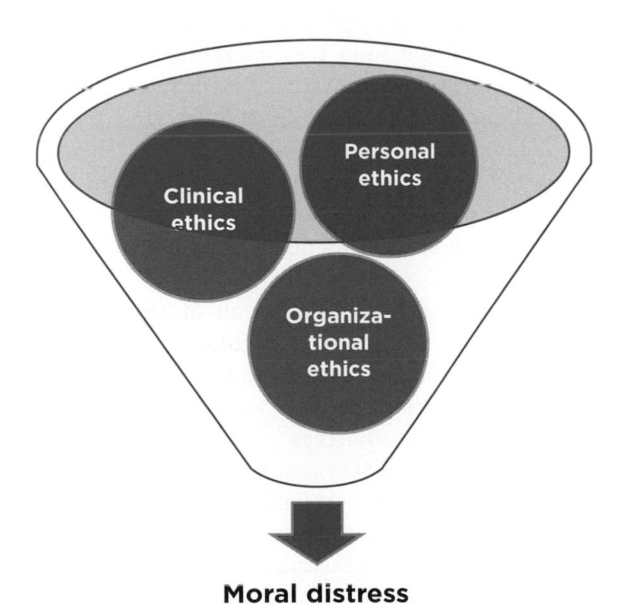

Figure 18-2. Moral distress and ethical conflict. (Adapted from Moffat, M. 2014, Reducing moral distress in case managers. *Professional Case Management, 19*(4), 173–186.)

BOX 18-3 Moral Distress: Case Scenarios

1. A case manager is asked to engage in independent assessment, an act that is outside of the scope of his or her professional level of licensure. "Oh just do it to get the job done." The case manager is told by his or her director that there are a flock of candidates who can be hired instead.
2. The case manager has documented suspicion that a pediatric patient is being abused and neglected by his parents, though is told by the patient's physician not to contact the authorities or report the case to child protective services. The physician claims to know the parents well and says, "I'll talk to them. You don't have anything to worry about."
3. A case manager is reviewing the electronic medical record documentation on several patients covered by the physician he or she is assigned to. Suddenly the case manager realizes the documentation is identical from patient to patient, and becomes concerned about cloned medical record documentation, something which an organization can be penalized for doing.
4. The case manager brings the issue to the attention of the medical director who says, "Don't worry about it. All the physicians are getting the lay of the land with this new product. They will stop this copy and paste thing in time. Though you might want to try it to see what a time saver it can be to copy and paste your notes across patients. But don't tell anyone I told you to do so."
5. A case manager is working with a patient to be transferred to a subacute nursing home for rehabilitation. The only bed available is at the facility where the patient's husband died several years ago. The patient is medically ready to transition, and as the hospital is focused on a new length of stay initiative the case manager is given a choice by his or her director, either discharge the patient to the available nursing home bed or provide her a formal letter of denial (HINN).

TABLE 18-6 Ethical Conflict Realms With Added Legal Constructs

Ethical Realms	Explained	Potential Legal Concern
Organizational Ethics	Human reactivity of a community devaluing caregiving expertise because of financial constraints. Concern for institutional culpability for meeting contractual obligations and regulatory mandates.	May present as greater focus on these issues than patient care: • Contract scope and adherence • Regulatory mandates and fiscal imperatives
Clinical Ethics	Advocacy to alleviate patient pain and suffering becomes irrelevant in bureaucratic regulations. Based on moral principles about indications (treatment available), patient preferences, quality of life, patient advocacy, and other contextual features.	May present as a greater focus on length of stay, cost of care than issues such as clinical appropriateness and/or futility of care, or patient self-determination.
Personal Ethics	Unequal power hierarchy of higher authority, diverting, underfunding, or denying funding for the "best" advocacy. Values and self-worth are included, with unique dilemmas based on human reactivity, unequal power hierarchy, advocacy, and professional competency.	May present as organizational priority for compliance with policies and procedures, regulations trumps focus on or attention to patient and/or caregiver. Overexposure to ethical conflicts cause a creative professional care planner to become instead a messenger of underfunded benefit plans, regulation mandates, or under-resourced care providers.

Adapted from Moffat, M. (2014). Reducing moral distress in case managers. Professional Case Management, 19(4), 173–186; Jonsen, A., Siegler, M., & Winslade, W. (2010). Clinical ethics: A practical approach to ethical decision-making (7th ed.). New York, NY: McGraw Hill; O'Donnell, L. (2007a). Ethical dilemmas among nurses as they transition to hospital case management: Implications for organizational ethics. Part I. Professional Case Management, 12(3), 160–169; O'Donnell, L. (2007b). Ethical dilemmas among nurses as they transition to hospital case management: Implications for organizational ethics. Part II. Professional Case Management, 12(4), 219–231; Rittenmeyer, L., & Huffman, D. (2009). How professional nurses working in hospital environments experience moral distress: A systematic review. Critical Care Nursing Clinics of North America, 24, 91–10.

By virtue of a case manager's role and position on the care team, he or she is made to feel like they are accountable for so much of what occurs in the practice setting. However, at the end of each day, case managers can only be accountable for their own practice. This includes possessing the current requisite knowledge base of ethical and legal parameters for professional case management practice, which are firmly grounded in the defined laws, professional standards, tenets, and ethical codes for the industry.

Technology Innovation and Licensure Portability

Case managers are faced with technology's unparalleled evolution across the health care industry. The impact is felt in every environment of practice, whether through a new product, program, process, or policy. Conversely, innovation's vast promise is often accompanied by concerns regarding the potential ethical and legal implications for case management practice (Fink-Samnick, 2013a).

One of the most challenging ethical and legal areas of focus involves the critical connection between state-to-state licensure and technology and innovation that now allows for diagnosis, assessment, and treatment intervention across via remote and telehealth means. Yet, despite the ongoing challenges related to licensure portability and how treatment providers will be reimbursed, a majority of health care providers still view telemedicine as a top priority in their operations, with some 90% reporting that they have already begun developing or implementing a telemedicine program (Oliva, 2014).

Case managers are involved in all of these initiatives through implementation and expansion of remote health programs, video-teleconferencing, and a steady influx of new and exciting products to connect with patients who might not otherwise be able to access a health care professional. The first thing any provider considering telehealth practices and technologies must thoroughly grasp is the payment model (Manos, 2014). Yet this can often be forgotten in lieu of the industry excitement regarding the anticipated revenue gains. Research predicts that the global telehealth market is expected to double from $11.6 billion in 2011 to about $27.3 billion in 2016. In addition, the telehospital/clinic market alone is expected to grow to $17.6 billion, and telehome segment is expected to reach $9.7 billion (Dolan, 2012). It is also expected that these numbers will continue to grow with the next generation of products scheduled to hit the market.

In recent studies across health care organizations, 64% currently offer remote monitoring of patient, and 52% report using real-time interaction with patients. However, as of the time of this writing, Medicare regulations require that the real-time telehealth visits be conducted while a patient is at a medical facility. This creates a situation where sick, home-bound patients must first be transported from their homes—sometimes by ambulance—to receive teleheath care (Manos, 2014). Strong advocacy to change the regulations and laws guiding these technologies continues with full forth across all health care professions involved in rendering care, especially case managers.

There is no doubt of case management's role in this genesis of health care delivery across the various transitions of care. These technologies are critical to the future success of their organizations, especially considering the biggest driver of this programming: the Patient Protection and Affordable Care Act (PPACA) (Oliva, 2014). Conversely, innovation's vast promise is often accompanied by concerns regarding the potential ethical and legal implications for case management practice (Fink-Samnick, 2013b).

Being paid for telemedicine remains an uphill battle for the bulk of health care professionals, especially those in case management. Some studies indicate as high as 41% of respondents note they are not reimbursed at all for telemedicine services, and 21% report receiving lower rates from managed care companies for telemedicine than for in-person care (Oliva, 2014). Case managers are reminded that practicing across state lines and in states and jurisdictions where they are not licensed or viewed as licensed (factoring in states involved with the nurse licensure compact) is potentially illegal as well as unethical.

Case managers must assure a proactive stance to stay abreast of new laws and regulations, as well as the expanded body of new and revised ethical codes. They must engage in the strong advocacy efforts underway to impact the legislative changes necessary to allow for legal practice that syncs with the practice reality of the times and populations in need. Otherwise, reactive practice will surely result in a greater potential for errors, miss-steps, and reactionary practice at best. Lack of understanding and adherence to current regulations puts all health care stakeholders at potential ethical and legal risk (Fink-Samnick, 2013a).

SUMMARY

The ethical and legal domains of a case manager's professional practice forge a powerful partnership, each with the implicit potential to invade any and all interventions. The times are complex, as are the patient populations which case managers are tasked to intervene with. There are dynamic factors which spiral around every circumstance case managers are tasked to engage in. The diverse scope of a case manager's professional expertise is sought out with increasing frequency. Although attention to separate ethical and legal influencers of practice is an important start, focus on these realms alone are insufficient to assure proficient case management intervention. Though adherence to a combined ethical–legal competency, professional case managers will find the success mandated, for them to engage in competent practice moving forward.

References

Allen, K. (2012, Spring). What is an Ethical Dilemma? *The New Social Worker Online*. Retrieved January 5, 2015, from http://www.socialworker.com/feature-articles/ethics-articles/What_Is_an_Ethical_Dilemma%3F/

American Case Management Association. (2013). *Standards of practice and scope of services for health care delivery system case management and transitions of care professionals*. Little Rock, AK: Author.

American Nurses Association. (2001). *Code of Ethics for nurses with interpretive statements*. Silver Spring, MD: Author.

American Nurses Association. (2010). *Scope and standards of practice: Nursing*. (2nd ed.). Silver Spring, MD: Author.

American Nurses Association. (2012). *Principles for social networking and the nurse*. Retrieved November 28, 2014, from http://www.nursingworld.org/socialnetworkingtoolkit

American Telemedicine Association. (2014). *Standards and guidelines*. Retrieved November 29, 2014, from http://www.americantelemed.org/resources/standards/ata-standards-guidelines/practice-guidelines-for-video-based-online-mental-health-services#.VHnhUIvF-JU

Astreja, A., Bellam, N., & Levy, S. (2005). Strategies to enhance patient adherence: Making it simple. *Medscape General Medicine*, 7(1), 4. Retrieved November 28, 2014, from http://www.ncbi.nlm.nih.gov/pmc/articles/PMC1681370/

Banja, J. (2008). Ethical issues in case management practice. In S. Powell & H. Tahan (Eds.), *CMSA Core Curriculum for Case Management* (2nd ed., pp. 594–607). Philadelphia, PA: Lippincott Williams & Wilkins.

BusinessDictionary.com. (2014). Conflict of interest. Retrieved November 28, 2014, from http://www.businessdictionary.com/definition/conflict-of-interest.html

Case Management Society of America. (2010). *CMSA standards of practice for case management* (Rev.). Retrieved April 25, 2013, from http://www.cmsa.org/portals/0/pdf/memberonly/StandardsOfPractice.pdf

Certification of Disability Management Specialists. (2010). *Code of professional conduct*. Retrieved November 29, 2014, from http://www.cdms.org/uploads/files/CDMS_Code_of_Professional_Conduct.pdf

Chadwick, R. (1998). Professional ethics. In *Routledge encyclopedia of philosophy*. Retrieved April 30, 2013, from http://www.rep.routledge.com/article/L077

Commission for Case Manager Certification. (2009). *Code of professional conduct for case managers*. Retrieved October 31, 2014, from http://www.ccmcertification.org/content/ccm-exam-portal/code-professional-conductcase-managers

Commission on Rehabilitation Counselor Certification. (2010). *Code of ethics*. Retrieved November 29, 2014, from http://www.crccertification.com/filebin/pdf/CRCCodeOfEthics.pdf

Congress, E. P. (1999). *Social work values and ethics: Identifying and resolving professional dilemmas*. Belmont, CA: Wadsworth Group/Thompson Learning.

Dolan, P. (2012). Where growth is coming in telemedicine. *American Medical News: Business Section*. Retrieved November 30, 2014, from http://www.amednews.com/article/20121113/business/311139997/8/

Dolgoff, R., Loewenberg, F. M., & Harrington, D. (2009). *Ethical decisions for social work practice*. (8th ed.). Belmont, CA: Thomson Higher Education.

Ethics Resource Center. (2012). *Values*. Retrieved November 28, 2104, from http://www.ethics.org/resource/definitions-values

Fink-Samnick, E. (2012) Aligning professional ethics with innovation: Licensure portability's predicament. *CMSA Today* (2), 10–13.

Fink-Samnick, E. (2013a). Case management's ethical eight: Preparing for the next wave. *Case in Point*, *11*(11), 1–5.

Fink-Samnick, E. (2013b). Duty to act: A comprehensive process in proceeding with duty to warn. *Professional Case Management, Legal and Regulatory Column*, *18*(3), 151–153.

Garner, B. (2014). *Black's law dictionary*. (10th ed.) San Francisco, CA: Thomson West.

Gottlieb, H. (2014). Medication nonadherence: Finding solutions to a costly medical problem. *Medscape*. Retrieved November 28, 2014, from http://www.medscape.com/viewarticle/409940_5

Gould, E., & Mitty, E. (2010). Medication adherence is a partnership, medication compliance is not. *Geriatric Nursing*, *31*(4), 290–298.

Jameton, A. (1984). *Nursing practice: The ethical issues*. Englewood Cliffs, NJ: Prentice Hall.

Jonsen, A., Siegler, M., & Winslade, W. (2010). *Clinical ethics: A practical approach to ethical decision-making* (7th ed.). New York, NY: McGraw Hill.

Manos, D. (2014). Telehealth and the realities of reimbursement. *Government Health IT*. Retrieved November 30, 2104, from http://www.govhealthit.com/news/telehealth-and-realities-reimbursement

Merriam-Webster's online dictionary. (2014a). Legal. Retrieved November 28, 2014, from http://www.merriam-webster.com/dictionary/legal

Merriam-Webster's online dictionary. (2014b). Morality. Retrieved November 30, 2014, from http://www.merriam-webster.com/dictionary/morality

Merriam-Webster's online dictionary. (2014c). Adherence. Retrieved November 28, 2014, from http://www.merriam-webster.com/dictionary/adherence

Merriam-Webster's online dictionary. (2014d). Compliance. Retrieved November 28, 2014, from http://www.merriam-webster.com/dictionary/compliance

Merriam-Webster's online dictionary. (2014e). Liability. Retrieved December 1, 2014 from, http://www.merriam-webster.com/dictionary/liability

Merriam-Webster's online dictionary. (2014f). Tenet. Retrieved November 30, 2014, from http://www.merriam-webster.com/dictionary/tenets

Moffat, M. (2014). Reducing moral distress in case managers. *Professional Case Management*, *19*(4), 173–186.

Mosby's Medical Dictionary. (2009). *Risk management*. (8th ed.). Philadelphia, PA: Elsevier.

Muller, L. S. (2008). Legal issues in case management practice. In S. Powell & H. Tahan (Eds.), *CMSA Core curriculum for case management* (2nd ed., pp. 571–593). Philadelphia, PA: Lippincott Williams & Wilkins.

Muller, L. S. (2011a) Contracts in case management: An updated view. *Professional Case Management. Legal and Regulatory Issues*, *16*(6), 311–315.

Muller, L. S. (2011b). Editor's commentary. *Professional Case Management, Legal and Regulatory Issues*, *16*(5), 258.

Muller, L. (2013). Duty to warn: The case manager's role. *Professional Case Management, Legal and Regulatory Column*, *18*(3), 144–151.

National Association of Social Workers. (2008). *Code of ethics*. Retrieved November 26, 2014, from http://www.socialworkers.org/pubs/code/code.asp

National Association of Social Workers. (2013). *Standards of practice for social work case management*. Retrieved November 21, 2014 from http://www.socialworkers.org/practice/naswstandards/CaseManagementStandards2013.pdf

National Association of Social Workers & Association of Social Work Boards. (2005). *Technology standards of practice for social workers*. Washington, DC: NASW Press.

National Council of State Boards of Nursing. (2014). *Social media guidelines for nursing*. Retrieved November 29, 2014, from https://www.ncsbn.org/347.htm

O'Donnell, L. (2007a). Ethical dilemmas among nurses as they transition to hospital case management: Implications for organizational ethics. Part I. *Professional Case Management*, *12*(3), 160–169.

O'Donnell, L. (2007b). Ethical dilemmas among nurses as they transition to hospital case management: Implications for organizational ethics. Part II. *Professional Case Management*, *12*(4), 219–231.

Oliva, J. (2014). Telemedicine remains top priority, despite ROI uncertainties. *Senior Housing News*. Retrieved November 30, 2014, from http://seniorhousingnews.com/2014/11/16/telemedicine-remains-top-priority-despite-roi-uncertainties/

Pronovost, P., & Vohr, E. (2010). *Safe patients, smart hospitals*. New York, NY: Hudson Street Press.

Random House Unabridged Dictionary. (2014). Bioethics. Retrieved April 30, 2012, from http://dictionary.reference.com/browse/bioethics

Reamer, F. (1995). *Social work values and ethics*. New York, NY: Columbia University Press.

Rittenmeyer, L., & Huffman, D. (2009). How professional nurses working in hospital environments experience moral distress: A systematic review. *Critical Care Nursing Clinics of North America*, *24*, 91–10.

SECTION 3

Positioning for the Paradigm Shift

19 PREPARING FOR CHANGE

OBJECTIVES

After studying this chapter, you will be able to:

1. Recognize the importance of methodical approaches to organizational change.
2. Recognize the importance of communication, influence, and planning in ensuring project success.
3. Identify and apply tools to facilitate individual readiness for change.
4. Evaluate important assessments points to understand your organization's readiness for change.
5. Assist direct reports and yourself in understanding and accepting the necessity for change.
6. Recognize the scope of work required to prepare for COLLABORATE implementation.
7. Identify options for modifying productivity expectations for individuals on the COLLABORATE implementation team.

KEY TERMS

Ability
ADKAR
Awareness
Commitment
Desire
DICE
Disruptive self-expression
Duration
Effort
Integrity
Knowledge
Opportunities
Reinforcements
Strategic alliance building
Strengths
Tempered radicals
Threats
Variable-term opportunism
Verbal jujitsu
Weaknesses

Shifting to the COLLABORATE practice model may be undertaken on by an individual or organization level. For the individual seeking to improve his or her professional practice, the competencies detailed in section 2 provide benchmarks on which to set personal goals. The department facing change must approach with a comprehensive strategy that informs and prepares case management staff and those working with them throughout the process. The result of these upgrades is enriched practice, which ultimately improves customer satisfaction and service quality.

Changing a practice paradigm requires a management strategy that enables employees to adopt new behaviors and expectations while simultaneously discarding old ones. Carefully managing the change process contributes to the realization of the business objectives, clearly defined from the project's outset. This creates synergy between theoretical solutions and tangible results (Hiatt & Creasey, 2012). The bottom line is that whether at an organizational level or on an individual basis, process change requires people to change. Section 3 focuses on preparation for COLLABORATE model implementation.

PREPARING FOR THE PARADIGM SHIFT

There is agreement that change management is a challenging undertaking. However, disagreement abounds as to the factors influencing transformation initiatives. Some of these factors include the time required to institute it, the number, expertise and ability of staff required to execute it, and the impact achieved because of it (Sirkin et al., 2005). When organizations do not take these foundational issues into account, change initiatives often run amuck and break down before really getting off the ground.

CHANGE AT THE ORGANIZATIONAL LEVEL

Preparing for change is both an individual and an organizational effort. Managing change comprehensively enables the transition beyond a starting point theory through its implementation to the endpoint of adoption. Business objectives are realized when a proposal is embedded into organizational bedrock. A variety of assessment points are useful to understand during the preimplementation phase of significant change, including the following:

- Scope of change
- Readiness for change
- Project resources
- Project sponsorship

Refer to Table 19-1 for considerations regarding each of these details (Hiatt & Creasey, 2012).

CHANGE MANAGEMENT EXPERTISE

With regard to case management, it is not unusual for individuals to rise into management positions for reasons other than proven competence and qualifications. Such is the case when convenience is the driver of promotions. It may be that filling a management position was of a critical nature. Often in those instances, expediency drives decision making based on subjective judgment of available staff rather than a thorough talent search for the best person to fill the vacancy. Even in situations when a promotion is based on qualifications and proven capabilities, the formal education and skills required to effectively manage change are different from those needed for day-to-day operational management.

It behooves senior management to perform a critical evaluation of its current employee roster. The point of this review is to understand the existing staff capability for taking on a significant change management process. It may prove beneficial to bring in the designated project manager as part

TABLE 19-1 Getting Ready for Change Considerations

Action	Considerations
Scope of change	How big is the change?
	How many staff are affected by the change?
	Is the change gradual or radical?
Readiness for change	What are the value systems and backgrounds of the affected staff/groups?
	How much change is already taking place?
	What degree of resistance to change is anticipated?
	What is the staff/group history of dealing with change?
Project resources	What is required to acquire project team resources?
	What are team member strengths and weaknesses?
Project sponsorship	Does a project sponsor coalition exist?
	What is required to enable project sponsors to lead the change process?

Adapted from Hiatt, J. M., & Creasey, T. J. (2012). Change management: The people side of change (2nd ed.). Loveland, CO: Prosci.

of this **knowledge** and skills review. Use of the **ADKAR** methodology, discussed later in this chapter, is valuable for assessing all staff members' knowledge, skills, and capabilities.

THE HARD ELEMENTS OF CHANGE

When undertaking significant change, it is essential that there be an authentic commitment to see a project through to its successful conclusion. Many efforts start with the simple realization that change is necessary. This **awareness** begins with an individual or small group noticing movement in the competitive environment, market position, technology advances, or financial performance (Kotter, 1995) or a combination of these and other factors. Recognizing the need for change is a first step toward making a commitment to the process that will bring about the change itself. However, those seeking change must be prepared to follow the entire process through to its conclusion, encompassing, but not limited to, defining the need, creating goals/desired outcomes, communication, assembling a project plan, implementing the change, measuring progress, and formalizing the new approach into lasting expectations pertaining to behaviors and performance.

There are elements to be addressed prior to as well as throughout the change management process. At an organizational level, when these factors are not paid attention to, there is often a breakdown of the change process itself. These hard elements, as identified by Sirkin et al. (2005) are Duration, Integrity, Commitment, and Effort. The **DICE** acronym applies to these variables because each can be loaded to favor project success.

Duration

The **duration** of a project, how long a project takes from start to finish, is not the determiner of success or failure. However, projects that roll on for prolonged period of time without sufficient oversight and review are more apt to run amuck. Organizations should define and conduct specific intervals of formal project review. The length of time between reviews is dependent on the organization's capability and project complexity. The probability that a change initiative will run into trouble rises exponentially when the time between reviews exceeds 8 weeks (Sirkin et al., 2005).

The change management plan should include achievable milestones and scheduled assessment meetings to facilitate project oversight, risk assessment, gap identification, and resource allocation. Milestones should describe major actions or achievements that enable the project lead team to confirm that progress has been made in the time since the last meeting. Examples of useful milestones include "Technology assessment completed" and "Benchmarking interviews completed." In situations where a milestone is not achievable, it is the responsibility of the project leader and team to assess the situational risk, identify the reasons for anticipated shortfall, enact corrective actions to avoid a failure, and incorporate take-away lessons to avoid repeating the same problem in the future (Sirkin et al., 2005).

To facilitate this level of organizational learning, the project team must provide consistent, clear, and concise progress reports to the oversight team. The lead team's responsibilities include assessing whether or not the project activities are having their intended effect on operations and understand how the project's progress to date impacts subsequent goals and communications. The lead team must have the power to address weaknesses or failures to achieve intended results through a variety of means (e.g., resource diversion, goal modification, change in project team makeup). The key activities of the lead team in these milestone meetings are to monitor project team dynamics, assess changes in the organization's perceptions of the initiative, and incorporate executive input into the project going forward (Sirkin et al., 2005).

Integrity

Integrity refers to the project team's performance and ability to achieve project goals within the defined timeline. Integrity is dependent on each individual team member's skills, behaviors, experience, and traits as each relates to the project's requirements and desired outcomes (Sirkin et al., 2005).

Maintaining integrity through a careful team member selection is a determining factor in overall project success. It is rare that an organization has a sufficient number of ready employees available to serve on a project team; managers are loathe to free up their best and brightest staff from day-to-day duties because of the risk it poses to regular operations.

Commitment

Commitment is the dedication level of leaders to a change initiative. The level of commitment, or lack thereof, must be apparent across the organization undertaking change. However, it is essential that influential leaders demonstrate visible support of the change in order for it to embed in the company culture. For those in leadership positions, the recommended rule of thumb is to visibly support and talk up the change initiative at least three times more than is felt to be necessary (Sirkin et al., 2005). Executives should not rely on self-gauged frequency but rather should validate with managers and frontline staff to ensure one's perception matches their reality.

Communication serves as a proxy for demonstrating commitment. Assuming a leadership role requires stepping up to the harder tasks associated with change. The **ability** to communicate the urgency of need for change as well as the implications associated with the undertaking is critical. Employees should equate the rationale for change as necessary to the organization's success. They must also be cognizant of the downside of change, including modification to and possible loss of jobs. True leaders do not shy away from taking on these difficult topics. Communications must be both well-timed and carefully considered because messaging that is inconsistent results in staff confusion and feeds into mistrust and absence of support for the change process. These negative influencers plant seeds of doubt in the minds of employees, which subsequently contribute to project failure because of the absence of staff commitment.

Never underestimate the effort required to build staff support for changing the manner in which they work. An informational campaign relying solely on written messaging creates a sense of remote leadership. The perception of distance infers a lack of commitment or concern, which lacks a certain gravitas for communication of such critical information. If memoranda and emails are the sole means of communication, it is unlikely that employees will grasp the urgency or necessity of changing the manner in which their work must change. This ultimately leads to project failure because of a lack of employee enthusiasm. Rather than wait for the inevitable failure, senior leaders should build in face-to-face communication sessions that include middle managers and staff. These sessions should emphasize two-way conversations, not simply standing in front of a group to announce changes. Focusing on project objectives, impact on employees, and the rationale behind the change should include reasons why the organization may well fail in the absence of planned changes (Sirkin et al., 2005). Providing time for questions from employees will help to build rapport and create an environment of transparency with regard to the project.

Effort

Effort refers to the overall impact on project team members and employees over and above their usual day-to-day work responsibilities. When launching process-change projects, few companies take into consideration the level of current staff exertion to complete existing responsibilities. When asked to take on even more tasks, employees are apt to resist, will not give sufficient attention to the new work, or will simply resist and become less productive in the completion of all tasks. For example, the degree of overwork becomes clear when discussing feedback on documents circulated in advance of a meeting. A quick glance around the room shows many project team members are busily scanning the documents for the first time and are unable to give constructive input on the impact of the proposed changes. The reason for this lack of preparedness has more to do with the fact that their managers have not lightened up on any of their regular duties. Project team members are expected to carry their full workload as well as additional project tasks. This hardly provides an incentive for becoming involved on a process improvement team.

It is helpful to provide guidance as to how much time an employee will need to spend on project-related work. It is recommended that 10% be considered the maximum workload increase because over that the project is likely to run into difficulties due to human resource overload (Sirkin et al., 2005). In addition to compromising project deliverables, productivity for regular duties and morale will likely also decline. When project team members begin to complain of conflict between regular versus project-related workload, those negative inferences are absorbed by their coworkers. It is likely that this negativity will result in the formation of negative opinions about the anticipated changes before staff receives formal communication about the project.

Companies must anticipate this and decide whether project team members will have some of their regular duties temporarily reassigned, starting with discretionary and nonessential responsibilities. Consideration should also be given to bringing in temporary staff or outsourcing work during the project's critical timeline (Sirkin et al., 2005). For project teams to function efficiently, members must have sufficient time to devote to their assigned deliverables.

In addition to project team considerations, organizations must also assess the impact of work processes modifications on already overburdened staff. While a period of adjustment to new processes (often referred to as the learning curve) is assured, has it also been acknowledged that the improved process may require more effort to complete than did the former processes? Has that increased level of effort (measured according to former standards) been deemed worth the change? Have measurements of productivity and effectiveness been evaluated for applicability to the new case management approach and new ones created? These are critical questions for senior leadership to contemplate as part of project preparation. Failing to consider the long-termed implications of process change raises a question as to whether an organization is truly committed to changing the approach to case management delivery. Existing productivity and effectiveness measures need to reflect and distinguish the new approach. A committed organization will include creating new measures to assess the new processes as integral to the project plan rather than continue to rely on former measures.

DICE Scoring

When applied to project preparation, the DICE framework includes a scoring system which management may utilize to identify staff strengths, weaknesses, and abilities pertaining to each hard element. Although the scores are a subjective determination of each rater, the framework allows for a more objective process to determine an initiative's prognosis for success. Each of the DICE factors is graded on a scale of 1 to 4. Scores signify each factor's contribution to success. The resulting score is categorized as a Win, a Worry, or a Woe. Using this approach, an organization gets a heads up as to which areas require additional attention on an individual basis. Box 19-1 provides guidance for utilizing the DICE scoring system.

PREPARING FOR CHANGE AT THE EMPLOYEE LEVEL

There will always be a range of employee reaction to change. The array spans those considered early adopters who enthusiastically incorporate new ways of doing things all the way through to the resistors who balk at any change to their status quo. These laggards can stall process improvement efforts to the point of serious disruption. Hence, expectations and performance implications must be clearly stated and

BOX 19-1 The DICE Scoring Framework

Scoring Process			
Factors	**Considerations and Scoring**		
Duration	Questions	Do formal project reviews occur regularly? For projects anticipated to last more than 2 months to complete, what is the average time between reviews?	
	Scoring (for projects over 2 months in length)	**If**	**Score**
		period between reviews is less than 2 months	**1**
		period between reviews is 2–4 months	**2**
		period between reviews is 4–8 months	**3**
		period between reviews is 8 months	**4**
Integrity	Questions	— Is the team leader capable? — How strong are the team members' skills and motivations? — Do team members have sufficient time to spend on the project?	
	Scoring	**If**	**Score**
		project led by highly capable leader, team members have skills and motivations to complete project within timeframe and the company has assigned at least 50% of team member time to work on the project	**1**
		team members lack dimensions of skill and motivation	**4**
		team member dimensions of skill and motivation fall in the mid-range	**2–3**
Commitment (C_1 = Executive level)	Questions	— Does executive management regularly communicate the reason for change and its importance to success? — Are these communications convincing? — Are communications consistent over time and across top-level management? — Has executive management devoted appropriate resources to the change initiative?	
	Scoring	**If**	**Score**
		executives, through actions and words, clearly communicated the need for change	**1**
		executives appear neutral as to the nature of change	**2–3**
		middle managers perceive executive managers to be reluctant to support change	**4**
Commitment (C_2 = Middle/ lower managers)	Questions	— Do employees most affected by the change understand the reason for it and believe that change is worthwhile? — Are employees enthusiastic and supportive or worried and obstructive?	
	Scoring	**If**	**Score**
		eager to take on the change	**1**
		simply willing to take on the change	**2**
		reluctant	**3**
		strongly reluctant	**4**

Scoring Process			
Factors	**Considerations and Scoring**		
Effort	Questions	— What is the percentage of increased effort that employees must make to implement the change? — Is the incremental effort in addition to heavy workload? — Have employees strongly resisted the increased demand placed on them?	
	Scoring	**If**	**Score**
		project requires less than 10% additional effort	**1**
		project requires 10%–20% additional effort	**2**
		project requires 20%–40% additional effort	**3**
		project requires over 40% additional effort	**4**

Calculation and Interpretation

DICE Formula = **D** + (**I** × 2) + (**C**1 × 2) + **C**2 + **E**

In this 1 to 4 scoring system, the formula produces a score ranging from 7 to 28.

Comparing the current project score with those of past project scores (and the outcomes of those projects) provides insight as to the probable success or failure of the current project.

Scoring Range and Interpretation

Range	Interpretation
Score between 7 and 14	This is the Win zone. The project very likely to succeed.
Score >14 but <17	This is the Worry zone. Risks to the project's success are rising, particularly as the score approaches 17.
Score 17 or more	This is the Woe zone. The project is extremely risky if score 17 to 19. Any score above 19, the project is unlikely to succeed.

Adapted from Sirkin, H. L., Keenan, P., & Jackson, A. (2005). The hard side of change management. Harvard Business Review, 83*(10), 108–118.*

understood from the outset, including integration of individual performance management goals. On an individual level, use of the ADKAR model helps diagnose and manage individuals through the change process. This model separates the individual change management process into phases, which are described in Table 19-2.

In addition to the phases of individual change, there are four objectives achievable using ADKAR methodology (Hiatt, 2006), including:

- In Managing Transitions, individuals self-assess their own progress through the change process, thus enabling the identification of personal barriers to progressing through the change process.
- In Focusing Conversations, communication is tailored to an individual level, making it more effective, and addresses specific areas of identified conflict and interest.
- In Diagnosing Gaps, aggregating employee input allows management to address similar categories and provides rationales for why the change process is failing or not progressing as anticipated.

TABLE 19-2 The ADKAR Model for Individual Change Management

Stage	Description
Awareness	Individual awareness of the need for change
Desire	Individual desire to participate and support the change
Knowledge	Individual knowledge regarding how to change
Ability	Individual ability to implement new skills and behaviors
Reinforcement	Individual-level reinforcement for keeping newly acquired skills and behaviors in place

Adapted from Hiatt, J. (2006). ADKAR: A model for change in business, government, and out community. Loveland, CO: Prosci.

- Through Identifying Corrective Actions, management constructs a framework for identification of activities needed to ameliorate the gaps and failures associated with change implementations.

Hiatt and Creasey (2012) provide an exercise that may be helpful in working with employees on an individual basis throughout the change process. The ADKAR approach is broken into steps as follows:

- Step 1: Write a brief description of the change project.
- Step 2: List all reasons why the change is necessary and rate the degree of Awareness of the need for change.
- Step 3: List the positive and negative factors or consequences related to the change affecting the level of **Desire** to adopt the change. Consider all of these factors/consequences, including the conviction in each, and then rate the overall desire to change.
- Step 4: Create a list of new Knowledge and skills needed to support the change. Consider if there is a clear understanding of the change, the knowledge and skills needed to work effectively and efficiently within the new work environment, and whether there has been education and training in relative to the knowledge and skill areas. Rate the proficiency level for the needed knowledge and skills.
- Step 5: Evaluate the employee's Ability to perform the new skills, knowledge, and behaviors.
- Step 6: Create a list of **Reinforcements** (incentives) needed to bolster retention of the change and rate the ability to support incorporation of the change into a standard pattern of behavior.
- Step 7: Review all scores, highlighting those rated 3 or lower. The first instance of this score is the place to begin working with the individual regarding the change.

Worksheets to complete each of the above steps are found in Boxes 19-2 through 19-8.

BOX 19-2 ADKAR Step 1 Worksheet

Supervisor/Manager—Briefly describe the change that is being implemented at your company.

____
____
____
____
____
____
____
____
____
____
____
____
____
____
____
____
____
____
____
____

Adapted from Sirkin, H. L., Keenan, P., & Jackson, A. (2005). The hard side of change management. Harvard Business Review, 83*(10), 108–118.*

RECOGNIZING ORGANIZATIONAL DRIVERS

Changing a professional paradigm is not something to be initiated lightly. As Kotter (1995) noted "the most general lesson to be learned from the more successful cases is that the change process goes through a series of phases that, in total, usually require a considerable length of time. Skipping steps creates only the illusion of speed and never produces a satisfying result." The degree of change required to institute the COLLABORATE model into standard practice is dependent on variables that are highly applicable to each organization. These variables include, but are not limited to, competitive market forces, organization type, adjacent department impacts, existing staff maturity (e.g., education, experience, proficiency), and technology (e.g., sophistication, user expertise). Completion of an environmental assessment is strongly encouraged to identify actual and potential danger zones. Once identified, it is possible to develop strategies in advance in order to stem the disruption of ongoing business processes.

Change within organizations is influenced by the structure and scope of the business itself. For case management departments attempting to implement significant operational change, recognizing how the actions within one department affect other departments within larger organization is important. Difficulties arise due to variable levels of recognition and support for the process change as well as in lack of preparing other departments for the impact of change. When the paradigm shift in one area goes unaddressed in other business units, the up- and downstream business process connections tend to misfire. Critical synapses become sluggish, if not clogged, ultimately disrupting existing business processes in multiple areas. For example, when medical management adjusts the manner in which case managers conduct provider outreach, the provider

BOX 19-3 ADKAR Step 2 Worksheet

Focuses on Awareness

List all reasons why the change is necessary and then rate the degree of your awareness of the need for change.

____

Circle the applicable rating: 1 2 3 4 5

Rating key:

A rating of 1 signifies the lowest degree of awareness of the need for change.

A rating of 5 signifies the highest degree of awareness of the need for change.

Adapted from Sirkin, H. L., Keenan, P., & Jackson, A. (2005). The hard side of change management. Harvard Business Review, 83*(10), 108–118.*

BOX 19-4 ADKAR Step 3 Worksheet

Focuses on Desire

List the positive and negative factors or consequences related to the change affecting the level of desire to adopt the change. Consider all of these factors/consequences, including the conviction in each, and then rate the overall desire to change.

____

Circle the applicable rating: 1 2 3 4 5

Rating key:

A rating of 1 signifies a low desire to change.

A rating of 5 signifies a high desire to change.

Adapted from Sirkin, H. L., Keenan, P., & Jackson, A. (2005). The hard side of change management. Harvard Business Review, 83*(10), 108–118.*

relations representatives notice an increase of incoming calls from provider office staff. The call-volume increase affects monthly provider report production. The delay in report compilation causes an interruption in processing reports used to calculate incentive payments and subsequently, a delay in issuing these bonus payments. Call volume in provider relations increases yet again as these payments are not received as anticipated. Hence, a case management process change, perceived to be an improvement in one department, is overshadowed by the upheaval and discord it causes in another area. It is highly advisable to conduct a thorough impact evaluation in order to obtain cross-functional support prior to undertaking the initiative. This allows forecasting to take place in adjacent work areas, and impacts can then be included in the overall project plan.

Change management should be undertaken with a strong belief that change is necessary for the continued success of the business. Although it may appear impossible to gain 100% enthusiastic support, failing to garner a consensus of opinion that an organization needs to change may prove a

BOX 19-5 ADKAR Step 4 Worksheet

Focuses on Knowledge

Create a list of new knowledge and skills needed to support the change. Consider if you have a clear understanding of the change and the skills you need to work effectively and efficiently within the new work environment and if you have received education and training in these skills? Rate your proficiency level with the identified knowledge and skills.

Circle the applicable rating: 1 2 3 4 5

Rating key:

A rating of 1 signifies a low degree of familiarity with the knowledge and skills needed for the change.

A rating of 5 signifies a high degree of familiarity with the knowledge and skills needed for the change.

Adapted from Sirkin, H. L., Keenan, P., & Jackson, A. (2005). The hard side of change management. Harvard Business Review, 83*(10), 108–118.*

BOX 19-6 ADKAR Step 5 Worksheet

Focuses on Ability

Consider the knowledge and skills identified as needed to implement the changes and evaluate the overall ability to change.

Circle the applicable rating: 1 2 3 4 5

Rating key:

A rating of 1 signifies a low degree of ability to change.

A rating of 5 signifies a high degree of ability to change.

Adapted from Sirkin, H. L., Keenan, P., & Jackson, A. (2005). The hard side of change management. Harvard Business Review, 83*(10), 108–118.*

fatal blow to long-term success. A good stepping-off point is highlighting common beliefs, starting with the organization's mission, vision, and values. However, leveraging outdated foundational statements to support an argument for present-day change may not be as powerful as anticipated. Challenge the organization's executives to evaluate and renew these pivotal statements regularly. Current mission, vision, and values statements that support consumer-centric professional health care and are committed to high-quality customer service and delivery excellence align well with the COLLABORATE model. Performing an assessment of the business environment serves useful in laying the groundwork for change.

BOX 19-7 ADKAR Step 6 Worksheet

Focuses on Reinforcements

Create a list of reinforcements (incentives) needed to bolster retention of the change. Are there reinforcements (incentives) in place to facilitate the incorporation of the change into a standard pattern of behavior?

Circle the applicable rating: 1 2 3 4 5

Rating key:

A rating of 1 signifies that reinforcements are inadequate to sustain the change.

A rating of 5 signifies that reinforcements are appropriate and in place to sustain the change.

Adapted from Sirkin, H. L., Keenan, P., & Jackson, A. (2005). The hard side of change management. Harvard Business Review, 83*(10), 108–118.*

BOX 19-8 ADKAR Step 7 Worksheet

Review all scores and transpose findings from steps 2 through 6 into worksheet.

Brief description of the change:

ADKAR Step	Score
Awareness of the need to change. Notes:	
Desire to make change happen. Notes:	
Knowledge about how to change. Notes:	
Ability to change. Notes:	
Reinforcement to sustain the change. Notes:	

Interpretation:

1. Highlight each score rated a 3 or lower.
2. Consider a score of 3 or lower as a starting point for addressing individual transition planning to ensure individual success through the change process.

Adapted from Sirkin, H. L., Keenan, P., & Jackson, A. (2005). The hard side of change management. Harvard Business Review, 83*(10), 108–118.*

CONDUCTING AN ENVIRONMENTAL ASSESSMENT

Evaluating the environment in which an organization operates is an important predecessor of change management. One approach to environmental assessment is the SWOT analysis. In this methodology, evaluation of Strengths, Weaknesses, Opportunities, and Threats takes place in an organized manner. A SWOT analysis is scalable to service, product, project, and industry as well as useful at an individual level as part of self-improvement or career management. As part of a COLLABORATE implementation, SWOT is helpful for identifying internal and external factors that is influential on case management practice in its present state.

Use of the 2 × 2 matrix (shown in Figure 19-1) facilitates visualization of situational issues, appropriateness, and implications of a change in the service-delivery model. Ultimately, the analysis sheds light on variables pertinent to an

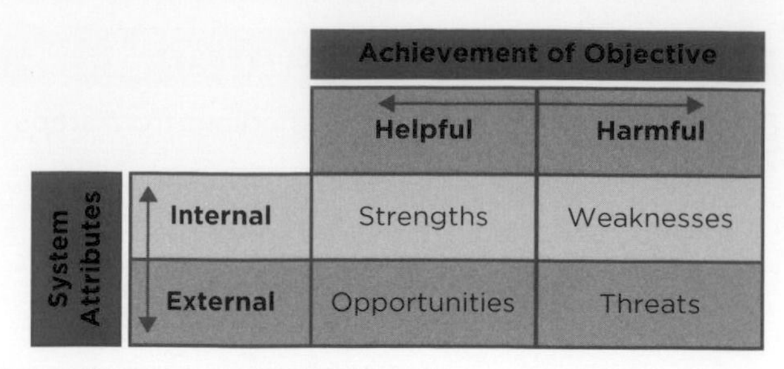

Figure 19-1. The 2 × 2 SWOT matrix.

organization's positional strengths, weaknesses, opportunities, and threats for the purpose of creating a competitive advantage through adoption of the COLLABORATE model. Due to the subjectivity of factor ratings, participants in the SWOT exercise should be well-versed in case management theory and practice.

Creating a question or proposition statement begins the SWOT analysis. The statement must be clear and concise as to the purpose of the project. For the purpose of changing the case management delivery model, an example of a prefacing project statement is:

> Deltawide Case Management is a long-standing champion of patient-centered care coordination. Over the years, Deltawide has enjoyed success demonstrated through achieving three-year accreditation approvals and receiving countless letters of thanks from its members. Although it has achieved past success, the last three years have seen a decline in overall membership, lower selection and qualification of numbers for case management intervention, and an increase in the average length of case management engagement. These trends are accompanied by membership gains in competitor health plans. Deltawide is undertaking this analysis as a means of identifying the factors contributing to recent declines and development of a strategy to halt and reverse these issues.

Strengths and Weaknesses

Strengths are considered attributes weighed as positive to an organization's internal environment. These characterizations range in degree of their help or harm to an organization, much the same as assets and liabilities on a balance sheet. Harmful or negative qualities are classified as **weaknesses**. When considering organizational strengths and weaknesses, posing the following questions will evoke thoughtful debate:

- What are the advantages of the proposed model change?
- What are our known capabilities within the organization?
- What are the resources and assets of our organization?
- How has our organization capitalized on the experience, knowledge, and skills of its employees?
- How does COLLABORATE provide us with unique marketing distinguishers?
- How does geography factor into changing our service model?
- How does changing the service model affect our pricing, value, and quality for better or worse?
- How does changing the service model affect our staff morale and commitment?
- What are the risks of changing the service model relative to our turnaround timeliness and quality ratings?
- How does changing the service model impact our accreditations, qualifications, and certifications?
- How do our current IT systems contribute to or detract from service delivery?
- How does our organizational culture influence new model adoption?
- Has current management been successful in implementing past changes?
- Does our organizational mission, vision, and values support new model adoption?
- Are our financial reserves adequate to carry the operation during transition?
- What are the implications of this service model change to our members/patients?

Opportunities and Threats

Opportunities are external factors considered to be favorable to an organization. **Threats** are external factors perceived to be adverse or unfavorable. When considering opportunities and threats, the following questions will spur discussion:

- How are market developments affecting critical business functions?
- Are market developments causing competitor vulnerabilities?
- Are industry trends changing market conditions?
- Have changes in lifestyle affected our membership or market?
- Has our technology kept pace with current market demand?
- Are any regional or national trends affecting our industry?
- Are we leveraging vertical or horizontal business opportunities?
- Have our competitors announced surprising or disruptive business changes?
- Are new products or services in the pipeline that will disrupt existing business practice?
- What is industry research telling us?
- Will a model change facilitate or disrupt any of our partnerships?
- How will the model change affect our ability to be competitive within the market?
- Will pending legislation or regulatory changes pose problematic to the existing or new model?
- How will the COLLABORATE model impact productivity and effectiveness?
- Does our current case management model fully engage eligible members and will COLLABORATE improve engagement of members and employees?
- Does our current case management model provide career advancement opportunities to our employees? Will COLLABORATE do so?
- Is our current case management model driven more by business priorities or membership needs?

CHANGE AT THE INDIVIDUAL LEVEL

Much attention has been devoted to making change at the organizational or departmental level. Unfortunately, many organizations are unable or unwilling to take on a significant change effort. Reasons for this include, but are not limited to, lack of desire, failure to recognize the need for process improvement, failure to recognize case management as a professional practice, and lack of resources to devote to a major change process. Although there is always the option to look for a position in a company that presents a better "fit" with an individual's values and practice approach, it is not always an option to risk a job change to find that perfect working environment. For individual's facing such circumstances, the desire and motivation to improve one's professional practice must come from within.

Meyerson's (2001) work in examining change recognizes individuals who enjoy their current jobs, wish to continue performing them successfully, but see things differently than the organizational norm. Rather than angrily challenging leadership, these **tempered radicals** serve as change agents to effect change with a moderate approach. These individuals embody the COLLABORATE leadership competency in that they exert influence through their professional knowledge and conduct.

There are four embodiments of tempered radicalism, including **disruptive self-expression**, **verbal jujitsu**, **variable-term opportunism**, and **strategic alliance building**. How each evidences itself varies. An individual demonstrates disruptive self-expression through the congruence of their personal, internal compass in which that cause others to take notice. Verbal jujitsu is a technique in which otherwise insensitive statements, actions, or behaviors are reversed back on themselves. Variable-term opportunism involves spotting, creating, and capitalizing on change opportunities. Finally, through forming strategic alliances these individuals facilitate change with more power than would be otherwise possible (Meyerson, 2001).

Tempered radicals present a puzzlement to organizations and colleagues because of the paradoxes in their conduct. They are firm, yet flexible, want change, yet are patient as it unfolds, seek alliances rather than pick fights, and unite people as they continue to work alone. The result is powerful, progressive, yet relentless evolutionary change (Meyerson, 2001).

Demonstrating Change: A Commitment to Self

The tactics employed through tempered radicalism present clear opportunities to case managers seeking the means by which to power-up their professional practice and embody the COLLABORATE practice model. Although examples of these approaches are provided herein, the beauty of individual expression is that it presents infinite possibilities for the professional case manager to shine.

Disruptive Self-Expression

At the most tempered end of the change continuum is the kind of self-expression that quietly disrupts others' expectations (Meyerson, 2001). Simple demonstrations of individualism are made with one's appearance, the manner and tone of communication with colleagues, or with decorative items at one's desk or workstation. When these things are outside of the norm, people take notice and eventually begin to talk about it with others.

Consider the example of Penny Nichols, a 35-year-old case manager working at General Health Care Systems in Racine. Unlike her colleagues who often wear blue jeans and jersey tops, Penny's concept of the company's business casual dress code includes chino trousers paired with a sweater set or a tweed blazer with oxford collared striped shirts. Her workspace is adorned with educational event announcements from the professional organization of which she is a member and a nicely framed case management certificate she received 2 years ago. Penny organized a small personal library consisting of contemporary reference books on pathophysiology and evidence-based care guidelines. She answers incoming phone calls rather than allowing them to go to voicemail, and speaks clearly but softly when communicating with her clients and colleagues. She maintains an organized, uncluttered workspace and is able to find things quickly due to her efficient document filing system.

Verbal Jujitsu

Verbal jujitsu is a martial art in which an attacking force is redirected. In the same spirit, the tempered radical does not return demeaning or insulting comments with the same but instead uses them as opportunities to demonstrate noticeable change (Meyerson, 2001).

Take Randy Bigen, a new case manager at a large-urban teaching facility in Boston. He is getting ready to visit a person who was admitted over the weekend. Marilin is a 55-year-old woman admitted for congestive heart failure. For no apparent reason, Marilin takes an instant dislike to Randy as he enters her hospital room. Abruptly, she indicates that she does not wish to speak to him. When he offers to return at a more convenient time, she cuts him off and asks him to leave.

Perplexed by the patient's behavior, Randy returns to the central station and reviews Marilin's medical record. He notices a medication discrepancy and just before the staff nurse administers the incorrect dose, he returns to the patient's room and discretely notifies her. A new medication order is obtained and the correct dose given. When Marilin learns of the problem, she thanks to staff nurse profusely to which she responds, "Don't thank me, thank your case manager. He is the person who discovered it."

That afternoon, Randy returns to speak with Marilin. He apologizes for coming in at an inconvenient time earlier and asks if she is able to talk to him now. Marilin responds, "It is I who needs to apologize for being so abrupt this morning. Thank you for being so understanding and for catching the problem with my medication. I have all the time in the world! What would you like to talk about?" Although Randy never learns why the patient was so negative toward him initially, his calm approach and professionalism won her over, enabling a successful transition to her home.

Variable-Term Opportunism

Individuals who exhibit variable opportunism have been compared to jazz musicians who improvise beautiful harmonies. On-the-fly situations present as opportunities to create solutions. There are two levels of this behavior, short-term and long-term. Short-term opportunism requires an individual to be prepared in order to capitalize on them as they happen. In the long-term, the tempered radical must be more purposeful and proactive (Meyerson, 2001).

Jana Preston is a 35-year-old case manager working at a busy rehabilitation hospital in coastal Virginia. She is very adept in using technology and is sometimes frustrated by the lack of support given to case management functions by the information services department. She is burdened by the oversized three-ring binder of reference materials she is required to carry around to the various units she covers. Because there is no plan to provide case management with laptops or tablets, she begins to scan and save all of her reference documents on a shared drive. The drive is accessible from every workstation in the facility and she will no longer have to carry everything from unit to unit. In addition, she realizes this will likely have a positive impact on infection transmission because of not carrying the binder from unit to unit, room to room. A few days later, Jana's colleagues notice she is not carrying her binder around. When her supervisor comments about it, Jana shares her new approach and the rationale for it. Immediately, she enlists Jana's support in organizing the shared drive resource. She had been challenged to come up with a way for all team members to access the same resources at the last manager's meeting. This perfect solution would not cost anything except a bit of Jana's time.

Within a month, none of the case managers is carrying a bulky binder and each enjoys access to the same resources and reference materials. Jana continues to add resources for her colleagues and keeps the shared drive updated and organized. Ultimately, when it is the case management department's turn to design and install a module in the electronic medical record, Jana is selected to assist in the development process.

Strategic Alliance Building

The individual who is motivated to enact change through tempered radicalism is clearly capable of making valuable contributions by working quietly and persistently. But why would a person who experiences success working alone bother work with others? For the same reasons that coalitions form—to garner more power and influence. Instead of contributing to an opposing camps mentality which makes finding compromise more difficult, tempered radicals look for commonalities of beliefs on which to build consensus and enact change (Meyerson, 2001).

Martina is a single mother of three, working as a case manager at a local health plan in eastern Pennsylvania for the past 10 years. Her children, ages 8, 9, and 11 years, are very active in afterschool programs. She relies on her sister for transportation and staying with the children until she is able to get home from work. This arrangement has worked well for the last year, but recent news of her brother-in-law's transfer to an office in California presents a major challenge. She tries to speak with her manager about job-sharing work-modified work hours but feels stonewalled because of a previous trial that ended badly. Rather than getting mad, Martina learns many other single parents are having similar difficulties. She investigates and finds out there are staff members in the provider support department who work-modified schedules, as well as member services staff who job-share.

On building a strong base of support and gaining a better understanding of the pros and cons associated with the various schedules, Martina and her coworkers develop a proposal allowing work schedule flexibility. They approach management and request a meeting to sit down and discuss it, inviting human resources to participate. When management learns of the scope of work–life balance issues facing the employees, the inconsistency of flexible work hours across various departments, and the possibility of losing high-performing staff because of the currently inflexible environment, a work group is formed to design and implement a uniform approach to nontraditional work hours. Within 6 months, the program is rolled out across the entire organization.

Although no single right way to initiate change applies in all circumstances, motivated individuals serve as quiet agents of change through their words and deeds. Case management needs more tempered radicals to set the example of professional practice and invoke evolutionary change even in environments that seem to be immovable bastions of bureaucracy. Adopting the COLLABORATE paradigm as one's professional framework sets the stage for growth and development. It also cuts a clear path onto which one's colleagues may follow.

SUMMARY

When appropriately considered and implemented, COLLABORATE provides a practice model to transcend the variety of professional disciplines engaged in case management practice across the health care continuum. Existing delivery models are frequently predicated on assumed business priorities and hiring convenience rather than for the purpose of leveraging practitioner competencies and educational backgrounds that are essential to effective and efficient practice, which lead to quality patient outcomes. As a result, the change process to the COLLABORATE paradigm requires careful preparation and planning prior to its implementation.

Although there is inherent value in the skills and knowledge brought to the care team by various professional disciplines, the advanced COLLABORATE model realigns disciplines behind a framework of unified, strengths-based professional case management identity. Suboptimal results come from forcing new competencies into an established practice model predicated by the long-standing divisions of professional discipline, work setting, credentials, and population served. Thoughtful preparation and planning in advance of undertaking this magnitude of change maximizes the potential impact of the model.

References

Hiatt, J. M. (2006). *ADKAR: A model for change in business, government, and out community*. Loveland, CO: Prosci.

Hiatt, J. M., & Creasey, T. J. (2012). *Change management: The people side of change* (2nd ed.). Loveland, CO: Prosci.

Kotter, J. P. (1995). Leading change: Why transformation efforts fail. *Harvard Management Review*, *73*(2), 59–67.

Meyerson, D. E. (2001). Radical change: The quiet way. *Harvard Business Review*, *79*(9), 92–100.

Sirkin, H. L., Keenan, P., & Jackson, A. (2005). The hard side of change management. *Harvard Business Review*, *83*(10), 108–118.

20 THE MANAGEMENT OF CHANGE

OBJECTIVES

After studying this chapter, you will be able to:

1. Identify Kotter's stages of change management.
2. Craft specific approaches aimed at the political, marketing, and military mind-sets within an organization in order to support a change project.
3. Recognize the importance of maintaining a sense of urgency to support case management model change.
4. Avoid the risk of losing project momentum by proactively addressing complacency risk.
5. Build coalition-like support for changing the case management model.

KEY TERMS

Coalition
Complacency
Culture
Kotter's eight-stage process
Marketing campaign
Military campaign
Political campaign
Short-term wins
Urgency

As recognized in chapter 19, the process of change is complex. However, when undertaken in an organized and methodical manner there presents an excellent opportunity for obstacles to be minimized, if not eliminated. Although leading up to change sometimes focuses too much on the negative aspects of why it is not worthwhile (e.g., cost, lost productivity, internal politics), failing to address issues that obstruct change will surely lead to the demise of any initiative.

The degree of support accorded to professional case management services is frequently associated with how case management is viewed by organizational leadership. In its purest form of practice, case management is a framework through which qualified, competent clinical professionals address the access, quality, and cost associated with health care through partnerships with individuals facing complex illnesses and injuries and members of their health care team. Case management is accomplished using a series of assessments and interventions, which leverage the practitioner's clinical and business knowledge. Case managers build on an individual's strengths while concurrently educating and fostering the development of new skills aimed in order to improve her or his self-management capabilities. The desired outcomes of case management are to facilitate meeting health care needs during an individual's vulnerable periods of infirmity and to enable health care consumers to effectively manage health and wellness care.

From this launching point, the COLLABORATE model focuses on competency-based practice. Organizations that consider health care throughput as being similar to manufacturing widgets, will likely not find value in this approach to case management practice. However, those seeking to establish and maintain a culture of high-quality health care and informed consumerism must provide an environment, which attracts knowledgeable, competent, motivated, and outcomes-driven health care professionals to facilitate its mission, vision, and values. This chapter provides change management process considerations for organizations and case management professionals seeking to shift the paradigm of case management service delivery from that of grinder-like production to one of innovative, quality-driven care coordination excellence.

SUCCESSFULLY MANAGING CHANGE

When we were children, our parents may have paid us a sum of money on a weekly basis for being responsible and completing assigned tasks or chores. We referred to this as our allowance. With regard to project management, organizations must accord the individuals involved in change initiatives similar consideration. The effort associated with implementing change is substantial and frequently underestimated. When considering that project team staff are responsible for their usual workload in addition to the project deliverables, it is a miracle when these projects are fully completed (Appelbaum et al., 2012).

Research indicates that failure rates range from 33% to as high as 80% (Beer & Nohria, 2000; Higgs & Rowland, 2000; Hirschhorn, 2002; Knodel, 2004; Sirkin et al., 2005; Kotter, 2008). The reality is that the reasons some projects fail is frequently due to project team fatigue. Team members carry project-related work in addition to their regular work. For a project to be successful, project team members must be paid an allowance of a reduced workload. This permits each person the time necessary to appropriately attend to project-related work.

A METHODICAL APPROACH FOR CHANGE

An organized methodology must be applied to optimize change initiatives: this text follows **Kotter's eight-stage process**. This eight-stage change process is leveraged in order to provide a framework for case management delivery model change. In light of today's evidence-based practice mind-set, one could be persuaded to not use an approach that had not been scientifically proven. Kotter's change management model appears to derive its popularity more from its direct and usable format rather than from any scientific consensus on the results. However, following an extensive review of literature no evidence was found against Kotter's change management model; it remains a recommendable reference (Appelbaum et al., 2012).

Although change management is a process unto itself, there are interlocking practices that when used successfully, facilitate the forward movement and completion of any change project. For example, chapter 19 discussed ADKAR and DICE as practices useful in preparing for change. As part of active change management, Hirschhorn (2002) describes campaigns that overlay and interconnect throughout the project's life cycle. These campaigns highlight political, marketing, and military mind-sets. In a larger organization, the case management department is often understood differently depending on whether the definer has more of a business or clinical perspective. Understanding these "campaigns" is key to gaining and maintaining the support of senior business leaders and management colleagues. Each adds value to and facilitates the case management model change process within the business environment of an organization.

Political Campaign

Successful project managers understand how to mount and conduct the **political campaign** in support of their project. These managers recognize the candidate with the most votes gets into office and so they forge coalitions to lead and sustain change initiatives just as winning politicians leverage coalitions supporting their candidacy or issue positions. Coalitions serve to broaden the base of support, increase credibility of the project leader, and deliver more resources to ensure reaching project objectives (Hirschhorn, 2002). A broad-based, yet flexible, approach to building support for change is important. Simply announcing that a change is going to happen will inevitably result in the formation of tribal communities. At either end of the spectrum, one will be totally resistant to change, whereas another will jump on the bandwagon in full support of it. This polarizing mentality makes the adoption of change highly unlikely.

In government, coalitions serve as powerful forces that support passage or defeat of legislative initiatives. Although not everyone in a coalition agrees on every single issue, consensus is reached in order to build support of the larger issues. Within organizations, leaders conduct political campaigns through the formation of management and worker coalitions, which lead to win-win situations. Astute project leaders acquire and maintain the broad-based support to ensure projects succeed.

Just as there are champions willing to fall on the sword of change, there will be opponents seeking to sink the ship. A perceptive project leader understands this range of support and utilizes her or his communication and consensus-building skills to bolster agreement on the necessity of change. It is essential to understand the senior leadership perception of case management. Who sees it as a professional practice? Who supports continuing professional education and development? Who considers case management as simply a position focused on cost control? The answers to these and other questions help form the strategic approach to changing the hearts and minds of those who just do not see the tremendous value of truly professional practice. Aligning with sympathetic leaders is important, but understanding the perspective of those who do not see the value-add of case management is even more critical as these people are more likely to undermine change efforts through active opposition or passive disregard.

Marketing Campaign

The **marketing campaign** is about influencing the opinions of others through promotion of an agenda, service, or product. Images, words, and actions spotlighting the fabulousness of a product or service are the implements of marketing. Real change agents are skilled in using these tools to reinforce their promotional messaging. Although seemingly disconnected, the chatter of ground-level employees contains important details from which spring key messages and symbols of influence which are weaved into project collateral in the form of posters, rallies, intradepartmental contests, and trinkets distributed across an organization (Hirschhorn, 2002).

For example, when a national health-related product and service provider underwent rebranding, project champions wanted all employees to get on the same page and commit to implementing the new way of conducting business. During a company-wide meeting, the image of the yellow school bus was repeatedly displayed in conjunction with the talking points about working together for customer satisfaction. The significance was a symbol of a "get-on-the-bus" mentality. On returning to their respective business offices, employees found little yellow school buses made of soft squeezable foam all over their departments. The trinket was a marketing tool with the purpose of reinforcing the "working in the same direction" messaging so that employees felt they were part of a solution.

Military Campaign

Change will not endure without an intentional effort to overcome pockets of resistance. Negative forces make logical arguments against change, which usurps the impact of the change itself. When in a battle to enact a new approach, leaders must tackle resistance with the precision of a carefully choreographed **military campaign**. Successful project leaders understand that employee time is scarce and that change initiatives often fail due to a lack of attention. Rather than begin an entirely new project, examine existing initiatives to determine if adding on to its scope can accomplish the same objectives.

For example, the Case Management Department of Good Health Accountable Care Health System is next in line for implementation of a module in the electronic medical record (EMR) system. As each of the preceding departments has done, a review and update of all workflow processes is underway. In order to incorporate the COLLABORATE model, the director decided to piggyback the process redesign on to the EMR project. As a result, the new documentation, workflow, and performance processes will be COLLABORATE-centric. The manager and staff assigned to the EMR project work concurrently with the director in order to incorporate the new practice paradigm into the computer system's design motif.

Management of the three campaigns is a simultaneous effort, although there will be times in which one becomes an overriding concern. However, a project leader would be naïve if she or he allowed each to become an island unto itself. Constant monitoring of each campaign identifies obstacles on which one must focus a bit more attention. Successful campaigns build winning coalitions, tap into people's thoughts and feelings, and deploy the right amount of resources at the right time. When one element lacks enthusiastic dedication, the overall initiative is very likely going to fail (Hirschhorn, 2002).

THE EIGHT STAGES OF CREATING CHANGE

Anyone who has worked in health care for more than 5 minutes has likely to have gone through at least one process change. It is as much a basic concept as that of taking someone's vital signs at a provider office visit. However, simply because someone has been a party to change, it should not be assumed that the process itself was well conducted or ultimately successful. People who have suffered through a poorly organized or introduced change carry with them very real memories, which continue to color their opinions and reactions of subsequent projects. The list of emotions likely to be stirred up with announcing a change includes worry, anger, confusion, pessimism, suspicion, mistrust, and resentment. For these reasons, change initiatives must be clearly associated with positive outcomes and conducted with an organized and methodical implementation plan. The process of change continues to be complex and challenging for organizations.

Organizations distinguish themselves as unique environments. From a 10,000-foot perspective, the mechanics of care delivery are largely similar. Arguably, it is the people who make an institution special. For the purpose of this book, Kotter's eight stages of change (shown in Figure 20-1) are discussed from a place of commonality. It is impossible to address every possible nuance relating to all populations, settings of care, or other polarizing factors.

Stage 1: Establish a Sense of Urgency

Establishing a sense of **urgency** as the impetus for change is critical to gaining the needed cooperation at all levels of an organization (Kotter, 2012). Without a sense of urgency, it is near impossible to garner sufficient influence and support for making changes. This commitment does not rest on the shoulders of a single person. Even when only a small group believes there is a need for change, this is where ideas as to the capacity, direction, and resources required start to well up.

Perhaps the biggest challenge to establishing a sense of urgency is overcoming organizational complacency. **Complacency** can be described in various ways, such as the belief that nothing can be done to effect change, change is too hard, change would be totally overwhelming in light of the current overworked environment, or even that an organization does not need to change because it is fine and dandy as it currently exists. At its foundation, complacency is a change killer.

In case management, complacency arises from a variety of sources (see in Figure 20-2). One should never underestimate the forces that reinforce complacency in order to maintain the status quo (Kotter, 2012). These forces may be so firmly entrenched that removing them become projects unto themselves. If possible, it is helpful to utilize the poor circumstances to create a sense of urgency around change. Sometimes, it may be necessary to create a crisis in order to highlight areas of risk if business continues as usual. Table 20-1 includes scenarios created to illustrate a need for urgent change.

Virtually every organization has champions of excellence. Begin a dialogue with these leaders; ask for help to confront the source of the problem. If senior leaders are unrealistically optimistic, focus honest conversations on the reality of your

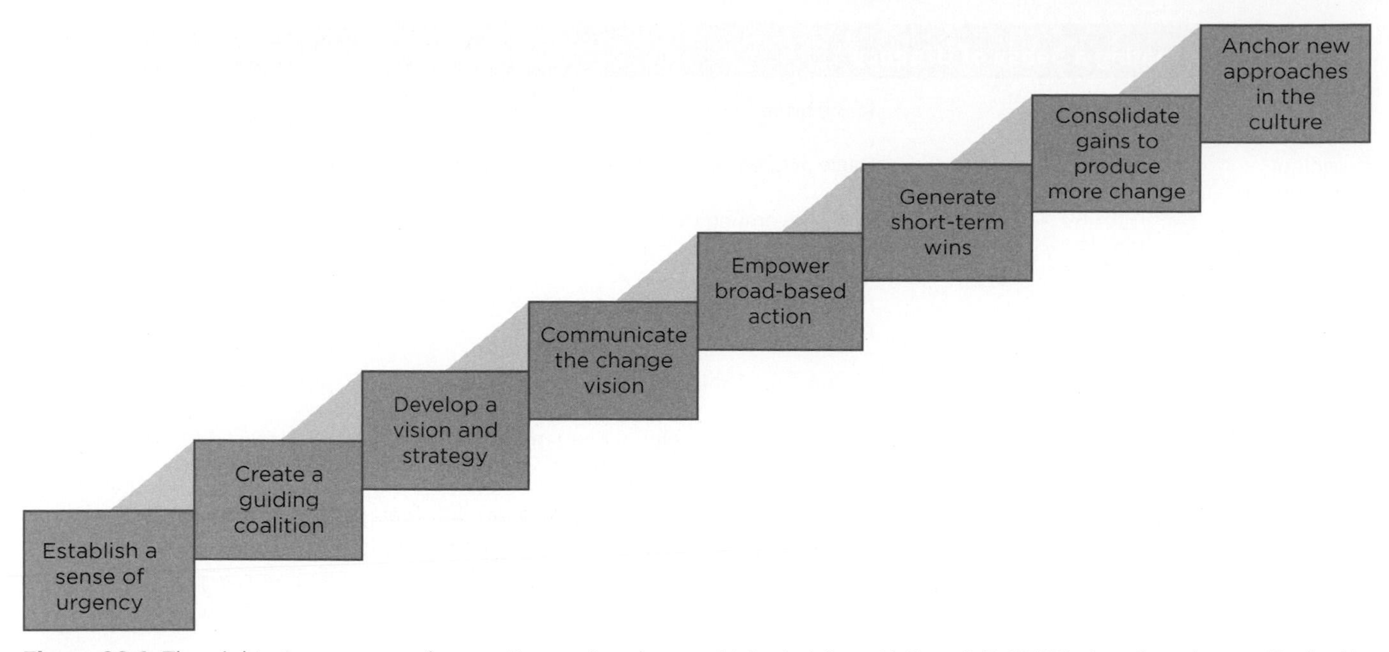

Figure 20-1. The eight-stage process for creating major change. (Adapted from Kotter, J. P. (2012). *Leading change* (2nd ed.). Boston, MA: Harvard Business Review Press.)

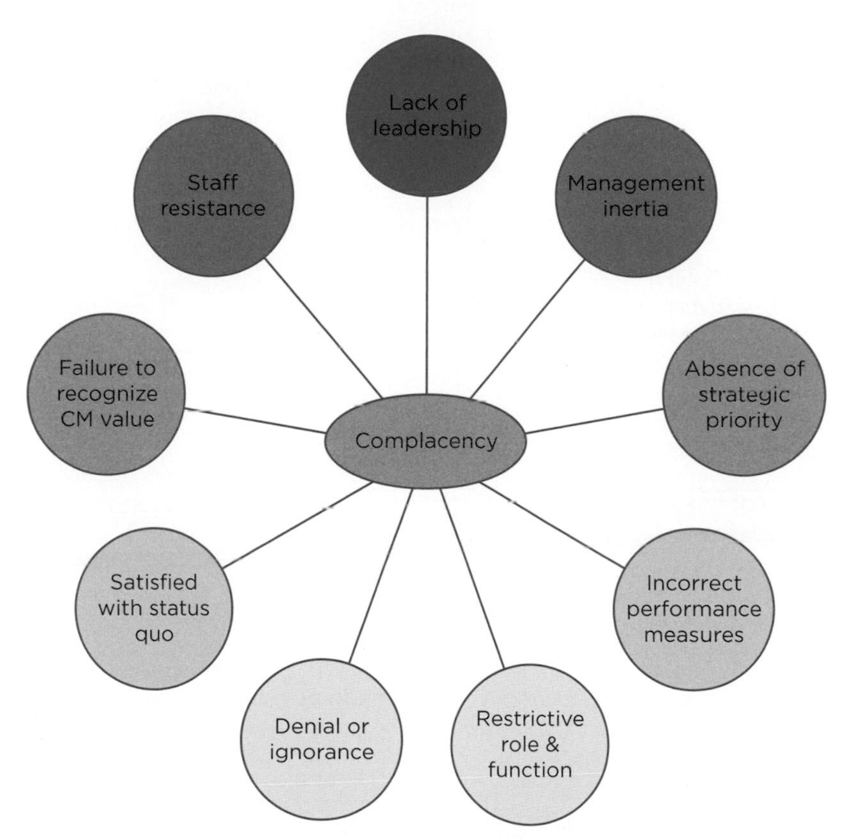

Figure 20-2. Sources of complacency in case management.

work situation and insist on stopping the baseless happy talk (Kotter, 2012).

Stage 2: Create a Guiding Coalition

A single individual is not often able to accomplish change, but a strong **coalition** can guide a change project from start to finish. Referred to as the Lead Team or Project Champions in some organizations, it may simply be the Implementation Team in others. Whatever title applies, this team must be comprised of the right mix of individuals who commit to a shared vision, agree on the project's ultimate outcome, and work together toward a successful execution. Project team members must have a decision-making authority as to the

TABLE 20-1 Creating a Sense of Urgency

Example	Situation	Response
Lack of leadership Management inertia Satisfied with status quo	Senior leader within 1 year of retirement refusing to initiate new long-term projects	Raise awareness of case management professionalism Circulate among colleagues or post articles from professional journals in common areas Request in-house continuing education programs focusing on professional practice Request medical staff to incorporate grand rounds on complex clients Seek ally within quality management department and address accreditation and credentialing requirements for staff and workflows Approach human resources with case management proposal closer to retirement date Request involvement in hiring replacement for retiring leader
Absence of strategic priority	Leaders are overly focused on network expansion to the exclusion of maintaining current business relationships	Research competitor initiatives Share journal articles pertaining to case management outcomes within similar organizations Identify and address credentialing and accreditation requirements and shortcomings pertaining to case management
Incorrect performance measures	Productivity as the sole driver of performance evaluation	Research competitor metrics Share journal articles pertaining to measuring case management-specific performance
Restrictive role and function Failure to recognize CM value Denial or ignorance	Belief system that case management is solely a cost-control tool Lack of understanding as to professional case management practice Continual job title changes blurring the lines of job distinction to the point that all positions substantially perform the same functions and tasks	Research competitor job descriptions Share journal articles pertaining to case management roles and functions Share pertinent case management practice standards Post success stories and client praise letters (redacted) in common areas Nominate high-performing case managers for company-wide recognition awards Share news of passing certification examination and use credentials in correspondence Encourage membership in pertinent professional organization
Staff resistance	Staff actively obstruct a manager's attempt to introduce process improvements, circumvent the manager, and complain about the changes to the department director and human resources.	Research competitor job descriptions Share journal articles pertaining to case management roles and functions Share pertinent case management practice standards Encourage membership in pertinent professional organization Work with human resources on performance management plans and updates to job descriptions Do not hesitate to use performance improvement plans when appropriate

project's activities and implementation. If not authorized to make decisions or commit time or resources, the project development and execution process bog down unnecessarily.

There are four characteristics essential to assembling a guiding coalition, which are position power, expertise, credibility, and leadership (Kotter, 2012). See Table 20-2 for definition of each characteristic. To enable case management change, project team members should be selected in order to represent from the perspectives of professional case management process and value, human resources, communication skill, member relations, provider relations, and contractual business agreements. The mix of leaders and managers present is also important. When there is a lack of leadership, the project team lacks the vision of potential impact and will not be able to adequately communicate the need for and direction of change. The result will be a plan to control rather than to empower people ultimately responsible for implementation. In order to ensure appropriate team leadership, an organization may opt to bring in someone from outside, promote an individual from within, or encourage someone from within to accept the challenge (Kotter, 2012).

There is also the question as to the number of members on a project team. The team should be comprised of individuals who are knowledgeable, respected, and are supported by senior leaders to make project decisions that affect various areas of the business. The size of a project team should reflect the size of the business affected by the scope of the project. However, teams of excessive size risk the potential for success because they become difficult to keep on track. It is difficult to recommend a specific number of team members, but it is advisable to examine past projects to determine if the number of team members influenced the initiatives' success or failure. If large project teams fail more often than small ones, consider limiting the size of the project team accordingly. It may also be helpful to use a secondary team approach in situations where highly specialized tasks are required. Secondary teams report to a designated primary team member serving as a mini-project manager with a clearly defined scope.

Kotter recommends avoiding the inclusion of certain types of people. The first type is the individual with an oversized ego, the second is the passive-aggressive "snakes," and the third is the underenthused participant. Oversized egos and snakes kill, whereas reluctance results in slow suffocation. Someone with a big ego does not recognize his or her own weaknesses or the strengths of other team members. The "snake" creates mistrust across the project team through her or his quiet commentaries regarding other team members. A reluctant individual can slow project implementation with indecision. These personality types create team tension ultimately leading to failure.

TABLE 20-2 Guiding Coalition Characteristics

Characteristic	Description
Position power	Support change to overcome dissenters
Expertise	Represent points of view to enable informed decisions
Credibility	Add gravitas to be taken seriously
Leadership	Proven capable of driving change

Adapted from Kotter, J. P. (2012). Leading change (2nd ed.). Boston, MA: Harvard Business Review Press.

The mixture of trust and sharing a common goal in combination with the right people has the potential for being a powerful team. The resulting sum of coalition power and influence has the capacity to make needed change happen despite the forces of inertia within an organization (Kotter, 2012). The axiom of the whole being greater than the sum of its parts applies in that the right combination of individuals working as a team has a greater potential to empower change.

Stage 3: Develop a Vision and Strategy

Transformation requires transparency and trust. For change initiatives to succeed, they must be grounded in vision, which clarifies the direction of change, motivates people to take action in that direction, and coordinates the people's actions.

In change situations, employees tend to become confused in the absence of the rationales for change. Explaining the current environment and connecting compelling reasons for change provides employees with motivations to change. The manner in which change is defined and implemented provides an organized framework for employees to undertake the required modifications (Kotter, 2012). For successful change to occur, time-consuming organizational noise is quieted through the development of an effective vision and implementation strategy. In order for a vision to be effective, it must be something that people can imagine as being possible, desirable, feasible, focused, flexible, and communicable (Kotter, 2012). Figure 20-3 expands each of these characteristics.

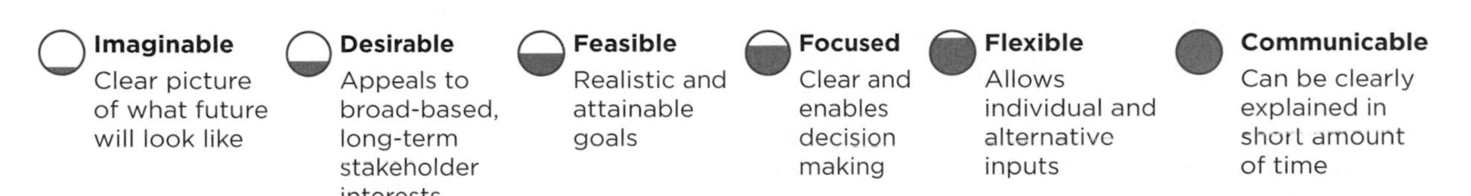

Figure 20-3. Characteristics of effective vision. (Adapted from Kotter, J. P. (2012). *Leading change* (2nd ed.). Boston, MA: Harvard Business Review Press).

When a case management department sets out to completely change its approach to service delivery, there is bound to be pockets of dissenters focused on keeping things the way they have always been for fear of the change itself, having to exert more effort into their work, or for other reason(s) specific to the person or team. It could be that past changes were not well developed when the project was undertaken, which resulted in many changes and confusion during the subsequent roll out. Always keep in mind that new is not always perceived as better. A well-conceived and clearly articulated rationale for change that is based in evidence, competitive market change, and other concrete motivator will speak volumes louder than a vague "feel-good-about-what-you-do" theory or worse yet, change based on no good reason.

Stage 4: Communicate the Change Vision

The manner in which the vision and strategy are communicated is as important as the actual development process. When changes are undercommunicated or inconsistent messaging takes place, transformation stalls (Kotter, 2012). Widespread acceptance of a conceptual vision of the future is rather difficult for some people, often generating more questions as a result of the information shared. This challenges the guiding coalition because not every question will have a firm answer at that point. Many questions arise out of a more emotional response to the announcement of impending change. One of the worst ways of responding to questions is that of becoming defensive and coming across in a condescending manner. The absence of leader comfort with communicating change contributes to the problem of undercommunication. To counter this potential, there are characteristics of effective communication (shown in Table 20-3), which should be attended to in the preparation of both the message and the messenger.

Chapter 11 touched on the accountable communication concept as it applied to leadership. This same approach provides a model applicable to process change situations. By consistently using an accountable communication style model, the project team maximizes accurate, timely, and complete information transfer. Rather than making one-way announcements regarding project status, the project manager and team members craft communications that are more handover in nature. In this situation, the sender (project team) verifies that the receiver (employees) not only gets the messages but also ensures an understanding of the message content. When questioning the degree of understanding, the project team asks questions to gauge the level of understanding. Address and broadcast incoming questions as quickly and frequently as possible to ensure maximum retention.

Stage 5: Empower Broad-Based Action

Arguably, the word *empowerment* has been beaten into the dirt with a rather large bat. However, the concept it conveys is still an important one, perhaps even more so in light of the relentless changes within the health care sector. Both clinical and business professionals working in health care are acutely aware of the shifting dynamics involving quality metrics, slipping reimbursement, clinical research, evidence-based care developments, therapeutic and pharmaceutical advancements, and business models applied to delivering and financing care.

TABLE 20-3 Characteristics of Effective Communication

Element	Intent	Example
Simplicity	Avoid jargon and techno-speak	Instead of saying "Using remote placement to optimize practice integration," simply say "We are placing case managers within medical practices."
Use of imagery and example	Create relatable images	In addition to writing a detailed description of an optimal communication process, create a graphic or flow chart illustration enhanced with arrows, colors, and brief labels.
Use multiple forums	Use a variety of mediums	Instead of a constant stream of email communiques, present at department meetings, go to the lunch room to meet with staff informally, and/or place a story in the organization's newsletter.
Be repetitive	Messages sent repeatedly	Enhance the potential for information to sink in by sending the same message multiple times.
Lead by example	Behave in a way consistent with the desired change.	Be the change you wish to see in others.
Address inconsistencies	Unless clarified, inconsistency will undermine credibility	When asked questions regarding previously shared information, construct a consistent manner of addressing them and widely broadcast the clarification.
Give-and-take	Two-way communication	Don't just send out announcements, but be sure to provide a means for questions to be asked. Have conversations, not just presentations.

Adapted from Kotter, J. P. (2012). Leading change (2nd ed.). Boston, MA: Harvard Business Review Press.

Unfortunately, qualified case managers are devalued by the practice of chipping away integral functions, which are then reassigned to less-qualified technicians or administrative staff. These individuals have neither the clinical education nor experience to appreciate the implications of their actions on client health and well-being. A common reason for this practice is that of reducing the expense of conducting business. All case management stakeholders should be asking whether this reduction in cost is worth the risk of diminishing the quality of care. Continuing to allow erosion at case management's practice foundation will ultimately translate to its demise.

Addressing incremental devaluation requires insistence on continuous educational achievement and improvement in knowledge, skills, and overall practice quality. By uniting behind the ideals of professional practice, case managers lessen the potential of being usurped by nonclinical technicians and administrative staff. Initially, veteran case managers may balk at the idea that their longstanding work habits are not good enough.

It is also important to evaluate barriers to empowerment, such as the following:

- A supervisor who discourages continuing education efforts because clinical experience requires time off from work
- Lack of expertise with computer technology which contributes to a lack of confidence in conducting searches for evidence-based practices
- Organizational restrictions on Internet access and other sources of clinical and quality information

Appealing to a sense of professionalism may not work in situations where individuals do not consider themselves as more than an employee. However, taking a progressive approach to developing a renewed sense of pride in one's work helps move these individuals toward adoption of a practice approach that undereducated, unqualified staff cannot replicate.

Another tool of empowering action is to embed the needed change into performance management strategy. When change is in the best interest of an individual, motivation to make that change is swayed. A review of the existing performance management program may reveal gaps in planning, monitoring, evaluation, promotion, and compensation incentives. In addition, the approach to recruitment, hiring, and job classification processes comes into question when a significant number of case management staff are highly resistant to practice improvement. Could it be that individuals working under the title of case manager are unqualified to do so? Yes, it could be. In fact, it is highly likely to be the case. This presents the perfect opportunity to evaluate job titles, descriptions, and qualifications to ensure the right people are in the right positions to serve the organization's best interest.

Empowering people to make needed change requires providing a supportive and engaging environment. Additional ways in which to empower case management staff are discussed in Figure 20-4.

Stage 6: Generate Short-Term Wins

Being part of positive change can be exhilarating. This is especially true when change comes to an organization in which employees withered under a morass of cumbersome workflows, requiring unnecessary effort for little to no satisfaction. Sometimes, the parties to change get lost in the spirit of a newly energized environment and forget the importance of showing measurable results. This is the point of stage 6. It is essential that specific **short-term wins** are identified and realized in order to justify ongoing support for change. If there are no proofs demonstrating that changes have reaped tangible benefits, cracks begin to erode the initial base of support. Eventually, support crumbles like termite-ridden wood.

Major change efforts require time ... sometimes lots of it. As has been discussed, there will be varying levels of support in any given change initiative. A passionate believer in the change will stay the course regardless of any bumps in the road. Those whose support is tempered by pragmatism

Communicate vision that makes sense

- Sharing a common and relatable vision of the future makes it easier to initiate change.
- Leverage practice standards and credentials in support of professionalism.

Structure an organization that is compatible with the vision

- If not supportive of change, organizational structure will obstruct it.
- Evaluate job titles and descriptions; institute changes which distinguish case management positions.

Provide education and training necessary to change

- In the absence of knowledge and skill necessary for new process, individuals will struggle and feel inadequate.
- Support in-house educational sessions providing continuing education credit toward licensure and certification.

Align information systems with vision

- A system which slows progress will obstruct change.
- Upgrade computer programs to facilitate the case management process and evidence-based decision making.

Confront individuals that undermine effort

- A bad boss disempowers people to change.
- Incorporate empowerment goals into individual performance plans.

Figure 20-4. Empowering case managers toward change. (Adapted from Kotter, J. P. (2012). *Leading change* (2nd ed.). Boston, MA: Harvard Business Review Press.)

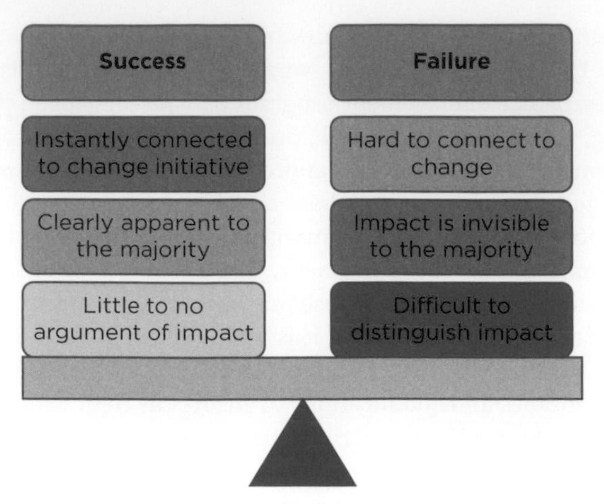

Figure 20-5. The success-versus-failure scale. (Adapted from Kotter, J. P. (2012). *Leading change* (2nd ed.). Boston, MA: Harvard Business Review Press.)

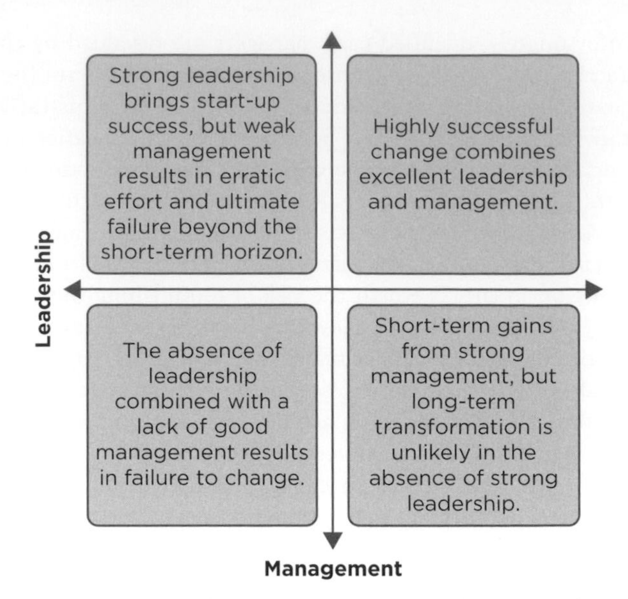

Figure 20-6. The relationship between leadership and management in transformations. (Adapted from Kotter, J. P. (2012). *Leading change* (2nd ed.). Boston, MA: Harvard Business Review Press.)

or who are not fervent followers require a higher standard of proof to sustain their enthusiasm. This is neither the time for subtlety nor minimally impactful results. Proof must be delivered in the form of clear and objective data proving that the changes are having their intended effect (Kotter, 2012). Because of this hazard, project team members must include incremental milestones and metrics in order to demonstrate improvement. Figure 20-5 highlights the balance between successfully demonstrating short-term wins on continued project support. Clearly, the support scale can tip either way.

The importance of short-term wins on a change project is many, but how wins are demonstrated needs to be unequivocal to a vast majority of stakeholders. The measures and milestones used must be of sufficient weight to make up for the interval sacrifices (e.g., number of newly opened cases, number of support service referrals). The project team can leverage information gained as a result of change can even be used to tweak process improvements. Success quiets the resistance, making it harder to continue arguing against change. It also adds to the momentum behind initiatives, converting centrists into proponents. In any event, the pressure to demonstrate change-driven success provides incentive for continuing the level of project urgency.

Although leadership has been the topic in previous chapters, the function of management of project oversight cannot be understated. Managers are essential to maintaining focus on project objectives, budget constraints, organization, and controlling in order to keep the plan on track. Although leadership is important, solid management is also essential (Kotter, 2012). Both functions and their interrelationship are at the crux of the make-or-break point for many transformative initiatives (see Figure 20-6).

Stage 7: Consolidate Gains and Produce More Change

There is a danger that comes with success and it can return an organization all the way back to stage 1. The danger is that of complacency with the progress already achieved. In realizing short-term wins, the spectra of satisfaction looms over what remains of the project's scope. Failing to anticipate and avoid this self-congratulatory smorgasbord contributes to the loss of momentum to finish the job.

Major change takes a long time, especially in large organizations. There are a multitude of forces with the capability of stalling forward progress well short of a project's finish line. Even as short-term wins add buoyancy, the associated gains can turn into ship-sinking torpedoes if the sense of urgency is overtaken by contentment (Kotter, 2012).

There are managers and leaders alike who support change efforts for a time. However, their taste for it dries up because of the stress that said change places on an organization. This is because organizations are deeply interrelated. Changes in one department have impact in others. It is virtually impossible to keep change limited to a distinct team or department. Consider the organization where case management resides within the medical management department. Changes within case management will certainly affect not only adjacent teams but will also bleed beyond the borders of that department. For instance, changes in how case managers relate to clients result in calls to member service agents. These comments may not all be complimentary. When call volume and dissatisfaction increases, the member services manager may very well demand that further changes be placed on hold while member service representatives attempt to repair client relationships. In the absence of gaining momentum and additional wins, those who were initially supportive can bring change projects to a grinding halt.

It is the nature of interdependency within large organizations that is often overlooked by the project team. Within

More Support for Change	More Hiring	Less Interdependence
• Short-term win: Improvement in rate of client goal achievement • Leveraged to raise level of staff support for further process improvement	• Short-term win: Improvement in service referral engagement rate • Leveraged to hire additional support staff needed to speed up referral completion	• Member service managers target processes originally enacted to address client complaints regarding case management • Representatives leverage gained time to undertake further process improvement review

Figure 20-7. Successes in case management change. (Adapted from Kotter, J. P. (2012). *Leading change* (2nd ed.). Boston, MA: Harvard Business Review Press.)

prior experience, the reality is that in highly interrelated organizations, almost every has to change (Kotter, 2012). The stress resulting from change must be counterbalanced by the sense of urgency that the change is absolutely necessary. The fact is progress may need to be slowed in order to address and manage the stressors brought on by change. Project scope may expand, or other projects identified. The net effect is that there will be more change than imaginable (Kotter, 2012). Figure 20-7 identifies successes associated with stage 7.

Stage 8: Anchor New Approaches in the Culture

The months, perhaps years, of work that goes into substantially changing an organization are hardly a linear progression. Change comes through surviving the cycles of highs and lows, with the knowledge that not every intervention is going to produce the desired result. However, when lessons are learned, each incremental step of the journey should be considered a great victory over passive acceptance of the status quo and a gain on behalf of truly client-centered health care.

Kotter (2012) defines **culture** as the normative behaviors and shared values across a group of people, and normative behavior as the accepted mannerisms and ways of acting within a group of people. Organizational culture is an extremely potent influencer of intraemployee behavior and client relationships. When organizational culture does not support employees to work at optimal levels of quality and customer service, even the best employee is at risk of disempowering coworkers and clients because of the manner in which she or he behaves. If one believes that it is the intent of the health care industry to provide evidence-based interventions in order to increase patient empowerment toward achieving improved levels of health and wellness, how will that be possible if organizations do not provide employees an environment that supports professional care coordination and case management? The bottom line is, on balance it will not.

Organizations must solidify the COLLABORATE model within an authentic culture that supports the professional practice of case management. An organization's culture is powerful for three reasons (Kotter, 2012):

- Employees are well-selected and indoctrinated.
- The environment exerts itself through the actions of hundreds, if not thousands, of employees.
- The effort associated with demonstrating behaviors and embodying values does not require much conscious effort.

These expectations must be formally and thoroughly embedded in every aspect of employee recruitment, onboarding, training, performance management, and support. If the model is laid over an existing culture that is not supportive of case management professionalism, there is a good chance that the entire project will have been an exercise in futility. Anchoring a new set of practices into organizational culture is difficult enough when consistent with the core of the culture. When they aren't, the challenge is much greater (Kotter, 2012). When installing the culture change, managers should:

- Talk frequently about the evidence supporting practice change,
- Link performance management new practice,
- Avoid talking-down the previous culture. Recognize that culture had value to the organization for the period it was the norm and highlight the reasons why it was no longer helpful or applicable,
- Work with human resources to identify and offer early retirement to appropriate individuals not accepting of the new model,
- Put in additional effort to retain employees who embrace the change,
- Ensure new hires are being thoroughly indoctrinated using new screening and interviewing, and on-boarding techniques focusing solely on the new model, and
- Avoid promoting employees into management positions who did not embody the new practices.

(Kotter, 2012)

It is essential to recognize that culture change is difficult to change. It happens only after people successfully embrace the new expectations. Figure 20-8 provides a few ways to anchor change into company culture.

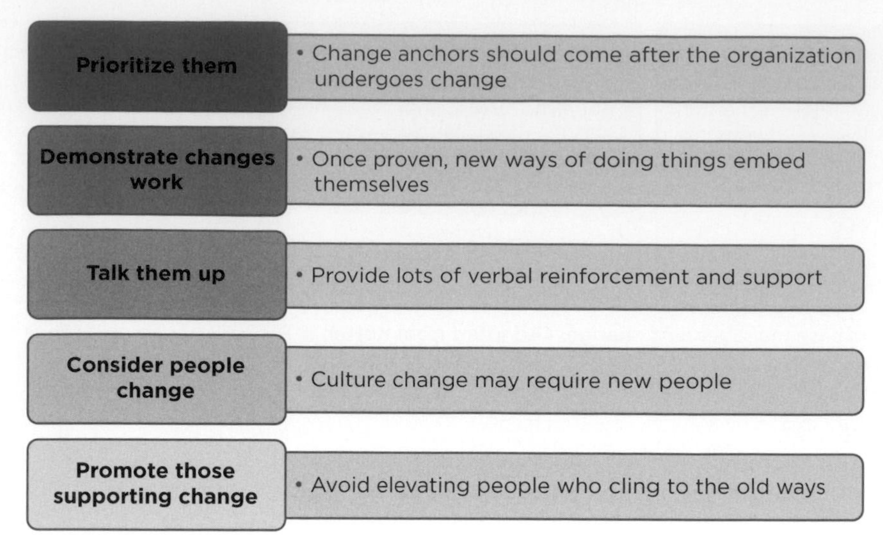

Figure 20-8. Anchoring culture change. (Adapted from Kotter, J. P. (2012). *Leading change* (2nd ed.). Boston, MA: Harvard Business Review Press.)

SUMMARY

There is no reason to think that health care change is going to slow down in an appreciative way any time soon. However, a change in the balance of political power may alter or even cancel initiatives scheduled to roll out. Regardless of the politics which influence public policy, people deserve high-quality health care and professional care coordination delivered by professional case managers. COLLABORATE provides a competency-based framework for client-centered case management.

References

Appelbaum, S. H., Habashy, S., Malo, J-L., & Shafiq, H. (2012). Back to the future: Revisiting Kotter's 1996 change model. *Journal of Management Development*, *31*(8), 764–782. doi 10.1108/02621711211253231

Beer, M., & Nohria, N. (2000). *Breaking the code of change.* Boston, MA: Harvard Business School Press.

Higgs, M., & Rowland, D. (2000). Building change leadership capability: The quest for change competence. *Journal of Change Management*, *1*(2), 116–130.

Hirschhorn, L. (2002). Campaigning for change. *Harvard Business Review*, *80*(7), 98–104.

Knodel, T. (2004). Preparing the organizational 'soil' for measurable and sustainable change: Business value management and project governance. *Journal of Change Management*, *4*(1), 45–62.

Kotter, J. P. (2008). *A sense of urgency*. Boston, MA: Harvard Business Review Press.

Kotter, J. P. (2012). *Leading change* (2nd ed.). Boston, MA: Harvard Business Review Press.

Sirkin, H. L., Keenan, P., & Jackson, A. (2005). The hard side of change management. *Harvard Business Review*, *83*(10), 108–118.

21 CREATING MEANINGFUL CASE MANAGEMENT PERFORMANCE

OBJECTIVES

After studying this chapter, you will be able to:

1. Define terms relevant to performance management.
2. Understand the elements of a job description.
3. Apply the systematic approach to performance management.
4. Detail the prerequisites to strategic performance management planning.
5. Identify the steps of performance management.
6. Identify the importance of career ladders to case management.
7. Connect COLLABORATE to performance management.

KEY TERMS

Appraisal
Best practice
Career ladder
Competency modeling (CM)
Core competencies
Goals
Great Eight competencies
Job-focused
Maximum performance
Mission
Objectives
Performance
Performance management (PM)
Performance management system
Performance measurement
Person-focused
Role-focused
Strategic planning
Traditional job analysis
Vision

Within the COLLABORATE paradigm, meaningful performance requires successful implementation of competency-based performance management (PM). This requires all involved parties to have a solid comprehension of the distinct moving parts that comprise the complex and often misunderstood concept of PM, as it aligns with the employee evaluation process.

Business organizations are demanding new and agile PM systems to replace traditionally passive employee evaluation approaches. A satisfaction survey of existing PM systems demonstrates a less than enthusiastic endorsement, with 58% of respondents giving their own organization's systems a grade of "C" or below (Vorhauser-Smith, 2012). Devising effective ways of managing and boosting employee performance is a cornerstone of organizational development, especially in the past decade (Cheng & Dainty, 2005). In fact, PM is considered a strategic human resource management activity, one to which competence and competency frameworks can be applied (Cheng & Dainty, 2005).

The factors that cross social and cultural contexts to influence PM make a strong case for the implementation of COLLABORATE, independent of practice setting, discipline, role, level, and classification of the position (e.g., full-time, part-time, per diem) (Cheng & Dainty, 2005). Add the diverse benchmarks by which a case manager's performance can be measured, and the benefits of a formal competency-based PM product for the workforce become more evident.

This chapter provides guidance for building a framework for competency-based PM, which ties the COLLABORATE competencies to innovative PM theories, concepts, and strategies. Individuals who assume PM occurs only at the annual evaluation should pay close attention to learn how this relates to the lifelong learning competency. To professionals who understand that high-quality PM begins prior to hiring an individual, you are ahead of the curve but prepare to learn more and enhance your proactive PM approach.

DEFINITIONS

It is paramount for case managers and those responsible for managerial oversight to level-set regarding definitions pertaining to PM. This begins with the word **performance** itself. Performance refers to behavior or what employees do (Aguinis, 2013). It is also defined as something accomplished, such as a deed or a feat (*Merriam-Webster's Online Dictionary*, 2014), which is a way in which a case manager refers to the tasks for which he or she is responsible to complete within a work period.

Performance management is an approach to appraising an employee, process, equipment, or other element in order to gauge progress toward predetermined goals. It is known by the names of organizational development, performance appraisal, and application PM among other titles (BusinessDictionary.com, 2014a). Another term often associated with PM is performance **appraisal**. This refers to a systematic and periodic process that assesses an individual employee's job performance and productivity in relation to certain preestablished criteria and organizational objectives (Abu-Doleh & Weir, 2007).

Daniels and Bailey (2014) identify several reasons why PM is valuable to organizations:

- It is practical and works since it is a set of specific actions for increasing desired performance and decreasing undesired performance.
- It produces short-term as well as long-term results.
- It requires no formal psychological training as it is supported by thousands of experimental and applied research studies, especially across the health care industry.
- It is a system for maximizing all kinds of performance.
- It creates an enjoyable place in which to work. When employees do something that is enjoyed, they are more likely to perform better than if they dislike what they are doing.
- It can be used to enhance relationships at work, home, and in the community.
- It is an open system, as motivation for positive performance on the job comes from all aspects of work. Employees across the organization share the accountability for performance; managers influencing employee performance as readily as employees influence the performance of managers.

Goal is a term burdened by misunderstanding across the professional community. It is defined as an observable and measureable end result having one of more objectives to be achieved within a more or less fixed time frame (BusinessDictionary.com, 2014b). Goals are often long on direction, but short on the specific tactics. However, goals have the potential to serve as powerful impetus to change the mind-set and direction of the employee's focus. For example, a goal of PM is that it should bring out the best in people while generating the highest value for the organization (Daniels & Bailey, 2014). Consider how a goal of this type would impact your perspective of your current employer. Examples of specific case management goals include reducing the acute level of care avoidable days by 50%, or improving appropriate classification of observation status by 60%.

An **objective** refers to smaller concrete steps by which the goals are achieved. Objectives are specific and thus easier to measure than goals. Objectives may be thought of as the basic tools that underlie all planning and strategic activities for organizations (BusinessDictionary.com, 2014c). Examples of a managed care case manager's objectives associated with the previously noted goals are to attend treatment team rounds and to discuss member care with hospital case managers.

Organizations use the terms **maximum performance** and **best practice** when referring to an expected level of optimal performance. Amid the diversity of perspectives and the immense body of literature that exists, it is important to note two major points on which agreement exists.

First, an emerging term in PM circles is maximum performance. Amid the literature review undertaken for this topic, no universally consistent interpretation was found for what a maximum performance means across all organizations or what it takes to achieve it. Although an exhaustive number of businesses and coaching entities promote their ability to assure maximum performance of employees, consistent definitions prove to be evasive in spite of the vast resources of the World Wide Web. In the face of this disparity, each organization is left to define the term within its own four walls.

Second, best practice is overused and warrants critical evaluation in the context of each organization, particularly when used in a PM perspective. Best practice is formally defined as a method or technique that has consistently shown result superior to those achieved with other means, and that is used as a benchmark (BusinessDictionary.com, 2014d). What works for one entity does not work for all in the huge landscape of practice, especially when one is referring to case management. There is far too much disparity in terms of access to resources and technology. In addition, as has been discussed throughout this text, the evolution and advancement of the health care industry at its swift rate makes today's best practice good only for a fixed moment in time, as it is quickly replaced by yet another best practice appearing around the next corner.

PERFORMANCE MANAGEMENT AND THE COLLABORATE CONNECTION

Performance appraisal and management are considered to be essential to an organization achieving its mission, as well as to ensure staff competence and environmental safety. This belief extends to all organizations, and not only those in health care (Bensing, 2011). Another perspective is that of a staunch criticism of performance appraisals being a waste of time and having a destructive impact on the relationship between managers and subordinates (Lawler, 2012). It is important to note that some of these oppositional views spout from foci heavily on performance appraisals as the primary driver or focus of PM, instead of being a component of it.

Lawler (2012) suggests that rather than debating the merits of the appraisal system and whether to eliminate performance appraisals, effort should be undertaken to make them more effective. It has also been identified in the literature that one way to have more successful performance appraisals is to include them as part of a more complete PM process, if not system (Bensing, 2011; Lawler, 2012), as is posed in this chapter. Equally relevant is the role that competencies play in assuring more effective performance appraisals.

Chapter 5 presents how the competencies appear across accreditation, state boards, and regulatory entities as well as how these are being integrated into performance appraisals and job descriptions. The COLLABORATE paradigm, with its competencies and key elements, is directly applicable to job description elements and PM frameworks as well as to the individual seeking to improve her or his professional performance, whether within or outside of organizational PM conventions.

THE JOB DESCRIPTION

A job (or position) description is a general statement written from a rather broad perspective. It is intended to capture the essence of a job and should be, but is not always, based on the findings of a job analysis.

Job Description Elements

A job description usually starts with a header, which highlights the job's title, internal coding classification, pay grade or rate, organizational rank, salary range, and tax classification (e.g., exempt, nonexempt). The header may also include the job's department hierarchy and/or reporting relationships (e.g., supervisor, subordinate) and other key working relationships. Figure 21-1 displays usual job description header items.

The body of the job description follows the header section. This includes a purpose, objective or summary statement,

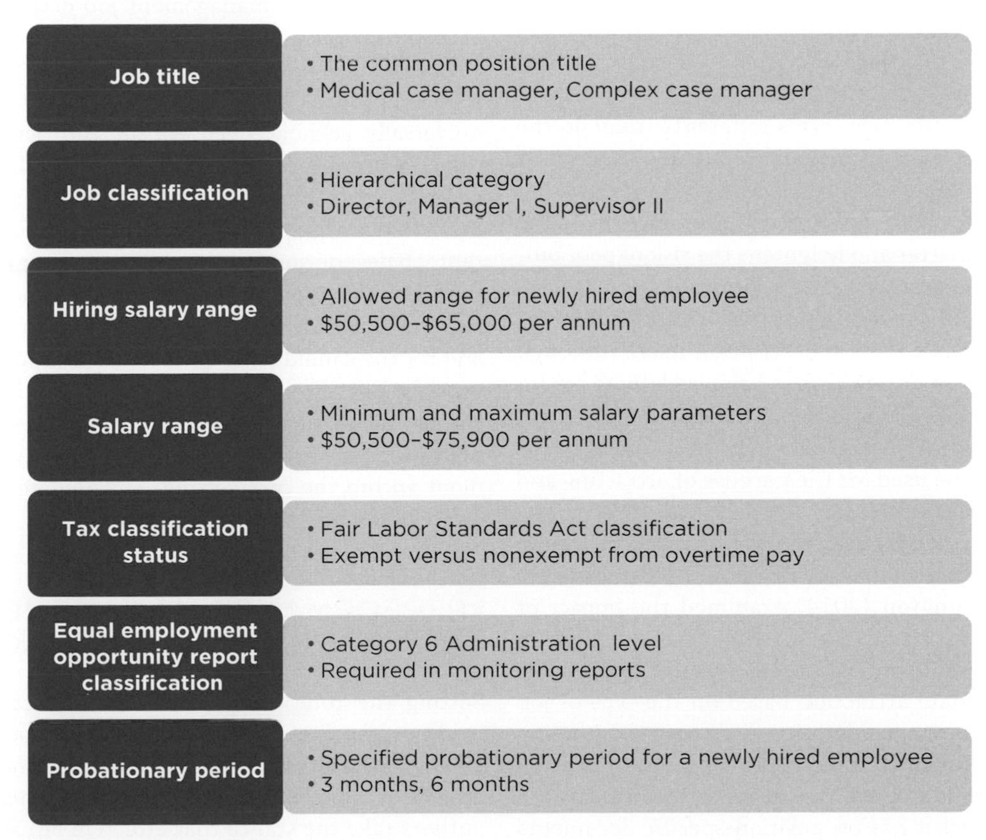

Figure 21-1. Job description header elements.

qualifications, preferred credentials, tasks, functions, activities, and working conditions. Other requirements of the position (e.g., physical capabilities, driver's license, reliable transportation) round out the document.

As straightforward as this may sound, an effective case management job description may be harder to come by than expected because the template used may have originated years previously, the new job description was based on one created within a different organization or one for an entirely different position or the author is not sufficiently familiar with case management to construct a meaningful document. These generic job descriptions do not capture the demands of case management in the present-day health care environment. In order to develop a meaningful case management job description, it may be best to begin with a blank page.

Developing a Job Description

The job description is a launching point from which PM documents are derived; hence its importance to expectation setting cannot be dismissed. When staff responsibilities are not well defined, important aspects of the overall organizational mission and department goals may be compromised. In addition, when there is significant overlap between positions, individuals become frustrated and competitive in a way that does not enhance the overall work product (Congressional Management Foundation, 2014).

There are many ways by which to develop a job description. Start with defining the key terms of each position (e.g., case management, utilization review, population health management). As pointed out in chapter 3, there are a multitude of definitions for case management applied across the entirety of health care as well as within respective care settings. If an executive with responsibility for the case management department defines terms differently than do the manager and staff, only happenstance creates synergy or the chance to align department goals with the organization's overall mission and vision. Leaving this to chance belies the importance of the matter and heightens the risk of poor outcomes, relative to each stakeholder's definition.

Once basic definitions are agreed on, consider the current and future uses of the job description itself. Although it may be that the job description is being redefined for internal purposes (e.g., salary alignment, department reorganization, COLLABORATE implementation), ultimately the job description will be used for the purpose of attracting and hiring new employees.

The question as to whether the job description should focus on tasks versus competencies should be considered. Hawkes and Weathington (2014) examined the impact of a competency-based versus task-based job description on candidate attraction. Although there was no appreciable difference in candidate attraction based on the type of job description, important considerations were raised, including the fact although organizations are moving toward a competence focus, candidates are not necessarily with this approach or the impact it has on position-specific documents and PM.

Another important point of the study was to point out that people choose jobs for a variety of reasons and that the job description may not have been central to their decision-making process. Openness to experience impacted the job seeker. The candidate with a higher openness to experience found the competence-based job description more attractive. Finally, the study evaluated the specific point of the love of learning (akin to the lifelong learning competency discussed in chapter 10) and job description preference. Interestingly, a greater love of learning did not translate to a preference for a competency-based job description for studied positions. Based on the present lack of significant evidence that a competence-based job description attracts more desirable candidates, it is advisable to consider that presenting only competencies or only tasks within a job description may not enhance favorable results in candidate attraction (Hawkes & Weathington, 2014).

COLLABORATE COMPETENCIES AND THE JOB DESCRIPTION

Although case management job descriptions are present in the literature, considerably more emphasis is required to a competency-based approach that is applicable across professional disciplines. With the industry so heavily focused on interprofessional initiatives, it is essential to develop job descriptions which are reflective of case management workforce diversity.

One way to incorporate the COLLABORATE competencies into a case management job description is to align each competency and their respective key elements with organizational goals and objectives. In this way a more consistent approach to professional case management can be universally acknowledged within and across practice settings. With regard to implementing COLLABORATE, the need for including practice setting–specific information in a job description is dependent on an organization's current job description format and content. It is suggested that the job description not be expanded to such lengths that it becomes difficult for the organization to manage updates and for the candidate to review and comprehend the job essentials. There are a variety of documents in which practice-specific details may be incorporated. However, if there is a highly unique characteristic(s) associated with case management within the care setting, a candidate should be made aware of it early in the hiring process.

PERFORMANCE MANAGEMENT AS A SYSTEMATIC APPROACH

Setting the tone for performance expectations does not begin on the first day of work. PM is about far more than simply a case manager's performance appraisal and the frequency by which it is completed. It is for this reason that the authors take the stance that effective PM should be viewed as a broader and more complex system as opposed to a single, fixed moment in time or a specific employee evaluation. This is consistent with views across the industry that PM is a process that is ongoing and continuous (Aguinis, 2013; Daniels & Bailey, 2014; Management Study Guide [MSG], 2014). It takes into account a series of components (Aguinis, 2013). PM is a comprehensive set of activities including but not limited to the following (MSG, 2014):

- Joint goal setting;
- Continuous progress review and frequent communication;
- Feedback and coaching for improved performance; and
- Implementation of an employee development program that acknowledges and rewards achievements.

Lawler identifies the components of goal setting, development, compensation actions, performance feedback, and a goals-based appraisal of performance (Lawler, 2012). The feedback should optimally occur quarterly, if not semiannually. Figure 21-2 presents a framework for a PM system.

When PM is viewed as a more global system opposed to a single linear process, it sets the platform for rewarding excellence by aligning the individual employee's accomplishments with the organization's mission and objectives. Through this interaction, clear performance expectations are established with the help of the employee to understand what is expected out of their assigned role.

Aguinis (2013) identifies six steps that must be accounted for in the PM process as shown in Figure 21-3.

Each step includes mandatory components, which align with the **performance management system** perspective discussed in this chapter. Of critical importance is the emphasis on the **strategic planning** employed in PM. The two terms, strategic planning and PM, are often viewed as synonyms; however, they are not. Strategic planning should be viewed as a distinct process that is used to guide a PM system. It is defined as a systematic process of envisioning a desired future, and translating this vision into broadly defined goals and a sequence of steps to achieve them. Strategic planning begins with the desired-end and works backward to the current status (Business Dictionary.com, 2014g):

- At every stage of long-range planning the planner asks, "What must be done here to reach the next (higher) stage?"
- At every stage of strategic planning the planner asks, "What must be done at the previous (lower) stage to reach here?"

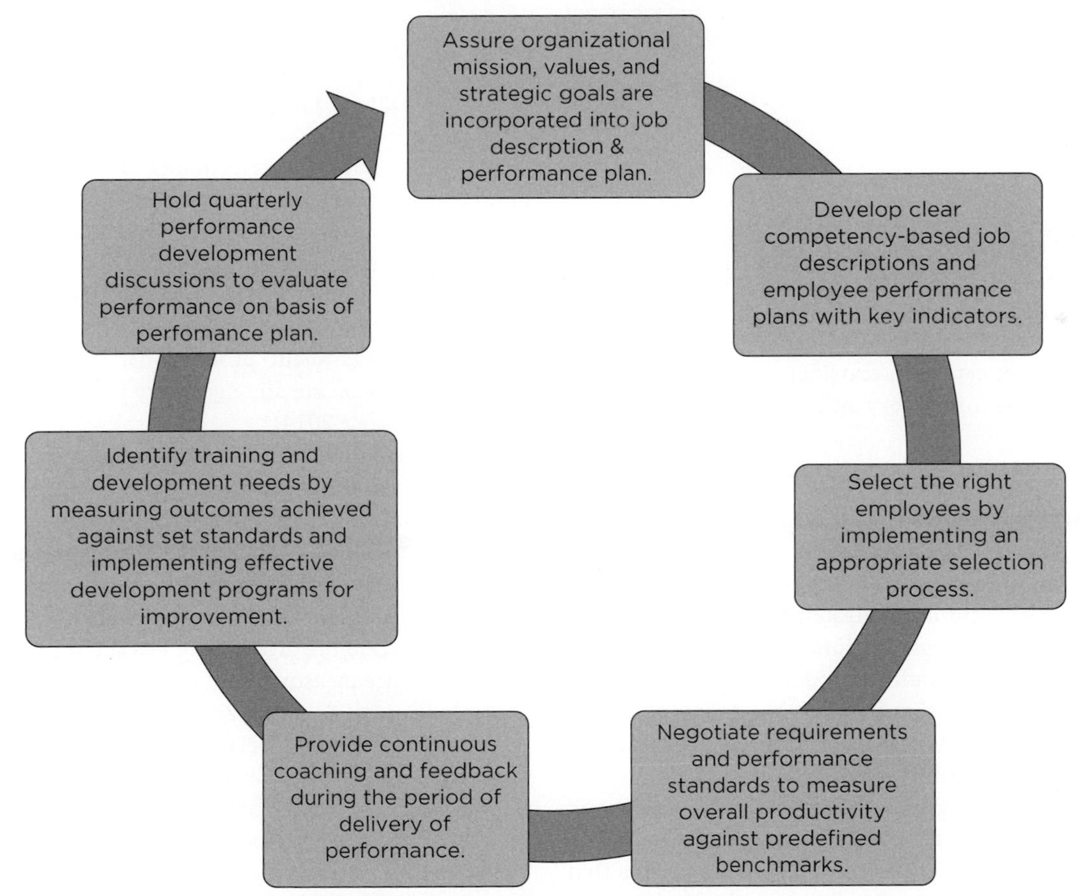

Figure 21-2. Performance management systematic approach. In addition (1) design effective compensation and reward systems for recognizing employees who excel in their jobs by achieving the set standards in accordance with the performance plans or exceed the performance benchmarks; (2) provide promotional/career development support and guidance to the employees; and (3) perform exit interviews for understanding the cause of employee discontent and exit from the organization. (Adapted from Aguinis, H. (2013). *Performance management* (3rd ed.). Upper Saddle River, NJ: Pearson Education; Lawler, E. E. (2012). *Performance appraisals are dead: Long live performance management; Leadership*. Retrieved, December 4, 2014, from http://www.forbes.com/sites/edwardlawler/2012/07/12/performance-appraisals-are-dead-long-live-performance-management/; Management Study Guide. (2014). *Performance management-meaning, system and process*. Retrieved, December 4, 2014, from http://managementstudyguide.com/performance-appraisal.htm)

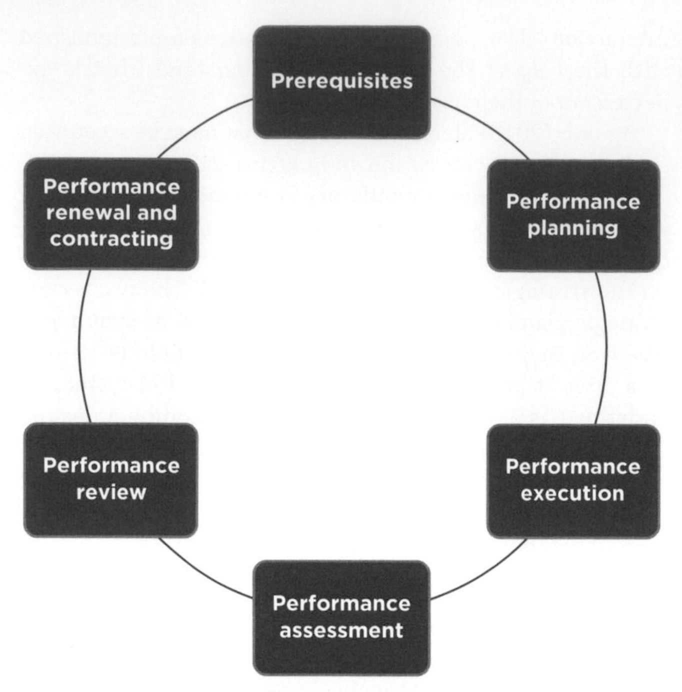

Figure 21-3. Six essential steps for performance management. (Adapted from Aguinis, H. (2013). *Performance management* (3rd ed.). Upper Saddle River, NJ: Pearson Education.)

THE PREREQUISITES OF STRATEGIC PERFORMANCE MANAGEMENT PLANNING

Before a PM system can even consider to be implemented, two prerequisites are mandatory and both are in the realm of strategic planning:

1. Knowledge of the organization's mission, vision, and strategic goals and
2. Knowledge of the job in question.

In these times of ever-evolving organizational ownership courtesy of mergers and acquisitions, and C-suite changes, it is essential that the organizational mission, vision, and strategic goals are clearly defined and shared across the entity. All management levels must solicit input from all people with units to create unit-level mission and vision statements, goals, and strategies (Aguinis, 2013).

The **mission** statement summarizes the organization's most important reason for its existence (Aguinis, 2013). The health care industry is flooded with organizations that share the mission statement, "to improve the health, well-being, and security of those we serve," or "to improve lives though providing cost-effective health care products and services." In contrast, an organizational **vision** is a statement of future aspirations. It is traditionally brief and concise, such as the vision statement for the Alzheimer's Association (2014), which is, "our vision is a world without Alzheimer's."

PERFORMANCE EXECUTION: THE RESPONSIBILITY FOR PERFORMANCE MANAGEMENT

To that end, there must be clear accountability by all involved in PM system. Although policies and procedures defining the PM process are beneficial, there are other means to assure accountability for implementation. Most models include a step to address how the performance plan and appraisal process will be executed, and who will have accountability for those components (Aguinis, 2013; Daniels & Bailey, 2014; MSG, 2014).

It is essential that the following factors be present from start of the development of the job description. Active input by the employee is a vital part of this stage, as it is during the development of performance standards, the creation of any rating form used, plus the evaluation process itself through two-way communication (Aguinis, 2013).

Grote (1996) notes the importance of assigning accountability for specific actions to supervisors and employees from the start of the PM process, and especially the performance review stage. Each of these actions is elaborated on in Box 21-1.

PERFORMANCE MEASUREMENT

Just as organizational performance is managed by the data, human performance is managed by it as well (Daniels & Bailey, 2014). Case managers understand the value of data, a topic discussed in chapter 9. Data is tangible and provides validation of otherwise subjective observations. It also increases the probability that managers will make correct decisions about promotions, suspensions, performance appraisals, and any necessary positive reinforcement (Daniels & Bailey, 2014).

Proper use of data guides performance improvement efforts and develops new programming. The use of data serves an equally powerful function in the PM system. **Performance measurement** allows managers to see smaller changes in performance than can otherwise be seen through casual observation. Seeing these small improvements allows managers to reinforce more often. Here lies the foundational value of performance measurement, as measurement is the key to progress (Daniels & Bailey, 2014).

Traditional views of performance measurement systems include measures of behavior (what an employee does) as well as results (the outcomes) (Aguinis, 2013). Measuring behaviors and competencies increases the credibility of case manager's performance appraisal, reduces emotionalism (e.g., emotional reaction), and fosters the means to increase constructive problem solving by the use of unbiased data on performance. Otherwise, the process is reduced to an opinionated, subjective, and irrational effort (Daniels & Bailey, 2014).

It is ironic that the definition of performance speaks to measures of behavior only, and does not include the emphasis on outcomes. Newer foci on performance measurement amplify the importance of weaving of these concepts

BOX 21-1 Employee and Supervisor/Managerial Primary Responsibilities for Performance Execution

Employee

1. Commitment to goal achievement: The employee must be committed to the goals that were set. One way to enhance commitment is to allow the employee to be an active participant in the process of setting the goals.
2. Ongoing performance feedback and coaching: The employee should not wait until the review cycle is over to solicit performance feedback. Also, the employee should not wait until a serious problem develops to ask for coaching.
3. Communication with supervisor: Supervisors are busy with multiple obligations. The burden is on the employee to communicate openly and regularly with the supervisor.
4. Collecting and sharing performance data: The employee should provide the supervisor with regular updates on progress toward goal achievement, in terms of both behaviors and results.
5. Preparing for performance reviews: The employee should not wait until the end of the review cycle approaches to prepare for the review. On the contrary, the employee should engage in an ongoing and realistic self-appraisal so that immediate corrective action can be taken if necessary. The usefulness of the self-appraisal process can be enhanced by gathering informal performance information from peers and customers (both internal and external).

Supervisory/Managerial

1. Observation and documentation: Supervisors must observe and document performance on a daily basis. It is important to keep track of examples of both good and poor performance.
2. Updates: As the organization's goals may change, it is important to update and revise initial objectives, standards, and key accountabilities (in the case of results) and competency areas (in the case of behaviors).
3. Feedback: Feedback on progression toward goals and coaching to improve performance should be provided on a regular basis certainly before the review.
4. Resources: Supervisors should provide employees with resources and opportunities to participate in developmental activities. Thus, they should encourage (and sponsor) participation in training, classes, and special assignments. Overall, supervisors have a responsibility to ensure that the employee has the necessary supplies and funding to perform the job properly.
5. Reinforcement: Supervisors must let employees know that their outstanding performance is noticed by reinforcing effective behaviors and progress toward goals. Also, supervisors should provide feedback regarding negative performance and how to remedy the observed problem. Observation and communication are not sufficient. Performance problems must be diagnosed early.

Adapted from Grote, D. (1996) in Aguinis, H. (2013). Performance management (3rd ed.). Upper Saddle River, NJ: Pearson Education.

together. Behavior performance can be viewed from an evaluative stance. This means the behaviors are judged as negative, neutral, or positive for the employee and organizational effectiveness (Motowidlo et al., 1997). The question becomes whether or not the behavior contributes to or hinders the accomplishment of the defined organizational or unit/department goals (Aguinis, 2013). How does the behavior of a case manager who is unable to lead team rounds impact the reduction of avoidable days?

Another way in which behavior performance can be viewed is multidimensional, which means there are two or more different kinds of behaviors that have the capacity to advance or hinder the defined organizational or unit/department goals (Murphy & Shiarella, 1997). A case manager, who contributes to the ability of the organization to decrease avoidable days, accomplishes this by his or her ability to build consensus across teams, plus the ability to engage and establish rapport with patients and families. The two behaviors identified may each be accounted for through evaluative means such as according to a numeric or text-based scale to demonstrate levels of competence.

Experts cite the frequency of which barriers to measuring performance will manifest. Reasons range from:

- Concern that some jobs cannot be measured.
- Measurement is hard work.
- Measurement is ineffective for it just signals punishment.
- There is insufficient time to measure.

(Daniels & Bailey, 2014)

The literature notes a number of methods how performance should be measured (Cheng & Dainty, 2005; Daniels & Bailey, 2014). Holmes and Joyce (1993) characterized three different approaches, which are grounded in different job role contexts (Cheng & Dainty, 2005). Expanded definitions of each appear in Table 21-1:

- **Job-focused**: Key tasks are functional in approach.
- **Person-focused**: Key tasks relate to the personal background, values, and personality.
- **Role-focused**: Key tasks are assigned based on how employee performance is impacted by environmental demands.

Although all three of the above approaches support the competency-based PM movement, clear benefits have been attributed to the use of the role-focused approach (Cheng &

TABLE 21-1 Types of Approaches to Measure Performance

Approach	Qualities	Competence Expressed
Job-Focused	Identifies key tasks of the work. Job exists independent of who holds the job.	In terms of the job performance and standards of performance expected to be achieved
Person-Focused	Considers the job holder's performance in terms of how it relates to the employee's personal background, personality, values, and motivation.	Macro in nature and distinct from the task-specific micro competencies of the job-focused approach. Competencies are intangible and dynamic.
Role-Focused	Focuses on the social context in which performance is undertaken. Job performance is viewed as the enactment of a role, which emerges through interaction between the role holder and others in the social situation, subject to their varying perceptions and expectations.	Emphasizes the various demands, which are made of the individual employee by others and the extent to which he or she accepts them. Examines the degree to which the employee's performance meets the demands imposed by both himself or herself and others. The role approach is grounded in the reality of the individual employee's situation, rather than in an abstract model of what any that person should be doing.

Adapted from Holmes and Joyce in Cheng, M. I., &. Dainty, R. I. J. (2005). Toward a multidimensional competency-based managerial performance framework: A hybrid approach. Journal of Managerial Psychology, 20, 380–396.

Dainty, 2005; Fowler et al., 2000, Holmes & Joyce, 1993). It goes further than either the job or person focus perspectives given its emphasis on the unique level of interaction that occurs between the individual, those working with them, and the environment (Cheng & Dainty, 2005). By examining the various demands and expectations made on the individual employee by others and the extent to which the employee accepts those demands, the role-focused approach acknowledges the extent to which the employee's performance meets demands imposed on him or her (Holmes & Joyce, 1993).

The role-focused approach also recognizes a variety of factors that can impact job performance (e.g., actions of coworkers, a leader's behavior, organizational culture and values). This results in the enhanced ability to assess and manage the performance of the employee by grounding the reality of his or her situation. The challenge in the role-focused approach is that it can lend a subjective quality to performance measurement, which is not consistent with how other experts view the stage (Daniels & Bailey, 2014).

Nonetheless, the role-focused approach can be valuable in the environment of a case manager's world, particularly given the fluid rate at which assignments change. Consider the number of times your own job roles and responsibilities have been altered, whether due to the emergence of new target populations of focus for your practice setting, or even new or revised reimbursement that impacts how the identification of clients and manifesting intervention unfold.

PERFORMANCE REVIEW

It is through a formal process that the performance review, also known as appraisal, is discussed and reviewed. Experts refer to this as the Achilles Heel of the process, mostly because of the discomfort managers and supervisors experience when providing feedback (Shore et al., 1998). This can present as anxiety during the discussion, if not avoidance to schedule or conduct the meeting. Providing feedback must be done effectively so that it leads to performance improvement as needed, plus employee satisfaction (Aguinis, 2013). Recommended steps for conducting productive performance reviews are provided in Box 21-2.

MOVING BEYOND THE PRESENT: DEFINING NEW GOALS AND COMPETENCIES

Building the bridge is only part of the process, for the bridge must be maintained over time. The same can be said for successful PM. All of the stages framed heretofore have a powerful role in measuring the overall competence of the case manager. This final stage appears across the literature by several names, from performance renewal and contracting (Aguinis, 2013), to feedback and coaching stage (MSG, 2013). Of particular importance is that there is no real final

BOX 21-2 Six Recommended Steps for Conducting Productive Performance Reviews

1. Identify what the case manager has done well and then present what has been done poorly. Cite both specific positive and negative behaviors.
2. Solicit feedback from the case manager about these behaviors. Listen for reactions and explanations to what you have presented.
3. Discuss the implications of changing, or not changing, the behaviors. Positive feedback is best, but the case manager must be made aware of what will happen if any poor performance continues.
4. Explain to the case manager how skills used in past achievements can help him or her overcome any current performance problems.
5. Agree on an action plan. Encourage the case manager to invest in improving his or her performance by asking questions, such as
   - What ideas do you have for _______?
   - What suggestions do you have for _______?
6. Set up a meeting to follow up and agree on the behaviors, actions, and attitudes to be evaluated.

Adapted from Aguinis, H. (2013). Performance management (3rd ed.). Upper Saddle River, NJ: Pearson Education.

stage or end of the PM process. It is why this section of the chapter is titled as it is.

The performance renewal and contracting stage is similar to the performance planning stage identified early on. Both of these stages engage the supervisor and case manager in defining goals and objectives based on those which were established in the prerequisite stage for the organization or unit/department. However, a difference emerges for the latter stage in that reflective processing takes over as the case manager engages insight and all of the information gained from the other stages (Aguinis, 2013). This action allows for the disparities between goals and objectives to be discussed, explored, and potentially revised. It is where the competency-based approaches discussed through this text and the COLLABORATE paradigm seize their opportunity for implementation.

CONNECTING COLLABORATE TO PERFORMANCE MANAGEMENT

As discussed in chapter 5, the competency movement emerged in the health care industry over the later part of the 20th century courtesy of influence and emphasis by a number of experts and organizations (Dreyfus & Dreyfus, 1980; Institute of Medicine, 1999, 2001, 2003; Lundberg, 1972; Prahalad & Hamel, 1990; The Joint Commission on Accreditation of Healthcare Organizations, 2000). These models have continued to advance as newer understandings of competencies, and how those competencies should be used populate the human resources and PM realm (Cheng & Dainty, 2005; Sanchez & Levine, 2009). This emphasis further sets the stage for the application of COLLABORATE as a vehicle to support the PM process.

In the PM arena, competencies and the concept of **competency modeling** (CM) have replaced the more **traditional job analysis**. A traditional job analysis focuses on describing and measuring the requirements of work (Sanchez & Levine, 2009). It can be viewed as more rigorous than CM in regard to data collection, level of detail, assessment of reliability of results, and documentation of the research process. On the other hand, CM involves the process of analyzing and describing types and ranges of abilities, knowledge, and skills present in an organization, or which it need to acquire to gain a competitive advantage (BusinessDictionary.com, 2014e). It is a more strategic process, which creates a conduit to influence day-to-day employee performance along strategic lines (Sanchez & Levine, 2009). This is far more consistent with the structured and strategic focus of PM defined by Aguinis (2013), for it links results to business goals.

Organizations will often identify specific or **core competencies** for attention by employees. These refer to the unique abilities that a company acquires from its founders, or develops and that cannot be easily imitated. They give a company one or more competitive advantages, in creating and delivering value to its customers in its chosen field (BusinessDictionary.com, 2014f). Examples of core competencies include fostering teamwork, managing change, and managing performance.

Reconsider the case scenario discussed during the performance renewal and contract stage. The supervisor and case manager are discussing the disparity goals and objectives, and the inability of the case manager to obtain a consistent outstanding rating across the competencies included in the performance plan. What staffing retention issues impacted the case manager's ability to complete the outcomes assigned to her for her unit? The attainment of a poor rating for the outcomes competency was the result. Both the case manager's efficiency and effectiveness were hampered and contributed to this rating. The supervisor assessed that pressures of the case management job requirements impacted the case manager's proficiency with the critical thinking competency; the individual was challenged with the creativity expected to develop treatment plans for patients and received a poor rating as well.

There are models similar to COLLABORATE, which pose a defined number of competencies for the workforce (Bartram, 2005; Ferguson, 2013; Kurz & Bartram, 2002). Kurz and Bartram (2002) developed the **Great Eight competencies** as work behaviors that promote employee effectiveness in 21st-century organizations. Aligned with each of the eight major sets of behaviors are additional clusters of competencies, which total 112 component competencies at the finest level of detail (Bartram, 2005). The Great Eight competencies appear in Table 21-2.

TABLE 21-2 The Great Eight Competencies

Competency Domain	Domain Definition
Leading and Deciding	Takes control and exercises leadership. Initiates action, gives direction, and takes responsibility.
Supporting and Cooperating	Supports others and shows respect and positive regard for them in social situations. Puts people first, working effectively with individuals and teams, clients, and staff. Behaves consistently with clear personal values that complement those of the organization.
Interacting and Presenting	Communicates and networks effectively. Successfully persuades and influences others. Relates to others in a confident, relaxed manner.
Analyzing and Interpreting	Shows evidence of clear analytical thinking. Gets to the heart of complex problems and issues. Applies own expertise effectively. Quickly takes on new technology. Communicates well in writing.
Creating and Conceptualizing	Works well in situations requiring openness to new ideas and experiences. Seeks out learning opportunities. Handles situations and problems with innovation and creativity. Thinks broadly and strategically. Supports and drives organizational change.
Organizing and Executing	Plans ahead and works in a systematic and organized way. Follows directions and procedures. Focuses on customer satisfaction and delivers a quality service or product to the agreed standards.
Adapting and Coping	Adapts and responds well to change. Manages pressure effectively and copes well with setbacks.
Enterprising and Performing	Focuses on results and achieving personal work objectives. Works best when work is related closely to results and the impact of personal efforts is obvious. Shows an understanding of business, commerce, and finance. Seeks opportunities for self-development and career advancement.

Adapted from Kurz, R., & Bartram, D. (2002). Competency and individual performance: Modeling the world of work. In I. T. Robertson, M. Callinan, & D. Bartram (Eds.), Organizational effectiveness: The role of psychology (pp. 227–255). Chichester, England: Wiley.

TABLE 21-3 The Great Eight Competencies Aligned With COLLABORATE Competencies

Great Eight Competencies (Kurz & Bartram, 2002)	COLLABORATE Competencies
Leading and Deciding	Critical Thinking, Leadership
Supporting and Cooperating	Transdisciplinary, Advocacy
Interacting and Presenting	Transdisciplinary, Advocacy
Analyzing and Interpreting	Critical Thinking, Outcomes-Driven
Creating and Conceptualizing	Lifelong Learning, Big-Picture Orientation
Organizing and Executing	Anticipatory, Organized, Resource Awareness
Adapting and Coping	Anticipatory, Lifelong Learning
Enterprising and Performing	Outcomes-Driven, Organized, Lifelong Learning

The Great Eight model is consistent with COLLABORATE's 11 competencies and the corresponding 27 total elements assigned to the main competencies, as discussed in chapter 7. A comparison of the major competencies for the two models and how they align with each other appears in Table 21-3.

CAREER AND CLINICAL LADDERS FOR CASE MANAGEMENT

A **career ladder** is a structured sequence of positions through which a person progresses within an organization (BusinessDictionary.com, 2014g). As pointed out by Knowles (2008), a career ladder lays the groundwork for professional and personal growth which is a foundational concept of the COLLABORATE paradigm. However, it is important to note that there are two terms used to describe ladder programs: career ladder and clinical ladder are used inconsistently in the research literature. Understanding the difference facilitates the construction process.

A ladder framework provides a path on which individuals may embark as a means of career development. The concept of a career ladder in case management has been a disjointed and organization-driven venture. However, the complexity of health care and care systems across practice settings demands that the professional case manager of today and tomorrow establish and maintain an organized, long-term progression of knowledge acquisition and career development. The ladder concept that is inclusive of competency-based practice proficiency addresses this need.

There are two types of career ladders frequently mentioned in nursing literature: One is a career advancement model and the other focuses on role expansion. The career ladder is an advancement system that rewards accomplishment through promotional opportunities. A clinical ladder construct is a voluntary program designed to enhance and reward role expansion (Nelson & Cook, 2008). The ladder framework may be descriptive rather than evaluative, and progress through the ladder may be task-oriented versus outcomes-based or driven by accomplishment of milestones versus requiring objective evaluation.

There are additional considerations important for the implementation of an effective ladder framework. One such consideration was that of eligibility. This was important to a Kaiser Permanente ladder used in Colorado. Participating nurses were only eligible to participate in the career ladder program after 1 year of service within the organization and had to maintain at least half-time work status (Nelson & Cook, 2008). Organizations designing a ladder should clearly define its eligibility requirement(s).

Establishing a sustainable case management-specific framework requires a clear understanding of case management as well as definition of a skill and experience levels. The Dreyfus model (1980) defines proficiency stages as novice, competence, proficiency expertise, and mastery (presented in Table 21-4). This model argues that skills are attained through monitoring, instruction, and experience and that an individual normally passes through five developmental stages, which designate novice, competence, proficiency, expertise, and mastery.

Although further study is required to classify case management activities according to proficiency level, the role and function studies undertaken by the Commission for Case Manager Certification (CCMC) may provide a suitable platform from which to launch this inquiry. CCMC captured the activities and knowledge areas necessary for effective case management practice intermittently over a period of years. The findings of this longitudinal study may offer a platform from which to launch further study required to define a cross-continuum hierarchy of proficiency as a basis for case management-specific career ladders.

TABLE 21-4 Dreyfus' Five Stages Model of Skills Acquisition

Novice	Competent	Proficient	Expert	Mastery
• The novice is given rules for determining an action based upon the presence or absence of certain factors. • The novice requires monitoring, by self-observation and/or instructor feedback to align behavior with existing rules.	• Competence comes with significant hands-on experience coping with real situations. • The individual learns or an instructor points out recurrent meaningful component patterns.	• Increased experience exposes the individual to many of typical situations. For the first time, situations have meaning. • The individual uses a memorized principle to determine the appropriate action.	• Accumulated experience is so comprehensive that a specific situation dictates an intuitively appropriate action. • The individual has reached the final stage in the improvement of mental processing.	• Mastery only takes place when the individual can cease to pay conscious attention to performance. • The individual channels mental energy into pzoducing the appropriate perspective and action rather than monitoring.

This is an original table derived from Dreyfus and Dreyfus.

Dreyfus, S.E., and Dreyfus, H.L. (1980). A Five- Stage Model of the Mental Activities Involved in Directed Skill Acquisition. (Supported by the U.S. Air Force, Office of Scientific Research (AFSC) under contract F49620-C-0063 with the University of California) Berkeley. (Unpublished study). Retrieved December 7, 2014 from http://www.dtic.mil/cgi-bin/GetTRDoc?AD=ADA084551

SUMMARY

A manager is responsible for the application and performance of knowledge (Drucker, 2001). PM is not an activity that should be left to chance, or limited to an annual evaluation. It is a purposeful activity which must be conducted through a strategic, meaningful, and systematic approach.

Use of the COLLABORATE framework as a guide for PM facilitates adoption of consistent professional practice and behavioral expectations across practice settings. Subsequently, case management outcomes contribute to evidence, which is mandatory to establish case management's transition from advanced practice to professional practice.

References

Abu-Doleh, J., & Weir, D. (2007). Dimensions of performance appraisal systems in Jordanian private and public organizations. *International Journal of Human Resource Management, 18*(1), 75–84.

Aguinis, H. (2013). *Performance management* (3rd ed.). Upper Saddle River, NJ: Pearson Education.

Alzheimer's Association. (2014). *Homepage*. Retrieved December 5, 2014, from http://www.alz.org/index.asp

Bartram, D. (2005). The great eight competencies: A criterion-centric approach to validation. *Journal of Applied Psychology 90*, 1185–1203.

Bensing, K. (2011). Nurse performance appraisals: What purpose do they serve? *NursingAdvance*. Retrieved December 4, 2011, from http://nursing.advanceweb.com/Regional-Content/Articles/Nurse-Performance-Appraisals.aspx

BusinessDictionary.com. (2014a). Performance management. Retrieved November 25, 2014, from http://www.businessdictionary.com/definition/performance-management.html

Business Dictionary.com. (2014b). Goals. Retrieved December 4, 2014, from http://www.businessdictionary.com/definition/goal.html

Business Dictionary.com. (2014c). Objectives. Retrieved December 4, 2014, from http://www.businessdictionary.com/definition/objectives.html

Business Dictionary.com. (2014d). Best practice. Retrieved December 4, 2014, from http://www.businessdictionary.com/definition/best-practice.html

Business Dictionary.com. (2014e). Competency modeling. Retrieved December 5, 2014, from http://www.businessdictionary.com/definition/competency-modeling.html

Business Dictionary.com. (2014f). Core competency. Retrieved December 5, 2014, from http://www.businessdictionary.com/definition/core-competencies.html

Business Dictionary.com. (2014g). Strategic planning. Retrieved December 5, 2014, from http://www.businessdictionary.com/definition/strategic-planning.html

Cheng, M. I., &. Dainty, R. I. J. (2005). Toward a multidimensional competency-based managerial performance framework: A hybrid approach. *Journal of Managerial Psychology, 20*, 380–396.

Congressional Management Foundation. (2014). *How to develop job descriptions*. Retrieved December 6, 2014, from http://www.congressfoundation.org/component/content/article/135

Daniels, A. C., & Bailey, J. S. (2014). *Performance management: Changing behavior that drives organizational effectiveness*. Atlanta, GA: Performance Management Publications.

Dreyfus, S., & Dreyfus, H. (1980). *A five-stage model of the mental activities involved in directed skill acquisition*. Washington, DC: Storming Media.

Drucker, P. F. (2001). *The Essential Drucker*. New York, NY: Collins Publishing.

Ferguson, R. (2013). *Finally! Performance assessment that works: Big 5 performance management*. North Charleston, SC: Create Space Independent Publishing Platform.

Fowler, S. W., King, A. W., March, S. J. & Victor, B. (2000). Beyond Products: New Strategic Imperatives for Developing Competencies in Dynamic Environments. *Journal of Engineering and Technology Management, 17*, 357–77

Grote, D. (1996). *The complete guide to performance appraisal*. New York, NY: American Management Association.

Hawkes, C. L., & Weathington, B. L. (2014). Competency-based versus task-based job descriptions: Effects on applicant attraction. *Journal of Behavioral and Applied Management, 15*(3), 190–211. Retrieved December 7, 2014, from http://search.proquest.com/docview/1548423667?accountid=458

Holmes, L., & Joyce, P. (1993). Rescuing the useful concept of managerial competence: From outcomes back to process. *Personnel Review, 22*(6), 37–52.

Institute of Medicine. (1999). *To err is human: Building a safer healthcare system*. Washington, DC: The National Academies Press.

Institute of Medicine. (2001). *Crossing the quality chasm: A new health system for the 21st century*. Washington, DC: The National Academies Press.

Institute of Medicine. (2003). *Health professions education: A bridge to quality (The Quality Chasm Series)*. Washington, DC: The National Academies Press.

The Joint Commission on Accreditation of Healthcare Organizations. (2000). *Hospital accreditation standards* (vol. 261–263, pp. 219–225, 319). Oakbrook Terrace, IL: Author.

Kurz, R., & Bartram, D. (2002). Competency and individual performance: Modeling the world of work. In I. T. Robertson, M. Callinan, & D. Bartram (Eds.), *Organizational effectiveness: The role of psychology* (pp. 227–255). Chichester, England: Wiley.

Lawler, E. E. (2012). *Performance appraisals are dead: Long live performance management; Leadership*. Retrieved, December 4, 2014, from http://www.forbes.com/sites/edwardlawler/2012/07/12/performance-appraisals-are-dead-long-live-performance-management/

Lundberg, C. C. (1972, Fall). Planning the executive development program. *California Management Review, 15* (1), 10–15.

Management Study Guide. (2014). *Performance management-meaning, system and process*. Retrieved, December 4, 2014, from http://management studyguide.com/performance-appraisal.htm

Merriam-Webster online dictionary. (2014). Performance. Retrieved December 4, 2014, from http://www.merriam-webster.com/dictionary/performance

Motowidlo, S. J., Borman, W. C., & Schmit, M. J. (1997). A theory of individual differences in task and contextual performance. *Human Performance, 10*, 71–83.

Murphy, K. R., & Shiarella, A. H. (1997). Implications of the multidimensional nature of job performance for the validity of selection tests: Multivariate frameworks for studying test validity. *Personnel Psychology, 50*, 823–854.

Nelson, J. M., & Cook, P. F. (2008). Evaluation of a career ladder program in an ambulatory care environment. *Nursing economics, 26*(6), 353–360.

Prahalad, C. K., & Hamel, G. (1990). The core competence of corporation. *Harvard Business Review, 68*(3), 79–91.

Sanchez, J. I., &. Levine, E. L. (2009). What is (or should be) the difference between competency modeling and traditional job analysis? *Human Resource Management Review, 19*, 53–63.

Shore, T. H., Adams, J. S., & Tashchian, A. (1998). Effects of self-appraisal information, appraisal purpose, and feedback target on performance appraisal ratings. *Journal of Business and Psychology, 12*, 283–298.

Vorhauser-Smith, S. (2012). Three reasons performance management will change in 2013. *Forbes*. Retrieved December 4, 2014, from http://www.forbes.com/sites/sylviavorhausersmith/2012/12/16/the-new-face-of-performance-management-trading-annual-reviews-for-agile-management/2/

SECTION 4

Epilogue: The Crystal Ball

If you always do what you've always done, you'll always get what you've always got.

Anonymous

EPILOGUE

In moving forward, the one fact that rings true is there will be constant change in our industry. As the health care terrain shifts and new influences continually surface, there will be consequences for case management practice. These impacts require nimble clinical professionals in possession of recognized and firmly established competencies. They must be agile to frame (and reframe) their professional practice to facilitate the best possible outcomes for their patients. This is exactly why the definition of a competency-based case management model's time has come, one sufficiently fluid to fit into any setting of care (Treiger & Fink-Samnick, 2014).

In the time since the COLLABORATE articles were originally published in professional case management, we received spirited feedback about the model from the professional community. Themes of these comments include, but are not limited to:

- Implementation potential across practice settings, with particular use for ambulatory care and community-based programs;
- Value to human resources with application to hiring and performance appraisals;
- Clear focus on performance metrics as outcomes;
- Worth as an integral tool to measure and validate overall case management returns on investment; and
- Framing that recognizes the value of competency-based performance in the highly competitive health care environment.

We are inspired by industry recognition of the positive impact that a competency-based model provides for the future of professional case management. As has been noted, a quality-improvement implementation of COLLABORATE requires top-down organizational alignment in combination with the full commitment of all stakeholders.

CONSIDERATIONS FOR MAKING THE PARADIGM SHIFT

Change is the law of life and those who look only to the past or present are certain to miss the future.

John F. Kennedy

Perhaps you are thinking, "How do I know if a paradigm shift is needed?" While prior generations of case managers might have entered their first day of employment hoping for long-term career stability, a different reality emerged over the past several decades. The health care environment has been fraught with continuous change. Steadiness and status quo quickly became regarded as stagnation. In fact, how many organizations in the 21st century have you seen promote their constancy as opposed to status quo? (Cameron & Quinn, 2011) There is never a really bad time at which to reconsider work-flow process and make changes that will improve operations, but more importantly—patient care.

The shift in health care's business culture framing of the 1980s into the 1990s saw increased competition. This was fueled in part by expansion of medical knowledge from biomedical research and manifesting technology, yielding expanded care options and longer lives for health care consumers (Fink-Samnick, 2008). In tandem, a tidal wave of mergers and acquisitions (M&As) occurred as free-standing hospitals consolidated and became part of larger systems, some forming care continuums. There were 310 M&As at the height of these actions in 1997 (Cuellar & Gertler, 2003). Those of us employed in the health care industry during these years endured significant occupational fluctuations as a result of these events. For some individuals working in case management, this translated to simultaneously managing their own changing titles, jobs, roles, and functions along with expanding clients, members, and benefit plan structures, often with little or no warning or training for taking on new responsibilities. However, case managers adapted to ensure both their own employment as well as the delivery of health care.

Fast-forward to the present and the influence of advancing information technology (e.g., electronic health records, case management software), the use of personal computers and the Internet, health care reform legislation, and innovation of delivery models (e.g., accountable care, patient-centered medical homes, transition of care initiatives). The result is an interweaving of intricate fabric that wraps around every care setting like a Christo installation (Christo and Jeanne-Claude, 2013). Suffice to say, change is a constant across the health care continuum.

URGENCY FOR A UNIFYING MODEL

The world hates change, yet it is the only thing that has brought progress.

Charles Kettering

In addition to the historical grounding provided in section 1, the urgency for adopting a practice model that may be applied across the care continuum benefits from a few more points of reference. The Affordable Care Act took aim at many targets in order to open up access, lower cost, and improve quality of health care across the nation. However, during the same time period as numerous efforts to implement improvements in care delivery met with variable success (and resistance), spending for health care increased from 13% to almost 19% of gross domestic product (Hernandez & Shewchuk, 2011). Ironically, diminished performance on many indicators of health system efficiency, declining population health metrics, and more pronounced health disparities have been observed despite these dramatic spending increases (Commonwealth Fund, 2011).

Case managers have a key role to play in managing change of our professional development and work settings if these efforts are to ultimately result in care that is more consumer-centric and continuity-conscious. However, we must first address our individual and collective shortcomings in order to push the needle in a positive direction. A consistent model of practice that deemphasizes setting of care and focuses on personal accountability to specific behaviors and skills takes a giant step forward in that direction.

The lack of professional unity is ultimately concerning. Over recent decades, case management has failed to coalesce in a manner that demonstrates the likelihood of lasting cohesion. As a result, case management may not be perceived as an organized force within health care. Although some of this may be related to the disjointed nature of the U.S. health care system, many professional disciplines in the health and human services sector have managed to develop both umbrella entities as well as numerous specialty practice groups, without it being seen as divisive; this includes, but is not limited to, medicine, nursing, social work, etc. Why does case management not follow this same path for professional advancement and sustainability?

There is also the point that case management developed as a dependent rather than a parent figure. In other words, case managers are generally task-oriented employees within large organizations rather than employers or contractors of their own services. This seems to be significantly affecting the ability to see case management develop beyond current limitations enforced by legislation, regulation, or organizational policy and procedure.

The collective "we" have failed to communicate and cooperate across the various stakeholder entities, which represent case/care management practice. In a desire to emphasize the uniqueness of a given setting of practice or population, additional professional, accreditation, and certification bodies were established. This ultimately divides our numbers and results in far less powerful political influence. At times, stakeholders appear to be working at odds with each other while contributing to what presents as Case Management's Identity Disorder (Treiger & Fink-Samnick, 2013a).

General confusion as to the differences and distinctions between professional organizations, certification entities, and commercial enterprises continues. There has not been a lasting concerted effort to address this confusion, perhaps because it may be viewed as beneficial to maintain the lack of clarity? Rather than leaving the issue unaddressed, a more constructive approach is to develop a professional career path that includes involvement in professional development activities, continuing education, and certification.

When we overlay industry-specific issues onto system-wide obstacles, it is a testament to dogged determination that case management still exists. However, in the absence of recognizing and acting on the deleterious impact of these multiple factors, quasi-case management roles continue to proliferate within the industry. Now, no single entity appears to have the support of the case management majority. These issues should be considered as priorities to industry stakeholders. The clock is ticking on the critical need for concerted professional advocacy, a competency integral for all case managers to master.

RESISTANCE + CHANGE = GROWTH

The greatest danger in times of turbulence is not the turbulence – it is to act with yesterday's logic

Peter Drucker

It is important to be cognizant of the reasons why change in a health care-related field has been so problematic. Simply put, it is difficult to push a rope and the U.S. health care system has proven to be especially rope-like due to special interests associated with politics, economics, and public perception. Blank (2012) summarized this issue well, "Forces in opposition [to change] include politicians who over promise; drug companies, big medicine and a medical research community whose lifeblood is continual expansion of profit-making medical technologies; physicians who will not say no to patients and are paid more to provide more care; tort lawyers who argue negligence when not all that is possible is done for their client; and patients and their families who demand everything that might help be done because cost should be of no concern if a third party is paying for it."

Another point to reconcile as we forge into the future of health care is that of the shift in point of care delivery. McDeavitt, Wade, Smith, and Worsowicz (2012) point out "health care is increasingly delivered by large organizations. As payment constraints tighten, it is likely that consolidation of providers will accelerate, with smaller hospitals being absorbed into larger systems."

Business change affects case management in a number of ways, including the consolidation of case management roles and functions into existing staff positions and the use of unlicensed, nonclinical staff to address specific tasks. This is problematic because identifying and addressing barriers to care and health should not be moving further away from discovery during a comprehensive bio-psycho-social-spiritual assessment. As the use of checklists providing specific intervention activities expands, so does the risk of overlooking vital information which may not be collected by these efficiency-focused tools. When a barrier assessment is reduced to an oversimplified transaction, why would an organization pay for a clinical profession to do it when a less qualified person will simply do as they are instructed?

There is also a risk of offshoring case management services. As pointed out in a Remington Report article, "As the education, skill set, and sophistication of case management progresses, it is increasingly likely that there will be a rise in compensation. One risk associated with higher salary expense is the consideration by healthcare organizations to outsource case management responsibilities, in some cases to offshore entities. This potential scenario is another valid argument in favor of officially codifying case management into legislation and regulation to prevent the performance of activities requiring a specific level of clinical education and competency to individuals without adequate knowledge gained through licensure, certification, education, or training within the United States healthcare system" (Treiger, 2011).

If case management is to remain relevant in the future, our combined leadership must work synergistically to achieve the following:

- Define professional case management practice and career paths;
- Define case management's value proposition;
- Identify case management best practice; and
- Define optimal consumer and organization-specific outcomes.

We achieve this by defining competencies for professional practice, which are agnostic to educational background, professional training, practice setting, population served, and licensure and/or certification. Although there are certainly specialty-specific requirements to be clearly documented, there should be touchstones on purposeful career paths geared to formal higher-education degrees and certifications. A single-level certification may have been a giant leap forward 20 years ago, but today's health care environment demands a more robust and organized framework to recognize knowledge, skill, and professional achievement.

CHANGE AND BEST PRACTICE

Because professional case managers are big-picture-oriented, examining practices outside of case management is vital. It has become too easy for some to embrace a defined best practice model simply because it is held up as such. The choice of a methodology should not come at the expense of a clear vision as to the implication of making significant changes within any organization. Hallencreutz and Turner (2011) raise interesting considerations pertaining to use of best practice, the first of which is not having an accepted definition of best practice [within one's organization] and the second being the lack of organization consensus on a best way to implement change. A lesson learned in the business sector was how overreliance on best practice may lead to complacency in approaching change: "Not taking advantage of what change management has to offer, will almost certainly delay the project further, whereas systematic change management throughout the project can significantly speed up the project" (Garde, 2010). Finding a change management approach best suited for your organization may require additional time prior to initiating the project. Although Kotter's eight-stage approach is considered a reliable model, others exist and may be used as a project management framework.

ORGANIZATIONAL CULTURE AMIDST OTHER INTEGRAL INFLUENCES

Culture does not change because we desire to change it. Culture changes when the organization is transformed the culture reflects the realities of people working together every day.

Frances Hesselbein

Navigating the culture of your environment is never easy. Transformation is difficult even if you managed to get through similar efforts undertaken in the past. However, some level of cultural change is likely to be required in order to implement COLLABORATE. Although this may present as a foreboding task, you may achieve greater clarity as to how to strategically position this effort by acknowledging the following three issues:

1. Distinguish between and understand the concepts of organizational culture and organizational climate. Both serve to define the entity you are employed for by influencing how the industry stakeholders' view it.

   By definition, organizational culture is enduring and entrenched for it refers to the overt, observable attributes of an organization. These attributes include its mission, core values, and core characteristics. On the other hand, organizational climate is a far more fluid dynamic which consists of the temporary attitudes, feelings, and perceptions of the individuals employed by the organization. It takes into account any perspectives that are modified as situations change based on new information. In a nutshell, organizational culture refers to the way things are as opposed to the organizational climate that encompasses the attitudes employees have about the culture (Cameron & Quinn, 2011).

   With respect to case management, an example of organizational culture might be to promote the belief that all engage in best practice to meet the needs of their target patient population. This is operationalized by the expectation that case managers achieve specialty certification, attend requisite continuing education programs, plus strive for advanced degrees. However, the organizational climate finds that although employees want to embrace the culture, they are, in reality, resentful of it because professional education benefits were cut as part of budget reduction. As a result, case managers must pay out of pocket for the very education that the organization hired them for, and relies on them to maintain. This has resulted in significant personal financial impact for all clinical employees.

Some may contend that both organizational culture and climate are subjective and nebulous, though as Bellot (2011) frames "Organizational culture exists. To that end it can't be avoided. It can be ambiguous, but it is unique to each institution and malleable." Every organization has a unique and distinct culture; each inherently fuzzy for they incorporate contradictions, paradoxes, ambiguities, and confusion.

2. Recognize the underlying challenges, which accompany any change to organizational culture. As Denning (2011) discusses, changing an organization's culture is one of the most difficult leadership challenges, due, in part, to its complex composition of factors. Organizational culture is comprised of an interlocking set of factors including goals, roles, processes, values, communication practices, attitudes, and assumptions; each subject to the individual input of an array of involved stakeholders who bring their unique belief systems of best practice to the effort. Although stakeholders present with best intent, the mutual competing and conflicting agendas meet the reality of the organization and a huge disconnect occurs. Implementation of the cultural transformation effort proceeds, hoping to yield profitable return on investment. This is accomplished through the grand efforts that come with any restructuring and streamlining of department operations, including, but not limited to:

- Reframing job roles and functions;
- Developing new titles for some, if not all of these jobs;
- Reallocating staff; and
- Generally overhauling overall service delivery.

Of course no one is quite sure if the outcomes will yield the return on investment estimated or if so, over what timeframe, including those who developed the plan. After several fiscal quarters if that long, the plug is pulled on a cultural change effort that is no longer responding to life support despite massive resuscitation efforts. Everyone in the organization now breathes a huge sigh of relief, until the next great organizational culture change moment is recognized and the process being anew. Consider your own employer and how many such restructuring efforts you can recall? Perhaps, you developed situational amnesia or simply lost count.

Over the past 30 years, health care has endured its own cultural shift from care of the patient's health to the care of the business of health care (Fink-Samnick, 2008). Case managers lived through the ongoing shift by being flexible and accommodating evolving roles and functions that resulted from reorganization initiatives during their employment tenure. In fact, it should give pause to consider that 75% of reengineering, total quality management, strategic planning, and downsizing efforts fail entirely or create problems serious enough to threaten the survival of the organization (Cameron & Quinn, 2011).

3. Assessing and diagnosing organizational culture is critical to moving forward. Case managers are trained to break down the complexities before them, whether organizational culture, interpersonal dynamics, or patients. A frequently used model is Cameron and Quinn's Organizational Culture Assessment Instrument (OCAI), based on their competing values framework (Cameron & Quinn, 2011). The OCAI's purpose is twofold; it is designed to help identify an organization's current culture. Then by using the same instrument, works to identify the culture that employees believe should be developed, one to match future demands and opportunities anticipated over the next 5 years. Just as there is no right or wrong culture, the OCAI supports the same premise by noting there are no right or wrong responses. Imagine the OCAI as the meeting of a strengths, weaknesses, opportunities, and threats (SWOT) analysis with a crystal ball.

The OCAI is one of many options available to assess and diagnose cultural change. Although it might present as an easy one to recommend, it is far from the only one. Given the diversity that underlies both the organizational culture and climate of each unique employer, readers are encouraged to explore assessment methodologies to ascertain an appropriate match. Much like the art of diagnosing patients, ask any 10 case management leaders to identify the assessment tools that have worked for them, and you will likely get 10 different recommendations.

THE LEADERSHIP OF CHANGE

There is nothing more difficult to take in hand, more perilous to conduct, or more uncertain in its success, than to take the lead in the introduction of a new order of things.

N. Machiavelli

There is a clear distinction between change management and change leadership, "Change management, which is the term most everyone uses, refers to a set of basic tools or structures intended to keep any change effort under control. The goal is often to minimize the distractions and impacts of the change. Change leadership, on the other hand, concerns the driving forces, visions, and processes that fuel large-scale transformation" (Kotter, 2011). Both are integral principles for case managers to reconcile.

As a case manager, you are a leader. It matters not whether you are in a formal leadership role in that 'C-Suite' because case management leadership happens in every aspect of practice and professional identity (Treiger & Fink-Samnick, 2013b). Discussions with countless corporate directors of case management find an increasing trend: recognition of case managers as the drivers, if not team leaders, of the care coordination processes in their respective organizations. This is consistent with efforts by regulatory entities and initiatives, such as those framed by The Joint Commission (2012) and the Institutes of Medicine's (IOM) Future of

Nursing (IOM, 2010). The Patient Protection and Affordable Care Act also emphasizes case management's opportunity to lead the health care team (Treiger & Fink-Samnick, 2013a).

The hot topic of hospital readmissions for Medicare beneficiaries within 30 days in October 2012 alone, supports case management's powerful role on the transdisciplinary health care team as a facilitator of both change leadership and change management. Some in health care's transdisciplinary workforce predicted early on, which foretold the need to reframe discharge planning and care coordination interventions. Zander (2010) stated, "If case management is not given the authority to be the central coordinator of the multiple activities involved to prevent readmissions, responsibilities will remain divided and never be totally effective."

The fines ensued with an initial $280 million in 2012 (Rau, 2012). As of August 2013, an additional $227 million in fines were levied against hospitals in all but one state as part of a second go-round, impacting some 2,225 facilities (Rau, 2013). Dr. Eric Coleman, a national expert on readmissions and director of the Care Transitions Program at University of Colorado, offered clear messaging to the industry, "People are starting to recognize that renaming discharge planning does not actually improve your readmissions rate" (Rau, 2013).

Case managers bring value to this arena by virtue of their education and training, including assessing and engaging in proactive interventions toward facilitation of the care process. Through operationalizing the key elements identified in COLLABORATE's outcomes, leadership, advocacy, and anticipatory competencies (Treiger & Fink-Samnick, 2013b), case managers are primed to support the organizational imperatives and take on the challenges of committed quality management and performance improvement.

OBSTACLES TO CHANGE

All progress is precarious, and the solution of one problem brings us face to face with another problem.

Martin Luther King Jr.

Understanding the barriers to change is a task undertaken by case managers every day. However, it is a task performed in the context of identifying obstacles faced by health care consumers, not by employers and not by those obstructing personal and professional advancement. Probably one the most significant influencer of incongruity is that one involves taking measure of someone else's problem rather than focusing in one's own backyard. However, if one is to honestly appraise the current state of case management practice, it requires critical examination of individual and collective performance. It is one thing to point and say "this is what you should be doing" or "this is how you should be doing it" or "if you don't do it this way, you aren't really doing it." However, it is quite another matter to step up and take on the issue of professionalization of case management. Consider this, is it time for naysayers to give up the wheel and allow those with clearer vision of what lies ahead to drive?

Some may argue that a more measured approach is advisable. Let's stop and assess where we are now after taking decades of measured steps. Has the conversation changed that much from where it was last month, last year, or last century? If you think not, take a moment to mull over the fact that case managers continue to be manipulated by the structures they work within. Bemoaning the lack of recognition of case management's value to the health care equation does not advance the practice. We can debate which credential is superior. We can divide our strength by splitting off into professional organizations that focus exclusively on practice setting or population served. Yes, we can continue to do those things and more but it won't move case management forward toward recognition as a professional clinical practice. Case management will continue in neutral unless stakeholders across academia, professional organization, and certification/accreditation bodies agree to work together in taking on the challenges of transforming case management practitioners from mid-level functional technicians to warriors on a mission to transform health care delivery.

The time has come to collaborate, no pun intended. One is hard-pressed to see the benefit of continuing mutually exclusive efforts to advance recognition of case management. Working as partners will certainly improve the likelihood of attaining a consensus-driven definition and career paths for professional practice, defining our value proposition across the health care continuum, and identifying best practices, and leveraging meaningful outcomes. Why? Perhaps, it is because individual efforts favor the needs of the few rather than benefits for the many.

In 2013, the Effective Health Care Program (EHCP) issued its report addressing key questions regarding case management. The project entitled Comparative Effectiveness of Case Management for Adults With Medical Illness and Complex Care Needs intended to determine the effectiveness of case management. However, the definition of case management that was used for the project was "a process in which a person (alone or in conjunction with a team) manages multiple aspects of a patient's care" (2013). It does not resemble any of the established definitions of case management. One hazards to guess that this verbiage was used because there is not a unified definition that the entirety of case management stands behind. Various organizations offer up a definition as a way to distinguish themselves. If case management leaders cannot agree on a definition, it is not reasonable to expect others to select one over another.

The research that was selected and evaluated by the expert panel, was identified as case management, but researchers recognized that heterogeneity of the included studies was problematic to ascertaining effectiveness due to the variance in factors such as practice scope, roles, functions, and activities. EHCP acknowledged, "Case managers typically performed multiple functions. These included but were not limited to assessment and planning, patient education, care coordination, and clinical monitoring. In general, emphasis on specific functions varied according to patients' conditions and the primary objectives of specific CM interventions. For example, interventions among patients with cancer typically focused on coordination and navigation, while interventions for patients with diabetes and CHF focused more on patient education (for self-management) and clinical monitoring. Most studies did not carefully measure the amount of effort case managers devoted to different functions, making it difficult to discern the degree to which emphasis on different case manager functions impacted CM effectiveness" (Hickam et al., 2013).

The lack of strong and consistent evidence demonstrating case management interventions as a valuable asset in health care management is disappointing. Positive report findings would have provided a solid platform on which to catapult future work in the field. However, the findings that were uncovered could be leveraged as a tremendous opportunity to unite case management stakeholders, critically evaluate the findings, and use the lessons learned as a springboard for charting a course for the future of collective practice improvement and success.

The distractions to unified practice improvement need to be carefully evaluated because they may prove themselves to be inconsequential in hindsight. It is time to be audacious. It is time to take a stand within the health care community. We must put aside any longstanding debates about case management and place professional survival on the fast track. Failing this, case management may be doomed to remain in the shadows, unable to maintain its relevance as health care delivery continues to progress.

IN CONCLUSION

As we strive to ensure consistent high quality of professional case management practice in an evolving health care environment, any attempt to wrap this book up with a neat bow would discount the emphasis we have placed on flexibility in response to ongoing challenges and dedication to lifelong learning. This book is the first volley over the bow of case management practice.

We challenge you, our valued colleagues, to engage in the important dialogues that impact your career, to pursue performance excellence in your professional practice, and to never forget that the medical record you touch, the computer screen you look at, and the telephone call you make or receive in some way affects the health and well-being of a human being. Although some of our tasks may seem rather rote by their very nature, it is critically important that we undertake our responsibilities with professionalism and pride. The COLLABORATE competency-based model provides a framework for delivering high-quality case management service. One question remains, are you ready to make the paradigm shift?

References

Bellot, J. (2011). Defining and assessing organizational culture. *Nursing Forum, 46*(1), 29–37.

Blank, R. H. (2012). Transformation of the US healthcare system: Why is change so difficult? *Current Sociology 60*, 415. doi:10.1177/0011392112438327

Cameron, K., & Quinn, R. (2011). *Diagnosing and changing organizational culture* (3rd ed.). San Francisco, CA: Josey-Bass Publishing.

Christo and Jeanne-Claude. (2013). *Artist website*. Retrieved September 6, 2013, from http://www.christojeanneclaude.net

Commonwealth Fund. (2011). *Why not the best? Results from the national scorecard on U.S. health system performance, 2011*. The Commonwealth Fund Commission on a High Peformance Health System, Washington, DC.

Cuellar, A. E., & Gertler, P. J. (2003). *Trends in hospital consolidation: The formation of local systems*. Health Affairs. Retrieved September 4, 2013, from http://content.healthaffairs.org/content/22/6/77.long

Denning, S. (2011). *How do you change an organizational culture*. Retrieved August 31, 2013, from http://www.forbes.com/sites/stevedenning/2011/07/23/how-do-you-change-an-organizational-culture

Fink-Samnick, E. (2008). Developing a resilience accountability continuum: Workplace resilience, part 2. *Professional Case Management, 13*(6), 338–343.

Garde, S. (2010). Change management—An overview. *Studies in health technology and Informatics*, 151, 404–412.

Hallencreutz, J., & Turner D. M. (2011). Exploring organizational change best practice: Are there any clear-cut models and definitions? *International Journal of Quality and Service Sciences, 3*(1), 60–68. Retrieved September 1, 2013, from http://www.emeraldinsight.com.ezproxy.apollolibrary.com/journals.htm?articleid=1911744&show=abstract#sthash.IQEWrJ6D.dpuf

Hernandez, S. R., & Shewchuk R. M. (2011). Working toward effective change in healthcare. *The Journal of Health Administration Education, 29*(3), 253–258.

Hickam, D. H., Weiss, J. W., Guise, J-M., Buckley, M., Motu'apuaka, M., Graham. E., . . . Saha S. (2013, January). *Outpatient case management for adults with medical illness and complex care needs*. Rockville, MD: Agency for Healthcare Research and Quality. Retrieved June 15, 2013, from http://www.effectivehealthcare.ahrq.gov/reports/final.cfm

Institutes of Medicine. (2010). *The future of nursing: Leading change, advancing health*. Washington, DC: National Academies Press.

The Joint Commission. (2012). *Hot topics in health care, transitions of care: The need for a more effective approach to continuing patient care*. Retrieved August 29, 2013, from http://www.jointcommission.org/assets/1/18/Hot_Topics_Transitions_of_Care.pdf

Kotter, J. (2011). *Change management vs. change leadership: What's the difference, Forbes*. Retreived August 30, 2013, from http://www.forbes.com/sites/johnkotter/2011/07/12/change-management-vs-change-leadership-whats-the-difference

McDeavitt, J. T., Wade, K. E., Smith, R. E., & Worsowicz, G. (2012, February). Understanding change management. *Physical Medicine and Rehabilitation*, 4, 141–143. doi:10.1016/j.pmrj.2011.12.001

Rau, J. (2012). Medicare to Penalize 2,217 hospitals for excess readmissions. *Kaiser Health News*, Retrieved September 9, 2013, http://www.kaiserhealthnews.org/Stories/2012/August/13/medicare-hospitals-readmissions-penalties.aspx

Rau, J. (2013). Armed with bigger fines, medicare to punish 2,225 hospitals for excess readmissions. *Kaiser Health News*, Retrieved September 8, 2013, from http://www.kaiserhealthnews.org/stories/2013/august/02/readmission-penalties-medicare-hospitals-year-two.aspx

Treiger, T. M. (2011). Case management: Prospects in definition, education, and settings of practice. *The Remington Report 19*(1), 46–48.

Treiger, T. M., & Fink-Samnick, E. (2013a). COLLABORATE©: A universal, competency-based paradigm for professional case management practice. Part I. *Professional Case Management, 18*(3), 122–135.

Treiger, T. M., & Fink-Samnick, E. (2013b). COLLABORATE©: A universal, competency-based paradigm for professional case management practice. Part II. *Professional Case Management, 18*(5), 219–243.

Treiger, T. M., & Fink-Samnick, E. (2014). COLLABORATE©: A universal, competency-based paradigm for professional case management practice. Part III. *Professional Case Management, 19*(1), 4–15.

Zander K. (2010). Case management accountability for safe, smooth, and sustained transitions. *Professional Case Management, 15*(4), 188–199.

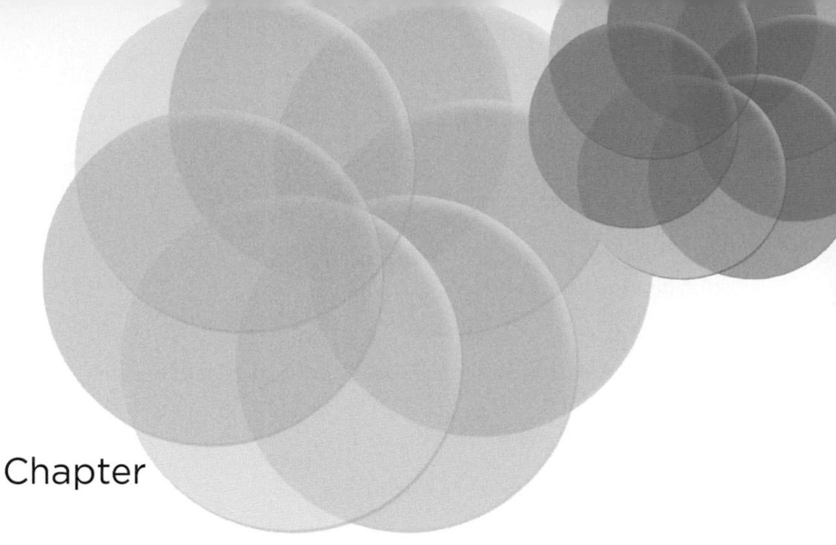

APPENDIX

Additional Website Resources by Chapter

Chapter 1

Boards of Charity
http://www.1856.org/socialhistory.html
http://archives.lib.state.ma.us/actsResolves/1863/1863acts0240.pdf

Settlement houses
http://www.encyclopedia.chicagohistory.org/pages/1135.html

Charitable Organization Societies
http://www.socialwelfarehistory.com/organizations/charity-organization-societies-1877-1893/

Social Security Administration
http://www.ssa.gov/history/35act.html
http://www.ssa.gov/OP_Home/ssact/ssact-toc.htm
http://en.wikipedia.org/wiki/Social_Security_Amendments_of_1965
http://www.socialsecurity.gov/OP_Home/ssact/title02/0201.htm#ft3

Older Americans Act
http://www.gpo.gov/fdsys/granule/STATUTE-79/STATUTE-79-Pg218/content-detail.html

Health Maintenance Organization Act
http://www.law.cornell.edu/uscode/text/42/300e

Medicare/Medicaid Waiver Programs
http://www.piperreport.com/blog/2008/08/12/medicare_and_medicaid_demonstration_waivers_primer/

Education for All Handicapped Children Act
http://college.cengage.com/education/resources/res_prof/students/spec_ed/legislation/pl_94-142.html

History of Social Work
http://en.wikipedia.org/wiki/History_of_social_work

NASW Encyclopedia of SW Charity Organization Societies
http://www.oxfordreference.com.libdata.lib.ua.edu/view/10.1093/acref/9780195306613.001.0001/acref-9780195306613-e-371?rskey=A0UJcc&result=3

Jane Addams
http://en.wikipedia.org/wiki/Jane_Addams

Florence Nightingale
http://en.wikipedia.org/wiki/Florence_Nightingale

Mary E. Richmond
http://www.socialwelfarehistory.com/people/richmond-mary/
http://en.wikipedia.org/wiki/Mary_Richmond
http://www.socialwelfarehistory.com/people/richmond-mary/,

Lillian Wald
http://special.lib.umn.edu/findaid/xml/sw0058.xml
http://www.henrystreet.org/about/history/

Annie Warburton Goodrich
http://en.wikipedia.org/wiki/Annie_Goodrich

Chapter 3

American Rehabilitation Counseling Association
http://www.arcaweb.org

American Board of Occupational Health Nurses
http://www.abohn.org

American Case Management Association
http://acmaweb.org

Association of Rehabilitation Nurses
http://www.rehabnurse.org
http://www.rehabnurse.org

National Association of Professional Geriatric Care Managers
http://www.caremanager.org

American Association of Nurse Credentialing
http://www.nursecredentialing.org

Commission on Case Management Certification
http://ccmcertification.org

Commission on Rehabilitation Counsellor Certification
http://www.crccertification.com

Chapter 4
Credentialing:
Case Management Society of America: Accreditation and Certification Listing
http://www.cmsa.org/individual/education/accreditationcertification/tabid/209/default.aspx

Credentials
Academy for Healthcare Management/American Health Insurance Professionals
http://www.ahip.org/ciepd/ahm/

American Case Management Association
https://www.acmaweb.org

American Board of Disability Analysts
http://www.americandisability.org

American Board of Quality Assurance/Utilization Review Physicians
http://www.abqaurp.org

American Association of Occupational Health Nurses
http://www.aaohn.org

American Nurses Credentialing Center
http://www.nursecredentialing.org

Association of Rehabilitation Nurses
http://www.rehabnurse.org/certification/content/Index.html

Center for Case Management
http://www.cfcm.com/wordpress1/

Certified Disability Management Specialists
http://www.cdms.org

Commission for Case Manager Certification
http://ccmcertification.org

Commission on Rehabilitation Counselor Certification
http://www.crccertification.com

Insurance Education Association
http://www.ieatraining.com

National Association for Health Care Quality
http://www.nahq.org/certify/content/index.html

National Academy of Certified Care Managers
http://www.naccm.net

National Association of Social Workers
www.socialworkers.org

Credentialing Oversight:
Association of Social Work Boards
http://www.aswb.org

Institute on Credentialing Excellence
http://www.credentialingexcellence.org

National Council of State Boards of Nursing
https://www.ncsbn.org/index.htm

Case Management Certificate Programs:
Rutgers School of Social Work
Certificate Program in Case Management
http://socialwork.rutgers.edu/continuingeducation/ce/certificateprograms/certcasemanagement.aspx

Seton Hall University College of Nursing
Certificate in Case Management
http://www.shu.edu/academics/nursing/case-management-certificate.cfm

University of California, San Diego/Extension
Case Management Certificate Program
http://extension.ucsd.edu/programs/index.cfm?vAction=certDetail&vCertificateID=13

University of California, Riverside
Medical Case Management Certificate
http://www.extension.ucr.edu/academics/certificates/case_management.html

University of Southern Maine Professional Development Programs
Certificate Program in Case Management
https://usm.maine.edu/pdp/certificate-program-case-management

Chapter 5
Competency-Based Accreditation:
American Association of the Colleges of Nursing
http://www.aacn.nche.edu

Council on Social Work Education: EPAS
http://www.cswe.org/Accreditation/EPASImplementation.aspx

Quality and Safety Education Nurse Initiative
http://qsen.org

Competency-Based Professional Initiatives:
Canadian Interprofessional Health Collaborative (CIHC)
http://www.cihc.ca

Interprofessional Education Collaborative (IPEC)
http://IPECollaborative.org

Institute of Medicine
http://www.iom.edu

Competency-Based Examinations:
Council for Aid to Education
CLA+, CWRA+
http://cae.org/performance-assessment/category/home/

Institute of Medicine
http://www.iom.edu

Competency-Based Degree Programs:
Excelsior College
http://www.excelsior.edu

Western Governors University
http://www.wgu.edu

University of Wisconsin
Flexible Option
http://flex.wisconsin.edu

Chapter 9
Agency for Healthcare Research and Quality
http://www.ahrq.gov

The Centers for Medicare and Medicaid Innovation Center
http://innovation.cms.gov

Critical appraisal:
Delfini
http://www.delfini.org

Evidence-based healthcare:
The Cochrane Collaboration
http://www.cochrane.org/about-us/evidence-based-health-care

Institute for Healthcare Improvement
http://www.ihi.org

Patient-centered Outcomes Research Institute (PCORI)
http://www.pcori.org

Chapter 10
Experiential Learning—Foundation:
Experience Based Learning Systems, Inc.
David and Alice Kolb
http://learningfromexperience.com/about/

Fifth Discipline:
Society for Organized Learning
Peter Senge
http://www.solonline.org/?page=PeterSenge

Health Literacy:
Agency for Healthcare Research and Quality
http://www.ahrq.gov/research/findings/factsheets/literacy/healthlit/index.html

Centers for Disease Control and Prevention (CDC)
Health literacy
http://www.cdc.gov/healthliteracy/

CDC resource listing
http://www.cdc.gov/healthliteracy/Learn/Resources.html

Health Literacy Fact Sheet
http://www.health.gov/communication/literacy/quickguide/factsbasic.htm

HIPAA HITECH
HHS.Gov: Health Information Technology for Economic and Clinical Health Act (HITECH)
http://www.hhs.gov/ocr/privacy/hipaa/administrative/enforcementrule/hitechenforcementifr.html

Mental Health Parity
Mental Health Parity and Addiction Equity Act (MHPAEA) of 2008: United States Department of Labor
http://www.dol.gov/ebsa/mentalhealthparity/

Multiple Intelligences: Learning Styles
Howard Gardner
http://howardgardner.com

VARK: A Guide to Learning Styles
http://www.vark-learn.com/english/index.asp

Nursing Education:
National League for Nursing
http://www.nln.org

Patient Protection and Affordable Care Act (PPACA)
http://www.hhs.gov/healthcare/rights/index.html

21st Century Skills:
The Partnership for 21st Century Skills
http://www.p21.org

Chapter 11
American Association of Colleges of Nursing (AACN)
Leadership for academic nursing (LANP)
http://www.aacn.nche.edu/lanp

American Case Management Association (ACMA)
Standards of practice and scope of services for health care delivery system case management and transition of care professionals
http://www.acmaweb.org/Standards

American Nurses Association (ANA)
Leadership Institute
http://www.ana-leadershipinstitute.org

American Nurses Credentialing Center (ANCC)
Magnet recognition program model
http://www.nursecredentialing.org/Magnet

American Organization of Nurse Executives (AONE)
Nurse executive competencies
http://www.aone.org/resources/leadership%20tools/nursecomp.shtml

Case Management Society of America
CMSA standards of practice for case management
http://www.cmsa.org/portals/0/pdf/memberonly/StandardsOfPractice.pdf

Center for Creative Leadership
http://www.ccl.org/Leadership/index.aspx

Council on Social Work Education (CSWE)
Leadership Institute
http://www.cswe.org/CentersInitiatives/CSWELeadershipInst.aspx

Forbes Leadership Forum
http://www.forbes.com/sites/forbesleadershipforum/

Forbes Magazine
http://www.forbes.com
Search term: leadership

Harvard Business Review
http://hbr.org/

National Association of Social Workers (NASW)
NASW standards for social work case management
http://www.socialworkers.org/practice/naswstandards/CaseManagementStandards2013.pdf

National League for Nursing (NLN)
NLN Leadership Institute
http://www.nln.org/facultyprograms/leadershipinstitute.htm

National Transitions of Care Coalition (NTOCC)
Model for Accountable Communication within Transition of Care Measures white paper
http://www.ntocc.org/Portals/0/PDF/Resources/TransitionsOfCare_Measures.pdf

Network for Social Work Management (NSWM)
Human services management competencies
https://socialworkmanager.org/competencies

Society for Social Work Leadership in Health Care (SSWLHC)
http://www.sswlhc.org/html/publications.php

Chapter 16
Boards of Nursing Interactive Map and Contact Information
https://www.ncsbn.org/contactbon.htm

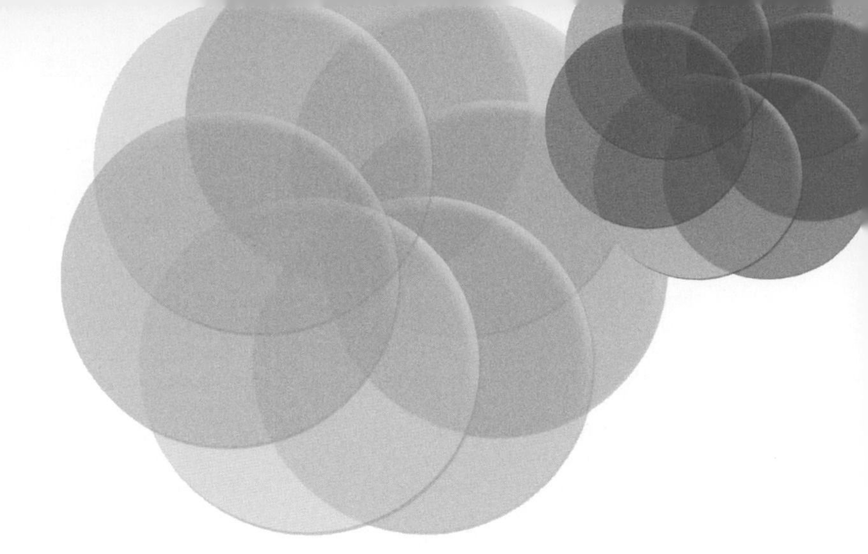

INDEX

Note: Page numbers followed by "*f*", "*t*" and "*b*" denote figures, tables and boxes, respectively.

L

M

N